Joseph C. Masdeu, M.D.

CURRENT THERAPY IN

NEUROLOGIC DISEASE–3

Medical Titles in the Current Therapy Series

Bardin:
Current Therapy in Endocrinology and Metabolism
Bayless:
Current Management of Inflammatory Bowel Disease
Bayless:
Current Therapy in Gastroenterology and Liver Disease
Brain, Carbone:
Current Therapy in Hematology–Oncology
Callaham:
Current Therapy in Emergency Medicine
Charles, Glover:
Current Therapy in Obstetrics
Cherniack:
Current Therapy of Respiratory Disease
Dubovsky, Shore:
Current Therapy in Psychiatry
Dzau:
Current Management of Hypertension
Eichenwald, Ströder:
Current Therapy in Pediatrics
Foley, Payne:
Current Therapy of Pain
Garcia, Mastroianni, Amelar, Dubin:
Current Therapy of Infertility
Glassock:
Current Therapy in Nephrology and Hypertension
Horowitz:
Current Management of Arrhythmias
Hurst:
Current Therapy in Cardiovascular Disease
Jeejeebhoy:
Current Therapy in Nutrition
Johnson:
Current Therapy in Neurologic Disease
Kacmarek, Stoller:
Current Respiratory Care
Kass, Platt:
Current Therapy in Infectious Disease
Kassirer:
Current Therapy in Internal Medicine
Lichtenstein, Fauci:
Current Therapy in Allergy, Immunology, and Rheumatology
Nelson:
Current Therapy in Neonatal–Perinatal Medicine
Nelson:
Current Therapy in Pediatric Infectious Disease
Parrillo:
Current Therapy in Critical Care Medicine
Provost, Farmer:
Current Therapy in Dermatology
Rogers:
Current Practice in Anesthesiology

CURRENT THERAPY IN
NEUROLOGIC DISEASE–3

RICHARD T. JOHNSON, M.D.

Professor and Director of Neurology
Professor of Microbiology and Neuroscience
The Johns Hopkins University School of Medicine
Neurologist-in-Chief
The Johns Hopkins Hospital
Baltimore, Maryland

B.C. Decker Inc. • Philadelphia • Toronto

Publisher

B.C. Decker Inc.
3228 South Service Road
Burlington, Ontario L7N 3H8

B.C. Decker Inc.
320 Walnut Street
Suite 400
Philadelphia, Pennsylvania 19106

Sales and Distribution

United States and Puerto Rico
Mosby-Year Book Inc.
11830 Westline Industrial Drive
Saint Louis, Missouri 63146

Canada
Mosby-Year Book Ltd.
5240 Finch Avenue E., Unit 1
Scarborough, Ontario M1S 5A2

Australia
McGraw-Hill Book Company Australia Pty. Ltd.
4 Barcoo Street
Roseville East 2059
New South Wales, Australia

Brazil
Editora McGraw-Hill do Brasil, Ltda.
rua Tabapua, 1,105, Itaim-Bibi
Sao Paulo, S.P. Brasil

Colombia
Interamericana/McGraw-Hill de Colombia, S.A.
Apartado Aereo 81078
Bogota, D.E. Colombia

Europe
McGraw-Hill Book Company GmbH
Lademannbogan 136
D-2000 Hamburg 83
West Germany

France
MEDSI/McGraw-Hill
6, avenue Daniel Lesueur
75007 Paris, France

Hong Kong and China
McGraw-Hill Book Company
Suite 618, Ocean Centre
5 Canton Road
Tsimshatsui, Kowloon
Hong Kong

India
Tata McGraw-Hill Publishing Company, Ltd.
12/4 Asaf Ali Road, 3rd Floor
New Delhi 110002, India

Indonesia
P.O. Box 122/JAT
Jakarta, 1300 Indonesia

Italy
McGraw-Hill Libri Italia, s.r.l.
Plazza Emilia, 5
1-20129 Milano MI
Italy

Japan
Igaku-Shoin Ltd.
Tokyo International P.O. Box 5063
1-28-36 Hongo, Bunkyo-ku,
Tokyo 113, Japan

Korea
C.P.O. Box 10583
Seoul, Korea

Malaysia
No. 8 Jalan SS 7/6B
Kelana Jaya
47301 Petaling Jaya
Selangor, Malaysia

Mexico
Interamericana/McGraw-Hill de Mexico, S.A. de C.V.
Cedro 512, Colonia Atlampa
(Apartado Postal 26370)
06450 Mexico, D.F., Mexico

New Zealand
McGraw-Hill Book Co. New Zealand Ltd.
5 Joval Place, Wiri
Manukau City, New Zealand

Panama
Editorial McGraw-Hill Latinoamericana, S.A.
Apartado Postal 2036
Zona Libre de Colon
Colon, Republica de Panama

Portugal
Editora McGraw-Hill de Portugal, Ltda.
Rua Rosa Damascono 11A–B
1900 Lisboa, Portugal

South Africa
Libriger Book Distributors
Warehouse Number 8
"Die Ou Looiery"
Tannery Road
Hamilton, Bloemfontein 9300

Southeast Asia
McGraw-Hill Book Co.
348 Jalan Boon Lay
Jurong, Singapore 2261

Spain
McGraw-Hill/Interamericana de Espana, S.A.
Manuel Ferrero, 13
28020 Madrid, Spain

Taiwan
P.O. Box 87-601
Taipei, Taiwan

Thailand
632/5 Phanolyothin Road
Sapan Kwai
Bangkok 10400
Thailand

United Kingdom, Middle East and Africa
McGraw-Hill Book Company (U.K.) Ltd.
Shoppenhangers Road
Maidenhead, Berkshire
SL6 2QL England

Venezuela
McGraw-Hill/Interamericana, C.A.
2da. calle Bello Monte
(entre avenida Casanova y Sabana Grande)
Apartado Aereo 50785
Caracas 1050, Venezuela

NOTICE

The authors and publisher have made every effort to ensure that the patient care recommended herein, including choice of drugs and drug dosages, is in accord with the accepted standards and practice at the time of publication. However, since research and regulation constantly change clinical standards, the reader is urged to check the product information sheet included in the package of each drug, which includes recommended doses, warnings, and contraindications. This is particularly important with new or infrequently used drugs.

Current Therapy in Neurologic Disease–3

ISBN 1-55664-265-2

Library of Congress catalog card number: 89-81912

10 9 8 7 6 5 4 3 2 1

CONTRIBUTORS

HAROLD P. ADAMS, Jr., M.D.

Professor of Neurology, and Director, Division of Cerebrovascular Diseases, University of Iowa College of Medicine; Attending Neurologist, University of Iowa Hospitals and Clinics; Consultant Neurologist, Iowa City Veterans Administration Hospital, Iowa City, Iowa
Transient Ischemic Attack
Temporal Arteritis and Vasculitis of the Central Nervous System

GREGORY W. ALBERS, M.D.

Assistant Professor of Neurology and Neurological Sciences, Stanford University Medical Center, Stanford, California
Principles of Pain Management

JAMES W. ALBERS, M.D., Ph.D.

Professor, Department of Neurology, University of Michigan Medical School, Ann Arbor, Michigan
Bell's Palsy

GARRETT E. ALEXANDER, M.D., Ph.D.

Associate Professor of Neurology, The Johns Hopkins University School of Medicine, Baltimore, Maryland
Torticollis

JAMES F. BALE, Jr., M.D.

Associate Professor, Division of Pediatric Neurology, Departments of Pediatrics and Neurology, University of Iowa College of Medicine, Iowa City, Iowa
Congenital Viral Infection

JOSEPH R. BERGER, M.D.

Associate Professor of Neurology and Internal Medicine, University of Miami School of Medicine, Miami, Florida
Neurosyphilis

JOSÉ BILLER, M.D.

Associate Professor, Division of Cerebrovascular Diseases, Department of Neurology, University of Iowa College of Medicine; Attending Neurologist, University of Iowa Hospitals and Clinics; Consultant Neurologist, Iowa City Veterans Administration Hospital, Iowa City, Iowa
Transient Ischemic Attack
Temporal Arteritis and Vasculitis of the Central Nervous System

PETER McL. BLACK, M.D., Ph.D.

Franc C. Ingraham Professor of Neurosurgery, Harvard Medical School; Neurosurgeon-in-Chief, Children's Hospital and Brigham and Women's Hospital, Boston, Massachusetts
Congenital Hydrocephalus

CECIL O. BOREL, M.D.

Assistant Professor of Anesthesia/Critical Care Medicine and Neurology, The Johns Hopkins University School of Medicine; Co-Director, Neurosciences Critical Care Unit, The Johns Hopkins Hospital, Baltimore, Maryland
Normal-Pressure Hydrocephalus
Acute Ventilatory Failure in Neuromuscular Disease

GEORGE J. BREWER, M.D.

Professor, Departments of Internal Medicine and Human Genetics, University of Michigan Medical School, Ann Arbor, Michigan
Wilson's Disease

MARK B. BROMBERG, M.D., Ph.D.

Assistant Professor, Department of Neurology, University of Michigan Medical School, Ann Arbor, Michigan
Bell's Palsy

MARK J. BROWN, M.D.

Professor of Neurology, University of Pennsylvania School of Medicine, Philadelphia, Pennsylvania
Subacute Combined Degeneration and Other Vitamin B_{12} Deficiency-Induced Disorders

ALASTAIR BUCHAN, M.D., FRCPC

Assistant Professor of Neurology, University of Western Ontario; Staff Neurologist, University Hospital, London, Ontario, Canada
Atherothrombotic Cerebrovascular Disease

DAVID W. BUCHHOLZ, M.D.

Assistant Professor of Neurology, The Johns Hopkins University School of Medicine; Director of the Neurological Consultation Clinic and Ambulatory Services, Clinical Neurosciences, The Johns Hopkins Hospital, Baltimore, Maryland
Neurogenic Dysphagia

THOMAS H. BURNSTINE, M.D.

Fellow in Epilepsy and Clinical Neurophysiology, Department of Neurology and the Epilepsy Center, The Johns Hopkins Hospital, Baltimore, Maryland
Focal Seizure Disorders

IAN J. BUTLER, M.B., F.R.A.C.P.

Professor of Neurology and Pediatrics, and Director, Divisions of Pediatric Neurology and Developmental Pediatrics, University of Texas Medical School at Houston, Houston, Texas
Migraine in Childhood

PETER L. CARLEN, M.D., FRCPC

Professor of Medicine, Division of Neurology, University of Toronto Faculty of Medicine; Head, Neurology Program, Addiction Research Foundation; Director, Playfair Neuroscience Unit, The Toronto Hospital, Toronto, Ontario, Canada
Wernicke's Encephalopathy and Alcohol-Related Nutritional Disease

PAUL CHAMBERS, M.D.

Senior Resident in Pediatrics, Albert Einstein College of Medicine, Bronx, New York
Myelomeningocele

LORA L. CLAWSON, R.N., B.S.N.

ALS Research Coordinator, The Johns Hopkins University School of Medicine, Baltimore, Maryland
Amyotrophic Lateral Sclerosis

BRUCE A. COHEN, M.D.

Assistant Professor of Clinical Neurology, Northwestern University Medical School; Associate Attending Physician, Northwestern Memorial Hospital, Chicago, Illinois
Postinfectious and Acute Transverse Myelitis

MONROE COLE, M.D.

Associate Professor of Neurology, Case Western Reserve University School of Medicine, Cleveland, Ohio
Intracerebral Hemorrhage

DAVID R. CORNBLATH, M.D.

Associate Professor of Neurology, The Johns Hopkins University School of Medicine, Baltimore, Maryland
Acute Inflammatory Polyneuropathy

ROBERT D. CURRIER, M.D.

Professor of Neurology, The University of Mississippi School of Medicine; McCarty Professor and Chairman, Department of Neurology, University of Mississippi Medical Center, Jackson, Mississippi
Inherited Ataxia

ROBERT H. DAILEY, M.D.

Clinical Professor of Medicine, University of California, San Francisco, School of Medicine, San Francisco, California
Alcohol Intoxication and Withdrawal

LARRY E. DAVIS, M.D., F.A.C.P.

Professor of Neurology and Microbiology, University of New Mexico Medical School; Chief, Neurology Service, Albuquerque Veterans Administration Medical Center, Albuquerque, New Mexico
Neurocysticercosis

GERARD M. DEBRUN, M.D.

Professor of Radiology, The Johns Hopkins University School of Medicine; Director of Interventional Neuroradiology, Department of Radiology, The Johns Hopkins Hospital, Baltimore, Maryland
Brain Arteriovenous Malformation

MAHLON R. DeLONG, M.D.

Professor of Neurology and Neurosciences, The Johns Hopkins University School of Medicine, Baltimore, Maryland
Parkinson's Disease
Torticollis

ROBERT J. DeLORENZO, M.D., Ph.D., M.P.H.

Professor and Chairman of Neurology, and Professor of Pharmacology and Biochemistry and Molecular Biophysics, Medical College of Virginia; Neurologist-in-Chief, Medical College of Virginia Hospitals, Richmond, Virginia
Status Epilepticus

J. RAYMOND DePAULO, Jr., M.D.

Associate Professor of Psychiatry, The Johns Hopkins University School of Medicine; Director, The Affective Disorders Clinic, The Johns Hopkins Hospital, Baltimore, Maryland
Depression

DARRYL C. De VIVO, M.D.

Sidney Carter Professor of Neurology and Professor of Pediatrics, Columbia University College of Physicians and Surgeons; Attending Neurologist, Attending Pediatrician, and Director of Pediatric Neurology, The Presbyterian Hospital in the City of New York, New York, New York
Reye's Syndrome

IVAN DIAMOND, M.D., Ph.D.

Vice Chairman and Professor of Neurology, and Professor of Pediatrics and Pharmacology, University of California, San Francisco, School of Medicine; Attending and Consulting Physician, Moffitt Hospital, Long Hospital, and San Francisco General Hospital; Director, Ernest Gallo Clinic and Research Center, San Francisco, California
Alcohol Intoxication and Withdrawal

MICHAEL N. DIRINGER, M.D.

Instructor of Anesthesia/Critical Care Medicine and Neurology, The Johns Hopkins University School of Medicine, Baltimore, Maryland
Disturbances of Sodium and Osmolality

EDWARD J. DROPCHO, M.D.

Assistant Professor, Department of Neurology, University of Alabama at Birmingham School of Medicine; Director, Neuro-Oncology Program, University of Alabama Comprehensive Cancer Center, Birmingham, Alabama
Glioma

ROSWELL ELDRIDGE, M.D.

Head, Clinical Neurogenetic Studies, Neuroepidemiology Branch, National Institute of Neurologic Disease and Stroke, and Senior Attending Physician, Clinical Center, National Institutes of Health, Bethesda, Maryland
Neurofibromatosis 2

LARRY EMPTING-KOSCHORKE, M.D.

Instructor, Department of Neurology, The Johns Hopkins University School of Medicine; Director, Blaustein Pain Treatment Center, The Johns Hopkins Hospital, Baltimore, Maryland
Chronic Low Back Pain and Failed Back Syndrome

GERALD ERENBERG, M.D.

Director, Learning Assessment Clinic, and Child Neurologist, The Cleveland Clinic Foundation, Cleveland, Ohio
Tourette's Syndrome

PETER J. FAGAN, Ph.D.

Assistant Professor, The Johns Hopkins University School of Medicine; Director, Sexual Behaviors Consultation Unit, The Johns Hopkins Hospital, Baltimore, Maryland
Sexual Problems in Spinal Cord Disease

STANLEY FAHN, M.D.

H. Houston Merritt Professor of Neurology, Columbia University College of Physicians and Surgeons; Attending Neurologist, Neurological Institute, Presbyterian Hospital in the City of New York, New York, New York
Dystonia
Hemifacial Spasm

LINDA M. FAMIGLIO, M.D.

Senior Fellow, Regional Epilepsy Center, Department of Neurological Surgery, University of Washington School of Medicine, Seattle, Washington
Acute Hepatic Porphyria

JOSEPH H. FRIEDMAN, M.D.

Associate Professor of Neurology, Brown University Program in Medicine; Director, Parkinson's Disease and Movement Disorder Center, Roger Williams General Hospital, Providence, Rhode Island
Neuroleptic Toxicity

GERHARD H. FROMM, M.D.

Professor of Neurology, University of Pittsburgh School of Medicine; Attending Physician, Presbyterian-University Hospital, Pittsburgh, Pennsylvania
Trigeminal and Glossopharyngeal Neuralgia

WILLIAM GAILLARD, M.D.

Fellow, Department of Neurology, The Johns Hopkins University School of Medicine, Baltimore, Maryland
Tuberous Sclerosis

MARK R. GILBERT, M.D.

Instructor, Department of Neurology, The Johns Hopkins University School of Medicine, Baltimore, Maryland
Epidural Spinal Cord Compression and Carcinomatous Meningitis

BARRY GORDON, M.D., Ph.D.

Assistant Professor and Director, Cognitive Neurology, The Johns Hopkins University School of Medicine, Baltimore, Maryland
Postconcussional Syndrome

PAUL GREENE, M.D.

Assistant Professor of Clinical Neurology, Columbia University College of Physicians and Surgeons; Assistant Attending Neurologist, Neurological Institute, Presbyterian Hospital in the City of New York, New York, New York
Dystonia
Hemifacial Spasm

JOHN E. GREENLEE, M.D.

Professor of Neurology, University of Utah School of Medicine; Chief, Neurology Service, Veterans Administration Medical Center, Salt Lake City, Utah
Brain Abscess and Parameningeal Infection

VLADIMIR C. HACHINSKI, M.D. D.Sc., FRCPC

Professor of Neurology, University of Western Ontario; Staff Neurologist, University Hospital, London, Ontario, Canada
Atherothrombotic Cerebrovascular Disease

EARL R. HACKETT, M.D.

Emeritus Head of Neurology, Louisiana State University School of Medicine in New Orleans, New Orleans, Louisiana; Clinical Professor of Neurology, University of Missouri–Columbia School of Medicine, Columbia, Missouri
Peripheral Nerve Injury

TIMOTHY C. HAIN, M.D.

Assistant Professor of Neurology and Otolaryngology, The Johns Hopkins University School of Medicine, Baltimore, Maryland
Vertigo

DANIEL F. HANLEY, M.D.

Assistant Professor, The Johns Hopkins University School of Medicine; Director, Neurosciences Critical Care Unit, The Johns Hopkins Hospital, Baltimore, Maryland
Normal-Pressure Hydrocephalus
Acute Inflammatory Polyneuropathy
Acute Ventilatory Failure in Neuromuscular Disease

DAN S. HEFFEZ, M.D., FRCS

Assistant Professor of Neurological Surgery, The Johns Hopkins University School of Medicine; Attending Neurosurgeon, The Johns Hopkins Hospital, Baltimore, Maryland
Spinal Injury

SUSAN HERDMAN, Ph.D.

Assistant Professor, Department of Otolaryngology—Head and Neck Surgery, The Johns Hopkins University School of Medicine; Physical Therapist, Department of Otolaryngology —Head and Neck Surgery, The Johns Hopkins Hospital, Baltimore, Maryland
Normal-Pressure Hydrocephalus

ROBERT M. HERNDON, M.D.

Professor of Neurology, Oregon Health Sciences University; Chief of Neurology, Good Samaritan Hospital and Medical Center, Portland, Oregon
Multiple Sclerosis

RICHARD A. HRACHOVY, M.D.

Associate Professor, Section of Neurophysiology, Department of Neurology, Baylor College of Medicine; Attending Physician, Neurophysiology Service, The Methodist Hospital, Houston, Texas
Neonatal Seizures and Infantile Spasms

OREST HURKO, M.D.

Associate Professor, Department of Neurology, and Assistant Professor, Center for Medical Genetics, Department of Medicine, The Johns Hopkins University School of Medicine, Baltimore, Maryland
Mitochondrial Encephalomyopathy

ALAN C. JACKSON, M.D., FRCPC

Assistant Professor of Medicine and Microbiology and Immunology, Queen's University; Attending Staff, Kingston General Hospital, Kingston, Ontario, Canada
Rabies

LISSETTE JIMENEZ, M.D.

Instructor, Department of Neurology, University of South Florida College of Medicine, Tampa, Florida
Pseudotumor Cerebri

RICHARD T. JOHNSON, M.D.

Professor and Director of Neurology, and Professor of Microbiology and Neuroscience, The Johns Hopkins University School of Medicine; Neurologist-in-Chief, The Johns Hopkins Hospital, Baltimore, Maryland
Herpes Zoster

MICHAEL V. JOHNSTON, M.D.

Professor of Neurology and Pediatrics, The Johns Hopkins University School of Medicine; Vice President of Medical Affairs, Kennedy Institute, Baltimore, Maryland
Intracranial Hemorrhage, Periventricular Leukomalacia, and Hypoxic-Ischemic Encephalopathy in the Neonate

BURK JUBELT, M.D.

Professor and Chairman, Department of Neurology, and Professor of Microbiology and Immunology, State University of New York Health Science Center at Syracuse College of Medicine; Neurologist, University Hospital, Crouse-Irving Memorial Hospital, and Syracuse Veterans Administration Medical Center, Syracuse, New York
Bacterial Meningitis

MERRILL C. KANTER, M.D.

Assistant Professor, Division of Neurology, University of Texas Health Science Center, San Antonio, Texas
Embolic Stroke of Cardiac Origin

PETER W. KAPLAN, B.Sc.(Hons), M.D., M.B., B.S., M.R.C.P.(London)

Assistant Professor, The Johns Hopkins University School of Medicine; Director of the EEG Laboratory and Attending Physician, Francis Scott Key Medical Center, Baltimore, Maryland
Generalized Seizure Disorders

JEFFREY R. KIRSCH, M.D.

Assistant Professor of Anesthesiology/Critical Care Medicine and Neurology, The Johns Hopkins University School of Medicine, Baltimore, Maryland
Disturbances of Sodium and Osmolality

WILLIAM C. KOLLER, M.D., Ph.D.

Professor and Chairman, Department of Neurology, University of Kansas Medical Center, Kansas City, Kansas
Essential Tremor

RALPH W. KUNCL, M.D., Ph.D.

Associate Professor of Neurology, The Johns Hopkins University School of Medicine; Co-Director, Neuromuscular Clinical Laboratory, The Johns Hopkins Hospital, Baltimore, Maryland
Amyotrophic Lateral Sclerosis

JOHN P. LAURENT, M.D.

Clinical Associate Professor, Baylor College of Medicine; Active Staff, Texas Children's Hospital, Houston, Texas
Syringohydromyelia

RONALD P. LESSER, M.D.

Associate Professor of Neurology and Neurosurgery, The Johns Hopkins University School of Medicine; Director, The Johns Hopkins Epilepsy Center and The Johns Hopkins EEG Laboratories, The Johns Hopkins Hospital, Baltimore, Maryland
Focal Seizure Disorders

THERA P. LINKS, M.D.

Fellow in Internal Medicine, University Hospital of Gronigen, Gronigen, The Netherlands
Periodic Paralysis

HOWARD L. LIPTON, M.D.

Professor and Vice Chairman of Neurology, University of Colorado School of Medicine; Attending Physician, University Hospital, Denver, Colorado
Postinfectious and Acute Transverse Myelitis

ROBERT P. LISAK, M.D.

Professor and Chairman, Department of Neurology, Wayne State University School of Medicine; Chief of Neurology, Harper-Grace Hospitals; Neurologist-in-Chief, Detroit Medical Center, Detroit, Michigan
Neurosarcoidosis

MARC MALKOFF, M.D.

Senior Clinical Fellow, The Johns Hopkins Hospital, Baltimore, Maryland
Acute Ventilatory Failure in Neuromuscular Disease

ELLIOTT L. MANCALL, M.D.

Professor and Chairman, Department of Neurology, Hahnemann University School of Medicine, Philadelphia, Pennsylvania
Cervical Spondylosis

KENNETH MAREK, M.D.

Assistant Professor of Neurology, Yale University School of Medicine, New Haven, Connecticut
Idiopathic Autonomic Insufficiency

ROBERT W. MARION, M.D.

Associate Professor of Pediatrics, Albert Einstein College of Medicine; Associate Attending Physician, Bronx Municipal Hospital Center; Director, Center for Congenital Disorders, Montefiore Medical Center, Bronx, New York
Myelomeningocele

BARBARA J. MARTIN, M.D.

Clinical Instructor, Department of Neurology, University of Pennsylvania School of Medicine, Philadelphia, Pennsylvania
Subacute Combined Degeneration and Other Vitamin B_{12} Deficiency-Induced Disorders

ROBERT L. MARTUZA, M.D.

Associate Professor of Surgery, Harvard Medical School; Director, Neurofibromatosis Clinic, and Associate Visiting Neurosurgeon, Massachusetts General Hospital, Boston, Massachusetts
Neurofibromatosis 2

JUSTIN C. McARTHUR, M.B., B.S., M.P.H.

Assistant Professor of Neurology, The Johns Hopkins University School of Medicine, Baltimore, Maryland
Neurologic Diseases Associated with HIV-1 Infection

PAUL R. McHUGH, M.D.

Henry Phipps Professor of Psychiatry, The Johns Hopkins University School of Medicine; Director and Psychiatrist-in-Chief, The Johns Hopkins Hospital, Baltimore, Maryland
Hysterical Behavior

GUY M. McKHANN, M.D.

Kennedy Professor of Neurology, The Johns Hopkins University School of Medicine, Baltimore, Maryland
Hepatic Encephalopathy

NEIL R. MILLER, M.D.

Frank B. Walsh Professor of Neuro-Ophthalmology, and Professor of Ophthalmology, Neurology, and Neurosurgery, The Johns Hopkins University School of Medicine, Baltimore, Maryland
Essential Blepharospasm and Meige's Syndrome

ELI M. MIZRAHI, M.D.

Associate Professor, Section of Neurophysiology, Department of Neurology and Section of Pediatric Neurology, Department of Pediatrics, Baylor College of Medicine; Staff Neurophysiologist, The Methodist Hospital and Children's Hospital, Houston, Texas
Neonatal Seizures and Infantile Spasms

JACEK L. MOSTWIN, M.D., D.Phil.

Assistant Professor of Urology, The Johns Hopkins University School of Medicine, Baltimore, Maryland
Urinary Problems in Multiple Sclerosis and Other Spinal Diseases

RICHARD T. MOXLEY III, M.D.

Professor of Neurology and Pediatrics, University of Rochester School of Medicine and Dentistry; Director, Neuromuscular Disease Center, Rochester, New York
Cramps

PATRICK A. MURPHY, M.D., Ph.D.

Professor of Medicine and Molecular Biology and Genetics, The Johns Hopkins University School of Medicine; Chief, Infectious Diseases, Francis Scott Key Medical Center, Baltimore, Maryland
Tuberculous Meningitis

SAKKUBAI NAIDU, M.D., B.S.

Associate Professor of Neurology and Pediatrics, The Johns Hopkins University School of Medicine; Director, Neurogenetics Unit, Kennedy Institute, Baltimore, Maryland
Inherited Neurodegenerative Diseases of Childhood

JACK NEIMAN, M.D., Ph.D.

Assistant Professor and Acting Head, Neuropsychiatry Division, Karolinska Institute, Stockholm, Sweden
Wernicke's Encephalopathy and Alcohol-Related Nutritional Disease

RICHARD B. NORTH, M.D.

Assistant Professor, Department of Neurosurgery, The Johns Hopkins University School of Medicine, Baltimore, Maryland
Acute Back Pain and Disc Herniation

CHAD K. OH, M.D.

Pediatric Resident, Rush Medical School; Associate, Rush-Presbyterian–St. Luke's Medical Center, Chicago, Illinois
Bacterial Meningitis

HANS J.G.H. OOSTERHUIS, M.D., Ph.D.

Professor of Clinical Neurology, University Hospital of Gronigen, Gronigen, The Netherlands
Periodic Paralysis

FREDERICK B. PALMER, M.D.

Associate Professor of Pediatrics, and Director, Division of Child Development, The Johns Hopkins University School of Medicine; Director, Developmental Pediatrics, The Kennedy Institute for Handicapped Children, Baltimore, Maryland
Cerebral Palsy

DILYS M. PARRY, Ph.D.

Geneticist, Clinical Epidemiology Branch, National Cancer Institute; Associate Director, Interinstitute Medical Genetics Program, Clinical Center, National Institute of Health, Bethesda, Maryland
Neurofibromatosis 2

ROY A. PATCHELL, M.D.

Assistant Professor of Neurology and Neurosurgery, University of Kentucky College of Medicine; Chief of Neuro-Oncology, University of Kentucky Medical Center, Lexington, Kentucky
Brain Metastasis

JOHN B. PENNEY, Jr., M.D.

Associate Professor of Neurology, University of Michigan Medical School, Ann Arbor, Michigan
Huntington's Disease

GEORGE DAVID PERKIN, B.A., FRCP

Consultant Neurologist, Charing Cross and
Hillingdon Hospital, London, England
Syncope

STEPHEN J. PEROUTKA, M.D., Ph.D.

Assistant Professor of Neurology and Neurological
Sciences, Stanford University Medical Center,
Stanford, California
Principles of Pain Management

PATTI L. PETERSON, M.D.

Assistant Professor of Neurology, Wayne State
University School of Medicine; Chief of Neurology,
Detroit Receiving Hospital, Detroit, Michigan
Mitochondrial Encephalomyopathy

PETER C. PHILLIPS, M.D.

Assistant Professor, Departments of Neurology,
Oncology, and Pediatrics, The Johns Hopkins
University School of Medicine, Baltimore,
Maryland
Brain Tumors in Children

LEON D. PROCKOP, M.D.

Professor and Chairman, Department of Neurology,
University of South Florida College of Medicine,
Tampa, Florida
Pseudotumor Cerebri

PETER V. RABINS, M.D., Ph.D.

Associate Professor of Psychiatry, The Johns
Hopkins University School of Medicine, Baltimore,
Maryland
Dementia

STEPHEN G. REICH, M.D.

Instructor in Neurology, The Johns Hopkins
University School of Medicine, Baltimore,
Maryland
Parkinson's Disease
Torticollis

LOUIS REIK, Jr., M.D.

Associate Professor of Neurology, University
of Connecticut; Attending Neurologist, University
of Connecticut Health Center, Farmington,
Connecticut
Lyme Disease

GERALD B. RICH, M.D., A.C.P.

Assistant Professor of Neurology, Oregon Health
Sciences University, Portland, Oregon
Sleep Disorders

ALAN I. ROSENBLATT, M.D.

Fellow, Developmental Pediatrics, The Johns
Hopkins University School of Medicine; Fellow,
Kennedy Institute, Baltimore, Maryland
Cerebral Palsy

ALLEN D. ROSES, M.D.

Jefferson Pilot Corporation Professor of Neurology
and Neurobiology, Duke University School of
Medicine; Chief, Division of Neurology, Duke
University Medical Center, Durham, North
Carolina
Muscular Dystrophy

JEFFREY D. ROTHSTEIN, M.D., Ph.D.

Instructor of Neurology, The Johns Hopkins
University School of Medicine, Baltimore,
Maryland
Hepatic Encephalopathy

WALTER ROYAL III, M.D.

Instructor, Department of Neurology, The Johns
Hopkins University School of Medicine, Baltimore,
Maryland
Drug Overdose and Withdrawal

ANDRES M. SALAZAR, M.D., Col., M.C.

Professor of Neurology, Uniformed Services
University of the Health Sciences; Director, Army
Head Injury Unit, Walter Reed Army Medical
Center, Bethesda, Maryland
Closed Head Injury

MARTIN A. SAMUELS, M.D.

Associate Professor of Neurology, Harvard
Medical School; Chief of Neurology, Brigham and
Women's Hospital, Boston, Massachusetts
Disorders of Consciousness

DONALD B. SANDERS, M.D.

Professor, Department of Medicine, Division of
Neurology, Duke University Medical School,
Durham, North Carolina
Lambert-Eaton Myasthenic Syndrome

LINDA F. SCHENDEL, P.N.P.

Staff Nurse, Blythdale Children's Hospital,
Valhalla, New York
Myelomeningocele

CHESTER W. SCHMIDT, Jr., M.D.

Associate Professor of Psychiatry, The Johns
Hopkins University School of Medicine; Chief of
Psychiatry, Francis Scott Key Medical Center,
Baltimore, Maryland
Sexual Problems in Spinal Cord Disease

MARTIN S. SCHWARTZ, M.D.

Consultant Clinical Neurophysiologist, St. George's Hospital, London, England
Paraneoplastic Syndromes

ROBERT J. SCHWARTZMAN, M.D.

Professor and Chairman of Neurology, Jefferson Medical College of Thomas Jefferson University; Chairman of Neurology, Thomas Jefferson University Hospital, Philadelphia, Pennsylvania
Reflex Sympathetic Dystrophy

DAVID G. SHERMAN, M.D.

Professor, Division of Neurology, University of Texas Health Science Center, San Antonio, Texas
Embolic Stroke of Cardiac Origin

SHLOMO SHINNAR, M.D., Ph.D.

Associate Professor of Neurology and Pediatrics, Albert Einstein College of Medicine; Director, Montefiore/Einstein Epilepsy Center, Montefiore Medical Center, Bronx, New York
Febrile Seizures

HARVEY S. SINGER, M.D.

Professor, Departments of Neurology and Pediatrics, The Johns Hopkins University School of Medicine, Baltimore, Maryland
Hyperactivity in Children: Attention-Deficit Hyperactivity Disorder

MARK STACY, M.D.

Clinical Instructor, Department of Neurology, Hahnemann University, Philadelphia, Pennsylvania
Cervical Spondylosis

GERALD G. STRIPH, M.D.

Clinical Assistant Professor of Ophthalmology, Medical College of Ohio, Toledo, Ohio
Essential Blepharospasm and Meige's Syndrome

S.H. SUBRAMONY, M.D.

Associate Professor of Neurology, University of Mississippi School of Medicine; Attending Physician, Department of Neurology, University of Mississippi Medical Center, Jackson, Mississippi
Inherited Ataxia

AUSTIN J. SUMNER, M.D.

Professor and Chairman, Department of Neurology, Louisiana State University School of Medicine in New Orleans, New Orleans, Louisiana
Brachial Neuritis

MICHAEL SWASH, M.D., FRCP, MRC Path

Senior Lecturer in Neuropathology, The London Hospital Medical College; Consultant Neurologist, The London Hospital, London, England
Paraneoplastic Syndrome

PATRICK J. SWEENEY, M.D., F.A.C.P.

Associate Clinical Professor of Neurology, Case Western Reserve University School of Medicine; Clinical Neurologist, Department of Neurology, The Cleveland Clinic Foundation, Cleveland, Ohio
Entrapment Neuropathy

RUP TANDAN, M.D., M.R.C.P.

Assistant Professor of Neurology, University of Vermont College of Medicine; Attending Neurologist, Medical Center Hospital of Vermont, Burlington, Vermont
Polymyositis

MARK L. TEITELBAUM, M.D.

Assistant Professor of Psychiatry and Medicine, The Johns Hopkins University School of Medicine; Director, Psychiatric Consultation-Liaison Service, The Johns Hopkins Hospital, Baltimore, Maryland
Hysterical Behavior

GIHAN TENNEKOON, M.D.

Associate Professor, Department of Neurology, The Johns Hopkins University School of Medicine, Baltimore, Maryland
Tuberous Sclerosis

KLAUS V. TOYKA, M.D.

Professor and Chairman, Department of Neurology, University of Wurzburg, Wurzburg, West Germany
Myasthenia Gravis

EILEEN P.G. VINING, M.D.

Associate Professor of Neurology and Pediatrics, The Johns Hopkins University School of Medicine, Baltimore, Maryland
Absence Seizures

REBECCA S. WAPPNER, M.D.

Associate Professor of Pediatrics, Indiana University School of Medicine, Indianapolis, Indiana
Aminoacidemia

DANNY F. WATSON, M.D., Ph.D.

Associate Professor of Neurology, Wayne State University School of Medicine, Detroit, Michigan
Chronic Neuropathy

LESLIE P. WEINER, M.D.

Chairman and Richard Angus Grant Senior Professor of Neurology, and Professor of Microbiology, University of Southern California School of Medicine, Los Angeles, California
Viral Encephalitis

DAVID O. WIEBERS, M.D.

Associate Professor of Neurology, Mayo Medical School; Head, Section of Neurology, Mayo Clinic and Mayo Foundation, Rochester, Minnesota
Intracranial Aneurysm

ASA J. WILBOURN, M.D.

Assistant Clinical Professor of Neurology, Case Western Reserve University School of Medicine; Director, EMG Laboratory, Department of Neurology, The Cleveland Clinic Foundation, Cleveland, Ohio
Entrapment Neuropathy

THOMAS N. WISE, M.D.

Associate Professor of Psychiatry and Medicine, The Johns Hopkins University School of Medicine, Baltimore, Maryland; Chief of Psychiatry, Fairfax Hospital, Falls Church, Virginia
Sexual Problems in Spinal Cord Disease

ANNE B. YOUNG, M.D., Ph.D.

Professor, Department of Neurology, University of Michigan Medical School, Ann Arbor, Michigan
Wilson's Disease

DEWEY K. ZIEGLER, M.D.

Professor of Neurology, University of Kansas School of Medicine, Kansas City, Kansas
Migraine and Cluster Headache

PREFACE

Current Therapy in Neurologic Disease was introduced in 1985 to supplement neurologic textbooks that emphasized etiology, pathophysiology, and diagnosis. Clear-cut therapeutic solutions were often hard to find in clinical texts; journals provided mainly new approaches and controversies; and pharmacology texts were usually filled with complex pharmacokinetics and alternative therapies. The purpose of this series was to ask an experienced clinician with specialized expertise in treating the disease in question to state simply and straightforwardly how he treats the patient with this particular ailment. These collections of second opinions have been well received.

As in the second edition, all authors have been changed. Some therapeutic approaches are quite new and others simply reflect a change of emphasis. Genuinely new information has become available during the past three years since the publication of the last edition, including the different clinical forms and management of neurofibromatosis; the better definition of HIV-associated disease including its intriguing interrelation with syphilis; the improved management of neurocysticercosis and Lyme disease; the much wider experience with botulinum toxin in blepharospasm, hemifacial spasm, and spasmodic torticollis; and the new practical issue of genetic counseling now feasible in Duchenne's and myotonic dystrophies.

In the second edition, we encouraged the use of treatment algorithms and added lists of patient resources, such as voluntary agencies that supply literature, support groups, or equipment sources. This has been continued. The principle of the series has been not to include references since all chapters are the personal opinions of the authors. Nonetheless, the most common criticism of the volumes, both personally and in reviews, has been the lack of references. Selected references related to therapy have been added to the chapters in this edition.

Drug doses have been checked, but the reader should scrutinize product information sheets for dosage changes or contraindications, particularly in new or infrequently used drugs.

I wish to express my sincere appreciation to the authors who share their expertise and experience with us. I also wish to thank Nancy Michel and Janice Fisher for their editorial assistance in preparing this volume, and to Brian Decker and his staff for their assistance and advice in continuing this series of therapy volumes.

Richard T. Johnson, M.D.

CONTENTS

PSYCHIATRIC CONDITIONS PRESENTING AS NEUROLOGIC DISEASE

DISORDERS OF CONSCIOUSNESS AND EQUILIBRIUM

DISORDERS OF CONSCIOUSNESS

MARTIN A. SAMUELS, M.D.

"Consciousness is a being such that in its being, its being is in question in so far as this being implies a being other than itself." (Sarte)

This impersonal concept of consciousness is the cornerstone of Jean-Paul Sartre's thought and represents one of the major principles underlying modern existentialism. Yet despite its profound importance, it has proved useless in the emergency department. Medical personnel require a more mundane definition—one capable of relating clinical phenomenology with anatomic and physiologic pathology. The concept of differential diagnosis fails when one is faced with a patient suffering from an altered level of responsiveness to external (and often internal) stimuli. The neurologist approaches the patient with a decreased level of responsiveness armed with a notion of consciousness which, although probably less profound than Sartre's, is practical and will allow one to localize the disorder, thereby reducing the plethora of possibilities to a realistic manageable number. To save time, some commonly encountered disorders may be treated simultaneously. The aim is to reach a diagnosis and or a definitive treatment within 1 hour of the patient's presentation.

AROUSAL AND AWARENESS

For our purposes, we shall assume that consciousness has two attributes, each of which has an anatomic substrate. These two attributes are arousal (or wakefulness) and awareness. Arousal (wakefulness) is that group of behavioral changes that occur when a person awakens from sleep. Of the array of changes that occur, the most conspicuous is that of opening of the eyes. Although one can be asleep with the eyes open or awake with the eyes closed, an organism with its eyes open is probably awake. Pathologic states associated with decreased respon-

siveness and closing of the eyes are therefore analogous to sleep in some respects. The neural system underlying this change in states is the fictitious ascending reticular activating system (ARAS), a conceptual array of nuclei and tracts, ascending in the core of the brainstem heading toward the nonspecific thalamic nuclei. These in turn relay information to the cerebral cortex. The inherent pacemaker rates of this centrocephalic system are the basis for the electroencephalogram. The ARAS is presumably part of the reticular formation in close proximity to other vegetative systems, such as those controlling respiration, cardiovascularity, eye movements, pupillary reaction, and cranial reflexes. Structural or metabolic processes that derange the function of the ARAS will probably have some effect on the neighboring systems that are dependent on reticular formation function. Thus, one cause of decreased consciousness would be failure of the ARAS. This category of decreased consciousness, also known as unarousal, is in a sense a state of pathologic sleep, and as such would share many of the behavioral manifestations of natural sleep, except that ordinary stimuli cannot arouse the patient.

Traditionally, the depth of unarousal is graded, largely to allow medical personnel to communicate with one another accurately in a shorthand fashion. Unfortunately, because the definitions of these grades have not been fully standardized, this has led to more rather than less confusion. It is best simply to describe the patient's appearance in plain English. For example: "Jones looks as if he were asleep. When I call his name he does not respond. When I pinch him he transiently awakens, curses, and falls back to sleep. I think he moves the left side less well than his right." This accurately describes the patient's state so that anyone can understand it. For those who must use shorthand, the following definitions of the various depths of unarousal may be used. *Confusion* (or inattention) refers to the inability to maintain a coherent stream of thought. This is the slightest abnormality in consciousness, and confused patients may appear to be awake or even hypervigilant with sympathetic hyperactivity (i.e., sweating with dilated pupils, tremor, and hypertension). This latter state, known as *delirium*, is generally seen in patients undergoing withdrawal from alcohol or sedatives or in states associated with excessive circulating sympathomimetic amines. *Drowsiness* is defined as a state of apparent sleep which can be overcome with a painful stimulus. For patients in a state of *stupor,* a simple pinch on the upper and lower extremities should elicit a response. If only reflex responses are elicited (e.g., decerebrate or decorticate posturing or triple flexion), one should not grade the state as stupor. *Coma* is defined as a state of apparent sleep in which there is only a reflex response (or no response at all) to a painful stimulus. Vague, undefined terms such as ''obtundation'' and ''lethargy'' should be avoided since generally no one, including the examining physician, knows what exactly they mean.

If a person is awake, does that mean that he or she is conscious? In humans, some aspects of consciousness are well beyond the brain stem's ken. It is these aspects of consciousness (which, for our purposes, we shall call ''awareness'') that are possibly unique to human beings. For the sake of our discussion, we will assume that the whole integrated function of the cerebral cortex is the anatomic substrate for awareness. We have learned from experience that in order to produce unawareness, there must be a diffuse bilateral lesion involving both sides of the cerebral cortex. Small lesions can produce profound deficits, such as aphasia, alexia, hemianopsia, and hemiparesis, but only a diffuse bilateral process, sparing the ARAS and diencephalic structures, can lead to unawareness or a vegetative state.

In summary, there are two kinds of unconsciousness: (1) unarousal caused by disease of the ARAS and (2) unawareness, caused by diffuse bilateral cerebral hemisphere disease. As far as we know, there are no other types of unconsciousness. Therefore, the problem of unconsciousness becomes a simple one for the physician. Is the trouble in the brain stem or is it diffusely present in the hemispheres? It should be obvious that failure of the arousal system renders it impossible to test the awareness system. Therefore, the question of whether there is consciousness when there is unarousal is a moot point.

MANAGEMENT OF THE UNCONSCIOUS PATIENT

Given this background, the evaluation of the unconscious person becomes simple. A few general practical rules should be kept in mind. The head or neck of the unconscious patient *must not be moved* until the cause of the loss of consciousness is determined. Head injuries are commonly associated with neck injuries. The latter may be the cause of the greatest permanent disability in an otherwise reversible concussion. At the scene of an accident, a collar should be placed on the neck in order to warn medical personnel not to move the head with respect to the torso until proper films can be taken. Naloxone, 0.01 mg per kilogram, administered by rapid intravenous (IV) infusion should be given immediately on the chance that an opiate overdose may be involved. Most adults should receive thiamine, 1 mg per kilogram, by rapid IV infusion in order to prevent exacerbation of possible Wernicke's encephalopathy. Dextrose, 1 g per kilogram, should be infused rapidly in order to reverse hypoglycemia. During the initial few minutes with the patient, a patent airway should be insured and the blood pressure measured. Most or all of the above maneuvers can be carried out in the field by emergency medical technicians.

When the patient reaches the emergency department, one should attempt to locate some person able to give a medical history. This is not always as easy as it sounds because often the unconscious patient has arrived in the emergency department unaccompanied. Family, police, ambulance personnel, or friends should be contacted and asked specifically about trauma, drugs (including alcohol, over-the-counter medications, and prescription drugs), headache, or other symptoms preceding the ictus, and whether such an attack has ever happened before. One good question to ask is: ''Do you have any theories as to what may have caused the trouble?''

Examination of the unconscious patient is aimed at determining whether the process is a brain stem disease or is diffuse in both hemispheres. One does this by examining brain stem structures that are in close proximity to the ARAS. These include those controlling cranial reflexes, respiratory control centers, pupillary reaction, and eye movements.

Certain cranial reflexes or automatisms are signs of relatively good brain stem function. These include sneezing and yawning, both of which are probably respiratory reflexes requiring a relatively intact reticular formation. Swallowing and hiccoughing, on the other hand, are probably mainly gastrointestinal reflexes that require only medullary function and do not carry the same good prognosis.

Both normal and Cheyne-Stokes respiratory patterns are relatively good signs in the unconscious patient, reflecting intact respiratory control centers in the pons and medulla. Hyperventilation in an unconscious person should always alert one to a search for a cause of metabolic acidosis. Such causes include diabetic ketoacidosis, lactic acidosis, methanol intoxication, ethylene glycol intoxication, and aspirin poisoning, and are usually also the cause of the unconsciousness. Hyperventilation without a metabolic cause (i.e., central neurogenic hyperventilation) is not a precisely localizing sign and as such is not particularly useful. Apneustic breathing (i.e., deep breaths with inspiratory cramps at the end of each deep breath) is a reliable sign of pontine damage. Ataxic (or Biot) respiration is the poorly coordinated, mechanically ineffective breathing seen in pa-

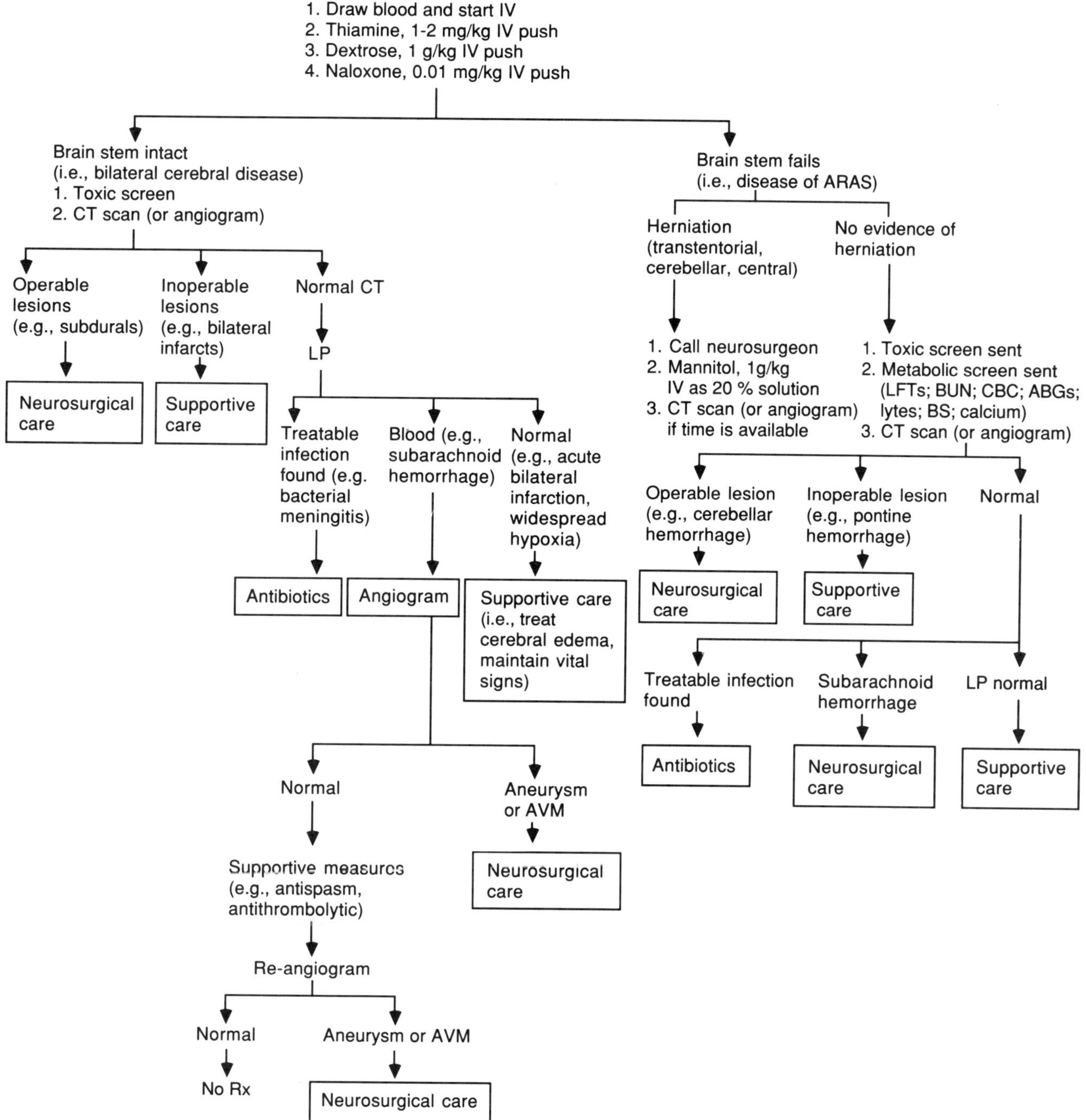

Figure 1 Diagnosis and treatment protocol in the comatose patient. LP = lumbar punctures; LFTs = liver function tests; ABGs = arterial blood gases; BS = blood sugar; AVM = arteriovenous malformation.
Republished with permission from Samuels MA, Aquino TM. Coma and other alterations of consciousness. In: Samuels MA, ed. Manual of neurologic therapeutics. 3rd ed. Boston: Little, Brown, & Co., 1986: 13.

tients with disease of the primary respiratory control centers in the medulla. In general, patients with apneustic and ataxic breathing should be intubated before the inevitable apnea occurs.

The pupils should be measured and the sizes recorded on the patient's chart. In general, sparing of the pupillary light reflex with simultaneous failure of other brainstem functions (e.g., breathing, eye movements) indicates a drug intoxication unless the drug in question has a direct effect on pupillary function (e.g., atropine). A dilating pupil in an unconscious patient with brain stem failure should be assumed to be caused by transtentorial herniation on the side of the large pupil. Such a patient should be hyperventilated (to a Pco_2 of about 25 mm Hg), and an imaging study (computed tomography or magnetic resonance imaging) should be performed while a neurosurgeon is called. Mannitol, 1 g per kilogram, may be given intravenously as a 20 percent solution if necessary. Unequal pupils in a conscious person is *never* caused by herniation of the brain. Most such patients are found to have a mydriatic drop in the eye, a migraine, or essential anisocoria. In no case should such a patient be treated for increased intracranial pressure.

The eye movements are examined to test the function of the brain stem from the level of the vestibular nuclei in the medulla to the oculomotor nuclei in the midbrain. There is no cause of brain stem unconsciousness—whether metabolic or structural—that does not also affect either the pupils, the eye movements, or both. First the patient is observed for spontaneous eye movement. If full conjugate eye movements occur without stimulus (so-called windshield-wiper eyes), this is strong evidence of a bihemisphere form of unconsciousness; the full-roving eye movements are prime fascia evidence of good brain stem function that has been disinhibited by the loss of input from the hemispheres above. If spontaneous eye movements are inadequate, the eyes should be stimulated to move using the vestibulo-ocular reflexes. The oculocephalic reflex cannot be used since, as I mentioned earlier, unconscious patients should not have their heads moved. The vestibulo-ocular reflex may be conveniently stimulated by infusing 20 to 50 ml of ice water into the ear. After a pause of a few seconds, the eyes should move conjugately and fully *toward* the side of the ice water infusion. If this occurs, the brain stem is partially functioning from the vestibular nuclei to the midbrain. If the hemispheres are functioning normally, they will issue a command to correct the vestibular-induced movement. This command probably comes from the frontal eye fields opposite the direction of the corrective fast eye movement. In physiologically explicable states of unconsciousness, there is always an abnormality in either the slow (vestibular) or fast (cortical) phase of the ice water–induced eye movement. If both phases are normal, the state of unconsciousness is caused by neither brain stem disease nor bilateral hemispheral disease. Because the traditional definition of unconsciousness attributes unconsciousness to only these two causes, this latter state is referred to as "functional" or "hysterical" unconsciousness. Unconsciousness is a relatively common conversion symptom, and is manifested by totally normal brain stem and hemispheral function as outlined above. It can usually be reversed through some type of strong suggestion that the patient will recover, thus allowing the patient a graceful way out of the emergency department.

Lastly, one should consider the presentation of a patient who is unresponsive but awake. In this case, the brain stem function is assumed to be intact, so the difficulty must be bihemispheral. If the ice water test shows intact slow (vestibular) phases but no fast (cortical) phases, one must conclude that the process is bilateral and diffuse in the hemispheres. This so-called vegetative state is distinct from brain death, since the latter includes brain stem death. The common processes leading to a chronic vegetative state are global hypoxic-ischemic damage such as cardiac arrest and chronic degenerative processes such as Alzheimer's disease. Other states in which patients appear to be awake but are unresponsive (akinetic mutism) include (1) the abulic state caused by bilateral prefrontal lobe disease (e.g., tumor, hemorrhage, hydrocephalus, degenerative disease, stroke), (2) the locked-in states (e.g., pontine hemorrhage), and (3) nonconvulsive status epilepticus, (4) catatonia, and (5) hysterical mutism.

Figure 1 shows a decision tree of the evaluation and treatment of unconscious patients based on the principles outlined in the text. It is designed so that the final diagnosis and/or definitive therapy is reached within 60 minutes.

SUGGESTED READING

Fisher CM. The neurological examination of the comatose patient. Acta Neurol Scand 1969; 45(suppl):5–56.
Levy DE, Caronna JJ, Singer BH, et al. Predicting outcome from hypoxic-ischemic coma. JAMA 1985; 253:1420–1426.
Plum F, Posner JB. The diagnosis of stupor and coma. 3rd ed. Philadelphia: Davis, 1980.
Ropper AH. Lateral displacement of the brain and level of consciousness in patients with an acute hemispheral mass. N Engl J Med 1986; 953–958.

SYNCOPE

GEORGE DAVID PERKIN, B.A., FRCP

Patients seldom use the term syncope to describe an episode of loss of consciousness. They are more likely to complain of experiencing blackouts or "passing out." A discussion of the management of syncope, restricting the term to episodes of altered consciousness triggered by a reduction of cerebral perfusion, is a relatively simple undertaking. In practice, however, many attacks of altered awareness cannot be so readily attributed to this cause, and their management becomes a more complex issue (Fig. 1). The problem is a common one. Between 1983 and 1987 I encountered 239 patients who had had one or more attacks of loss of consciousness that were not clearly epileptic in origin. The breakdown of their diagnoses is given in Table 1.

HISTORY

Patients usually appreciate that when they have had attacks of loss of consciousness, additional information about the episodes is required from a third party. If that information is not forthcoming at the first interview, the patient should be encouraged to bring a witness at their next visit. Close relatives are not necessarily best suited for this purpose. Often, concern over the attack limits their ability to give an accurate history. Estimates of the duration of the individual phases of the episode tend to be inaccu-

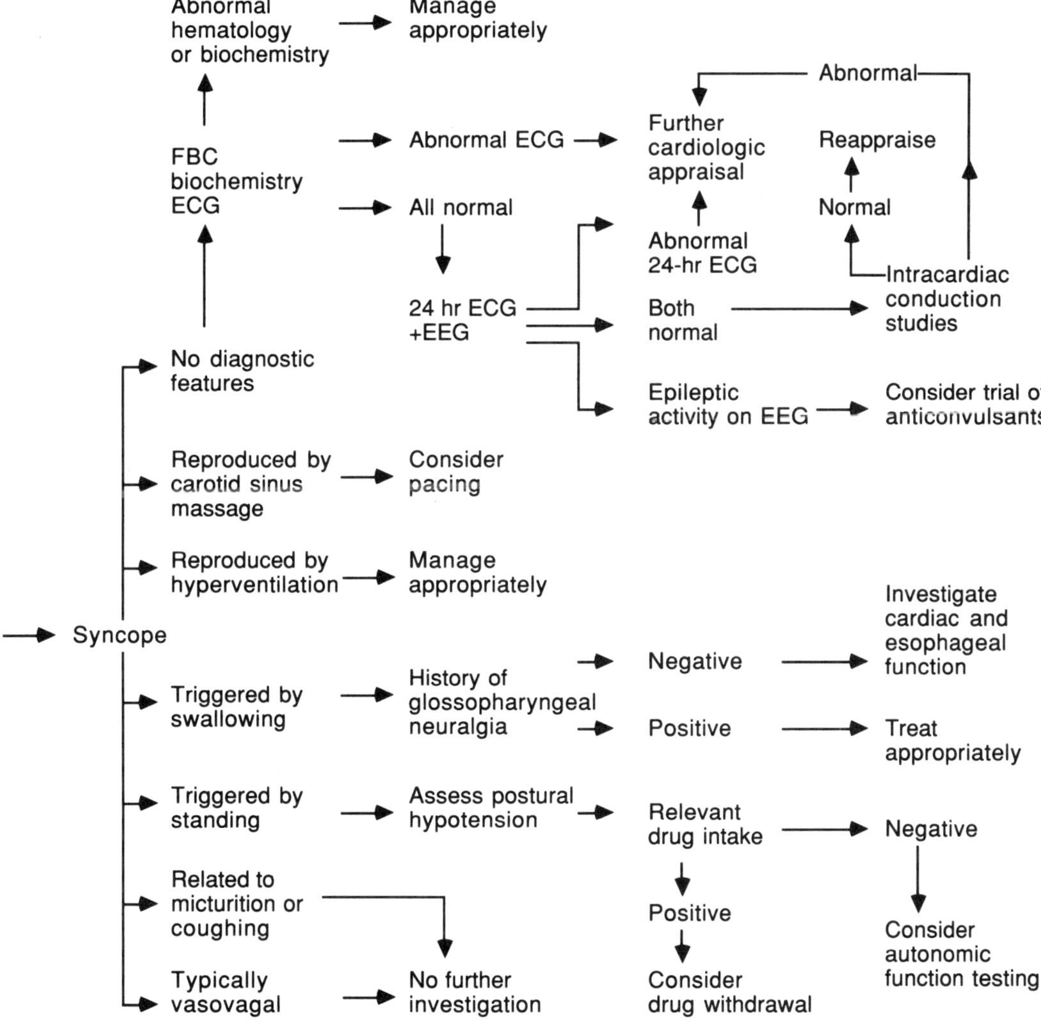

Figure 1 Evaluation and treatment of syncope. (Republished with permission from Perkin GD. Diagnostic tests in neurology. London: Chapman and Hall Medical, 1988:34.)

Table 1 Causes of Syncopal Attacks in a Series of 239 Patients

Causes	No. of Patients
Vasovagal attacks	76
Micturition syncope	6
Cough syncope	2
Vomiting syncope	1
Syncope secondary to anemia	1
Cardiac syncope	4
Orthostatic hypotension	1
Hyperventilation syndrome	21
Hysteria	7
Unknown	120
Total	239

rate, and elaborate descriptions sometimes owe more to the imagination of the witness than the reality of the event. Critical details aiding diagnosis include those describing the nature of any prodromal symptoms and the circumstances in which the attacks have occurred. Often these two pieces of information alone serve to establish the diagnosis. More problematic in terms of management is the group of patients in whom the initial history and examination fail to suggest a possible cause for the event.

VASOVAGAL ATTACKS

This is the most common form of diagnosable syncope encountered in clinical practice. The majority of attacks, which are more common in women than in men, occur during the 2nd and 3rd decades of life. There is a well-defined aura, with malaise, nausea, faintness, pallor, and sweating featuring prominently. The attacks are often triggered by specific events—for example, venesection or a stressful emotional experience. The loss of posture tends to be less abrupt than in epilepsy, and the patient lies quietly after such an attack. Patients giving a typical history do not require investigation. They should be advised to sit or (preferably) lie down as soon as symptoms appear. Loss of consciousness seldom occurs if the patient is already sitting, and never if they are lying, so that the effectiveness of posture change in influencing symptoms can serve as a diagnostic test. Individuals particularly liable to faint should lie down before having potentially painful procedures performed.

Under what circumstances may further investigation be necessary? Apparently typical attacks can occur in older patients; in my series, 5 percent were older than 40 years of age. The possibility of a cardiac dysrhythmia is higher in this group. If the cardiovascular system and electrocardiogram (ECG) are normal, I do not investigate further unless the episodes are recurrent. A brief tonic posture can occur during an attack of a vasovagal syncope but not clonic movements or a tonic-clonic progression, both of which suggest the diagnosis of a vasovagal syncope complicated by epilepsy. In this case, management depends on how closely related the attacks are to a specific stimulus; in some patients, avoidance of the relevant trigger may be a more rational approach than the use of anticonvulsants. Electroencephalography (EEG) is an appropriate means of investigation, but seldom computed tomography or magnetic resonance imaging scanning, since the occurrence of a vasovagal syncope complicated by epilepsy is rarely if ever the reflection of structural pathology within the central nervous system.

MICTURITION SYNCOPE

Attacks of micturition syncope are usually nocturnal, occur predominantly in men, and are more likely to occur after alcohol ingestion. Eyewitness accounts are seldom forthcoming and, when available, usually provide information only about the aftermath of the event. If the history is typical, no action is required other than that of suggesting to the patient (if male) that he be in a sitting position when micturating, particularly at night. Prostatic obstruction is seldom of importance in the genesis of this condition and should be investigated only if there are suggestive symptoms.

COUGH SYNCOPE

Cough syncope is rare. Typically, a bout of intractable coughing terminates in a syncope. I have encountered one patient in whom persistent retching had a similar effect. If the history is characteristic of patients with this condition, no further investigation is required. Management should be aimed at the underlying chest disorder. If the paroxysm of coughing that triggered the syncope was not particularly violent and if the attacks are recurrrent, it is advisable to perform ECG monitoring while the patient coughs. Sometimes this reveals that the syncope is caused by an atrioventricular block precipitated by coughing. If so, insertion of a pacemaker is required.

SWALLOW SYNCOPE

I have never seen a case of swallow syncope. Most patients with this complaint have structural disease of the esophagus readily revealed by barium swallow or endoscopy. Sometimes, however, the esophageal abnormality is subtle or even absent.

ECG monitoring should be performed while the patient swallows to identify the type of cardiac conduction defect responsible for the syncope. If there is overt esophageal disease, it is managed appropriately. If not, alternative treatments include either the use of anticholinergic drugs or cardiac pacing adjusted to the nature of the atrioventricular block. The latter approach is preferable.

CAROTID SINUS SYNCOPE

It has been suggested that this condition is underdiagnosed, although I have seldom encountered it in clinical practice. Cardioinhibitory and depressor forms are described in the literature, with the former producing a syncope by triggering asystole or atrioventricular block, and the latter by inducing hypotension. Reproduction of an attack by carotid sinus massage remains the cornerstone of diagnosis. ECG control is mandatory during this procedure. Symptomatic forms of the condition result from tumor invasion of the sinus, but the vast majority of cases are idiopathic. Therapeutic approaches include carotid sinus denervation and pacing. Theoretically, the former can deal with both the cardioinhibitory and depressor forms. Pacing, however, is probably the preferable option.

CARDIAC SYNCOPE

In some patients who experience syncope, a cardiac basis for the problem is suggested by a history of concurrent palpitations or by the presence of an abnormally slow heart rate on clinical examination. Additional support is provided if an observer is able to record an abnormal heart rate during subsequent attacks. A routine ECG may serve to establish a diagnosis, but if it does not, a period of Holter monitoring is justified. For patients with complete heart block or the sick sinus syndrome, the treatment of choice is cardiac pacing. Tachyarrhythmias are less likely to produce a syncope. If, on the basis of 24-hour monitoring or of clinical examination, I suspect a cardiologic abnormality, I refer the patient for an expert opinion. Other cardiac disorders sometimes presenting with syncope include aortic stenosis and atrial myxoma.

ORTHOSTATIC HYPOTENSION

Syncope caused by postural hypotension figures infrequently in a neurologist's case-load, but is a relatively common problem in the elderly. The history of attacks triggered by postural change is readily elicited, and the extent of the problem easily determined by measurement of blood pressure with the patient in the lying and standing positions. Drug therapy is often partly responsible; during the enquiry, one should look for ingestion of diuretics, hypotensive agents, phenothiazines and tricyclic antidepressants. Management should consist of either discontinuing the use of the offending agent or, if this is not possible, advice regarding changing posture. Full-length elastic stockings will help reduce venous pooling.

In some patients, orthostatic hypotension is the first manifestation of either pure autonomic failure or multisystem atrophy (Shy-Drager syndrome). The management of both conditions is unsatisfactory. The patient is advised to rise slowly from the sitting or recumbent posture. Micturition should be performed in the sitting position. The lavatory door must never be locked, as it may prevent access to the patient during a syncopal episode. Care-givers or relatives should be advised about what action to take if the patient complains of faintness. Therapeutic measures are of limited value. I advise patients to wear full-length elastic stockings, putting them on before rising in the morning, and prescribe fludrocortisone, 0.1 mg administered three times daily. The patients are encouraged to sleep at a slight ''head up'' tilt, slowly increasing to about 10 to 15 degrees. Beyond this, I have not been convinced that other forms of treatment influence the problem. Regimens advocated in the past have included administration of ephedrine, dihydroergotamine, a combination of tyramine and a monoamine oxidase inhibiter, and cardiac pacing at an artificially high rate. An antigravity suit successfully controls symptoms but is too cumbersome to be recommended.

HYPERVENTILATION SYNDROME

In most series, loss of consciousness has been an infrequent component of the hyperventilation syndrome. In my cases, encountered between 1983 and 1987, loss of consciousness occurred in one-fourth of patients, although for many of these, loss of consciousness was an isolated event despite multiple episodes of hyperventilation. The combination of a normal neurologic examination and the reproduction of an attack by overbreathing serves to establish the diagnosis, although some physicians also require the identification of hypocapnoea during the attack. Although rebreathing into a bag can rapidly terminate symptoms, I find many patients reluctant to use this measure. Where the symptoms are of recent onset and episodes are infrequent, discussion of the mechanism often helps alleviate the problem. In more chronic cases, formal breathing exercises are necessary. If there is evidence of an associated anxiety state, I favor psychiatric referral rather than simply prescribing anxiolytics.

CONVERSION HYSTERIA

Conversion hysteria is occasionally a cause of syncopal attacks. Pseudo-seizures are seen more commonly. The diagnosis can be difficult to establish and necessitates identification of other conversion reactions. Injuries sustained as a result of syncopal events do not exclude the diagnosis. The episodes are seldom brief, with the patient more often entering a fugue-like state lasting for hours. If the onset of conversion reactions has been relatively recent, and particularly if there are depressive features, I favor psychiatric referral. In my experience with patients who have longer-standing symptoms, attempts to modify their reactions have failed.

SYNCOPAL ATTACKS OF UNCERTAIN CAUSE

The protocol for the investigation and management of the conditions already described is straightforward (Fig. 1). There remains a substantial proportion of patients (almost exactly half in my series) in whom the cause of the syncopal event is not readily discernible. In other words, the attacks do not suggest epilepsy, nor are there the clinical characteristics that would identify one of the conditions discussed earlier in this chapter. Clinical examination is normal. In this case, the next step is to perform routine hematologic and biochemical investigations along with an ECG. In all likelihood, the results of these tests will be normal, but occasionally they suggest the probable basis for the events (as in the case of one of my patients with an unsuspected, but severe anemia). Further management should be influenced by whether the attack was isolated or recurrent. My policy is not to investigate further in patients who have had an isolated syncopal event with normal findings on the initial screening. If the attacks have recurred, I obtain an EEG and proceed to a 24-hour period of Holter monitoring. Unless they are very frequent, attacks rarely occur during the monitoring period, but certain abnormalities indicate the need for cardiologic appraisal. These include frequent or repetitive ventricular ectopy and periods of sinus arrest. In addition, high-resolution ECG monitoring, if available, should be performed in order to identify any low-amplitude signals in the terminal portion of the QRS complex or in the ST segment. Such potentials correlate with a susceptibility to spontaneous or inducible ventricular tachycardia and require cardiologic appraisal.

Remaining are a substantial number of patients with syncope whose investigations have yielded normal results. For these, the question of performing more invasive cardiologic procedures, including ventricular stimulation, arises. These techniques are not universally available and are more stressful for the patient. Furthermore uncertainty sometimes remains as to whether electrophysiologic abnormalities detected by such techniques necessarily explain the patient's attacks. I believe there is no justification for such investigation in patients who have had an isolated syncopal event or infrequently recurring events and in whom there are no cardiologic abnormalities. In patients who experience frequent syncope, the investigation is probably warranted, although further prospective studies in this field are required.

SUGGESTED READING

Morady F. The evaluation of syncope with electrophysiologic studies. Clin Cardiol 1986; 4:515–526.
Riley TZ, Roy A, eds. Pseudo-seizures. Baltimore: Williams and Wilkins, 1982.
Schellack J, Fulenwider JT, Olson RA, et al. The carotid sinus syndrome: a frequently overlooked cause of syncope in the elderly. J Vasc Surg 1986; 4:376–383.

VERTIGO

TIMOTHY C. HAIN, M.D.

Vertigo, the illusion of rotation, is nearly always caused by vestibular system dysfunction. Management of vertigo is easiest when an accurate localization and etiologic diagnosis are available. Unfortunately, however, an etiologic diagnosis cannot be established in the majority of patients with vertigo.

In cases where a specific treatment is not available, symptomatic relief may be provided by antiemetics and drugs that depress peripheral vestibular function. Unfortunately, all vestibular suppressant medications have side effects that limit their use. Furthermore, reduction of vertigo is accomplished by reducing vestibular function on *both* the normal and abnormal side. Thus, vestibular suppressants can induce ataxia.

The inability of available medications to suppress vertigo effectively without unacceptable side effects has led clinicians to attempt other modes of treatment. Recently, greater emphasis has been placed on vestibular rehabilitation therapy in which recovery is promoted by exercises aimed at facilitating central adaptive mechanisms.

This chapter concentrates on common conditions that account for most of the referrals to a vertigo clinic and defines the role of medication or vestibular exercises in treating these disorders.

PATHOPHYSIOLOGY

The peripheral vestibular apparatus, which consists of the semicircular canals and otolith organs, senses angular and linear acceleration. Angular acceleration is related to rotation of the head and is registered by the canals. Linear acceleration is related to translation of the head as well as changes in the orientation of the head to gravity and is registered by the otoliths. Accordingly, illusions of rotation, translation, or tilt and symptoms initiated or aggravated by head movement are the hallmarks of vestibular system disease.

Symptoms of semicircular canal disturbance include a sensation of rotation as if the body were spinning, cartwheeling, or tumbling. Symptoms of otolith disturbance include sensations of tilt, levitation, or impulsion. If an otolithic disturbance is severe enough, the patient may be precipitated to the ground (e.g., the "otolithic crisis of Tumarkin" experienced by patients with Meniere's syndrome). Symptoms of autonomic overactivity such as sweating, pallor, nausea, and vomiting nearly always accompany vertigo of labyrinthine origin.

Central vestibular lesions, which may also cause vertigo, usually involve structures in which afferent activity from both labyrinths have been combined. The resulting pattern of imbalance in vestibular activity may more closely resemble naturally induced sensations of rotation and is usually associated with milder symptoms than peripheral vestibular imbalance.

ACUTE PERIPHERAL VESTIBULAR IMBALANCE

Most peripheral causes of vertigo result in distress caused by sensation of movement, nausea, and malaise for only 2 to 3 days. Even patients with vestibular nerve section are usually up and about within 1 week. Accordingly, even untreated, most patients with symptoms caused by a transient and incomplete paresis of vestibular function on one side will be ready to go back to their regular activities after 1 week.

In treating this condition, the dilemma of the physician is that, although patients want to be treated with a medication that will completely suppress their vertigo and somatic responses to vestibu-

Table 1 Drugs Used for Nausea

Drug	Dose	Comments
Droperidol (Inapsine)	2.5 or 5 mg IM *or* sublingual q12h	May produce extra-pyramidal reaction
Prochlorperizine (Compazine)	10 mg IM or p.o. q4–6h *or* 25 mg rectal q12 h	May produce extra-pyramidal reaction
Promethazine (Phenergan)	25 mg p.o. q4–6h *or* 25 mg rectal q6h	Sedating

lar imbalance, such treatment can harm the patient, by denying his nervous system the ability to compensate for a vestibular lesion. If the vestibular imbalance is covered up by a vestibular suppressant medication, little repair activity may be initiated. Even bedrest may be contraindicated. Animal studies have clearly shown that when experimental vestibular lesions are made, immobilization delays recovery.

The strategy is therefore to use as few medications as possible and to encourage head movement and early ambulation. When there appears to be no alternative to medication, I prefer to use antiemetics such as prochlorperazine (Compazine) or promethazine (Phenergan). These may be prescribed as suppositories. Brief usage of Antivert (meclizine) may also be helpful. If the patient appears to be dehydrated, he should be admitted. Tables 1 and 2 list commonly available drugs and dosages.

In the acute phase, generally on the 1st day, patients should be warned that sudden head movements and changing the position of the head relative to the gravitational axis may cause increased vertigo. However, once the patient is able to sit up and navigate about the room, he should be encouraged to attempt as much normal activity as is possible without triggering emesis. Medications, particularly sedatives, should be discontinued as soon as possible, as they may retard eventual compensation. Most patients recover spontaneously without the need for a formal vestibular rehabilitation program,

Table 2 Drugs Used to Decrease Vertigo

Drug	Dose	Comments
Diazepam (Valium)	5–10 mg p.o., IM, or IV (1 dose) given acutely	Sedating respiratory depressant
Dimenhydrinate (Dramamine)	50 mg p.o. q4–6h	Sedating
Meclizine (Antivert)	25 mg p.o. q4–6h	Sedating
Scopolamine Transdermscop	patch q3d	Anticholinergic side effects

because their vestibular impairment is transient rather than permanent.

What about the patients who don't recover spontaneously? Usually they have a fixed vestibular paresis or loss. Such patients can benefit from an organized physical therapy program incorporating the gait training and visual-vestibular exercises outlined in Table 3. This ensures that they receive adequate sensory input for their impaired vestibular system and develop appropriate strategies to deal with sensitivity to head motion and disequilibrium.

BENIGN PAROXYSMAL POSITIONAL VERTIGO

Benign paroxysmal positional vertigo (BPPV) is the most common cause of vertigo in the elderly. The diagnosis is easily made if the patient has had a

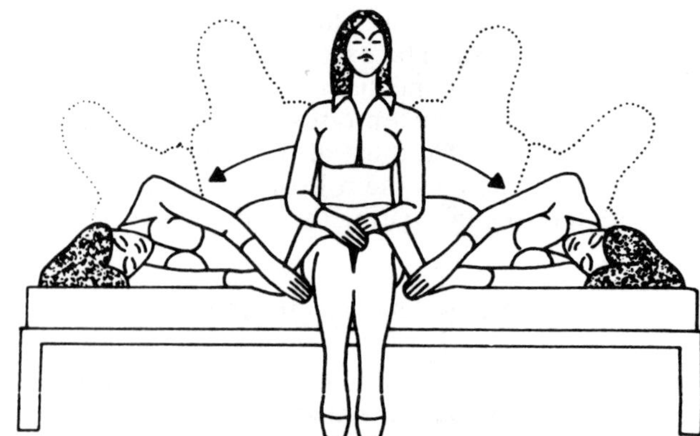

Figure 1 Positioning exercises for the treatment of benign paroxysmal positional vertigo (see Table 3 for details). (Republished with permission from Brandt T, Daroff RB. Physical therapy for benign paroxysmal positional vertigo. Arch Otolaryngol 1980; 106:484.

history of vertigo elicited by turning over in bed and if there is a typical nystagmus pattern that appears on positional testing. The cause is currently believed to be small bits of free debris that are loose in the labyrinthine system and which settle to the bottom of the ear, causing nystagmus for certain head positions. These patients are sometimes troubled by mild gait ataxia, but they are always most concerned by their inability to control vertigo that arises when they roll over in bed at night, or when they get up in the morning.

Drugs are not useful in treating BPPV because, although the vertigo is severe, it lasts only for a few seconds. There are two available approaches to treatment.

Most patients benefit from exercises for BPPV (see Table 3), which consist essentially of repeatedly inducing the symptoms of the vertigo for 2 weeks or until the symptoms can no longer be induced. This approach is often successful, presumably because either (1) the debris is moved to an insensitive portion of the labyrinth, (2) the patient learns to tolerate his symptoms, or (3) the disease process remits spontaneously. Because BPPV is fatigable, some patients induce their symptoms purposefully at the beginning of the day so that they can go about their activities without trouble. If the exercises provoke nausea, patients can be premedicated with antiemetics. If patients do not benefit from the exercises, the diagnosis should be reconsidered as central positional nystagmus can be mistaken for BPPV.

A second treatment option is to cut the nerve to the posterior semicircular canal—that is, to perform a singular neurectomy. This procedure should be considered only in patients who have been sympto-

---

Table 3 Vestibular Exercises

Gait-training exercises
    Begin walking with feet at a comfortable distance apart, progress to tandem position, eyes closed tandem, and head up tandem.
    Perform the above exercise while standing on a slab of foam rubber about 4 inches off the floor.
    Walk across the room with the eyes open and then with the eyes closed.
    Walk from heel to toe across the room with the eyes open and then with the eyes closed.

Visual-Vestibular exercises
    View a small target (about 2 in. × 2 in.) containing written material (e.g., a match cover). Fix the target to the wall or other solid object—do *not* use a hand held object. While trying to keep the words on the target in clear focus, move your head, first from side to side (approximately ± 45 degrees) and then up and down (approximately ± 30 degrees) at progressively higher speeds. The speed of the head movement should be increased until the words on the target can no longer be read.
    Perform the above exercise with a large-patterned target.
    Hold a small target or a patterned piece of cardboard at arm's length. While trying to keep the pattern or target in focus, move the head and target horizontally in opposite directions approximately 20 degrees to either side.
    Play any game involving simultaneous movement of the head and use of vision.

Exercises for BPPV
    Assume an upright sitting position in bed, with your legs on the floor (see Fig. 1). Close your eyes and suddenly tilt yourself to one side so that one side of your body is against the bed. Turn the head slightly upward and wait for the vertigo to subside. Sit back up and wait for 30 seconds before tilting to the opposite side. If vertigo occurs in this position as well, wait until it subsides and then sit up again. Perform this exercise five times in the morning and five times at night until 2 days have passed during which you do not experience vertigo.

matic for more than 2 years, in whom the side of lesion is certain, and who have not benefitted from the exercises. Most patients decide against neurectomy because of the risk of hearing impairment associated with this surgery.

MENIERE'S SYNDROME

The diagnosis of Meniere's disease should be considered in any patient who has both intermittent vertigo combined with a static or intermittent hearing deficit, or vertigo combined with an abnormal sensation in one ear. Meniere's syndrome is probable when a brisk spontaneous nystagmus is observed on at least one occasion, fluctuations in hearing can be documented on audiometry, and studies necessary to exclude structural lesions of the labyrinth have been performed.

Two levels of therapy may be considered. For patients who have infrequent episodes of vertigo, vestibular suppressants, possibly combined with an antiemetic, are used for the acute attack, and no medications are used in the interim. Oral meclizine and promethazine are the most useful agents for mild attacks. For patients with severe attacks who present in the emergency room, prochlorperazine (which can be given intramuscularly) and diazepam are the most useful agents. If patients appear dehydrated, they should be admitted to the hospital. Vestibular exercises are not used, as adaptations made during the period of transient vestibular imbalance are inappropriate when the patient has recovered. Over the long-term, salt restriction and use of a mild sodium-wasting diuretic such as hydrochlorothiazide may reduce the frequency of attacks.

For patients who are troubled by frequent attacks of vertigo and who have hearing loss confined to one ear, vestibular neurectomy or labyrinthectomy may be considered. These operations must be considered with caution, since many patients with Meniere's syndrome have bilateral disease; in such patients, surgery will be ineffective. Furthermore, even if patients have disease confined to one side at the time of treatment, they may develop Meniere's syndrome in the opposite ear in the future. Nevertheless, given the ineffectiveness of drug therapy, vestibular neurectomy or labyrinthectomy may be the only practical form of relief to offer.

OTOTOXICITY

Ototoxic antibiotics can cause oscillopsia, ataxia, and vertigo. Usually the diagnosis of ototoxicity can be made on the basis of the history alone; patients with this condition include those receiving peritoneal dialysis or those whose bone marrow transplant has recently become infected and who have begun receiving ototoxic antibiotics. After they recover from their infection and try to get out of bed, they discover their ataxia. On examination, these patients can read the vision chart with their head still, but drop two or more lines of acuity when their heads are gently oscillated.

These patients usually respond well to physical therapy. Several avenues of adaptation to their deficit are available. First, there is considerable plasticity of the vestibulo-ocular reflex, and by having the patient perform maneuvers that exaggerate the mismatch between their head movements and compensatory eye responses (i.e., activities that elicit oscillopsia), their symptoms may be diminished (see Table 3).

Cognitive strategies provide a second avenue of help. Patients can "spot" or fixate a reference traget before making a head movement, and use their intact visual pursuit mechanism to provide visual stability. Before walking across a room in the dark, patients should form a mental map of the room before turning out the lights.

It is also important to optimize nonvestibular methods of obtaining orientation information and to develop better motor programs for dealing with instability. Improving vision through wearing proper eyeglasses or through cataract removal if indicated, and the use of appropriate (low-heeled) shoes can be very useful. The gait-training exercises such as those outlined in Table 3 may be used. Of course, medications that are ototoxic or which suppress the vestibular system (such as those listed in Table 2) and their pharmacologic relatives should be avoided.

CENTRAL VERTIGO

Vertigo and disequilibrium occur in patients with lesions of the cerebellum or brainstem and particularly of the area of the vestibular nucleus and the floor of the 4th ventricle. The vestibular nucleus is a large structure that extends from pons to medulla. While patients with peripheral vestibular asymmetry typically recover within months, patients with central vertigo may continue to be distressed by ataxia, nausea, and illusions of motion for years. Presumably the persistence of their symptoms reflects a lesion in the central mechanisms that usually compensate for vestibular lesions.

Although vestibular suppressants such as meclizine or scopolamine are usually unsuccessful in the treatment of central vertigo, they are worth a try. Ativan (lorazepam) in a dose of 1 to 2 mg twice daily helps in some cases. Gait training and visual-vestibular exercises such as those outlined in Table

3 should be attempted. In patients with craniocervical junction abnormalities such as the Chiari malformation, a two-post cervical collar may be tried.

VERTIGO OF UNKNOWN ORIGIN

The last, most difficult to treat, and unfortunately, most common group of patients are those who experience vertigo for which we have no clue as to the origin. Some of these patients have psychogenic causes of vertigo, and others simply have disorders for which our diagnostic technology is not adequate. There are probably a large number of patients in the latter group; although there are three semicircular canals and two otolith organs on each side of the head, we have specific tests for the lateral semicircular canals only—we have no good way of assessing function of the vertical canals or of the otolith organs.

My approach to these patients is to manage them symptomatically and follow them at 3- or 6-month intervals. I refer patients disabled by their vertigo for vestibular physical therapy. Patients with intermittent symptoms are prescribed vestibular suppressants which they are to use only when symptomatic. All vestibular suppressants are discontinued in patients with chronic disequilibrium or vertigo.

I see these patients emergently when they are acutely dizzy, hoping to be able to establish the side of lesion through observation of a nystagmus or hearing loss. Often, a trial of salt restriction and diuretics is useful because it is generally impossible to exclude the possibility of Meniere's syndrome. In patients with frequent headaches, an attempt at migraine prophylaxis is worthwhile.

SUGGESTED READING

Baloh RW. Dizziness, hearing loss, and tinnitus: the essentials of neurotology. Philadelphia: F.A. Davis, 1984.
Brandt T, Daroff RB. Physical therapy for benign paroxysmal positional vertigo. Arch Otolaryngol 1980; 106:484.
Wood CD, Graybiel A. Evaluation of sixteen anti-motion-sickness drugs under controlled laboratory conditions. Aerospace Med 1968; 39:1342.

SLEEP DISORDERS

GERALD B. RICH, M.D., A.C.P.

Four major groups of sleep disorders are recognized: disorders of initiating and maintaining sleep, disorders of excessive somnolence, disorders of the sleep/wake schedule, and the parasomnias. Although a thorough history is important to the diagnosis of a sleep-related problem, the patient is often unable to contribute crucial information about his sleeping patterns for the very reason that he was asleep during the period in question. To help resolve this dilemma, I encourage the patient's spouse/bedpartner to complete questionnaires on sleep patterns and other personal historical features and to accompany the patient to the initial evaluation.

Various diagnostic aides are unique to the field. One is the sleep/wake diary, which the patient keeps for 2 weeks before the evaluation. The understanding of certain circadian rhythm disorders are particularly helped by this practice.

Also pivotal in diagnosis and therapeutic decision making is polysomnography. This continuous electrophysiologic monitoring process should be performed in a facility specializing in sleep disorders, with an accredited clinical polysomnographer available. Data collected should include the results of electroencephalography (EEG) and electromyography, cardiorespiratory measures of various types, and information on eye and extremity movements. Data must be collected at a time corresponding to the patient's sleep period during the light-dark cycle. The practice of brief diurnal "nap" studies in place of true polysomnography is fraught with diagnostic inaccuracy and should be avoided. The polysomnogram is critical to the discovery of the pathology producing altered alertness and to the quantification of sleep time and stage percentages. For the evaluation of the individual with irresistible "daytime" sleepiness, a polysomnogram is followed by a multiple sleep latency test. The latter consists of a series of structured naps performed during a patient's habitual period of wakefulness and is the only accurate method of establishing the presence of true *physiologic* sleepiness. The use of daytime, abbreviated EEG studies—even when eye movements are recorded—should no longer be considered an acceptable diagnostic method for patients with sleep disorders. I refuse to prescribe habituating, potentially abused medications, where otherwise appropriately indicated, unless objective verification of pathology has been completed by the above means.

DISORDERS OF INITIATING AND MAINTAINING SLEEP

Insomnia, often treated as a diagnostic entity, is comprised of a diverse group of disorders with psychological and organic etiologies. Defining an adequate amount of sleep is difficult, with a normal amount of sleep ranging between 4 and 10 hours and varying with age. Determining what constitutes sleep onset delay is also difficult, although a 30-minute interval can be considered reasonably normal. With a careful history, insomnia can be subdivided into three main categories with important treatment implications. Patients with sleep onset difficulties as the primary complaint most frequently have psychiatric difficulties and infrequently require polysomnography. The second group are those awakening uncharacteristically early, experiencing either an inability to return to sleep or light, fragmented sleep thereafter; such cases are often indicative of depressive disorders, although there can be important exceptions. The last group are those patients experiencing abnormal awakenings at night without obvious medical or psychological explanation; the frequency of organic disturbance in this group is high and diagnostic polysomnography typically essential. Age is another important clinical factor. The younger individual typically has sleep initiating disturbances; the elderly more often develop sleep maintenance problems.

Transient psychophysiologic insomnia, essentially a situational sleep disturbance, arises in response to an acute stress and is a universal human experience. The occasional night of poor sleep does not require specific intervention. The real goal of insomnia treatment is to provide a restorative sense to sleep and, even more crucial, to provide the patient with a normal degree of alertness during his scheduled waking hours. In those situations in which sleep deprivation may aggravate already existing anxiety or depression or the ability to deal with acute illness, the use of medication may be of benefit. Care should be exercised in selecting an agent relative to existing medical conditions, and with consideration given to the possibility that the agent may aggravate other sleep disorders that may be as yet undetected, such as sleep apnea. Eliminate pharmacologically active agents that may aggravate the insomnia. Caffeine and nicotine should be discontinued, and prescribed drugs should be scrutinized for possible involvement. Iatrogenic transient insomnia is associated with the use of corticosteroids, theophylline, L-dopa, and propranolol, among others. It may be alleviated by changes in dose, timing of the use of the drug relative to bedtime, and supportive explanation to the often frantic patient bewildered by the source of his problem and the possibility of its continuing over the long-term.

A variety of agents may be used transiently (usually for 1 to 3 weeks) which vary in efficacy. A sedating antihistamine such as diphenhydramine in doses of 50 to 100 mg is useful and is associated with little risk of daytime sedation or adverse effects on sleep structure. The amino acid L-tryptophan, a serotonergic precursor, in doses of 2 to 5 g, has been of benefit; its efficacy is said to be enhanced by vitamin B_6 (in low doses to avoid neuropathy) and a low-carbohydrate snack. Benzodiazepines may have value in transient cases.

For sleep onset disorders, triazolam is of clear benefit, having a rapid onset of action and elimination; however, the latter makes it unsuitable for long-term use or sleep maintenance problems. Doses of up to 0.25 mg are of benefit, with higher amounts potentially increasing the risk of diurnal sedation; this agent should also be watched for its potential amnestic side effect, although any of the agents in this class can cause similar problems. Temazepam, usually at doses of 15 to 45 mg, may be useful for patients with such problems. For sleep maintenance difficulties, oxazepam in typical doses of 10 to 40 mg has been found to be particularly helpful, with few residual effects, although it needs to be administered 1 to 2 hours before desired onset secondary to delayed absorption. Lorazepam in doses of 0.5 to 2 mg is also helpful in the treatment of awakening disorders. Clorazepate in doses of 7.5 to 22.5 mg is a useful hypnotic for sleep maintenance, and may be of particular value in those patients in whom an anxiolytic effect is desirable on the following day. A long-acting drug such as flurazepam, which tends to accumulate with continued use, is certainly an effective hypnotic but is best reserved for those patients in whom residual daytime sedation is desired or can be tolerated. Older hypnotic agents either have poorly established efficacy or are associated with an unacceptable risk of side effects. The use of phenothiazine is not recommended for insomnia unless a specific psychiatric indication is present, especially considering the potential for tardive dyskinesia. Sedating tricyclics may be somewhat efficacious in patients with transient insomnia, but they are not typically used and their anticholinergic reactions may be particularly problematic. Over-the-counter anticholinergic agents or alcohol may be helpful in inducing sleep onset, but efficacy is rapidly lost and the short half-life may lead to early morning awakening or can produce nocturnal confusion or even psychosis.

Although chronic insomnia may have a multitude of origins, one of the most common and least recognized is persistent psychophysiologic insomnia, which is highly treatable. This is an insomnia predominantly of sleep onset (although sleep maintenance problems may arise as well) that usually develops from an adverse experience and sometimes continues for years after the resolution of the inciting episode. It is frequently aggravated by the chronic use of sedative-hypnotics as a result of the development of tolerance for these drugs and the direct disruption of sleep they cause. Treatment should center around behavior modification. The *slow* tapering of sedative-hypnotics may substantially improve sleep quality; tapering over a period of weeks to months can generally avoid the physiologic withdrawal and anxiety caused by being without medication and which may undermine efforts. Central to treatment are the use of "sleep hygiene" measures (Table 1). Because consistency of effort is pivotal to success, frequent patient contact is often of benefit; simply reviewing measures and then seeing the patient 3 months later will generally result in failure. The sparing, intermittent use of benzodiazepine is acceptable as well as reassuring to the patient. The use of progressive relaxation exercises are of particular benefit in alleviating anxiety and the heightened muscle tension often experienced. Perseverance over an 8- to 12-week period is often successful in restoring normal sleeping patterns without pharmacotherapy.

Another behavioral technique that can be effective is the restriction of the amount of time spent in bed. The quality of sleep appears to be relative to the extent to which sleep is disrupted, which in turn is increased the longer one remains in bed. The amount of time spent in bed is limited to the esti-

mated total sleep time (even given the insomniac's tendency to significantly underestimate this) with a gradual increment of time as sleep improves. The patient continues to arise at his habitual time. Generally, a substantial consolidation of the fragmented sleep is noted, and the patient perceives the quality of his sleep as improved.

Other forms of chronic insomnia pose considerable dilemmas in management. Individualized approaches to diagnosis, including possible polysomnography, are needed. Psychotherapy may well be the most important modality. The use of comparatively low-dose, sedating antidepressants can sometimes be rewarding and do not cause the problems of tolerance or prominent risk of side effects that contribute to insomnia. Such agents include amitriptyline, doxepin, and trazodone, commonly in doses of 10 to 100 mg. Again, phenothiazine use is discouraged. In chronic medical/neurologic conditions in which the disease causes sleep disruption, these agents may also be of value. Chronic benzodiazepine use should generally be discouraged.

PERIODIC LEG MOVEMENTS

Of the organic insomnias, four etiologic factors are most common: chronic pain, gastroesophageal reflux, sleep apnea, and periodic movements associated with sleep. The latter encompasses two main disorders: nocturnal myoclonus and the "restless legs" syndrome. The last is a sleep onset and maintenance insomnia arising from relentless paresthesia consisting of an irresistible urge to move an extremity, usually the legs. Once the patient is asleep, highly periodic extremity movements with interevent intervals usually of 20 to 40 seconds occur, resulting in arousals from sleep of typically brief duration. Nocturnal myoclonus is a related disorder producing repetitive awakenings most commonly resulting from repeated episodes of rhythmical leg jerks. In neither disorder is the patient aware of the reason for his awakening. These disorders produce nonrestorative sleep, daytime fatigue, and even pathologic sleepiness.

Treatment begins with polysomnographic diagnosis, then the search for what one hopes is a treatable cause. Etiologic factors that have been implicated include (1) iron, vitamin B_{12}, and folate deficiencies, (2) renal failure, (3) diabetes, (4) electrolyte imbalances, (5) hepatic failure, (6) peripheral neuropathy and radiculopathy, (7) myelopathy, (8) alcohol and sedative-hypnotic withdrawal, (9) the use of some tricyclic antidepressants, and (10) caffeine.

The management of nocturnal myoclonus and the "restless legs" syndrome is similar. The deci-

---

Table 1 Sleep Hygiene

1. Identify and maintain a consistent arising time as well as bedtime. Do not try to retire early. This helps strengthen circadian factors.
2. Avoid late evening activities that are highly stimulating.
3. Avoid alcohol or caffeine within 3 hours of retiring, if used at all.
4. Organize the bedroom so that it is a quiet, cool, darkened area.
5. Obtain regular exercise in the afternoon or early evening.
6. Do not *try* to sleep.
7. Do not remain in bed wide awake for more than 30 minutes. Leave the bedroom and engage in quiet, relaxing (yet not any type of productive) activity, returning to bed as soon as drowsy.
8. To dispel intrusive thoughts, make a brief list of the anxiety-producing issues and review them the following day.
9. Use only the bedroom for sleep—do so nowhere else.
10. Maintain normal daytime interactions with others, and do not nap.

sion to begin treatment depends on symptom intensity, since withholding treatment does not alter the course of either disease. Considerable fluctuation in course is seen at times. Simple measures may benefit mild and more intermittent cases. Most important is restricting the patient's use of caffeine and related agents. Performing regular exercise and stretching maneuvers before bedtime is helpful for some. Wearing support stockings, even TED types, can be tried. For some patients, keeping the affected limbs warm at night and taking warm baths soon before retiring are helpful. Supplemental vitamins are of uncertain efficacy but are benign, and therefore for milder cases, I usually suggest a trial of calcium, magnesium, potassium, B-complex vitamins, and vitamin E in 400 to 800 U doses.

For most patients, however, prescription drugs will be necessary. Many agents appear to be symptomatically effective by suppressing arousals from sleep, not by eliminating the involuntary movement. (Such treatment therefore does not better enable the bed partner to tolerate sharing the same bed; however, this dilemma is sometimes solved by the use of separate mattresses contained in a common frame.) At bedtime, a benzodiazepine is most often employed. For most patients, oxazepam is used first, in doses ranging from 10 to 40 mg taken 1.5 to 2 hours before the patient retires. Clonazepam in doses of 0.5 to 2 mg has been used, but its tendency to cause diurnal sedation makes it less desirable. Other agents that may be of value include triazolam, lorazepam, and clorazepate at the dosages mentioned in the previous section of this chapter. With the "restless legs" syndrome, it is often necessary to dose at earlier intervals to allow onset of action to occur before the patient retires. Medication may even need to be used during the patient's waking hours if symptoms are noticeable while the patient is at rest during the day; in this case, a less sedating agent is best. An analgesic taken at bedtime can be helpful; even aspirin may be of value. Quinine sulfate is sometimes used in doses of 325 mg at bedtime. A wide range of other agents may also be beneficial. Diphenylhydantoin at doses of 200 to 400 mg may be of value in patients with diurnal restlessness. Similarly, carbamazepine in doses of 200 to 600 mg or valproic acid in doses of 250 to 500 mg at bedtime can be used, with waking hour doses if necessary. When administered in doses of 5 to 20 mg per hour, baclofen, a gamma-aminobutyric acid agonist in the spinal cord, can be useful, even diurnally when paresthesia during the daytime is prominent. Clonidine, a centrally acting adrenergic agonist may be of use in doses of 0.1 to 0.4 mg, although results can be highly variable. L-tryptophan in doses of 2 to 5 g has been of some limited benefit. Because some patients have complained of cool distal extremities, peripheral vasodilators have been tried; in this selected group, phen-oxybenzamine, a postsynaptic, alpha-adrenergic blocker in doses of 10 to 30 mg, is of value.

One of the most recent and promising developments in management centers around the use of dopaminergic drugs. Carbidopa/L-dopa combinations at a ratio of 1 : 4 has been found to be effective for the more severe and refractory cases, and particularly for patients with "restless legs" syndrome. Doses of one to two 25/100 tablets at bedtime is well tolerated, and is sometimes repeated part way through the night if symptoms recur. Use during the day has also proven effective. Bromocriptine, a dopamine agonist, also has been described as effective.

Finally, opiate medications can be employed for the most severely affected patients or those in whom other agents are unsuccessful or poorly tolerated. Codeine in doses of 30 to 60 mg or propoxyphene in doses of 65–100 mg have both been used effectively.

DISORDERS OF EXCESSIVE SOMNOLENCE

Sleepiness during the day is a universal human experience, and therefore deciding at what point it is pathologic is difficult. An abnormal process is considered when the experience is chronic, excessive, irresistible, and exists despite an estimated sleep time that is normal premorbidly for the individual and his age, as well as in the face of normal circadian factors. All individuals without *obvious* general medical or traditional neurologic disorders to explain the symptom should be strongly suspected of having an organic disorder. All such patients require polysomnography and multiple sleep latency tests to arrive at the specific diagnosis necessary to select treatment.

Narcolepsy is a disorder that usually initially occurs during adolescence and early adulthood and is of lifelong duration. Narcolepsy is a disorder of REM sleep and consists of a classic tetrad of symptoms. First is irresistible napping or frank sleep attacks (in virtually all cases), which are indicative of fully formed attacks of REM sleep. Occurring in clear consciousness, cataplexy is almost pathognomonic of narcolepsy and consists of attacks of weakness in response to emotional stimuli; they represent isolated attacks of the muscle hypotonia seen as a part of normal REM. Sleep paralysis is an inability to move that occurs at sleep/wake transition points. Hypnagogic and hypnopompic hallucinations emerge in the same state and are indicative of the dreams of REM sleep. The sleep of such individuals is typically fragmented and is sometimes secondary to other sleep-related disorders such as periodic leg movements.

Central nervous system hypersomnia is likewise a lifelong disorder of excessive daytime sleepiness that emerges at varying ages, continues without remission, and has a heredofamilial pattern. Prolonged periods of deep nocturnal sleep, difficulty in awakening, sleep drunkness, waxing and waning diurnal sleepiness, and unrefreshing, irresistible napping are seen. The etiology of this disorder varies widely, having several symptomatic causes.

Treatment is symptomatic and can be divided into that directed at the somnolence and that directed at the ancillary symptoms in the classic type. A variety of conservative measures may be employed such as careful sleep hygiene, ensuring that there is adequate sleep time, and planned or structured naps that coincide with peak sleepiness periods. The postprandial period can be particularly difficult for some, and it may be necessary to limit the amount of food ingested (particularly at midday) or employ a schedule of small frequent meals. Alcoholic beverages and some over-the-counter medications should be used with caution. The selection of occupation may require careful attention; individuals with a more prominent disorder may need to choose a job in which they can be more physically active.

Control of excessive daytime sleepiness almost always requires stimulant agents. Concern is always present about the potential for abuse, but in practice this is quite rare in those who have polysomnographically confirmed disease and who are closely monitored. Tolerance to the agents is a more common problem, necessitating gradual increases in dose. Having the patient take a periodic medication "holiday" (of approximately 1 week) is usually effective in restoring good response at acceptable doses. Many patients, however, have disease of sufficient intensity that this is not possible. When unacceptable dose levels are reached, the pattern of alternating one medication for a fixed period with an unrelated agent for the same length of time is a valuable strategy. The first few days of cross-over, however, can be difficult. Another general point to consider is the timing of doses relative to mealtime; experience has shown that better absorption and response is noted if medication is taken on an empty stomach. A variety of side effects are common to the stimulants and may interfere with their use, particularly sympathomimetic ones. Preparations or agents of sustained or slow release may help, but some individuals simply will not respond to slow-release drugs, suggesting that for these patients a threshold factor may be present. Slow-release preparations may be of value in patients who experience difficulty in awakening in the morning. These preparations are taken at bedtime and often do not result in excessive sleep disruption. Tablet agents, on the other hand, allow more selected timing of use, resulting in tailoring of doses to day-to-day fluctuations in disease intensity or to activities that occur irregularly and during which symptoms tend to be greater (e.g., while driving or watching a movie).

Pemoline is the drug most commonly used to initiate treatment because of its low rate of side effects and potential for abuse. The drug is usually administered in doses of 18.75 mg each morning, which is doubled if no response is seen, and a second dose taken before lunch is added if the response is too short in duration. Amounts of as much as 150 mg are used. This is generally a slow-release agent, allowing fewer dosing times and use at bedtime. Mazindol is another drug with relatively few sympathomimetic side effects and varying durations of action. Doses of 4 to 10 mg in divided amounts are commonly used. Methylphenidate in tablet or sustained-release forms is highly effective, although perhaps has a greater potential for causing side-effects. Amounts varying from as little as 5 mg (administered as necessary) to as much as 100 mg are used. Tablets contain 5 to 20 mg of the drug and the slow-release form, 20 mg. Dextroamphetamine and methamphetamine agents are both commercially available; although only the 5 mg tablet is available, sustained-release forms can be obtained in amounts of 5, 10, and 15 mg. The total dose per 24 hours for these agents is the same as that for methylphenidate. Propranolol has been described as successful in treating narcolepsy, but my experiences with it have been discouraging.

The "ancillary" symptoms of classic narcolepsy generally respond poorly to stimulant agents. The treatment of cataplexy is usually of the most importance; again, the decision to initiate therapy should depend on symptom intensity. The hallucinations, sleep paralysis, and often vivid and dysphoric dreaming are generally benign although unpleasant. Medications for cataplexy usually have a positive effect on these other symptoms, but as much as 20 percent of the time, these symptoms may remit. General improvement can be gained by administering a benzodiazepine at bedtime to consolidate the fragmented sleep; this is clearly appropriate in those patients in whom periodic leg movements are seen, although one should be cautious regarding the possible presence of apnea in sleep.

Certain tricyclic antidepressants (although not all) are useful in treating narcolepsy. Most are reasonably well tolerated. The first to be used was imipramine. Relatively sedating in most instances, it may be better to administer it at bedtime, although it may be administered twice per day in amounts of 25 to 100 mg. Imipramine may be particularly helpful in patients with troublesome nocturnal symptoms. Protriptyline is now the most commonly used tricyclic antidepressant; it can be helpful in the treatment of cataplexy as well as daytime sleepiness, although rarely is it successful by itself for the latter. Medication can be initiated in doses of as little as 2.5 mg and increased to as much as 60 mg, although the latter is rarely necessary. It is generally best if the medication is taken twice per day. Desipramine is another relatively stimulating tricyclic and is used in a manner similar to that of protriptyline. Dosages vary between 12.5 and 150 mg. Clomipramine in doses of as much as 200 mg has been used successfully. Monamine oxidase inhibitors can be useful for cataplexy; phenelzine in doses of up to 60 mg per day in divided doses is generally used. Contrary to the experience of some, we have found this drug reasonably well tolerated. Combining it with stimulants is of obvious concern, but can be cautiously done. The recent use of opiate compounds can be of distinct benefit for severe, relatively refractory cases of classic narcolepsy. Codeine has been helpful for both EDS and cataplexy, although rarely as a sole agent; doses of 30 to 150 mg per day have been given. More rarely, other opiates have been used.

Other medications are emerging that either are not yet readily available or remain available on an investigational basis only. These include viloxazine (a nontricyclic, noradrenergic uptake blocker without anticholinergic side effects) in doses of as much as 200 mg per day, fluoxetine (a serotonin uptake blocker without anticholinergic side effects) in doses of as much as 60 mg per day, zimelidine (a serotonin uptake blocker, not currently available), and gamma-hydroxybutyrate (GHB). The latter has limited availability in this country, but can have substantial positive effects on cataplexy, daytime sleepiness, and nocturnal sleep disturbance. Doses are generally 3 g administered at bedtime, with a second dose necessary halfway through the night; side effects are few.

SLEEP APNEA SYNDROME

Sleep apnea syndrome is defined as repeatedly interrupted breathing during sleep. Two main forms exist, the most common is obstructive; upper airway hypotonia results in the episodic apnea, with retained thoracic and diaphragmatic effort. Central apnea also produces repeated apneic disturbances, with the disappearance of all evidence of respiratory effort. The latter is quite infrequent, while mixed apnea is most frequent. By convention, apnea is pathologic if it lasts more than 10 seconds and occurs more than five times per hour or 30 times per night. Numerous problems emerge as a result of hypoxemia and sleep fragmentation: daytime sleepiness, personality and memory changes, nonrestorative sleep, morning headache, hypertension, cardiac failure and related conditions, among others. The patient often perceives his sleep as sound, while the bedpartner characteristically describes raucous snoring, apnea, and restless behavior, even nocturnal enuresis and seizures. Detailed polysomnographic investigations are essential to diagnosis and to selecting appropriate treatment.

Excess weight is an important factor in sleep apnea. Weight loss rarely normalizes nocturnal respiratory dysfunction but almost always results in improvement; it may allow much more conservative management. Restricting sleeping positions may be effective in some instances. Careful observation of the effects of position on apnea is made when the initial polysomnogram is taken; if restriction of sleeping position appears to be effective, retesting is necessary to confirm its efficacy. Both lateral decubitus and simultaneous reverse Trendelenberg positions may be used.

Pharmacologic agents have a limited role in the management of sleep apnea. Protriptyline may be highly effective, especially if the apnea occurs predominantly during REM sleep, and is more appropriate in milder cases. The dose should range from 5 to 40 mg, although amounts of more than 20 mg are of less clear efficacy. Medroxyprogesterone, a central respiratory stimulant, can be useful in the treatment of central apnea or as an adjunct in obstructive apnea. As primary drug in the latter, it may increase the respiratory rate without affecting airway muscle tone, thereby intensifying the disorder. Doses of up to 60 mg are applicable for most patients, especially to avoid complications such as gynecomastia. Administration of oxygen during sleep can be of benefit primarily in patients with disorders dominated by hypoventilation and in those with central apnea, sometimes if apnea is partial. Aminophylline has not been found to be of major value in treating adult apnea, nor has the use of decongestants to limit nasal congestion other than in patients with otherwise uncomplicated snoring.

Some important cautions should be exercised as well. Alcohol has a potent intensifying effect on sleep apnea. Similarly, the use of sedative-hypnotics or narcotic analgesics should be administered with caution in patients with this disorder. A particularly vulnerable time for such patients is after surgery.

Mechanical methods are central to the treatment of sleep apnea, particularly nasal continuous positive airway pressure. Levels of positive pressure (PEEP) at usually 5 to 15 cm H_2O are administered via a small nasal mask during sleep, creating a pneumatic splint preventing airway obstruction. It is completely effective in virtually all patients who can adapt to its use; 85 to 90 percent continue to use it at home on a long-term, if not necessarily permanent, basis. Tracheostomy is rarely needed, although it may be used by some patients during weight reduction, allowing upper airway surgery a greater likelihood of success later. Initiating treatment requires monitoring in the laboratory to establish the appropriate pressure under direct observation and to help the patient adjust to its use. Individuals should be seen frequently to increase success and compliance. Response can be dramatic, with a patient's incapacitating daytime sleepiness disappearing within a couple of days.

Several different types of oral orthotics advance the mandibule, stabilize the palate, and possibly reduce upper airway negative pressure. Such a device is of greatest benefit in patients with a shallow hypopharynx and can be effective in those with uncomplicated snoring as well. Problems in use have been few and tolerance good unless gag reflexes are particularly active.

Surgical therapy remains a cornerstone of management. Tracheotomy now is best reserved for life-threatening cases where nasal continuous positive airway pressure (CPAP) cannot be used. Tonsillectomy is efficacious if the tonsils are large and is particularly of value in children. Septoplasty generally is not of value unless the nasal obstruction is substantial. The most extensively performed procedure is now uvulopalatopharyngoplasty, in which excess palatal and pharyngeal tissue is removed. The serious complication rate is low: nasal speech is rare after surgery, although some nasal incompetence for swallowing is seen to a mild degree in as many as 25 percent of patients. Prediction of response is aided by the use of the lateral cephalometric film, although other imaging techniques of the upper airway have been employed. While figures vary, approximately one-third of patients who undergo this operation are normalized, another third are at least 50 percent better, and (rarely) patients' conditions are worsened from scarring causing nasopharyngeal stenosis. The elimination of snoring in 90 to 95 percent makes this procedure a consideration for its treatment. Finally, for patients with appropriate upper airway anatomy, maxillomandibular advancement procedures can be successful.

Sleep apnea is a chronic, dynamic disorder. No matter what treatment is used and regardless of the initial response, the patient must be followed on a long-term basis, and repeat polysomnography must be completed to confirm clinical impressions of success objectively. This is especially true after surgical procedures that may eliminate snoring but not necessarily apnea.

SLEEP/WAKE CYCLE DISORDERS

A variety of disorders are related to the disruption of circadian rhythms. Jet lag, irregular sleep/wake patterns, and the shift maladaptation syndrome are recognized. Perhaps the best described is the delayed sleep phase syndrome. It consists of a profound, persistent sleep onset insomnia (occasionally daytime sleepiness secondary to sleep deprivation and circadian factors). Sleep architecture itself is normal, and only sleep's timing relative to the light-dark cycle is disturbed. An organic disturbance in the circadian pacemaker is thought to result in a weak phase advance mechanism that yields the insomnia. Therapy has been a challenge. Sleep hygiene is of value. Chronotherapy is the primary modality used, consisting of the sequential phase delay of the time of retirement by 3 hours each day until the desired bedtime is reached. Although subject to some disagreement, benzodiazepines have been found of value during this process and for long-term control. Phototherapy, 2 hours of broad-spectrum light at the end of the sleep period, at approximately 2,500 lux, has met with some success; however, the exact intensity, spectrum "doses," and efficacy are not clearly established.

PARASOMNIAS

Sleepwalking, night terrors, and nocturnal enuresis fall in this group. These are thought to represent disorders of partial arousal from slow wave sleep, and are of generally uncertain etiology. Most are benign disturbances seen predominantly in childhood and requiring no specific therapy except parental reassurance. They often disappear in adolescence; should they persist or re-emerge in adult life, then consideration for psychiatric evaluation/therapy is important. Where behaviors are destructive or injurious, then pharmacologic intervention may be necessary. Benzodiazepine agents, with their tendency to suppress slow wave sleep, can be useful. Tricyclics are best avoided (except in enuresis where the mechanism of action is different), with their tendency to increase these stages and potentially symptoms.

The most recently discovered parasomnia is the REM behavior disorder. This syndrome's symptoms arise as a result of the loss of ability to generate the normally actively induced skeletal muscle atonia. Symptoms are primarily those of enacting the content of often dysphoric dreams, with often destructive or injurious results. A large proportion of cases are symptomatic. Diagnosis is established by polysomnography to confirm the REM pathology. If possible, treatment is aimed at correcting any underlying pathology; otherwise clonazepam has been found efficacious.

SUGGESTED READING

Kryger M, Roth, T, Dement W. Principles and practice of sleep medicine. Philadelphia: WB Saunders, 1989.
Riley TL. Clinical aspects of sleep and sleep disturbance. Stoneham MA: Butterworth Publishers, 1985.

PATIENT RESOURCES

Association of Professional Sleep Societies
604 Second Street S.W.
Rochester, Minnesota 55902

American Narcolepsy Association
Box 5846
Stanford, California 94305

IDIOPATHIC AUTONOMIC INSUFFICIENCY

KENNETH MAREK, M.D.

Autonomic failure causes a wide spectrum of symptoms, including prominent abnormalitites in regulation of blood pressure, heart rate, sweating and temperature control, gastrointestinal, bladder, sexual, and pupillary function, lacrimation, and salivary glands. Orthostatic hypotension is the most disabling feature of autonomic insufficiency. In this chapter, a multimodal approach to the management of blood pressure control in patients with autonomic failure is outlined. The goals of therapy are practical: to improve the patient's ability to stand for longer periods and to prevent syncope. Appropriate therapy frequently requires a combination of non-pharmacologic and pharmacologic treatment.

Disorders of the autonomic nervous system may be classified as either neurologic or non-neurologic. Non-neurologic etiologies remain the most common cause of autonomic dysfunction and are often treatable. An initial approach to any patient with orthostatic hypotension should include a thorough evaluation to determine whether there is volume depletion, cardiac dysrhythmia, or endocrine disorder (pheochromacytoma, adrenal insufficiency), and whether the patient is using hypotensive drugs (tricyclic antidepressants, antihypertensives, antiparkinsonians, alcohol). The neurologic causes of autonomic insufficiency may be characterized as either primary (generally involving the central nervous system) or secondary (generally part of a peripheral neuropathy). Common causes of secondary autonomic insufficiency include diabetes, amyloid, Guillain-Barré syndrome, porphyria, and paraneoplastic syndromes. In patients with these conditions, autonomic dysfunction may be improved by treating the underlying disease process. Primary autonomic insufficiency is most commonly caused by multisystem atrophy (MSA) or idiopathic orthostatic hypotension (IOH). In this chapter, I concentrate on the treatment of primary autonomic failure, but much of the treatment approach may be used to manage autonomic dysfunction of any cause.

APPROACH TO THERAPY

The first step in the treatment of autonomic insufficiency is to identify those patients with autonomic failure. While this may seem obvious, during the early stage of the disease, patients often report vague and intermittent symptoms. Orthostatic signs must be measured and autonomic insufficiency may be further confirmed at the bedside by measuring variability in heart rate caused by respiration or that follows a Valsalva maneuver. The degree of orthostatic hypotension that may evoke symptoms depends on both the absolute blood pressure and the rate of change of blood pressure. Therefore the goal of blood pressure management must be individualized. Early in the management of this problem, the patient's family or a friend should be instructed to take blood pressure measurements at home. Again, blood pressure values should serve only as a guide to disease, while the most important measure of disease progression and therapeutic response remains severity of symptoms.

Patients with autonomic failure develop hypotension in response to several stimuli in addition to that of standing. They may be sensitive to heat, exercise, large meals, or otherwise innocuous pharmacologic agents. In addition, they may develop supine hypertension. The therapeutic approach to these patients is multifaceted. Therapy begins with practical recommendations and continues with pharmacologic intervention, if necessary.

Nonpharmacologic Therapy

The initial management of mild orthostatic hypotension is based on several simple practical measures designed to optimize patients' functional capacity. The primary goal is to maximize circulating blood volume. Patient education is an essential component of therapy. Clear, specific instructions should be given regarding diet, activity, pressure garments, and nonprescription medications.

Patients should be encouraged to maintain adequate hydration with increased fluid and liberal salt intake. Salt tablets may be used to provide the patient with 3 to 4 g of sodium each day. The patient should be cautioned concerning fluid overload and the possibility of supine hypertension. The patient should eat several small meals since large meals may rapidly worsen orthostatic hypotension since blood flow shifts to the splanchnic bed and vasodilator substances may be secreted. Activity should be restricted after large meals to lessen symptoms. Patients rapidly learn to avoid sudden changes in posture and to avoid prolonged standing. Hypotension also may be worsened by prolonged bedrest. Tilting the head of the bed with 4-inch blocks may lessen orthostatic symptoms on rising in the morning. Supine hypertension may also be managed by tilting the head of the bed, thereby using the patient's orthostasis to reduce blood pressure. An alternative commonly used by patients is to sleep in a recliner, either during the day or night. A moderate-graded exercise program may be beneficial. Swimming is the best tolerated exercise, but patients should never be left alone and may experience hypotension on leaving the water. These patients should also avoid excessive heat, which they tolerate very poorly since increased temperature causes vasodilation that may be complicated by anhidrosis.

Pressure garments are a useful but poorly tolerated adjunct to therapy in patients with autonomic insufficiency. Generally, custom-fitted elastic stockings, either thigh-high or to the umbilicus (like panty hose) must be used. The stockings increase central blood volume by preventing pooling of blood in the legs. These stockings should be removed at night and put on before the patient arises from bed in the morning. However, these garments are difficult to put on (generally requiring the help of a family member or caretaker), are very uncomfortable in hot weather, and are quite expensive.

Patients should be advised to avoid all medications except those prescribed by a physician familiar with their autonomic disorder. These patients frequently have very poor regulation of blood pressure so that otherwise innocuous drugs may cause marked hypotension. Over-the-counter preparations such as cold remedies, allergy pills, diet pills, or nasal sprays are often problematic. Alcohol, a potent vasodilator, generally worsens symptoms substantially. Caffeine may lessen orthostatic symptoms, perhaps by reducing adenosine-induced vasodilation.

Pharmacologic Therapy

In patients with more severe autonomic insufficiency unresponsive to the practical measures detailed above, a variety of medications have been used to treat hypotension. These drugs are listed in Table 1. Most of the agents increase blood pressure through an increase in intravascular volume or a relative stimulation of vasoconstriction. Often these drugs are used in combination to manage severe symptoms. Patients may respond to therapy with marked fluctuations in blood pressure so that all changes in medications must be monitored carefully.

Treatment is generally initiated with fludrocortisone (Florinef) at a dose of 0.1 mg daily slowly titrated to approximately 1 mg daily. Fludrocortisone increases vascular volume and enhances the response of blood vessels to vasoconstrictors. Supine hypertension is often a limiting side effect. Hypokalemia frequently occurs but is easily managed with potassium supplementation. If symptoms persist in patients receiving adequate fludrocortisone, the next step is to add either indomethacin (Indocin) (25 mg three times per day) or ibuprofen (up to 800 mg four times per day). These drugs may increase blood pressure by inhibiting the vasodilator effects of prostaglandins. If the combination of Florinef and Indocin/ibuprofen is ineffective, the Indocin or ibuprofen should be discontinued.

The next strategy is to combine Florinef with a vasoconstrictor agent. The mechanisms of action of the vasoconstrictor drugs generally involve adrenergic stimulation of blood vessels either by direct release of norepinephrine, adrenergic receptor–mediated interactions, or inhibition of norepinephrine catabolism. The first approach is to combine Florinef with an alpha-adrenergic receptor agonist, either phenylpropanolamine (25 mg daily increased to 75 mg three times per day) or ephedrine (12.5 mg twice per day increased to 50 mg four times per day). Unfortunately these agents act for only a short period and may be poorly absorbed. Furthermore, small doses of alpha-agonists may precipitate marked hypertension possibly because of denervation supersensitivity in patients with postganglionic neuronal lesions. If treatment with alpha-agonists is ineffective, these drugs should be discontinued and an alternative receptor-active drug should be tried. However, treatment of hypotension with other adrenergic receptor-active drugs is complex and must be individualized. In some patients, either clonidine or yohimbine (an alpha-2-adrenergic receptor agonist and antagonist, respectively) may lessen hypotension. The paradox of two drugs with opposing actions that both improve hypotensive symptoms may be explained by a potential peripheral action of clonidine and a central action of yohimbine. Beta-adrenergic blockade may also be effective in some patients. Propranolol at low doses (10 to 40 mg twice per day) may improve hypotensive symptoms through predominant beta-2-adrenergic antagonism, but treatment is limited because at higher doses, the net effect of both beta-1- and beta-2-adrenergic antagonism may worsen hypotension. Specific beta-2-adrenergic antagonists currently being developed may prove more useful.

If vasoactive agents are ineffective, a number of other medications (listed in Table 1) that have been reported to improve hypotension may be used. Two additional agents should be mentioned. Caffeine (250 mg) may alleviate symptoms related to postprandial hypotension, but patients frequently develop tolerance to its effects. Vasopressin by nasal spray may be effective in reducing the nocturnal diuresis in these patients and thereby alleviate symptoms.

Special Therapeutic Considerations

Orthostatic hypotension may be caused by several syndromes. Ideally, as the mechanisms of these syndromes are elucidated, specific effective treatments may be developed. Current biochemical and physiologic evaluations of patients have already identified several subsets of patients who should be treated in a manner differing from the general guidelines outlined above.

A group of patients with primary orthostatic hypotension may be distinguished by their marked

Table 1 Drugs Used to Treat Orthostatic Hypotension

Drug	Dose	Comments
Volume expanders		
Fludrocortisone	0.1–0.5 mg t.i.d.	Supine hypertension, hypokalemia
Adrenergic agents		
Receptor agonists		
Phenylpropanolamine	25–75 mg t.i.d.	Supine hypertension
Ephedrine	25–50 mg t.i.d.	Supine hypertension
Phenylephrine	2–4 sprays q4h	Use only in nasal spray form
Midodrine		Experimental agent
Clonidine	0.2–0.6 mg b.i.d.	May worsen hypotension
Receptor antagonists		
Propranolol	10–40 mg q.i.d.	Higher doses may worsen hypotension, useful for orthostatic tachycardia
Pindolol	2.5 mg t.i.d.	Mixed agonist-antagonist
Yohimbine	5–10 mg b.i.d.	Central presynaptic receptor action
Increase synthesis		
L-threo-DOPS	100–600 mg/day	Use in dopamine beta-hydroxylase deficiency
Increase release		
Tyramine		Only bulk powder available
Decrease catabolism		
Monoamine oxidase (tranylcypromine)	10 mg t.i.d.	Potential severe hypertension
Vasodilator inhibitors		
Prostaglandin inhibitors		
Indomethacin	25–50 mg q.i.d.	GI distress, ulcers
Ibuprofen	400–800 mg q.i.d.	GI distress
Caffeine	250 mg before meals	Use for postprandial hypotension
Metaclopramide	10–20 mg t.i.d.	Dopamine receptor antagonist
Miscellaneous		
Vasopressin (DDAVP)	2–4 μg IM qhs	Prevents nocturnal diuresis

tachycardia associated with standing. This condition has been postulated to represent a relative preservation of beta-adrenergic versus alpha-adrenergic receptors. These patients should be treated with a combination of Florinef and propranolol.

Two additional unusual hypotensive syndromes should be mentioned. Hyperbradykininism is a familial disorder associated with elevated levels of the vasodilator bradykinin. This disorder has been responsive to treatment with propranolol. Recently a specific dopamine beta-hydroxylase (an enzyme necessary for the synthesis of norepinephrine) deficiency has been identified in some patients with severe orthostatic hypotension. These patients have responded to treatment with L-threo-DOPS, which increases norepinephrine.

GUIDELINES FOR MANAGEMENT

The treatment of autonomic insufficiency in general and of orthostatic hypotension in particular remains a difficult problem. However, a combination of practical measures and pharmacologic interventions may alleviate symptoms and enable patients to continue some normal activities. The goals of treatment are simply to increase the length of time a patient can remain standing, without the development of unacceptable side effects. An approach to management is outlined in Figure 1. The general guideline is that blood pressure should be approximately 80 to 100/60 to 70 when the patient is standing and 160 to 180/90 to 100 when the patient is supine.

Several principles of therapy should be emphasized. Therapy should be a multifaceted "stepped" approach beginning with nonpharmacologic recommendations and, if necessary, proceeding to the use of a medication or a combination of medications. Florinef remains the most useful drug in most cases. Other drugs should be used in conjunction with Florinef and discontinued if ineffective. Treatment must be individualized and the side effects of drugs carefully monitored. Patients with autonomic insufficiency are particularly susceptible to the potential side effects of these drugs on bowel and bladder control in addition to the common problem of supine hypertension. Treatment is designed to reduce symptoms, but current therapy is not likely to reverse progression of disease or to enable patients to return to their normal lifestyle. Many of these patients require extensive psychosocial support in

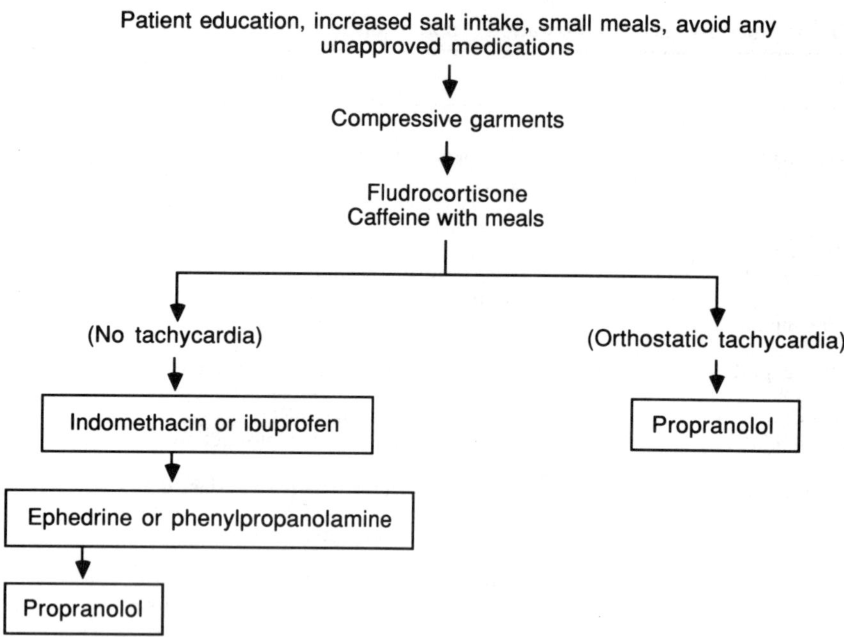

Figure 1   An ordered general strategy for the management of orthostatic hypotension. Management should be individualized to treat specific patient needs. Other drugs to treat orthostatic hypotension are listed in Table 1.

dealing with this enigmatic but disabling disease process. Finally, the value of the physician's role in educating patients by explaining their bewildering array of symptoms cannot be overestimated.

SUGGESTED READING

McLeod JG, Tuck RR. Disorders of the autonomic nervous system. Ann Neurol 1987; 21:519–529.
Onrot J, Goldberg MR, Holloster AS, et al. Management of chronic orthostatic hypotension. Am J Medicine 1986; 80:454–464.
Polinsky RJ, Kopin IJ, Ebert MH, Weise V. Pharmacologic distinction of different orthostatic hypotension syndromes. Neurology 1981; 31:1–7.
Schatz IJ. Orthostatic hypotension. Philadelphia: F.A. Davis Co., 1986.

PATIENT RESOURCE

Dysautonomia Foundation
270 Lexington Avenue
New York, New York 10017

SEIZURES

NEONATAL SEIZURES AND INFANTILE SPASMS

ELI M. MIZRAHI, M.D.
RICHARD A. HRACHOVY, M.D.

NEONATAL SEIZURES

Therapy for neonatal seizures is directed toward treatment of specific underlying etiologic factors and administration of antiepileptic drugs (AEDs) to stop the seizures. Although the principles that govern the medical and pharmacologic management of newborns with seizures have not changed significantly over the past several years, the basic clinical problems of seizure diagnosis and assessment of adequacy of AED therapy have recently been the subject of much investigation. As a result, concepts have been developed that have altered the traditional approach to the management of neonates suspected of having seizures.

Clinical and Electroencephalographic Characteristics

Recent investigations of neonatal seizures using time-synchronized, electroencephalographic (EEG)/polygraphic/video monitoring techniques indicate that there are two basic types of clinical seizures (Table 1): those closely associated with electrical seizure activity and those with no electrocortical signature. In addition, electrical seizures can occur without the presence of clinical seizure activity.

Clinical seizures that occur in association with EEG seizure activity include focal clonic seizures, focal tonic seizures (tonic eye deviation and asymmetric tonic posturing), some myoclonic seizures, and, rarely, apnea (usually associated with other motor manifestations). These clinical seizures (e.g., clonic limb movements) cannot be arrested by physical restraint and cannot be provoked by tactile stimulation. The seizures are usually seen in neonates who appear alert interictally. The interictal EEG usually shows normal background activity. The most common etiologic factors of these clinical seizures are focal structural lesions (infarction or hemorrhage), infection, and (less frequently) metabolic abnormalities.

Clinical seizures that may occur without electrical seizure activity include symmetric, generalized tonic posturing, certain myoclonic seizures, and a group of behaviors referred to as motor automatisms. Most motor automatisms have previously been described as subtle seizures and include oral-

Table 1 Electroclinical Classification of Neonatal Seizures

Clinical seizures with a consistent electrocortical signature
Focal clonic
Unifocal
Multifocal
Alternating
Migrating
Hemiconvulsive
Axial
Focal tonic
Asymmetric truncal
Eye deviation
Myoclonic
Generalized
Focal
Apnea
Clinical seizures without a consistent electrocortical signature
Myoclonic
Generalized
Focal
Fragmentary
Generalized tonic
Extensor
Flexor
Mixed extensor/flexor
Motor automatisms
Oral-buccal-lingual
Ocular signs
Progression movements
Pedaling
Stepping
Rotary arm movements
Complex purposeless movements
Electrical seizures without clinical seizure activity
Seizure discharges of the depressed brain
Partially treated clinical seizures with initial, consistent, electrocortical signature
Clinical seizures masked by paralysis

buccal-lingual movements, certain ocular signs, movements of progression (swimming, rowing, pedaling), and complex purposeless movements. These clinical behaviors may be arrested by restraint or repositioning of limbs, head, or trunk. They may be elicited by tactile stimulation, and the intensity of the response may increase with increasing rates (temporal summation) or sites (spatial summation) of stimulation. Increased intensity of stimulation may provoke movement in regions of the body distant from the site of stimulation (irradiation of the response). These clinical seizures are characteristically seen in infants who are lethargic or comatose. The EEG background activity is typically depressed and undifferentiated, often showing no electrical activity of cerebral origin. Hypoxic-ischemic encephalopathy is the etiologic factor most often associated with these seizure types. Because of the clinical and EEG characteristics of the seizures and their response to stimulation and restraint, we believe that their pathophysiology is primarily nonepileptic. They represent primitive reflex behaviors that are facilitated as a result of forebrain depression.

Electrical seizure activity not associated with clinical seizures may occur in infants who have been pharmacologically paralyzed, in infants with a markedly depressed level of consciousness, and in infants who have received AEDs.

Patient Evaluation and Classification

Neonatal seizures, whether ultimately classified as epileptic or nonepileptic, indicate the presence of significant central nervous system (CNS) dysfunction and call for prompt investigation and evaluation of potentially treatable etiologic factors. Some evidence suggests that prolonged, recurrent epileptic activity may be harmful to the immature brain; therefore, immediate steps should be taken to stop the epileptic seizures.

The first step in evaluation is the characterization and classification of the seizures. A detailed description of the suspected clinical event and how it is affected by stimulation and restraint provides the basis for seizure classification. For example, focal clonic contractions of a limb, which cannot be arrested by light restraint, must be presumed to be of epileptic origin. Generalized, symmetric tonic posturing that occurs spontaneously and can be suppressed by restraint or repositioning and elicited by tactile or proprioceptive stimulation may be considered to be of nonepileptic origin.

Diagnosis of the etiology underlying the seizures requires a detailed history (family history, illnesses contracted during pregnancy, maternal drug use, perinatal history) and physical examination (neurologic examination, ophthalmologic examination, general examination, and assessment of skin lesions and fontanelle). Initial laboratory studies include determination of levels of serum glucose, sodium, magnesium, calcium, bicarbonate, urea nitrogen, creatinine, ammonia, and blood gases. A lumbar puncture for assessment of infection and hemorrhage is essential. Depending on the clinical impression, additional laboratory tests may include urine for amino acids and organic acids, and maternal and infant titers for toxoplasmosis, rubella, cytomegalovirus, herpes virus, coxsackievirus, and syphilis. Bedside cranial ultrasonography may be used to investigate the presence of hemorrhage. If the infant is stable, and if it is clinically indicated, computed tomography (CT) is used to determine the presence of infarction, hemorrhage, malformations, or calcifications.

EEG is a valuable tool in the diagnosis and management of neonatal seizures; however, its use may be limited by availability, individual laboratory capabilities, and the expertise of the interpreting neurophysiologist or neurologist. In the EEG of a neonate, the only reliable evidence of epileptic activity is the finding of electrical seizure activity itself. In neonates, unlike in older children and adults, the finding of interictal sharp waves is nonspecific and is not believed to indicate an epileptic process. Although the interictal EEG is limited in providing evidence of an epileptic process, it is useful in diagnosing diffuse and focal injury, in determining conceptional age, and in assessing prognosis.

Recently, interest has been shown in the application of EEG/polygraphic/video monitoring to the diagnosis of neonatal seizures. However, this technique is currently available at only a few centers and is not essential for an accurate characterization and classification of many types of clinical seizures. Many seizures can be classified correctly based on bedside observation, on how the seizures respond to restraint and stimulation, on the infant's level of alertness, and if available, on the interictal background EEG activity.

Treatment

General Medical Management

The first step in the treatment of neonatal seizures is to ensure adequate ventilation and perfusion. Impairment of respiration and alterations in systemic blood pressure may be the result of the etiologic factors responsible for the seizures, may occur in the course of repeated seizures, or may result from vigorous AED therapy.

Etiology-Specific Therapy

Treatment is directed toward specific underlying causes, including CNS infection. Specific metabolic abnormalities are responsible for some types of seizures (most commonly, focal clonic seizures) and can be corrected. Hypoglycemia, diagnosed rapidly by Dextrostix determination, is treated initially with glucose, 2 ml per kilogram of D10W (0.2 g per kilogram) IV, followed by intravenous (IV) maintenance dosages of as much as 0.5 g per kilogram per hour. Hypocalcemia is treated with an initial IV dose of 4 ml per kilogram of 5 percent calcium gluconate solution followed by oral maintenance dosages of 500 mg per kilogram per day. Hypomagnesemia is initially treated with 50 percent magnesium sulfate solution, 0.2 ml per kilogram IM, with maintenance intramuscular (IM) dosages of 0.2 ml per kilogram per day. Pyridoxine deficiency is often cited as a major cause of neonatal seizures, particularly those resistant to AED therapy. We have found this etiologic factor to be extremely rare. The dosage of pyridoxine hydrochloride is 100 mg, administered intravenously.

Initiation of AED Therapy

The decision to start AED therapy is often difficult to make, even after the seizures have been accurately characterized and classified. Epileptic seizures may be harmful to the immature brain; however, AED therapy is not without risk to the neonate. Based on clinical information alone (without benefit of bedside EEG or EEG/video monitoring), four situations may arise in which one must decide whether or not to treat the patient with AEDs:

1. Focal clonic seizures that are prolonged and recurrent. These seizures, which are clearly of epileptic origin, are vigorously treated with AEDs.
2. Focal clonic seizures that are brief and infrequent. These seizures, also of epileptic origin, are likewise treated with AEDs. However, there is current debate as to whether this is desirable. These seizures are not believed to be harmful to the developing brain and are considered to be self-limited. Further investigations are required to resolve this clinically important issue.
3. Tonic seizures and motor automatisms that can be arrested by restraint or repositioning of limbs or trunk and elicited by stimulation. These are believed to be nonepileptic in origin and are not treated with AEDs.
4. Tonic seizures and motor automatisms that do not respond in the characteristic manner to restraint and stimulation; this may occur because of a variation in stimulation techniques. Investigations in which EEG/video monitoring is used suggest that these events are not epileptic in origin. However, if such monitoring techniques are not available, tonic posturing and motor automatisms that

do not respond to restraint and stimulation are treated with AEDs.

If bedside EEG and EEG/video monitoring are used, two additional situations may arise in which one must decide whether or not to treat the patient:

1. Clinical seizures that occur in the absence of EEG seizure activity. These events are not considered to be of epileptic origin and are not treated with AEDs.
2. EEG seizure activity without any signs of clinical seizures. When found in infants who have not been previously treated with AEDs or who, although previously treated, have subtherapeutic serum levels of phenobarbital and phenytoin, these electrical events are treated with AEDs.

Types and Dosages of AED Therapy

The initial AED administered is phenobarbital, and the loading dose is 20 mg per kilogram. Additional dosages may be required acutely to control the clinical seizures and to attain a therapeutic serum level between 20 and 40 μg per milliliter. Maintenance dosage, typically begun 24 hours after initial loading, is 3 to 4 mg per kilogram per day, given in two divided doses. Serum levels are followed closely, because phenobarbital may accumulate in the neonate and result in clinical intoxication. Intravenous administration of phenobarbital has been associated with respiratory depression, systemic hypotension, and (with high dosages) cardiovascular depression. Monitoring of these functions during and after infusion is warranted.

If phenobarbital levels of up to 40 μg per milliliter do not control the clinical seizures, phenytoin is added. The initial loading dose is 20 mg per kilogram. Therapeutic serum levels range from 15 to 20 μg per milliliter. Intravenous maintenance dosage is 3 to 4 mg per kilogram per day. Rapid IV phenytoin administration has been associated with cardiac arrhythmias; therefore, it is recommended that phenytoin be infused slowly, with cardiac monitoring.

Diazepam is used when the clinical seizures continue to be prolonged and persistent despite therapeutic levels of phenobarbital and phenytoin. The dosage for acute management is 0.1 to 0.3 mg per kilogram IV. Special attention must be paid to the infant's respiratory status during administration. In addition, systemic hypotension has been associated with use of IV diazepam, particularly when the diazepam is given after phenobarbital. Therefore, blood pressure is monitored during and immediately after diazepam infusion.

The use of other AEDs has been proposed when clinical seizures persist and continue to be prolonged. These include primidone (at a loading dose of 20 mg per kilogram, resulting in plasma levels of 8 to 15 mg per liter) and lorazepam (0.05 mg per kilogram IV), although the routine use of the latter drug in neonates has not yet been approved and may have adverse effects similar to those seen with diazepam. Paraldehyde, previously used for management of acute cases, is no longer commercially available.

Termination of AED Therapy

It may be difficult, in the acute phase of management, to determine the appropriate end point of AED therapy. When focal clonic seizures are treated in infants during EEG/video monitoring, the clinical seizures may be effectively controlled while the electrical seizure activity persists. Under these circumstances, the physician is faced with the decision of whether to consider the therapy sufficient, since the clinical seizures have been controlled, or to continue administering AEDs in an attempt to eliminate the electrical seizure activity. Unfortunately, this second goal may not be attained even with high-dose polypharmacy, or if it is attained, it is at the expense of a significant depression of brain function. This important issue in AED therapy has not yet been resolved. We treat the infant until the clinical seizures are controlled, and if the EEG seizure activity persists, until both phenobarbital and phenytoin serum levels are in the high therapeutic range.

Discontinuance of AED therapy is highly individualized; no specific guidelines have been established, despite rigorous investigations. In infants whose seizures are well controlled acutely, and who have a normal neurologic examination and a relatively normal EEG, maintenance AED therapy is usually discontinued within 3 months. Phenytoin is usually tapered and discontinued before IV lines are discontinued. Phenobarbital therapy is tapered and eventually discontinued, usually within a few weeks. Infants who are neurologically impaired and have a severely abnormal EEG receive longer courses of phenobarbital maintenance.

Prognosis

The prognosis for infants who experience seizures is determined primarily by the underlying etiology and the degree and duration of the brain injury as well as the time at which it was sustained. Some etiologic factors (e.g., hypoxic-ischemic encephalopathy) have a high incidence of morbidity and mortality, whereas others (e.g., hypocalcemia) have a generally favorable prognosis. Other factors that may assist in an accurate determination of prognosis include the neurologic examination and serial recordings of the EEG. The relationship of the development of epilepsy during later life to the occurrence of seizures during the neonatal period has not been established.

INFANTILE SPASMS

Infantile spasms are relatively rare seizures occurring during infancy and early childhood. Patients with this disorder have a high incidence of developmental retardation, and the seizure disorder is usually associated with the unique EEG pattern hypsarrhythmia. The seizures are generally refractory to standard anticonvulsants and unique in their response to hormonal therapy.

Clinical and EEG Characteristics

Onset of infantile spasms usually occurs during the first 4 to 8 months of life. There are three main types of infantile spasms, depending on whether the flexor or extensor muscles are predominantly affected and on the number and distribution of the muscle groups involved: (1) mixed flexor-extensor spasms, which occur most frequently; (2) flexor spasms, the next most common; and (3) extensor spasms, which occur least commonly. Most infants with this disorder have more than one type of spasm, and the type observed at any given moment may be influenced by body position. Clinical phenomena associated with the motor spasms include eye movements, consisting of deviation or deviation followed by rhythmic nystagmoid movements, and respiratory pauses; both occur in approximately 60 percent of motor spasms. Alterations in heart rate occur rarely. Many infants cry after a spasm, but a cry or scream does not appear as an ictal phenomenon. The majority of infantile spasms occur in clusters, and within a given cluster, the intensity of the spasms usually waxes and then wanes. Approximately the same number of spasms occur during the night as during the daytime. However, infantile spasms rarely occur when infants are actually asleep, tending to occur immediately upon arousal or soon thereafter.

A variety of interictal EEG patterns may be seen when patients are having spasms. These include diffuse slowing, focal slowing, generalized slow-spike and slow-wave activity, focal or multifocal spikes and sharp waves, and (rarely) normal background activity. However, the most common pattern seen is hypsarrhythmia or one of its various modifications (i.e., modified hypsarrhythmia).

Patient Evaluation and Classification

Patients with infantile spasms require a thorough evaluation at the time of presentation. This evaluation includes a careful developmental assessment, physical and neurologic examination, CT scan, and other laboratory tests as indicated (e.g., metabolic screening, chromosomal analysis). In approximately 60 percent of cases, various prenatal, perinatal, and postnatal etiologic factors can be

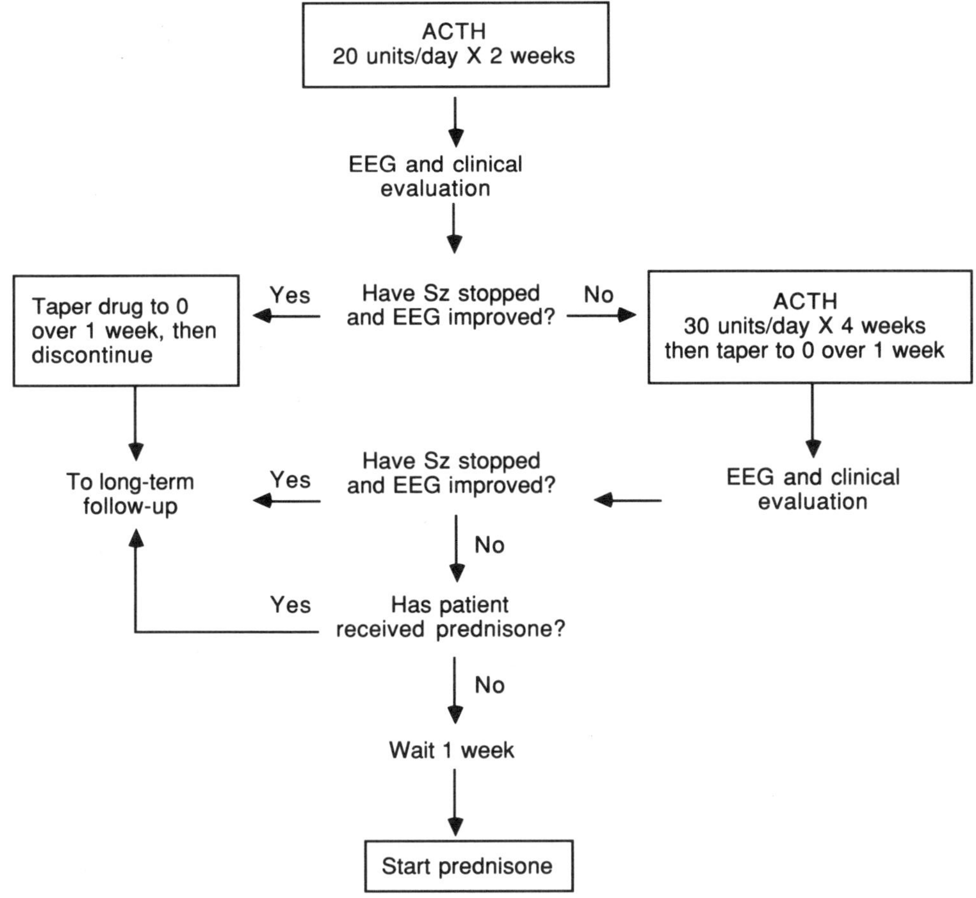

Figure 1 ACTH treatment regimen. Sz = seizures.

identified. Prenatal factors include intrauterine infection, prematurity, cerebral dysgenesis, hypoxia-ischemia, and genetic disorders. Perinatal factors include hypoxia-ischemia and traumatic delivery, while postnatal factors include head injury, inborn errors of metabolism, CNS infection, hypoxia-ischemia, and intracranial hemorrhage. Approximately 50 percent of patients have major neurologic deficits and another 40 percent have minor ones. Approximately 85 to 90 percent of patients with infantile spasms show some degree of mental and developmental retardation.

Using this information, one can divide patients with infantile spasms into two groups: those with a symptomatic condition and those with a cryptogenic condition. A patient is classified as having a cryptogenic condition if there is no known associated etiologic factor, development is normal before onset of the spasms, there is no abnormality on neurologic examination, and the CT scan is normal before institution of therapy. Approximately 10 to 15 percent of patients can be classified as having a cryptogenic condition; the remainder are classified as having a symptomatic condition. As discussed later in this chapter, the classification of patients as

cryptogenic or symptomatic is crucial for assessing long-term developmental outcome.

Treatment

Hormonal Therapy

Acute Effects. The only known means of effectively stopping infantile spasms and improving the EEG of the patient is therapy with adrenocorticotropic hormone (ACTH) or corticosteroids. The following treatment regimen is recommended for all patients with infantile spasms, regardless of age, treatment lag, or patient classification (cryptogenic versus symptomatic). Before institution of hormonal therapy, the clinical evaluation of the patient discussed previously (including CT scan) should be performed, and a baseline EEG, including a sleep tracing, should be obtained. Either ACTH or prednisone may be given initially, since the response rates to these two drugs do not differ significantly. If ACTH is chosen (Fig. 1), the initial dosage is 20 U per day. After 2 weeks of ACTH therapy at a dosage of 20 U per day, the EEG is repeated. If the patient has responded (defined as improvement in the EEG

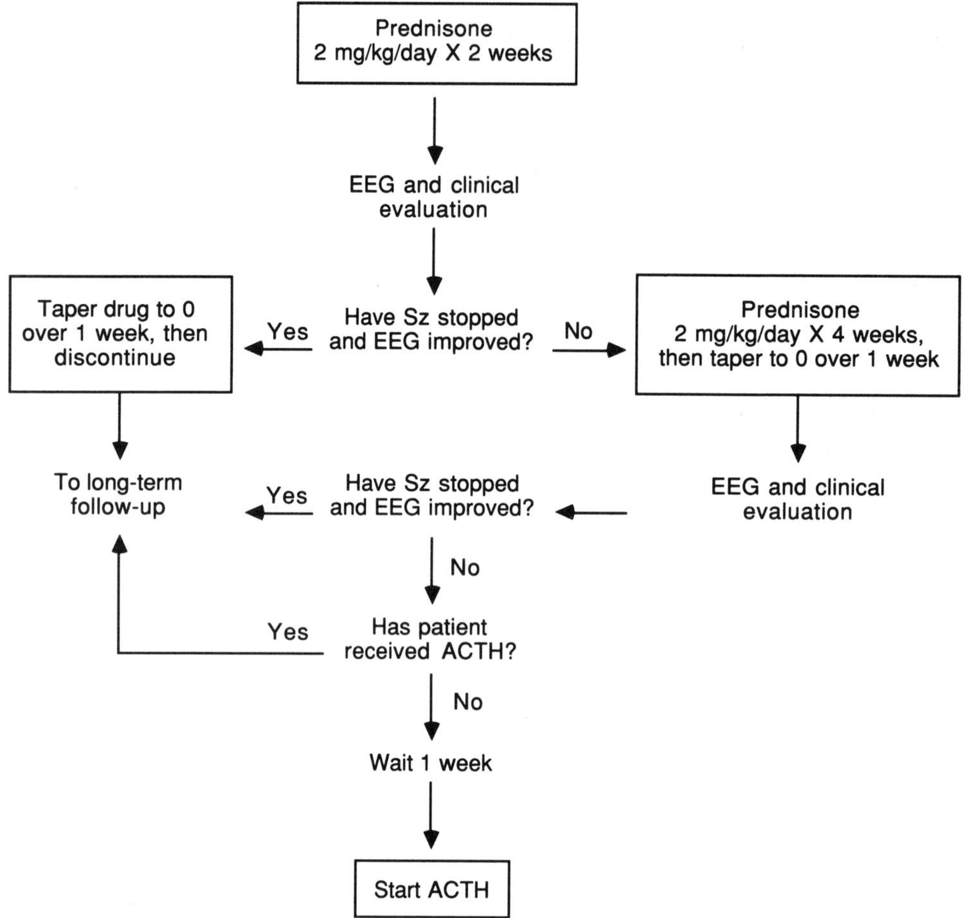

Figure 2 Prednisone treatment regimen. Sz = seizures.

and total cessation of spasms), ACTH is tapered and discontinued over a 1-week period, and the patient is followed in a routine clinical manner. If the patient has not responded after 2 weeks of ACTH therapy, the dose is increased to 30 U per day. ACTH is continued at this dosage for an additional 4 weeks, after which it is tapered and discontinued over a 1-week period. A repeat EEG is performed at this point. If the patient has responded to the ACTH, he or she is followed in a routine clinical manner. If a relapse occurs, the patient is given a repeat course of ACTH at the dose at which the initial response occurred. If the patient does not respond to ACTH and has not been treated with prednisone, prednisone is given after ACTH has been discontinued for 1 week.

If prednisone is administered (Fig. 2), it should be given in a dose of 2 mg per kilogram per day. The follow-up is similar to that of patients receiving ACTH. After 2 weeks of therapy, a repeat EEG is performed. If the patient shows a response at this time, prednisone is tapered and discontinued over a 1-week period, and the patient is followed routinely. If the patient has not responded after 2 weeks of

prednisone therapy, the drug is continued at a dose of 2 mg per kilogram per day for an additional 4 weeks, after which it is tapered over a 1-week period and discontinued. A repeat EEG is performed at this time. If the patient has responded, he or she is followed in a routine manner. If a relapse occurs, the patient is given a repeat course of prednisone. If the patient does not respond to prednisone and has not been treated with ACTH, administration of ACTH is begun after prednisone therapy has been discontinued for 1 week. Throughout the entire course of ACTH or prednisone therapy, the patient's blood pressure should be monitored closely, and serum electrolytes should be checked weekly.

Approximately 60 percent of patients with infantile spasms will respond to this therapeutic regimen; in most patients, the response is seen within 2 weeks of initiation of hormonal therapy. Approximately one-third of the patients will have a relapse, but a second course of therapy is usually effective. It is important to remember that relative normalization of the EEG may occur in approximately half of the patients who continue to have spasms after institution of hormonal therapy.

Side Effects. The most common side effect seen in patients with infantile spasms treated with ACTH or prednisone is hypertension; in our experience, it occurs in approximately 25 percent. Hypertension can be controlled by adding an antihypertensive agent or by reducing the dosage of ACTH or prednisone. Other side effects include electrolyte imbalance, suppression of the immune system, ocular opacities, gastrointestinal disturbances, hypertrophic cardiomyopathy (shown by echocardiography), myopathy, and transient brain shrinkage (shown on CT scan).

Long-Term Outcome. It has been believed that in the hormonal treatment of infantile spasms, ACTH and/or corticosteroids not only improve the EEG and control the spasms but also improve the outlook for mental and motor development. Whether hormonal therapy has any effect on long-term development is a controversial and unresolved issue. In our experience, the overall prognosis for patients with this disorder is poor; only 5 percent of patients with infantile spasm have normal outcomes, whereas almost 75 percent have severe or very severe impairment. Long-term outcome does not seem to be affected by whether the patient does or does not respond to hormonal therapy or whether the treatment lag is short or long. The only factor that seems to affect long-term outcome is whether the patient's condition is cryptogenic or symptomatic. In our studies, 38 percent of the patients with cryptogenic conditions were normal or had only mild impairment at follow-up, in contrast to 5 percent of the patients with symptomatic conditions; however, we have found no way to predict which of those patients with cryptogenic conditions will have normal outcomes and which will be retarded.

Anticonvulsant Therapy

Of the various traditional anticonvulsants that have been used to treat patients with infantile spasms, only valproic acid and the benzodiazepines, particularly nitrazepam, have been reported to be effective. The most effective dosages of nitrazepam have ranged from 0.3 to 1.0 mg per kilogram per day, whereas dosages of valproic acid have been variable, ranging up to 100 mg per kilogram per day. Our patients who failed to respond to ACTH and prednisone and were then given valproic acid or nitrazepam also failed to respond to these drugs.

ACKNOWLEDGMENTS

Supported by Grants NS25884 (to R.A.H.) and NS11535, and by Teacher-Investigator Development Award NS00810 (to E.M.M.), from the National Institute of Neurological Disorders and Stroke, National Institute of Health, United States Department of Health and Human Services.

SUGGESTED READING

Aicardi J. Infantile spasms and related syndromes. In: Aicardi J, ed. Epilepsy in children. New York: Raven Press, 1986:17.

Hrachovy RA, Frost JD Jr. Infantile spasms. Clev Clin J Med 1989; 56(suppl):S10.

Hrachovy RA, Frost JD Jr, Kellaway P, Zion T. Double-blind study of ACTH vs. prednisone therapy in infantile spasms. J Pediatr 1983; 103:641.

Kellaway P, Mizrahi EM. Neonatal seizures. In: Lüders H, Lesser RP, eds. Epilepsy: electroclinical syndromes. New York: Springer-Verlag, 1987:13.

Mizrahi EM, Kellaway P. Characterization and classification of neonatal seizures. Neurology 1987; 37:1837.

Painter MJ, Bergman I, Crumrine PK. Neonatal seizures. In: Pellock JM, Myer EC, eds. Neurological emergencies in infancy and childhood. Philadelphia: JB Lippincott, 1984:37.

FEBRILE SEIZURES

SHLOMO SHINNAR, M.D., Ph.D.

A febrile seizure is defined as a seizure associated with fever occurring in a child who does not have evidence of acute intracranial infection or electrolyte imbalance and without any prior history of afebrile seizures. Although fever is not always present at the time of the seizure, it must occur within 24 hours of the episode. Febrile seizures usually occur between 3 months and 7 years of age, the peak incidence being between 6 months and 3 years of age.

Febrile seizures are the most common form of childhood seizures. They occur in 2 to 5 percent of all children in the United States. Approximately one-third of all children who experience a febrile convulsion will have one or more recurrent febrile convulsions, and 10 percent will have multiple episodes. Following the nomenclature of the National Collaborative Perinatal Project and the National Institute of Health (NIH) Consensus Conference, febrile convulsions are classified as either simple or complex. The simple febrile convulsion is a single brief generalized tonic clonic convulsion lasting less than 15 minutes. A febrile convulsion is classified as complex if it is either prolonged, focal, or multiple. A prolonged febrile convulsion is one lasting more than 10 or 15 minutes, depending on the study. A focal febrile seizure is diagnosed either by a witnessed focal onset or by a Todd's paresis postictally. Children who have more than one seizure during the 24 to 48 hours of the same acute illness are classified as having one complex (multiple) febrile seizure. It is important to note that the presence of prior neurologic abnormalities and/or the presence of a family history of epilepsy do not enter into whether a febrile convulsion is defined as simple or complex. They are, however, important predictors of whether the child will develop epilepsy in the future.

INITIAL EVALUATION

All children who experience a seizure associated with fever require an emergency medical evaluation. The definition of a benign febrile convulsion implies that intracranial infection and acute systemic insults aside from fever have been excluded. The evaluation should focus on the cause of fever, with emphasis placed on excluding meningitis and encephalitis.

In all children who have a febrile convulsion, lumbar puncture should be seriously considered. The presence of any of the following risk factors for meningitis should mandate a lumbar puncture at any age: (1) a focal seizure, (2) an abnormal neurologic examination, (3) a seizure occurring after the child has arrived in the emergency room, or (4) prior medical care within 48 hours. Age is also an important consideration, as children younger than 18 months of age will not always exhibit meningeal signs. In children, meningismus is also often absent postictally. In general, my practice is to perform a lumbar puncture on all children younger than 12 months of age presenting with a first febrile convulsion, no matter how their condition seems. In children 1 to 2 years of age, lumbar puncture should be strongly considered, although it can occasionally be avoided in a child who has a brief generalized tonic clonic seizure and who, by the time he is seen in the emergency room, appears entirely normal except for his fever. In children older than 2 years of age, clinical judgment is usually adequate to distinguish the seriously ill child from the child with a benign febrile convulsion. When in doubt, one should always err on the side of performing a lumbar puncture.

Other laboratory evaluations should not be considered routine and should be directed at determining the source of the fever rather than the seizure. In the child younger than 2 years of age, blood cultures are helpful for ruling out bacteremia. An electroencephalogram (EEG) performed either soon after the seizure or more than 2 weeks later is of little use in predicting either seizure recurrence or the subsequent development of epilepsy. The common belief that an EEG performed 2 weeks after the initial febrile convulsion will separate children who have benign febrile convulsions from those with "epilepsy triggered by fever" has little factual basis. Computed tomography (CT) scans are rarely indicated in the evaluation of febrile seizures. I reserve CT scans for the patient with a persistent new neurologic deficit or what is clearly a focal seizure, especially a focal seizure associated with a Todd's paresis. Even in such cases the yield is low. When indicated, a lumbar puncture should not be delayed to obtain a CT scan, as the delay may be fatal in cases of meningitis.

TREATMENT OF INITIAL EPISODE

The majority of febrile convulsions are brief and self-limited. By the time the child is brought to medical attention, the seizure is usually over. In these cases, no specific treatment for the seizure is necessary. If a treatable cause of fever is found or if meningitis is suspected, appropriate antibiotic therapy should be given.

The usual definition of a "prolonged" febrile seizure is any febrile seizure lasting 10 to 15 minutes. While these would be atypical, a 15-minute seizure is not life-threatening. In rare cases, febrile convulsions are more prolonged, lasting more than 30 minutes. Such convulsions are classified as complex. They usually occur in the context of an acute insult or in a neurologically abnormal child. These episodes of febrile status epilepticus should be treated as life-threatening emergencies and treated vigorously according to the usual status epilepticus protocol. (A description of this protocol is outside the scope of this chapter.) Many, myself included, substitute intravenous phenobarbital for phenytoin for children with febrile status. In my experience, one can usually administer the phenobarbital without having to intubate the patient if the patient is being carefully monitored. Note that we are talking about true status epilepticus.

Somewhat more common is the case of a child with multiple febrile convulsions—i.e., more than one febrile seizure occurring on the same day. Typically, such a child is brought in for one or two brief febrile convulsions that occurred at home and then proceeds to have another one. As discussed earlier, these children should have a lumbar puncture to rule out meningitis. A phenobarbital loading dose of 10 to 15 mg per kilogram given slowly over 30 minutes intravenously, or orally if the patient is awake, is reasonable. The short-term administration of phenobarbital is unlikely to cause significant morbidity and will help control the seizures until the clinical situation is better defined. It is my practice to admit these children overnight. Note that initial acute treatment of a febrile seizure with a loading dose, either because the seizure was prolonged or multiple, in no way commits one to administering long-term prophylactic therapy with phenobarbital.

LONG-TERM MANAGEMENT

As febrile convulsions are usually benign, brief seizures without neurologic sequelae, lately there has been reluctance to give children long-term daily anticonvulsant therapy after an initial episode. At present in the United States there is no effective therapy for preventing a febrile seizure at the time of the illness. Aggressive management of the fever would appear to be a rational approach. However, febrile convulsions tend to occur as the fever rises. In as many as one-third of the cases, the convulsion itself is the first sign the parent has that the child has a fever. Indeed the actual temperature elevation may occur hours after the seizure. Therefore, while we usually advise the parents to administer acetaminophen at the first sign of fever, we also always tell them that it may not help.

A popular treatment several decades ago was to give intermittent phenobarbital therapy at the time of acute illness. Parents were instructed to give the phenobarbital only when the child was ill. Studies have shown that this therapy is no more effective than placebo. The problem with this therapy is twofold. As stated above, the febrile convulsion may be the parents' first indication that the child is ill. Second, unless one uses a loading dose, it will take several days to achieve an effective serum level of phenobarbital, by which time the child has either had a seizure or is no longer at risk during this acute episode. Most physicians would be justifiably uncomfortable instructing a parent to give the child 15 to 20 mg per kilogram of phenobarbital every time the child appeared ill.

There are recent reports that rectal diazepam administered at the time of onset of fever will reduce the chance of a subsequent febrile convulsion, especially in children with a high risk of recurrence. These reports also indicate that rectal diazepam will rapidly terminate a febrile convulsion. At present, rectal diazepam is not FDA approved in the United States. Some neurologists have used the intravenous form rectally. In my opinion, the routine use of rectal benzodiazepines in the treatment or prevention of febrile convulsions is not justified. One exception may be the rare child who has recurrent prolonged febrile convulsions and does not tolerate phenobarbital therapy or in whom phenobarbital therapy is not effective. Even in such a case, this treatment should be undertaken only if the parents are reliable and after a thorough discussion of the risks and benefits as well as the experimental nature of the therapy.

Daily phenobarbital therapy in doses similar to those used in the treatment of epilepsy will significantly reduce the chance of recurrence of febrile convulsions. This has been shown in several controlled clinical trials. Serum levels of greater than 15 μg per milliliter need to be achieved for efficacy.

Phenobarbital usage is associated with a wide variety of cognitive and behavioral side effects which in many cases are severe enough to necessitate discontinuation of therapy. The most common of these is a paradoxical hyperactivity that occurs in 30 percent or more of these children. Other common problems include irritability, sleep disorders, and changes in behavior. In school-age children and adults, one can demonstrate that even those who are having no overt problems have significant cognitive deficits, particularly those related to attention span, that are readily demonstrable on formal neuropsychological testing.

Phenytoin has not been shown to be effective in preventing recurrent febrile seizures. In addition, there are significant problems associated with its use in young children, both in terms of unreliable absorption in children younger than 2 years of age and the high incidence of gingival hyperplasia seen in preschool children, even those who have received preventive dental care. Carbamazepine also has not been shown to be effective in preventing recurrent febrile convulsions. In several studies, carbamazepine was ineffective in preventing recurrent febrile convulsions in children who did not respond to phenobarbital.

Valproic acid is effective in preventing febrile convulsions. The NIH Consensus Conference does mention it as a possible alternative treatment to phenobarbital. It has fewer cognitive side effects and is associated with a lower incidence of behavioral problems. However, one must keep in mind that the majority of febrile convulsions occur in children younger than 2 years of age. This is precisely the age group that has the highest incidence of the idiosyncratic fatal hepatotoxicity. In children younger than 2 years of age who are neurologically abnormal, the incidence of fatal hepatotoxicity may be as great as one in 500. This has considerably diminished early enthusiasm for the use of valproic acid sodium in the treatment of what is usually a benign, self-limited seizure disorder. I very rarely use valproic acid in treating febrile seizures.

SELECTION OF PATIENTS FOR PHENOBARBITAL TREATMENT

As discussed earlier in this chapter, the current standard treatment for preventing recurrent febrile convulsions consists of daily phenobarbital therapy in doses similar to those used in the treatment of epilepsy. Febrile seizures are usually benign and self-limited. Phenobarbital therapy carries with it a significant morbidity, particularly in terms of cognitive and behavioral side effects. In any decision making regarding therapy, one must carefully weigh the risks and benefits of the therapy in question. It is my bias that in most cases, the morbidity of therapy usually exceeds that of the disease and I therefore restrict therapy to a few situations. The indications for therapy are discussed below.

The NIH Consensus Conference on Febrile Seizures recommended that therapy "should be considered" in children with (1) complex febrile seizure (focal, prolonged, or multiple), (2) an abnormal neurologic examination (including presence of a static encephalopathy), (3) a family history of febrile or afebrile seizures, (4) recurrent febrile seizures, or (5) febrile seizure when younger than 1 year of age. These recommendations, however, do not identify a small group of children who would benefit from treatment. If every child who met at least one of the above criteria were treated, more than 50 percent of children would receive treatment.

The NIH Consensus Conference treatment recommendations simply do not make sense in light of the findings over the last decade. They fail to distinguish between risk factors for future epilepsy (complex febrile seizure, abnormal neurologic status, family history of afebrile seizures) and risk factors for recurrent febrile convulsions (patient's age at the time of the first febrile seizure). Although febrile convulsions are in certain cases a marker for future epilepsy, there is no evidence that the treatment of febrile convulsions prevents the development of epilepsy in the future. There is also little evidence to support the hypothesis that recurrent febrile convulsions cause epilepsy. Thus treatment with phenobarbital should be reserved for the prevention of further febrile convulsions.

Thirty to forty percent of children who experience an initial febrile convulsion will have a second one. Approximately half of these children will go on to have a third febrile seizure. Only about 10 percent will have more than three febrile convulsions. The most important risk factor appears to be the patient's age at the time of the first febrile convulsion. Approximately 50 percent of children younger than 1 year of age with a febrile convulsion will experience a recurrence. Attendance at a day-care center and a family history of febrile and afebrile seizures have also been implicated as risk factors for recurrence.

I recommend therapy for the following patients:

1. Those who have had at least two prolonged febrile convulsions within 1 year.
2. Those who have had two febrile convulsions prior to 1 year of age.
3. Those who have three or more febrile convulsions more frequently than every 6 months.
4. Those who have a coexisting disease causing a febrile convulsion to place the patient at high risk. (For example, a patient with congenital heart disease with significant cardiac impairment may not be able to withstand the stress of a febrile convulsion.)

This is clearly a small minority of the children with febrile convulsions. Over the years, I have become more and more convinced of the essentially benign nature of febrile convulsions and of the morbidity associated with therapy with phenobarbital and am treating fewer and fewer patients. If a child treated with phenobarbital has side effects from the medication, I usually discontinue the phenobarbital and tell the parents that having a few more febrile convulsions is associated with less potential morbidity than valproic acid therapy for patients in this age group. I reserve valproic acid therapy for the child older than 3 years of age who is still having more than three febrile convulsions per year and who does not tolerate phenobarbital. Even then, I am reluctant to administer valproic acid therapy.

Regardless of whether or not one treats the child with phenobarbital, one must take the time to explain to the parents the nature of febrile seizures, what to do in the event of the next seizure, and the uncertainty of the prognosis. Because febrile seizures are frightening events to the parents, they need reassurance and education. It is also important to emphasize that the decision to treat or not to treat at any given time is not absolute but based on an assessment of the relative risks and benefits of treatment at that time. That decision is subject to change if the child should experience further seizures or unacceptable morbidity from the medications.

SUGGESTED READING

Freeman JM. Febrile seizures: an end to confusion. Pediatrics 1978; 61:806–808. Editorial.

Knudsen FU. Recurrence risk after first febrile seizure and effect of short-term diazepam prophylaxis. Arch Dis Child 1985; 60:1045–1049.

National Institutes of Health. Febrile seizures: Consensus Development Conference summary. Bethesda, MD: National Institute of Health, 1980: Vol. 3, No. 2.

Nelson KB, Ellenberg JH, eds. Febrile seizures. New York: Raven Press, 1981.

Wolf SM, Forsythe A. Behavior disturbances, phenobarbital, and febrile seizures. Pediatrics 1978; 61:728–731.

ABSENCE SEIZURES

EILEEN P.G. VINING, M.D.

The therapy of classical absence seizures (previously referred to as petit mal seizures) is straightforward and generally successful. Typically these are seizures of childhood that begin and end abruptly and involve sudden, brief cessation of activity, staring, and slight movement of the eyes. The electrocephalogram (EEG) is generally normal between seizures and shows 3-per-second spike-wave activity during the seizure. They respond well to ethosuximide and appear self-limited; after a seizure-free period, medication can usually be discontinued without recurrence of seizures. Unfortunately, these classical or simple absence seizures are really quite rare (less than 10 percent of absence seizures are simple). Five other types of absence seizures (complex absence) are differentiated; although they share the critical elements of short duration, abrupt onset and termination, impairment of consciousness, and high frequency, they are classified on the basis of whether they involve mild clonic movements, atonic components, tonic components, automatism, or autonomic components. In addition, absence seizures can be a major component of many forms of epilepsy ranging from benign classical childhood absence epilepsy to the Lennox-Gastaut syndrome. They can be seen in association with tonic-clonic seizures, myoclonic seizures, atonic seizures, and even partial seizures. Therapy in these situations is more complex.

WHY DO WE TREAT ABSENCE SEIZURES?

Because of growing concerns about the potential side effects of antiepileptic drugs, with increasing frequency, physicians and patients are questioning the necessity of treating seizures. Frequently the parents are not even aware that their child is experiencing seizures until the school officials or teachers point out that the child is having attentional problems and request that he or she receive a medical evaluation. Patients and parents understand the impact of tonic-clonic seizures more easily than that of absence seizures. When tonic-clonic seizures are witnessed, the event is recognized, and often fear is engendered. Absence seizures, on the other hand, are by nature more insidious. They may go unrecognized for a significant period of time, with the child, family, and teacher believing that the child has a learning problem. Unless the child is experiencing academic difficulties, the parent may question how such a brief episode can be harmful. Occasionally it

is helpful to induce several of these seizures with hyperventilation, while asking a child to process information and recall it (a short rhyme or phrase). When parents see that the child is missing information during those moments, they can understand why he might be struggling in the classroom. Although the child is not at the same physical risk of injuring himself as during a tonic-clonic seizure, some physical risk exists if seizures occur during a ball game or while crossing the street. These seizures should be treated because they interrupt normal function and interfere with learning.

SIMPLE ABSENCE SEIZURES

If the child has clear cut simple absence seizures (brief staring spells, with minimal movement of the eyes and with an EEG that shows 3-second spike-wave complexes), I begin treatment with ethosuximide, 10 mg per kilogram per day administered twice daily, although with a half-life of 30 to 40 hours (50 hours for adults), single daily dosing is probably acceptable. In patients with dose-related side effects such as gastrointestinal distress and headaches, I split the dose to improve tolerance. Because seizures generally occur frequently, their incidence is a good measure of success and the dose should be increased every 10 to 14 days until seizures have been controlled or until side effects are observed. A wide therapeutic range exists for this drug, and some individuals require very high serum levels to achieve control of seizures. Frequently this can be accomplished without any evidence of toxicity; I have followed children with blood serum levels considerably higher than the therapeutic range, even reaching 150 to 200 μg per milliliter, without evidence of toxicity. Baseline laboratory studies should include a complete blood count (CBC), which is to be monitored after the initiation of therapy and intermittently thereafter (once or twice per year) as the patient is followed. Rare reactions to ethosuximide include allergic drug reactions, systemic lupus erythematosus, nephrotic syndrome, and bone marrow aplasia.

Since these seizures rarely begin in adulthood, I would carefully question my diagnostic evidence before beginning adult therapy with ethosuximide. In adults, absence seizures are generally associated with other seizures and require therapy with valproic acid.

The monitoring of patients with absence seizures presents some interesting challenges and some important potential dilemmas. How do you know that you have controlled all of their seizures? Absence seizures are subtle and it is difficult to know whether a person is seizure-free. This may be important in judging if seizures are contributing to learning problems or if there is an underlying learning disorder. For the person who wants to drive, should an

EEG be obtained to determine whether all the spike-wave activity has disappeared? Should medication be increased until the EEG is normalized even if no seizures are reported? What is the clinical significance of spike-wave activity seen in the EEG laboratory? Should vigilance testing be done on the individual with concomitant EEG to look for alterations associated with spike-wave complexes? On the other hand, would the patient have spike-wave complexes in real-life situations where vigilance is increased (e.g., classroom situations, driving)? Does ambulatory monitoring need to be done for all these individuals in order to determine if the spike-wave complexes exist in natural settings? There are no clear answers to these questions. If a child had frequent seizures and no longer has them while receiving therapy, I consider treatment successful and am not concerned about EEG activity. On the other hand, if that child continues to have problems in the classroom and his or her attention span is questioned, I use the EEG to gain more understanding. If the child has ongoing spike-wave activity, I increase the dosage of medication and attempt to optimize therapy, still trying to ascertain if he or she is doing better in school. If absence seizures have been controlled for 2 years and I consider discontinuing the medication, I use an EEG for guidance. If spike-wave complexes remain, I continue therapy and repeat the EEG at 1 year. The issue of ongoing spike-wave complexes and whether an individual is eligible to drive an automobile is much more complex and clear precedents do not exist. We have not reached a point where all persons must have a normal EEG before they are allowed to drive. However, if as the physician you believe that these brief bursts of activity are interfering with the patient's normal functions, you believe by definition that person has ongoing seizures. In this case, the patient should be advised not to drive and therapy should be adjusted.

ATYPICAL ABSENCE SEIZURES

If the seizures are atypical, more prolonged with myoclonic, atonic, and tonic features or automatism, with an EEG that does not show classical 3-per-second spike-wave activity and is often interictally abnormal, ethosuximide is less likely to be effective and valproic acid is the drug of choice. It is available in many forms, including enteric-coated capsules (Table 1).

Valproic acid is generally initiated at 10 mg per kilogram per day divided into two doses administered twice daily. Although the half-life is generally reported to be 8 to 12 hours, most individuals tolerate this dosage since plasma steady state may not be crucial to the efficacy of this drug. In fact, some report that the drug has been most effective when

Table 1 Therapy Preferences

Condition	Treatment
Simple absence seizure	Ethosuximide (Zarontin)
Atypical absence seizures	Valproic acid (Depakene, Depakote) Ethosuximide Benzodiazepines Clonazepam (Clonopin) Clorazepate (Tranxene) Lorazepam (Ativan)
Absence seizures associated with other seizures	Valproic acid Benzodiazepine Ethosuximide
Difficult-to-control absence seizures with or without other seizures	Always question diagnosis Ethosuximide + valproic acid Carbamazepine (Tegretol) Acetazolamide (Diamox) Ketogenic diet ACTH or prednisone Corpus callosotomy

given once per day, suggesting that peak levels of the drug produce a therapeutic response. Such a short half-life also would suggest that the steady state and thus the therapeutic efficacy at a given dosage should be seen within 3 to 4 days. However, many reports suggest that it may take as long as 2 weeks to judge efficacy at a given dosage and a similar period of time to judge whether decreasing the dose or discontinuing the drug will adversely affect seizures.

Physicians tend to be reluctant to prescribe valproic acid because of reported hepatotoxity and rare deaths from liver failure. In one report it was noted that children younger than 2 years of age who received polytherapy were particularly at risk for hepatic failure (one in 800 patients), whereas in patients older than 10 years of age who received monotherapy, there were no deaths. Another serious potential problem is thrombocytopenia and interference with platelet aggregation. Baseline liver function tests and platelet counts should be obtained. After the patient has been taking the medication for 2 to 3 weeks, these studies should be repeated. They should then be repeated if appetite loss, vomiting, nausea, or bruising develop or one to two times per year. Obviously if the patient is about to undergo surgery, platelet count and function should be assessed. Other significant problems include pancreatitis and changes in mental function associated with elevated ammonia levels. Other side effects, which may be dose related, include nausea, alopecia, sedation, and tremor. Weight gain is frequent. Neural tube defects have been reported in approximately 1 percent of babies whose mothers were taking valproic acid during pregnancy. Counseling regarding this complication is essential since prenatal testing is available.

I generally increase the dosage in increments of 5 to 10 mg per kilogram per day every 2 weeks until the seizures are controlled or side effects are seen. Generally children require 25 to 40 mg per kilogram per day. Only rarely do patients require as much as 60 to 80 mg per kilogram per day, and in isolated circumstances, I have used as much as 100 mg per kilogram per day without problems. Adults may require 4 to 5 g per day for seizures that are difficult to control, although the usual dosage is 2 to 3 g per day.

If valproic acid is not effective, I consider using ethosuximide; this may be especially useful if there is a myoclonic component to the seizures. The other major class of useful drugs are benzodiazepines. A major problem of these medications are their sedative-hypnotic nature and a tendency toward tachyphylaxis. Absence seizures are frequently exacerbated by drowsiness, a common side effect of these drugs. Diazepam generally is not a good long-term prophylactic drug. Clonazepam may be helpful, but side effects include personality change, irritability, and increased secretions. There is little long-term experience with lorazepam, although side effects may be less common. Clorazepate dipotassium may also be an effective agent, with perhaps less sedation and behavior change than is seen with clonazepam.

ABSENCE SEIZURES ASSOCIATED WITH OTHER SEIZURES

When absence seizures exist in tandem with other seizure types, in particular tonic-clonic seizures, myoclonic seizures, or atonic seizures, the therapeutic approach is different. If the person has absence seizures and isolated tonic-clonic seizures, I use valproic acid as a single agent. In the past, a combination of ethosuximide and phenobarbital was recommended. If the absence seizures are part of the Lennox-Gastaut syndrome, valproic acid is the drug of choice, with benzodiazepines as second-line agents. If the absence seizures are part of juvenile myoclonic epilepsy of Janz, again valproic acid is the drug of choice. Other drugs are rarely effective in treating this syndrome.

IF SEIZURES ARE NOT CONTROLLED

If seizures are not controlled by the time ethosuximide, valproic acid, and benzodiazepines are pushed to the point of toxicity, I give a final trial of a combination of ethosuximide and valproic acid. If that fails, I carefully re-examine my diagnosis. A critical question to consider at this point is whether these episodes are actually seizures. Unlike patients

with partial complex seizures and even generalized tonic-clonic seizures, it is the rare patient with absence seizures who does not have an abnormal EEG that is compatible with the clinical picture. However, if seizures are not successfully controlled, I wonder if the child simply has a severe attentional deficit disorder or perhaps a hyperventilation syndrome. Further history may give additional information and the EEG should be reevaluated.

A person who appears to have absence seizures may actually have partial complex seizures. This differentiation can be particularly difficult if the patient has episodes involving staring and automatism that last 1 to 2 minutes. Postictal confusion is one sign of a partial complex seizure. The EEG may also be helpful; a person with partial complex seizures may have only an occasional spike interictally on their EEG, rather than spike-wave complexes. If the "absence seizures" occur relatively infrequently and if they do not begin and end abruptly, I place the patient on carbamazepine.

If I conclude that I am dealing with absence seizures, two other medical therapies are tried. Acetazolamide is sometimes useful, either alone or in combination with other agents, and the ketogenic diet may be very effective in children. The latter involves an initial starvation into ketosis and the maintenance of ketosis using a diet in which 80 percent of the calories are generally apportioned to fats and the additional 20 percent to a combination of protein and carbohydrates. Another somewhat drastic alternative therapy for mixed seizure disorders is the use of ACTH or prednisone.

When absence seizures are intractable and associated with other seizure forms (tonic, atonic, myoclonic), it may be necessary to consider a surgical approach—in particular, corpus callosotomy.

Generally if patients fail therapy with ethosuximide or valproic acid, they are difficult to manage. Polytherapy can be complex because of drug interactions, and it may be helpful to refer those patients to specialists. The impact of these seizures on function and adjustment may require additional services to help the patient and family cope with the problem.

PATIENT ADJUSTMENT

Epilepsy is a disorder that requires many psychosocial and societal adjustments. Parents may feel guilty about thinking their child was "dumb" or poorly motivated. The child will need support and encouragement to understand how his attention has been constantly interrupted by seizures and that with medication, those interruptions should stop. He needs to know how important it is to tell his parents if he starts to feel that he is missing things again. He may need help in catching up with work that he missed or only poorly understood during the seizures. Teachers need to understand the physiologic nature of the problem so that they can help monitor for complete seizure control and be able to make certain that the child has fully mastered the material that was presented while the absence seizures were occurring. Often a child's friends need an explanation of the condition because they may have concluded that he or she is "flaky," "weird," or "strange." They, too, can be helpful in letting the child and family know whether seizures are completely controlled. The older child may have difficulty in sports (keeping the eye on the ball) or with video games. The adult may describe difficulties concentrating, and friends may wonder why he keeps missing aspects of their conversations. All of these individuals need to understand that these lapses in consciousness were seizures, that the person was not being "dumb" or intending to offend or ignore them. Parents need help in readjusting to a normal child, one whom they are not constantly prodding or yelling at to secure attention. There may also be questions concerning genetics—who else is at risk. Some absence seizure disorders do have familial tendencies, and therefore this must be addressed.

Much mythology concerning epilepsy remains in society, and I encourage patients and families to acquire as much information as possible and join with other families in combatting the stigma and improving the society's understanding of the problem. The Epilepsy Foundation of America has local affiliates in most states and large cities and is an excellent resource.

SUGGESTED READING

Braathen G, Theorell K, Persson A, et al. Valproate in the treatment of absence epilepsy in children: a study of dose-response relationships. Epilepsia 1988; 29:548–552.
Gastaut H, Zifkin B, Mariani E, et al. The long-term course of primary generalized epilepsy with persisting absences. Neurology 1986; 36:1021–1028.
Holmes G, McKeever M, Adamson M. Absence seizures in children: clinical and electroencephalographic features. Ann Neurol 1987; 21:268–273.
Sato S, White BG, Penry JK, et al. Valproic acid versus ethosuximide in the treatment of absence seizures. Neurology 1982; 32:157–163.
Snead OC, Benton JW, Myers GJ. ACTH and prednisone in childhood seizure disorders. Neurology 1983; 33:966–970.

PATIENT RESOURCE

Epilepsy Foundation of America
4351 Garden City Drive
Landover, Maryland 20785

Information and Referral Service (Professional and patient information): 1-800-EFA-1000

National Epilepsy Library (Searches and articles at no cost to professionals): 1-800-EFA-4050
(In Maryland call: 301-459-3700)

FOCAL SEIZURE DISORDERS

THOMAS H. BURNSTINE, M.D.
RONALD P. LESSER, M.D.

Focal epileptic seizures originate in one or more discrete areas of the cerebral hemispheres. They are classified under the following headings: simple partial seizures, complex partial seizures, partial seizures with secondary generalization, and secondarily generalized seizures, which are generalized seizures of focal origin. Simple partial seizures do not impair consciousness; they consist of motor, sensory, autonomic, or psychic symptoms. Complex partial seizures do impair consciousness, although they may begin as simple partial seizures (e.g., an aura) consisting of any of the previously mentioned symptoms. Complex partial seizures may be accompanied by automatisms, which are complex motor activities occurring after consciousness is altered during the ictal or postictal phases of which the patient is amnestic. Whatever their manifestations, seizures that impair cognition or sensorimotor coordination often curtail educational, employment, and social opportunities. Therefore the goals of treatment should include eliminating as much seizure activity as possible and minimizing the disruption of the patient's personal life that epilepsy causes.

DIAGNOSIS

It is often difficult retrospectively to differentiate epileptic seizures from other paroxysmal events. For example, in the differential diagnosis of complex partial seizures, one takes into consideration almost any cause of alteration of consciousness, some of which may be nonepileptic disorders (Table 1), or other types of epilepsy such as petit mal seizures (i.e., absence seizures) (Table 2). Coexistence of

Table 1 Nonepileptic Disorders That May Be Mistaken for Complex Partial Seizures.

Syncope
Hyperventilation syndrome
Psychogenic seizures
Intoxications
Metabolic derangements/delirium
Migraine
Transient ischemic attacks
Sleep disorders

more than one disorder is considered if more than one type of episode occurs. For instance, 10 to 20 percent of patients with psychogenic seizures also have epilepsy. However, when two diagnoses are suspected, each needs objective confirmation.

The clinical history is the most important initial diagnostic tool, since the physical examination usually is normal. The examiner should ask about the course of events during the seizure: the aura, the effect of the episode on consciousness, the duration of the episodes (including whether this duration was estimated or measured), and the number of different types of episodes that occurred. Such subgroupings may indicate the site or sites of onset or the etiology of the seizures. One should then ask more specifically about motor activity, including focal clonic or tonic movements, or forced versive deviations; autonomic activity, such as diaphoresis, dyspnea, and palpitations; simple sensations of smell, taste, pain, abdominal discomfort or rising, and vertigo, tinnitus, or photopsias; more complex sensory perceptions, including well formed hallucinations; and psychic symptoms, such as emotional, language, and memory disturbances. Reserve questions about these phenomena until the end of the history to make the patient more comfortable with the history taking process and to obtain a spontaneous account unaf-

fected by physician concerns. Also, some patients are reluctant to admit to having psychic and hallucinatory symptoms unless they are reassured that these experiences may be part of an epileptic seizure. One can then ask the patient or witnesses about occurrences that take place while the patient's awareness is decreased—e.g., facial expressions, repetitive or semipurposeful movements, altered speech, and the patient's reaction to being spoken to or touched. One should also assess the frequency of each seizure type, any cycling or clustering of seizures (e.g., during the perimenstrual period, ovulation, or pregnancy), and precipitating events, including stress and fatigue. Other clues to the etiology of the seizures may be in the history. One should ask about gestation and delivery, febrile seizures, head trauma, other central nervous system disorders, systemic illnesses, any medications that the patient is currently taking (including nonprescription preparations, alcohol, caffeine, and recreational drugs), sleeping habits, and a family history of seizures.

Ancillary tests may provide additional information. Since focal seizures arise from focal disease, computed axial tomography (CAT) studies or magnetic resonance imaging may show evidence of an underlying structural abnormality. Magnetic resonance imaging (MRI) may show small focal lesions or mesial temporal sclerosis not revealed by routine computed axial tomography. Occasionally, cardiac monitoring or echocardiography may be indicated if there is evidence for cardiogenic syncope.

The electroencephalogram (EEG) provides support for the diagnosis of epilepsy and aids in determining the appropriate anticonvulsant treatment, depending on the type of epileptiform discharges (focal onset versus primary generalized). Recordings should be obtained both while the patient is awake and asleep. The test may reveal epileptiform activity in either state, but sleep is often an activator of epileptiform discharges. An EEG obtained after a night of sleep deprivation also can increase the yield of epileptiform activity. Further abnormalities may occur with activation procedures such as hyperventilation and photic stimulation. These two techniques, useful for detecting generalized epileptiform activity, occasionally reveal focal epileptiform abnormalities as well. The yield also can be increased by adding extra electrodes: either over skin, especially over the temporal and orbito-frontal regions, or semiinvasively, using electrodes (sphenoidal, ethmoidal, and nasopharyngeal) which, again, record mainly from the anterior temporal or orbito-frontal regions. Only unequivocal spikes, polyspikes, sharp waves, and spike-and-slow-wave-complexes are indicative of epilepsy. Nonspecific abnormalities, such as focal or generalized slowing, may occur in patients with epilepsy, but also are seen in those with other conditions. Furthermore,

Table 2 A Comparison of Complex Partial Seizures and Absence Seizures

	Complex Partial Seizures	*Absence Seizures*
Aura	Usually	None
Duration	1–3 min	<30 sec
Automatisms	Often	Sometimes
Postictal phase	Usually	None
EEG findings	Focal epileptiform activity	Generalized 3/sec spike-and-slow wave complexes
Treatments	Carbamazepine	Ethosuximide
	Phenytoin	Valproic acid
	Phenobarbital	Clonazepam
	Primidone	
	Valproic acid	
	Clorazepate	
	Resective surgery	

several normal variants may be confused with epileptiform patterns: wicket spikes or rhythms; benign epileptiform transients of sleep or small sharp spikes; 14- and 6-Hz positive spikes; hyperventilation effects; hypnagogic and hypnopompic hypersynchrony; and slow wave transients of the elderly. Conversely, the EEG may be normal on repeated occasions in patients with epilepsy. In such cases, the diagnosis of epilepsy is not excluded by the normal EEG; additional recording, including prolonged monitoring, may be required.

TREATMENT

Once the diagnosis of a focal seizure disorder has been made, appropriate treatment is required. When prescribing antiepileptic medications, several principles should be considered:

1. Monotherapy is usually preferable to polypharmacy. Most patients with epilepsy can achieve seizure control through the use of a single anticonvulsant agent. Not only is monotherapy easier for the patient to use, there is a decreased risk of toxicity caused by drug-drug interactions: antiepileptic medications can potentiate each other's side effects and alter each other's serum concentration (Table 3).

2. In most cases, a single brand name antiepileptic drug should be used, since generic anticonvulsants are not necessarily bioequivalent, primarily because of differences in gastrointestinal absorption of the drugs. Therefore anticonvulsant levels may vary if the patient switches from one formulation to another. Also, differing preparations of the same brand may not have the same bioequivalency. For example, Dilantin capsules have a bioequivalency of approximately 90 percent, while Dilantin *tablets* have a bioequivalency of almost 100 percent. Therefore changing only the preparation, and not the dosage, of Dilantin could alter the amount of absorbed drug by 10 percent. Given the zero-order kinetics of phenytoin at higher blood levels, such an alteration could lead to a significant change in the serum concentration of the drug.

3. The dosage of an anticonvulsant should be gradually increased to the point at which seizure control or toxicity is reached. If a patient does not achieve seizure control with the maximal tolerated dose of the initial medication, treatment with another anticonvulsant should be initiated. When the patient is taking an appropriate dose of the second drug, the initial drug may be gradually tapered and often may then be discontinued. Anticonvulsant medications should be tapered gradually because of the possibility of rebound seizures occurring during an abrupt withdrawal period.

4. If monotherapy with several first-line antiepileptic medications for partial seizures has been unsuccessful, polypharmacy becomes appropriate.

5. Serum concentrations of the antiepileptic medications should be obtained when a steady state has been achieved, which occurs after approximately five and a half serum half-lives. The so-called therapeutic ranges do not apply to all patients. Many patients need serum concentrations that are either below or above these ranges, depending on the clinical circumstances (i.e., the degree of clinical toxicity or seizure control).

6. When interpreting serum drug concentrations, one should consider the various factors that could affect the values obtained, such as (1) compliance, body weight, and age, (2) drug interactions, (3) systemic illnesses, (4) medication absorption, excretion, metabolism, protein binding, and serum half-life.

7. The total serum concentration represents the sum of the protein-bound and nonprotein-bound fractions. Excluding ethosuximide, all major anticonvulsants are partially protein bound, but only the nonprotein-bound (free) fraction penetrates the blood-brain barrier and exerts an anticonvulsant effect.

8. The free serum concentration may be altered by conditions affecting protein binding of the medication such as systemic illnesses (e.g., renal failure) and drug interactions. An example of the latter occurs when valproic acid is added to a phenytoin

Table 3 Effect of Adding a Second Antiepileptic Drug on Serum Concentration of First Antiepileptic Drug

Initial Drug	Second Drug	Effect of Second Drug on Serum Concentration of Initial Drug
Carbamazepine	Phenobarbital	Decrease*
	Phenytoin	Decrease*
	Primidone	Decrease*
Phenobarbital	Carbamazepine	No change
	Phenytoin	Increase
	Valproic acid	Increase*
Phenytoin	Carbamazepine	Increase*
	Phenobarbital	Decrease, increase, or no change
	Primidone	No change
	Valproic acid	Decrease*
Primidone	Carbamazepine	Increased concentration of derived phenobarbital
	Phenytoin	Increased concentration of derived phenobarbital
	Valproic Acid	Increase
Valproic acid	Carbamazepine	Decrease*
	Phenobarbital	Decrease*
	Phenytoin	Decrease*
	Primidone	Decrease*

* Interactions particularly likely to be encountered in clinical practice. (Modified with permission from Brown TR, Feldman RG. Epilepsy: diagnosis and management. Boston: Little, Brown, and Co., 1983: 155.)

regimen. The free serum concentration of the phenytoin may rise since valproic acid is more tightly bound to serum proteins than phenytoin. Therefore the patients may have anticonvulsant toxicity because of an elevated free fraction while the total serum drug concentration is within or below the range usually employed.

Most antiepileptic medications cause similar signs and symptoms of neurologic dose-related toxicity. Higher cortical function and the vestibulocerebellar system are most commonly affected. If dose-related toxicity occurs, we try decreasing the dosage until the toxicity is no longer evident. We then gradually increase the dosage in small increments, using divided doses.

Certain anticonvulsants have nondosage-related hepatic and bone marrow toxicity. In patients using these agents, laboratory parameters such as the hepatic transaminases and complete blood counts should be monitored initially. Minor declines in values such as that of the white blood cell count should be expected. However, this decline should be maximal within the first few weeks of treatment, and partial recovery should occur by the end of the first few months. If there is a continuing trend of abnormalities in parameters such as the white blood cell count the responsible anticonvulsant drug should be discontinued and another one begun. Similarly, hepatic dysfunction usually occurs within the first few months of therapy. Again, the drug involved should be discontinued and another one begun. Of the first-line antiepileptic medications, carbamazepine is the one most often associated with bone marrow toxicity and valproic acid is the one most often associated with hepatic toxicity. However, fatalities from pancytopenia due to anticonvulsants, including carbamazepine, are extremely uncommon and do not constitute a contraindication to the use of carbamazepine in clinical practice. Rare cases of fatal hepatic necrosis have occurred, but almost all of these were in young children receiving polypharmaceutic therapy that included valproic acid. Therefore, valproic acid should be used with caution in young patients, especially those younger than 3 years of age.

Although antiepileptic medications have been associated with birth defects, much of the evidence is inconclusive. Valproic acid, however, has been associated with neural tube defects in as many as 1 percent of infants born to women who took this medication during the first trimester of pregnancy. Although the majority of infants born to such patients are normal, valproate is best avoided during pregnancy. Unfortunately, most women do not know that they are pregnant until after neural tube closure, which takes place at the end of the first month. Therefore, although most women taking valproate have offspring with no birth defects, whenever possible, substitution of another anticonvulsant for valproate should be considered if conception is likely.

The current consensus is that phenytoin and carbamazepine are the two best initial alternatives for the treatment of focal seizures, and some clinicians also report favorable results with valproic acid. Primidone and phenobarbital, although more sedating, may also be used. When monotherapy with these first-line antiepileptic drugs is unsuccessful, a second medication may be added. We usually prescribe either phenytoin or carbamazepine, depending on patient response, plus a second drug, usually valproic acid or clorazepate. It is generally better to administer two drugs with differing proposed mechanisms of action. However, there are occasional patients who respond best to combinations of medications with similar proposed mechanisms of action, such as the combination of phenytoin and carbamazepine. Other second-line anticonvulsants may be tried, but few patients respond well to them when the primary medications have been unsuccessful. These patients may be considered for enrollment in experimental drug protocols or for surgical therapy.

When treatment with antiepileptic drugs fails to control seizures or when the diagnosis is in doubt, the patient should undergo intensive monitoring that includes a video and EEG record of the patient over a period of hours or days. This may establish the diagnosis of epilepsy with certainty, determines the seizure type, and localizes the site or sites of epileptogenicity. Medication withdrawal initiated before admission or preferably on an inpatient basis is often necessary to increase the frequency of seizures. In addition, both sleep and sleep-deprivation studies arc easily obtained during inpatient recordings. Also, using other electrodes in addition to the standard electrodes of the 10-20 system may increase the yield and improve the localization of epileptiform activity. Scalp electrodes may be placed between and below the standard electrode positions. Additional skin surface electrodes may be placed over the face and cheeks. Finally, nasopharyngeal, sphenoidal, and ethmoidal electrodes may be added.

Alternatively, 24-hour ambulatory outpatient EEG monitoring may be considered. However, while less expensive than inpatient monitoring, it has several disadvantages. No video record or precise second-by-second correlation of EEG and clinical events is obtained. The clinician must rely on the patient to keep a detailed diary of potentially ictal events for clinical-neurophysiologic correlations. There are typically only three to seven EEG channels, plus one often used for electrocardiography (ECG), limiting the amount of data that can be obtained and the precision with which epileptiform activity can be localizcd. IIowever, one useful application of ambulatory EEG monitoring is as an event detector for the patient experiencing frequent episodes in a particular setting—for example, the patient's home or workplace.

Patients being considered for epilepsy surgery require an extensive preoperative evaluation, which begins with consistent localization of epileptic foci using prolonged video/surface EEG monitoring. If there is evidence of a potentially resectable epileptic focus and if the patient is willing to undergo a surgical procedure and understands the risks involved, further analysis is undertaken; this should include MRI of the head, neuropsychological testing, intracarotid sodium amobarbital (Wada) testing, and cerebral angiography in the context of the Wada testing. The neuropsychological and Wada tests are necessary to assess the integrity and lateralization of higher cortical functions such as memory and language. If the patient is a candidate for excisional epilepsy surgery, additional data obtained through the use of invasive (depth or subdural/epidural) electrodes may be required to delineate the epileptogenic region precisely.

Different types of invasive electrodes have somewhat different indications. If the issue is archicortical laterality, depth electrodes are usually employed since they can penetrate into the hippocampus or amygdala. These usually are excellent indicators of the side of seizure onset, but they provide limited sampling of the neocortex, and assessment of interictal epileptiform activity is difficult, in part because of the presence of normal variants that closely resemble seizure discharges. Alternatively, subdural strips or grids placed on the floor of the middle fossa can record similar information. When the laterality of a neocortical epileptogenic lesion is to be determined, either subdural/epidural or depth electrodes can be placed bilaterally to assess homologous areas of cortex. However, depth electrodes can record only from a few neocortical sites, and if more information beyond that of the laterality of a neocortical focus is required, subdural electrodes are preferable. Subdural grid, or strip, electrodes may aid in the planning of resective surgery by delineating the extent of epileptogenic cortex and by facilitating functional localization of primary speech, motor, and sensory regions.

The diagnosis and treatment of epilepsy often affects the lifestyle of the patient, many aspects of which must be discussed with the patient during the first visit. Patients should be cautioned to avoid situations that would be particularly dangerous to themselves or others if their consciousness or sensory-motor coordination should become impaired (e.g., operating a motor vehicle or machinery in certain working conditions). The laws pertaining to driving vary with each state and with the Interstate Commerce Commission. Physicians treating patients with epilepsy should be familiar with the regulations of the states in which they practice. Swimming and bathing should be discussed with the patient; because of the risk of drowning during an episode, others should be available to remove the patient from water if necessary, and showering may be preferable to taking a bath. One should inform the patient that his or her rights to employment and educational opportunities are not, in most cases, curtailed as a result of his disorder, and the patient should be counselled on how to minimize the disruption of their professional and personal lives that epilepsy causes.

The patient's family and/or friends need to be taught what to do when a seizure occurs. Patients often suffer oral injuries if a hard object, such as a spoon, is placed in their mouths during seizures in order to prevent the victims from "swallowing their tongues." Most non-health professionals need to be instructed to (1) remove the patient's eyeglasses, (2) remove furniture and potentially sharp objects from the immediate surrounding area, (3) loosen the patient's collar, (4) gently lay the patient on the side, if possible, and (5) place a pillow or rolled up jacket under the patient's head. The patient does not have to be taken to the emergency room unless the seizures are prolonged, repetitive, atypical, or of new onset.

Concerns about heredity should be dealt with. Many non-health professionals believe that all forms of epilepsy are primarily genetic in origin. It must be emphasized to the patients and their families that while there is strong evidence of a genetic component in certain types of primary generalized epilepsy, the vast majority of the children of epileptics do not have seizure disorders.

Aspects of reproduction that are affected by epilepsy and anticonvulsants also should be discussed. Patients using anticonvulsants need to be warned that the efficacy of birth control pills may be diminished, primarily because of the increased hepatic metabolism of hormones caused by many antiepileptic drugs. In practical terms, this means that low-dose formulations of birth control pills may become subtherapeutic. One should also stress the need for planning pregnancies, especially if the woman is taking valproate sodium, for the reasons stated earlier in this chapter. We warn patients that they may experience an increased frequency of seizures during pregnancy and caution them to monitor their serum medication concentrations closely. Although many women are worried about the possible deleterious effects of the anticonvulsant drugs on the fetus, they should be informed that most of the teratogenic effects have not been conclusively proven and occur in only a small minority of infants; seizure activity itself, because of either the hypoxia and acidosis of generalized tonic clonic seizures or the impaired motor coordination and consciousness of focal seizures, also poses a significant threat to the fetus. Finally, these risks appear to occur only when the mother (not the father) takes antiepileptic drugs.

SUGGESTED READING

Browne TR, Feldman RG. Epilepsy: diagnosis and management. Boston: Little, Brown and Co., 1983.

Dreifuss FE, Langer DH, Moline KA, Maxwell JE. Valproic acid hepatic fatalities. II. US experience since 1984. Neurology 1989; 39:201–207.

Engel J Jr. Surgical treatment of the epilepsies. New York: Raven Press, 1987.

Lesser RP. Psychogenic seizures. In: Pedley TA, Meldrum BS, eds. Recent advances in epilepsy–2. New York: Churchill Livingstone 1985; 273–296.

Levy RH, Dreifuss FE, Mattson RH, et al. Antiepileptic drugs. 3rd ed. New York: Raven Press, 1989.

Lüders H, Lesser RP. Epilepsy: electroclinical syndromes. New York: Springer-Verlag, 1987.

PATIENT RESOURCE

Epilepsy Foundation of America
4351 Garden City Drive
Landover, Maryland 20785
Telephone: 1-800-332-1000

GENERALIZED SEIZURE DISORDERS

PETER W. KAPLAN, B.Sc. (Hons), M.D., M.B., B.S., M.R.C.P.

A generalized seizure is the clinical expression of a bihemispheric paroxysmal electrical disturbance that usually affects consciousness. Generalized seizures may present with different clinical signs, varying from a motionless stare to unresponsiveness accompanied by convulsions. Many brain functions including those subserving sensation, movement, speech, and awareness may be affected during the course of a seizure, although the patient is usually normal interictally. The term *epilepsy* is used to describe recurrent seizures resulting from persisting disease of the brain.

The seizure type and its frequency determine treatment and decisions regarding when and for how long medications should be given.

SEIZURE TYPES

Primary generalized nonconvulsive (absence), convulsive (tonic-clonic), and myoclonic epilepsies are probably largely genetically determined. Tonic, clonic, and atonic (astatic) seizures are frequently seen with diffuse cortical damage acquired during the perinatal and neonatal period (Table 1).

Clinical Manifestations of Epilepsy

In primary generalized epilepsy, the seizure discharges appear virtually synchronously over both hemispheres, in contrast to secondary generalized seizures, which begin in a localized area of the cortex. Although both types may present with tonic-clonic movements, primary generalized seizures are more frequently genetically determined or stem from a diffuse cortical insult. When a focal onset, whether sensory, autonomic, or motor, is determined or focal epileptiform activity is noted on the electroencephalogram (EEG), secondary generalized seizures should be suspected. A family history of seizures with no clinical focal onset or aura would suggest a primary generalized seizure disorder.

Even when a diagnosis of generalized seizures has been made (Table 2) and the patient has begun taking anticonvulsant medication, the seizures may continue. One may question then whether the correct diagnosis has been made. Psychogenic seizures may resemble tonic-clonic seizures and inpatient evaluation with video and EEG monitoring may be helpful in determining the nature, site, and frequency of the events so that appropriate management may be instituted.

Primary Generalized Tonic-Clonic (Grand Mal) Epilepsy

Primary generalized tonic-clonic seizures may appear at any age, although usually before the patient is 35 years old. No focal onset is noted. With the immediate generalization of the electrical discharge, the patient may cry out, roll the eyes upwards, and stiffen. There is an immediate loss of consciousness and frequently a fall to the ground

Table 1 Classification of Generalized Seizures (Bilaterally Symmetrical and Without Local Onset)

International Classification	*Previous Terminology*
Absence seizures	Petit mal seizures
Myoclonic seizures	Minor motor seizures
Clonic seizures	Grand mal seizures
Tonic seizures	Grand mal seizures
Tonic-clonic seizures	Grand mal seizures
Atonic seizures (astatic)	Akinetic, drop attacks

Adapted with permission from Commission on Classification and Terminology of the International League Against Epilepsy. Proposal for revised clinical and electroencephalographic classification of epileptic seizures. Epilepsia 1981; 22:489–501.

Table 2   Classification of the Generalized
Epilepsy Syndromes

Idiopathic (age-related)
  Benign neonatal familial convulsions
  Benign neonatal convulsions
  West syndrome (idiopathic cases)
  Epilepsy with myoclonic-astatic seizures (Lennox-Gastaut
    syndrome)
  Childhood absence epilepsy (pyknolepsy)
  Epilepsy with (Myo)clonic absences
  Juvenile absence epilepsy
  Benign juvenile myoclonic epilepsy (impulsive petit mal)
  Epilepsy with generalized tonic-clonic seizures on awakening

Symptomatic
  Nonspecific etiology (age-related)
  Neonatal seizures
  Early myoclonic encephalopathy
  West syndrome (infantile spasms, Blitz-Nick-Salaam-
    Krampfe)

Special syndromes
  Occasional seizures
    Febrile convulsions
    Nonfebrile convulsions (in infancy or adolescence)

  Epilepsies characterized by specific modes of seizure
    precipitation

  Syndromes of chronic neuropsychologic suffering with
    status-like EEG activity
    Syndromes of limited course
      Epilepsy with continuous spike-waves during slow sleep

Adapted with permission from the Commission on Classification and Terminology of the International League Against Epilepsy. Proposal for classification of epilepsies and epileptic syndromes. Epilepsia 1985; 26:268–278.

with possible injury. An initial, predominantly symmetric, tonic contraction of musculature with cessation of breathing or forced expulsion of air with a ''cry'' is followed approximately one-half minute later by short, rapid, interrupted jerking movements of the limbs. This may be accompanied by foaming at the mouth and biting of the tongue. Urinary, and less frequently, fecal incontinence may follow the tonic or clonic phase. At the end of the clonic phase, limb contractions are less frequent, then cease and are followed by slow, labored breathing, lethargy, and amnesia. The patient may have a headache and sleep. The EEG, which is rarely obtained during the seizure, may show high-voltage, rapid, bilaterally synchronous spikes that decrease in frequency, stop, and are replaced by diffuse suppression of background activity.

Myoclonic Epilepsy

Seizures consist of brief, usually symmetric single or multiple jerks of the limbs or head. In the etiologically diverse progressive myoclonic epilepsies, the jerks are frequently stimulus-sensitive and may be induced by voluntary movements. They are associated with cognitive, cerebellar, and pyramidal tract abnormalities. More benign disorders, including essential myoclonus, tonic-clonic epilepsy with myoclonus (myoclonic epilepsy), and benign juvenile myoclonic epilepsy are not progressive. Myoclonic epilepsy may be photosensitive, with paroxysmal EEG abnormalities induced by photic stimulation. Essential myoclonus is usually not stimulus-sensitive and is not associated with convulsions or EEG abnormalities. The myoclonus may occur more frequently in the early morning and usually during wakefulness. Some patients have a family history of the disorder.

Clonic and Tonic Seizures

These seizures are rare and may represent a variation of generalized convulsive seizures, with one clinical characteristic predominating. Consciousness is usually lost during these seizures. In children, symmetric, bilateral tonic seizures frequently exhibit a slow hyperextension of the neck, torso, and legs with flexion of the arms. The EEG shows fast spikes at 9 to 10 Hz for both types. Clonic seizures may show spike-wave patterns.

Atonic Seizures

Atonic seizures are accompanied by a sudden loss of muscle tone with head or limb drop, frequently with falls to the ground and injury (drop attacks), and often a brief loss of consciousness. The EEG may show low-voltage fast activity, polyspikes, or voltage attenuation.

TREATMENT

General Management

Because of the frequent misperceptions regarding epilepsy, its causes, and its significance, it is essential to explain the nature of the disorder and lay to rest unwarranted feelings of guilt, inadequacy, and stigma (Table 3). The patient should be encouraged in every way to adapt to the disability and assume, as much as is possible, a normal life. General advice is aimed at regularizing the time and duration of sleep, as sleep deprivation may increase seizure tendency. Moderation in the use of alcohol and drugs with a central stimulant effect (amphetamines) or with possible epileptogenicity (antihistamines, tricyclic antidepressants, phenothiazines, theophylline) is also important (although when dosages are within the therapeutic range, these drugs may not significantly alter seizure threshold).

Adults, unless otherwise handicapped, should be able to maintain employment, although certain

Table 3 Treatment

1. Ascertain the diagnosis and type of seizure.
2. Discuss the diagnosis, implications, and therapeutic options with the patient or the patient's parent(s).
3. Based on the seizure type, select the most appropriate drug.
4. Increase the anticonvulsant dosage until seizures are controlled or until clinical toxicity appears.
5. If the anticonvulsant is ineffective at "toxic" levels, introduce a second anticonvulsant. When this drug produces a satisfactory blood level, gradually discontinue the first drug.
6. Monitor drug use frequently, as needed.
7. Provide information on local support groups, counseling, and educational materials.
8. After the patient has been without seizures for 2 to 5 years, consider tapering anticonvulsants.

occupations involving heights, dangerous machinery, working near or in water, or driving must be carefully evaluated with respect to patient and public safety. Although there are risks to many facets of daily living, it is difficult to foresee them all. Moderate exercise does not increase seizure frequency.

Patients with severe disability, inadequately controlled convulsive seizures, or mental retardation may require supervised home care or institutionalization. Most communities have care centers or a local chapter of a group that provides help for people with epilepsy (see *Patient Resources* at the end of this chapter).

In women with epilepsy, there is no formal contraindication to pregnancy, and although seizure control may vary during pregnancy, it usually can be adequately managed. All antiepileptic medications are thought to be potentially teratogenic during the first trimester of pregnancy, but valproate sodium and to a lesser extent phenytoin are most implicated. Neurotubular defects may be diagnosed antenatally with amniocentesis and measurement of alpha-fetoprotein levels. If at all possible, pregnancies should be planned and the physician alerted. Options for management without anticonvulsant medication or possibly with carbamazepine (which has a lower teratogenic potential) should be explored depending on seizure type and frequency. Although some epilepsies can carry a genetic component, it is not clear which pattern of inheritance predominates in a particular family. If inheritance can be assessed, this information may help prospective parents, but generally, a positive family history increases the risk two- to fourfold.

Management at Home

It is important that the family visit the physician to discuss the management of the patient at home. The family should be advised not to panic when a seizure occurs, but to turn the patient to the side or prone so as to avoid aspiration, and not to place any hard object or finger in the patient's mouth (the tongue cannot be "swallowed"). The family should also be asked to observe the seizure, as this may provide important information for determining the seizure type. They should seek acute medical attention if seizure activity continues for more than 10 minutes. In patients with known seizures and in the absence of fever and respiratory or cardiovascular problems, single or self-limited seizures probably do not warrant an emergency room evaluation.

Driving and Other Activities

The patient should be given specific advice regarding the driving laws in the state and a note should be placed in the patient's records to this effect. Most states prohibit individuals with generalized seizures from driving for periods of 3 to 24 months, depending on the locality, and some states require that all seizures be reported to the bureau of motor vehicles. All activities in which a momentary lapse of consciousness might endanger the patient or others, such as climbing, swimming, or working near moving machinery should be avoided if seizure control has not yet been achieved. Patients with nocturnal seizures only may be exempted from these restrictions.

Anticonvulsant Therapy

The Single Seizure

A single, idiopathic primary generalized tonic-clonic seizure does not necessarily imply a diagnosis of epilepsy or mandate chronic anticonvulsant therapy. Seizures associated with a precipitant cause (e.g., a toxic or metabolic disturbance) may be treated conservatively since the treatment of the underlying disturbance may suffice. When the patient has an "idiopathic" generalized convulsion, the decision to treat becomes more complex. About half of the patients in this group will have at least a second seizure. Those patients in whom further seizures pose significant social, employment, and driving problems might prefer the possible unpleasant side effects and bother of chronic medication. Conversely, some patients will wait until they have another seizure before deciding to take anticonvulsants. These concerns and treatment plans may vary from case to case and should be thoroughly discussed with the patient or the patient's family before planning therapy. Alcohol withdrawal seizures are difficult to manage, as frequently the patient discontinues both alcohol and anticonvulsants at the same time, thus precipitating seizures. In this group, resuming anticonvulsant therapy is often a futile experience.

Treatment of continued acute seizure activity will be addressed elsewhere in this text.

Recurrent Motor Seizures

The goal of therapy is to obtain optimal seizure control with the fewest medications and side effects. First-line therapy consists of the use of a single anticonvulsant (Table 4). Medication should be started at low doses and built up in gradual increments every 3 to 7 days. In order to reflect a steady state of the anticonvulsant, unless the patient is clinically toxic, serum anticonvulsant levels should be obtained no earlier than five drug half-lives after the full daily dose is reached or after changes in dosage have been made in order to reflect a steady state of the anticonvulsant. When either seizure control is reached or therapeutic levels are attained, I follow the patient monthly initially, and then at longer intervals while I monitor relevant hematologic or hepatic functions. Before considering changing to another single anticonvulsant or adding a second anticonvulsant, I gradually increase the dosage until "toxicity" appears (i.e., clinical side effects such as ataxia, somnolence, diplopia, marked malaise) or until seizure control is reached. The dosage, often above the therapeutic range, is then adjusted to be below the "toxic" dosage. Potential side effects should be fully explained, and the patient should understand that if skin rashes appear, the physician should be promptly notified.

If the initial anticonvulsant is unsatisfactory, the patient is prescribed a second anticonvulsant to be administered in a similar fashion, and the first agent is then discontinued. This may be repeated with three or four of the first-line agents before one progresses to multiple anticonvulsant therapy. During the overlap period, anticonvulsant drug interaction with resultant toxicity may develop and should be watched for.

First-Line Anticonvulsant Therapy

Valproic Acid (Depakene), Divalproex Sodium (Depakote)

Valproic acid is the drug of choice in patients with primary generalized tonic-clonic seizures, in patients with myoclonic seizures or seizures with a prominent myoclonic component. Depakote, somewhat more expensive, is believed to be better tolerated than Depakene, with less stomach upset. Depakote is available in 125-, 250-, and 500-mg tablets, and a common regimen is 250 to 500 mg taken orally two to four times per day. I start with 10 to 15 mg per kilogram per day and increase the dosage by 5 to 10 mg per kilogram per day at weekly intervals to a maximum dosage of 60 mg per kilogram per day, or 4,000 mg per day. The half-life is 8 to 12 hours, with peak blood levels reached within 1 to 4 hours after ingestion. A common goal is a level of 50 to 100 mg per liter, but higher levels are necessary in many patients. Common side effects include gastrointestinal upset, skin rashes, weight gain, ataxia, hyperactivity, drowsiness, tremor, headache, and hair loss. Serious side effects include liver failure, pancreatitis, and thrombocytopenia. Monitoring for marked changes in liver enzymes is important. When used as monotherapy in adults, fatal hepatic failure is virtually unknown.

Carbamazepine (Tegretol)

For cosmetic reasons, treatment with carbamazepine is preferable to that with phenytoin since gum hyperplasia (occurring in 10 to 30 percent of patients) is absent. Although more expensive than the nongeneric preparation, Tegretol avoids the wide spectrum of bioavailability and thus the problems of variable seizure control. An initial dosage of 100 to 200 mg administered once per day for 3 to 5 days, increased every 3 to 5 days to an initial plateau of 600 mg, may avoid some medication intolerance. The adult dosage may vary betwen 400 and 2,000 mg per day. The half-life is 10 to 25 hours, with the daily dosage divided into three to four doses. The therapeutic serum levels are approximately 4 to 12 mg per liter. Frequent side effects include fatigue, skin rashes, upset stomach, blurred and double vision, and ataxia as toxic levels are achieved. More serious side effects include the Stevens-Johnson syndrome, leukopenia, and thrombocytopenia, but a causal relationship to aplastic anemia is very rare.

Table 4 Anticonvulsants

Seizure Type	Drugs	Adult	Child	Usual Blood Levels*
Primary generalized tonic-clonic	Valproate sodium	1,000–3,000 mg	30–60 mg/kg	50–100 μg/ml
First-line therapy	Carbamazepine	600–2,000 mg	20–30 mg/kg	4–12 μg/ml
	Phenytoin	200–600 mg	4–7 mg/kg	10–25 μg/ml
Second-line therapy	Primidone	750–1,500 mg	10–25 mg/kg	6–12 μg/ml†
	Phenobarbital	90–250 mg	3–5 mg/kg	15–40 μg/ml
Myoclonic, atonic, tonic	Valproate sodium	1,000–3,000 mg	30–60 mg/kg	50–100 μg/ml
	Clonazepam	1.5–20 mg	0.01–0.2 mg/kg	0.013–0.072 μg/ml

* Higher levels are needed in some patients.
† With primidone monotherapy, primidone levels of approximately 20 μg/ml are frequently encountered.

Phenytoin (Dilantin)

Less expensive, but equally effective is Dilantin. Adult doses start at 100 mg administered once daily for 3 to 5 days, increasing gradually to an initial plateau of 300 mg per day. In urgent circumstances, an oral load of 1,000 mg may be given. The drug is absorbed within 4 to 8 hours and has a variable half-life of 7 to 42 hours (usually about 24 hours). Because it is protein-bound, low albumin levels may cause increased "free" levels and toxicity at lower dosages. The usual goal is to administer 10 to 20 mg per liter, but some patients may tolerate levels of 25 mg per liter or more without untoward effect. Although Dilantin is frequently administered three times daily, adequate control may sometimes be obtained with a once-daily regimen. Frequent side effects include coarsening of the facies caused by thickening of the subcutaneous tissue around the eyes and nose, facial and body hirsuties (occurring in 30 percent of young women), and gum hyperplasia (occurring in 30 percent of patients). Skin rashes (occurring in 2 to 10 percent of patients), stomach upset, mild drowsiness, and cognitive dysfunction are not unusual. Pseudolymphoma with arthralgia, fever, hepatosplenomegaly, and lymphadenopathy, as well as true lymphoma, have been described. Hepatitis, drug-induced lupus, peripheral neuropathy, folate deficiency, and osteoporosis are also seen. With 'toxic' levels, ataxia and behavioral disturbances may occur.

Second-Line Therapy

Primidone (Mysoline)

Primidone is less preferred as a first-line drug because of compliance problems caused by drowsiness and malaise, and less optimal seizure control. Advantages include a long half-life of the phenobarbital metabolite and low cost. After giving an initial test dose of 50 mg for hypersomnolence reaction, one should prescribe a dosage of 125 to 250 mg administered once daily, increasing this by 250 mg at 5- to 7-day intervals until a maximum of 1,500 mg, a therapeutic effect, or marked sedation is reached. The daily dosage is divided in two or three doses. These gradual increments are often necessary to avoid a marked sedative effect. Side effects include respiratory depression, confusion, behavioral and cognitive changes, and ataxia. Gastrointestinal upset and skin rashes may also be seen.

Phenobarbital

Phenobarbital is the least expensive of all anticonvulsants. Although it does not cause cosmetic side effects, it may cause behavioral problems, especially in children (it produces hyperactivity in 40 percent). With its prominent initial sedative effect and long half-life of 72 hours, it is best given once daily, at night. Peak blood levels are reached 10 to 12 hours after an oral dose with a therapeutic range of 15 to 40 mg per liter. I start with doses of 30 mg and increase these by 30 mg every 3 to 5 days until a total of 90 to 250 mg or 1 to 3 mg per kilogram per day is reached. Although excreted by the kidney, it is detoxified by the liver so that the dosage need only be slightly reduced in patients with renal insufficiency. These factors, as well as the interactions of phenobarbital with other medications and anticonvulsants, require that it be carefully monitored when changes in medication therapy are made. The side effects are much the same as those of primidone, although phenobarbital may be less sedating. Withdrawal of this anticonvulsant may be slow and problematic, as discussed later in this chapter.

Clonazepam (Klonopin)

This benzodiazepine is frequently used for myoclonic seizures. The serum half-life is 20 to 40 hours, with serum levels (5 to 70 ng per milliliter) correlating only approximately with clinical effectiveness. Side effects include drowsiness, dizziness, ataxia, personality changes, and drug tolerance. The drug is administered once daily, starting with a dosage of 0.01 to 0.03 mg per kilogram per day, which is then increased by 0.5 mg every 3 to 7 days to a maximum dosage of 0.1 to 0.2 mg per kilogram per day or 20 mg per day. Occasional exacerbation of other seizure types has been noted.

Interactions

All of the anticonvulsants may have interactions with each other and other intercurrent medications. (For interactions between anticonvulsants, see the chapter on partial seizures; for interactions between anticonvulsants and other drugs, see 1989 edition of The Medical Letter Handbook on Drugs and Therapeutics.)

Polypharmacy and Patients Who Are Difficult to Control

The most common cause of poor control is noncompliance. For patients with poor compliance, written schedules, diaries, and plastic, compartmentalized daily pill boxes (available at most pharmacies) are helpful. Compliance may be assessed from the history, the testimony of witnesses of the seizures, blood levels, and by counting the number of tablets that the patient has not taken. Fine tuning of the daily dosage, readjustment of the frequency, the timing of intake, and attempts at producing drug levels above the laboratory "therapeutic" level but below clinical toxicity may be necessary. After most medication readjustments, repeated blood therapeutic monitoring is needed at five to eight half-lives after the time of medication change. Careful follow-up of patients receiving high doses is required.

When seizures are frequent while the patient is receiving the highest tolerated dose of a single anticonvulsant (and after each first-line anticonvulsant has been tried), a second agent may be added. Adding one of the first-line drugs is preferred, although primidone or phenobarbital may be satisfactory. However, problems with concurrent use of two first-line drugs may lead to more severe side effects. For example, when taken together, phenytoin and carbamazepine may lead to marked ataxia. Combining phenobarbital and primidone contribute little actual or theoretical improvement in seizure control and sedation may be further increased. The best combinations may prove to be medications with different mechanisms of action, such as valproate sodium and either phenytoin or carbamazepine. Interactions between the two anticonvulsants and other drugs may greatly alter blood levels, and frequent monitoring may be necessary since anticonvulsant levels may rise or fall. For example, if valproic acid is added to the regimen of a patient receiving phenobarbital, central nervous system depression caused by a rise in phenobarbital levels may result (see appendix in chapter on complex partial seizures). Some combinations, such as that of valproic acid and clonazepam, may produce absence status epilepticus and therefore should be avoided. Patients should continue to take two anticonvulsants only if attempts to gradually wean the patient from one of the drugs leads to breakthrough seizures. In "brittle" (poorly controlled) patients, drug change-overs may necessitate hospitalization or intravenous loading of anticonvulsants. Most patients with primary generalized seizures are responsive to treatment with anticonvulsants, and epilepsy surgery is rarely helpful. If patients do not respond to anticonvulsants, the diagnosis should be re-examined for the possibility of secondary generalization, as poorly controlled seizures in patients with secondary generalization may make them eventual candidates for epilepsy surgery.

For clinic evaluation, a "seizure diary" is of great help in determining the frequency and type of seizures. If doubt persists, prolonged inpatient video and EEG monitoring or ambulatory monitoring helps determine the frequency, timing, and types of seizures, and helps distinguish these from other paroxysmal events such as syncope, panic attacks, or even pseudoseizures.

Anticonvulsant Withdrawal

After the patient has been without seizures for 2 to 5 years, I consider withdrawal of the single anticonvulsant. In patients who are seizure-free while receiving two anticonvulsants, one may attempt withdrawal of one of the anticonvulsants after 6 to 12 months. Even if the patient is seizure-free, however, caution should be exercised. Should seizures recur, medication should be resumed. The patient should be discouraged from driving an automobile during the months of anticonvulsant withdrawal. It is believed that epileptic discharges on a EEG obtained before withdrawal might herald an unfavorable outcome, but this is disputed. Although the seizure-free period is a good predictor of possible successful anticonvulsant withdrawal, previous unsuccessful attempts at withdrawal forebode a poor result. Rapid withdrawal of benzodiazepines or barbiturates may precipitate seizures even in a normal population and therefore should be withdrawn gradually. In the withdrawal of anticonvulsant medications such as phenytoin or carbamazepine, a common practice is to taper medications gradually, one at a time; however, there is little evidence to suggest that this forestalls withdrawal seizures. After initially reducing the dosage by one-third, one may decrease the phenobarbital dosage by 15 mg every 2 weeks in the most "brittle" patient. Sleep disturbances such as insomnia and anxiety are frequently encountered, especially in long-time users of anticonvulsants, and these problems should be anticipated and explained so that the patient can see the long-term benefit of an unpleasant withdrawal phase.

SUGGESTED READING

Drugs for epilepsy. Med Lett 1989; 31:1.

Fromm GH, Fisher RS, Dasheiff R, Hachinski V (discussants). Controversies in neurology: first seizure management reconsidered. Arch Neurol 1987; 44:1189–1191.

Laidlaw J, Richens A. A textbook of epilepsy. New York: Churchill Livingstone, 1982.

Ojemann LM, Baugh-Bookman C, Dudley DL. Effect of psychotropic medications on seizure control in patients with epilepsy. Neurology 1987; 37:1525–1527.

Solomon GE, Plum F. Clinical management of seizures: a guide for the physician. Philadelphia: WB Saunders, 1976.

PATIENT RESOURCES

Epilepsy Foundation of America
4351 Garden City Drive
Suite 406
Landover, Maryland 20785

Epilepsy International
Las Palmas C-160
2855 Apalachee Parkway
Tallahassee, Florida 32301

STATUS EPILEPTICUS

ROBERT J. DeLORENZO, M.D., Ph.D., M.P.H.

The International Classifications of Epileptic Seizures defines status epilepticus as a seizure lasting for more than 30 minutes or intermittent seizures lasting for more than 30 minutes from which the patient does not regain consciousness. Thus, any seizure that lasts for more than 30 minutes must be diagnosed as status epilepticus. The first step in treating status epilepticus is making the diagnosis.

Many physicians are not sensitive to the importance of diagnosing this condition and making appropriate treatment initiations to avoid complications. Great care should be taken in determining the duration of any prolonged seizure; this as well as the time of seizure onset should be ascertained from ambulance drivers or emergency room staff. The importance of this in determining the diagnosis cannot be overemphasized.

Persistent generalized tonic-clonic seizures are the most common form of status epilepticus and are associated with the major risks of morbidity and mortality caused by this condition, and therefore this chapter focuses on the treatment of generalized tonic-clonic status epilepticus.

MORTALITY ASSOCIATED WITH STATUS EPILEPTICUS

One major reason for promptly diagnosing status epilepticus is that this condition is associated with high morbidity and mortality rates. Studies over the last 20 years involving more than 100 patients indicate that the mortality rate of status epilepticus ranges from 8 to 50 percent. Even a mortality rate as low as 8 to 10 percent is a significant risk.

Status epilepticus must be considered a major medical and neurologic emergency. In our experience at the Medical College of Virginia Epilepsy Research Center, where a large community and university–based study of status epilepticus is being conducted, we find that the mortality rate associated with status epilepticus in the community study parallels that of the university study. Thus, the high mortality rate associated with status epilepticus noted in previous university studies has recently been confirmed by our findings in a community-university environment.

Although our recent investigations indicate statistically valid correlations among seizure duration, etiology, and mortality, it is still too soon to base clinical decisions of treatment on these indicators. We are currently developing and testing a mortality relative risk scale and hope that this scale may lead to the identification of high-risk patients.

Once I have determined that the patient has prolonged seizures lasting more than 30 minutes and make the diagnosis of status epilepticus, I become concerned. Since these are patients at risk for death or developing serious complications, there is no room for missing this diagnosis or for not treating these patients aggressively.

CAUSES OF STATUS EPILEPTICUS

Once a diagnosis of status epilepticus has been made, the clinician must immediately consider the possible cause of the prolonged seizures. Treatment of status epilepticus, although directed at the control of seizures, must also take into account the underlying cause since these conditions often require aggressive treatment. Figure 1 presents the breakdown of etiologies of 280 cases of the Medical College of Virginia (MCV) series. These etiologies are typical of several other large studies.

The causes of status epilepticus shown in Figure 1 have been broken down into ten major etiologic subgroups: (1) withdrawal from anticonvulsants, (2) anoxia, (3) hypotension, (4) alcohol-related status, (5) metabolic, (6) infectious, (7) cerebrovascular disease, (8) tumor, (9) hemorrhage, (10) other causes. As can be seen from Figure 1, the three major etiologies associated with status epilepticus are cerebrovascular disease, alcohol-related causes, and withdrawal from anticonvulsants. Each of these

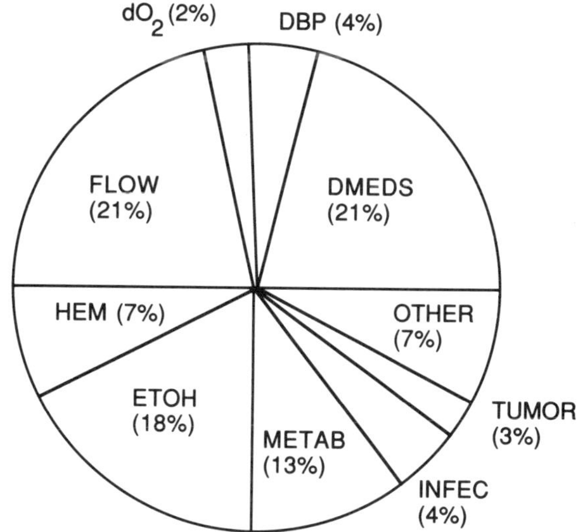

Figure 1 Etiologies of status epilepticus (percentage of patients). DMEDS = withdrawal from anticonvulsants; dO$_2$ = anoxia; DBP = hypotension; ETOH = alcohol-related causes; METAB = metabolic; INFEC = infectious; FLOW = cerebrovascular disease; HEM = hemorrhage.

categories represents one-fifth to one-fourth of the patients seen in most large series. Another major cause, representing anywhere from 10 to 15 percent of the cases, is metabolic disease.

Not all patients with status epilepticus have had previous seizures. Only about one-fifth of the patients who develop status epilepticus have a history of epilepsy. Many of the other causes of status epilepticus are of rather serious consequence, including central nervous system infection, vascular injury, tumor, and severe metabolic disease. Thus anytime a patient presents with status epilepticus, one should be greatly concerned because of the seriousness of the seizures and many of the underlying etiologies.

TREATMENT

Although it would be ideal to have a rigid protocol for the treatment of status epilepticus, this is not always possible because of the clinical variability in the presentation of status epilepticus, the patient's condition, and the possible idiosyncratic reactions to certain anticonvulsant drugs. Despite this inherent variability, we have developed a standard treatment plan for patients treated in the Greater Richmond Metropolitan area which includes care at the MCV Hospital Complex and surrounding community hospitals.

The protocol for treating adults with generalized tonic-clonic status epilepticus is based on years of clinical experience in treating this condition by physicians of the MCV Hospital and the surrounding community and on the protocols from other successful treatment plans. Thus by synthesizing the experience from our own patient population and that of the literature, we have developed a unified treatment plan that has been tested and utilized in both the MCV and community hospital. This standard recommended treatment protocol is summarized in Table 1.

The Diagnosis

As discussed earlier, the first major step in treating status epilepticus is to make the diagnosis. The most common error in missing the diagnosis is not obtaining a clear and detailed history of the duration of the seizures. Often the physician arrives in the emergency room or to the floor after the patient has been stabilized by the emergency room staff; the patient may have been undergoing a seizure for 20 to 30 minutes en route to the hospital and for another 20 to 30 minutes in the emergency room, but by the time the physician arrives, the seizures have been controlled with intravenous (IV) diazepam or phenytoin and the diagnosis of status epilepticus may not be made. Great care should be taken to avoid making this error.

Stabilizing the Patient

The second major treatment step is to stabilize the patient medically and to establish an IV line. Since a significant percentage of the causes of status epilepticus also produce severe cardiovascular and autonomic changes, it is essential that the patient's vital signs and medical condition be stabilized and the diagnosis or cause of status epilepticus be determined (see Table 1).

The IV line is ordinarily supported with normal saline containing vitamin B complex supplement. The only contraindication for the use of normal saline is a hypertensive patient or a patient requiring salt or fluid restriction. However, even in these situations, it is important to have a normal saline line piggybacked into the IV system so that phenytoin can be given with the normal saline in small volumes as needed. The MCV protocol recommends administration of a bolus of 50 ml of 50 percent glucose at this time. This is a routine emergency procedure. Once the line is obtained, the medical treatment of status epilepticus begins.

Figure 2, a decision tree for the initial treatment and stabilization of the patient, shows the basis for our diagnostic studies and hospitalized care. Most patients with status epilepticus arrive in the emergency room or present in the inpatient setting. After the stabilization of the patient, it is essential to obtain neurologic consultation whenever possible. The electroencephalogram (EEG) and computed tomography (CT) scan are invaluable in helping determine the etiology. Lumbar puncture (LP) is recommended for all status epilepticus patients if the CT scan and physical examination show no evidence of a mass lesion or other contraindications to performing the LP. If the patient stabilizes rapidly and regains consciousness during the diagnostic evaluation, admission to the neurology inpatient unit is recommended with good nursing care. If the patient does not regain consciousness or is medically unstable, admission to a neurological service intensive care unit (NSICU) is advisable. Careful observation and records of vital signs and the EEG are valuable in providing responsive care to these patients.

Anticonvulsants

The first anticonvulsant usually employed in the ambulance or emergency room setting is the IV injection of diazepam, administered at a rate not to exceed 2 mg/per minute until the seizures stop or a total of 20 mg has been given. The majority of our patients have received diazepam as the initial drug in this fashion. However, an alternative initial anticonvulsant that appears to be equally effective is lorazepam. Lorazepam is administered at a rate of 2 mg per minute (0.1 mg per kilogram) and repeated at 10- to 15- minute intervals if seizures persist. Experi-

Table 1 Status Epilepticus Treatment Protocol for Adults

Step	Time Frame of Intervention	Procedure
1	0–5 min	Determination of status epilepticus. As soon as the diagnosis is made, institute monitoring of blood pressure, temperature, pulse, respiratory ECG and EEG. Insert oral airway and administer O_2 if necessary. Insert an IV catheter and draw venous blood for levels of anticonvulsant, glucose, electrolytes, Ca, Mg, BUN, CBC. Draw arterial blood for ABG. Obtain urine for urinalysis and toxic screen if indicated. If necessary, nasotracheal suction is performed.
2	6–9 min	Place an IV line with normal saline containing vitamin B complex. Administer a bolus of 50 ml of 50% glucose.
3	10–30 min	Infuse IV lorazepam given at a rate of 2 mg/min (0.1 mg/kg) to a maximum dose of 5 mg or alternatively administer IV diazepam given at a rate not to exceed 2 mg/min until seizures stop or to a total of 20 mg. This is followed by IV phenytoin, 20 mg/kg at a rate no faster than 50 mg/min. If seizures are not controlled, a repeat bolus of phenytoin of 10 mg/kg can be given before one proceeds to Step 4. Monitor ECG and blood pressure.
4	31–59 min	If seizures persist, perform elective endotracheal intubation before starting a bolus infusion of phenobarbital at a rate not to exceed 100 mg/min until seizures stop or to a loading dose of 20 mg/ng.
5	60 min	If control is still not achieved, other options include: 1) Pentobarbital with an initial IV loading dose of 5–10 mg/kg with additional amounts given to produce a "burst suppression" pattern on EEG. Maintenance of pentobarbital anesthesia is continued for approximately 4 hours by an infusion of 1–3 mg/kg/hr. The patients are then checked for the reappearance of seizure activity by decreasing the infusion rate. If clinical seizures and/or generalized EEG discharges persist, the procedure is repeated; if not, the pentobarbital is tapered over 12–24 hrs. 2) Paraldehyde is given either intravenously or rectally at a dose of 0.1–0.15 ml/kg after being diluted in normal saline every 2 to 4 hours if necessary. 3) Diazepam (50–100 mg) is diluted in a solution of 500 ml 0.9% NaCl or D_5W and run as a continuous infusion to achieve blood levels of 0.2–0.8 mg/ml. The IV solution is changed every 6 hours as advised by certain authors and short-length IV tubing is used.
6	61–80 min	If seizures are still not controlled, call the anesthesia department to begin general anesthesia with halothane and neuromuscular blockade.

Continuous EEG monitoring is recommended in the obtunded patient to assure that status elipticus has not recurred. In the management of intractable status, a neurologist who has expertise in status elipticus should be consulted and advice from a regional epilepsy center should be sought.

ence with lorazepam is not as extensive as with diazepam. A potential advantage of lorazepam is that it may have a more long-lasting effect. However, there must be more widespread experience with this drug before its relative benefits compared with those of diazepam can be established.

Immediately after the completion of benzodiazepine treatment, the next step is to provide a major anticonvulsant therapy. Diazepam, although having a long half-life in the body, is only effective in treating status epilepticus for approximately 30 minutes, during which time it reaches its peak blood level after the IV injection. Immediately after this peak blood level has been reached, diazepam is distributed in the fat of the body and its level comes down to a baseline level. As the diazepam level rapidly decreases, it is no longer effective as an anticonvulsant in controlling status epilepticus. A small percentage of patients taking diazepam or lo-

razepam will stop having seizures. However, the majority of patients require further anticonvulsant treatment before seizures are arrested. In those patients with seizures that stop rapidly with benzodiazepine treatment, an alternative anticonvulsant is still initiated to maintain the anticonvulsant effect. Thus the alternative anticonvulsant must be initiated before the anticonvulsant effects of diazepam subside, usually 20 to 30 minutes after injection.

The anticonvulsant of first choice is phenytoin. In a dose of 18 mg per kilogram, it is administered at a rate not to exceed 50 mg per minute. A significant percentage of patients will stop having seizures after benzodiazapine and phenytoin treatment. Phenytoin has been shown to be as effective as any other anticonvulsant in controlling status epilepticus. In addition, phenytoin is relatively nonsedative in the doses used to treat status epilepticus. Thus the patient who

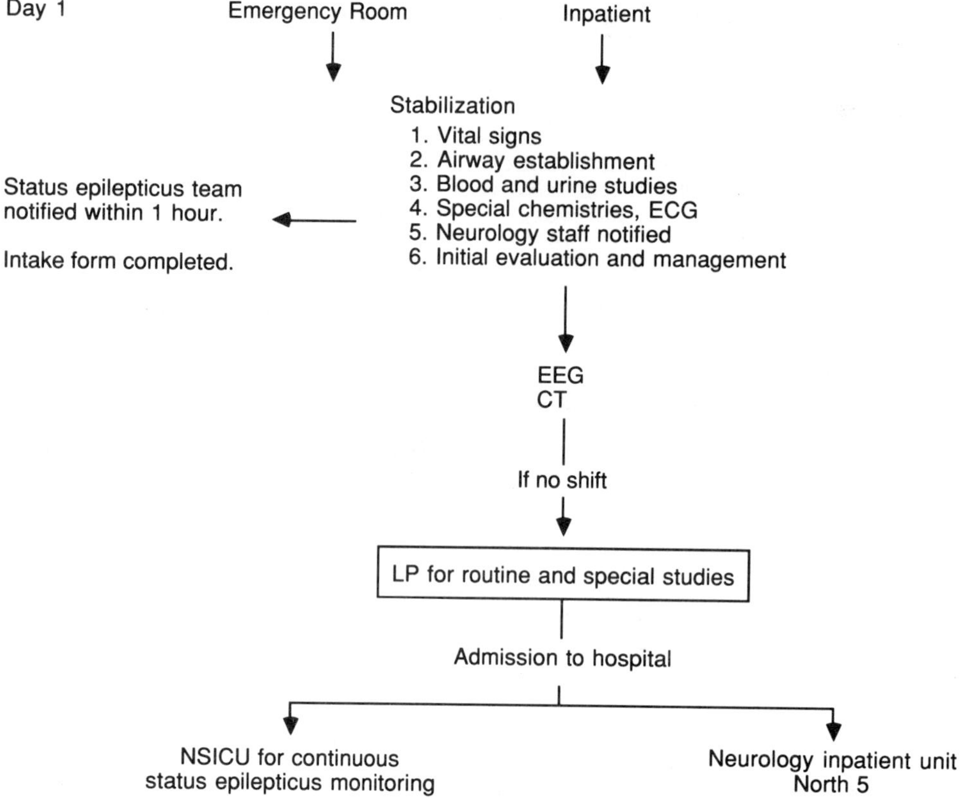

Figure 2 Flow chart for status epilepticus patients admitted to the Medical College of Virginia Hospital Complex.

is postictal will usually wake up after seizures depending upon the duration of the postictal coma. The lack of sedation caused by the phenytoin is a major advantage in patient care. Some patients successfully treated with diazepam and phenytoin will awaken within an hour or so after status epilepticus. Some patients may even wake up in the emergency room after status epilepticus.

Some disadvantages of employing phenytoin must also be addressed. Phenytoin is not soluble in 5 percent dextrose in water (D_5W) or other types of IV solutions that do not have a significant amount of normal saline. Normal saline is the preferred vehicle for IV infusion of phenytoin. If D_5W is used as the vehicle to infuse phenytoin, phenytoin crystals will immediately develop in the IV line as the phenytoin is injected. If one uses the recommended rate of injection, these crystals will form as the drug is administered and the clinician may not be able to see this in the IV line. In addition, mixing phenytoin with D_5W in a dripping reservoir will result in the patient receiving no drug at all since all of the phenytoin will precipitate out of the solution. When phenytoin comes out of solution during the injection, it has no significant anticonvulsant action.

It is essential that the clinician use the appropriate vehicle for IV phenytoin usage. If the patient cannot be administered saline because he requires salt restriction, D_5W can be run as the main IV line and normal saline solution can then be piggybacked into the system and opened into the system only when phenytoin is injected. After a limited injection of saline has been administered, the patient can be switched back to the appropriate IV treatment.

Care must be exercised in giving phenytoin to a patient who has epilepsy and may already have a therapeutic phenytoin blood level. Although this is an uncommon situation, it should be considered, since it can result in a high phenytoin blood level that in rare situations can cause cerebellar toxicity.

Another potential risk of phenytoin usage is hypotension and decreased cardiac output. In most normal healthy individuals, these side effects are not significant and are rarely of any consequence when the recommended dosage and rate of administration of phenytoin are used. However, more rapid rates of phenytoin administration can result in significant hypotension. In elderly patients with compromised cardiovascular status, phenytoin may produce hypotension and cerebrovascular collapse. Thus during phenytoin administration, electrocardiogram (ECG) or blood pressure monitoring is recommended, especially in the elderly patient.

Our protocol recommends that if a seizure persists after phenytoin infusion, elective endotracheal intubation be initiated before one starts a bolus infusion of phenobarbital. Phenobarbital is administered as a second anticonvulsant at a rate not to exceed 100 mg per minute until the seizures stop or until a loading dose of 20 mg per kilogram is reached.

Phenobarbital is an effective anticonvulsant in the treatment of status epilepticus. Before it was realized that phenytoin could be given rapidly through IV infusion, phenobarbital was widely used as the initial drug. Phenobarbital is effective and relatively safe in treating patients with status epilepticus. However, phenobarbital has a major side effect in that it is sedative and causes respiratory suppression. Most patients given a loading dose of 20 mg per kilogram of phenobarbital will be sedated for at least 24 hours. Thus this raises the difficulty of having to wait until the patient fully recovers from sedation before evaluation can begin. For this reason, phenobarbital is usually not given as the first major anticonvulsant and is a second-line agent after treatment with phenytoin.

Seizures Resistant to Treatment

In the more unlikely situation that seizure control is not achieved after benzodiazepine, phenytoin, and phenobarbital treatment, further anticonvulsant administration must be considered. At this time, either paraldehyde or a diazepam drip is used. Paraldehyde is preferably given rectally at a dose of 0.1 to 0.15 mg per kilogram after being mixed one-to-one with mineral oil. Paraldehyde can be conveniently mixed one-to-one part with mineral oil in a suspension and administered per rectum through a Foley catheter. The catheter is lubricated and carefully inserted into the rectum, and the catheter balloon is inflated. The paraldehyde and mineral oil mixture can be easily injected through the catheter. The catheter is then clamped. The paraldehyde is rapidly absorbed through the rectal route. Plastic containers should not be used for paraldehyde. Many forms of plastic are dissolved by this drug. Most IV tubing and Foley catheters are not soluble in paraldehyde.

The use of per rectal paraldehyde is also useful if an IV line cannot be placed. In the rare situation that an IV line cannot be started and benzodiazepine or phenytoin cannot be initially administered, per rectal paraldehyde is often the route of choice for obtaining initial control of status epilepticus. Paraldehyde can also be administered intravenously, but this is less desirable because of the potential complications. Unfortunately, it is becoming more difficult to obtain paraldehyde for patient use. This is a major obstacle for this useful treatment option.

If paraldehyde is not successful or if one prefers to use a diazepam drip initially, diazepam can be used again. Diazepam, 50 to 100 mg, is diluted in a solution of 500 ml of 0.9 percent sodium chloride or D_5W and run as a continuous infusion to achieve blood levels of 0.2 to 0.8 mg per milliliter. The use of diazepam has significant problems. For example, diazepam can come out of solution over time because it is not highly water soluble. Therefore the IV solution should be changed every 6 hours and short runs of IV tubing should be used. One must also be careful to control the continuous IV solution to avoid overdoses and rapid infusion rates. This procedure must be monitored in the intensive care unit setting so that overtreatment and resultant respiratory arrest do not occur.

In the rare patients in whom seizures are not controlled with this treatment protocol, a pentobarbital anesthetic is used with an initial IV loading dose of 5 mg per kilogram with additional amounts administered to produce a ''burst suppression'' pattern on the EEG. Maintenance of pentobarbital anesthesia is continued for approximately 4 hours by infusion of 1 to 3 mg per kilogram per hour. After this interval, the patient is checked for reappearance of seizure activity by decreasing the infusion rate. If clinical seizures and/or generalized EEG discharges persist, the procedure is repeated. If there are no repeat seizures, pentobarbital is tapered over the next 12 to 24 hours.

In remote cases in which this protocol is still not successful in controlling seizures, the anesthesia department is consulted and general anesthesia with halothane and neuromuscular blockade is initiated. This situation is extremely rare.

Treatment of Status Epilepticus in Children

Special considerations are often given to the treatment of children and infants with status epilepticus. Table 2 provides the status epilepticus treatment protocol for pediatric patients at the MCV Hospital Complex. This protocol is used in the same fashion as the adult protocol and has the same initial procedures. Table 2 gives the appropriate tests to be performed. After stabilization has been achieved, an IV line is placed with normal saline. A bolus of 2 ml per kilogram of 50 percent glucose is then given.

After the patient has been stabilized, initial anticonvulsant treatment is begun. The pediatric protocol recommends the use of IV lorazepam as the first-line treatment administered at a rate of 1 to 2 mg per minute to a maximum dose of 5 mg. The appropriate loading dose is 0.1 mg per kilogram.

After IV lorazepam has been administered, the patient is treated with IV phenytoin, 18 to 20 mg per

Table 2 Status Epilepticus Treatment Protocol for Children

Step	Time Frame of Intervention	Procedure
1	0–5 min	Determination of status elipticus. As soon as the diagnosis is made, institute monitoring of temperature, blood pressure, pulse, respiratory ECG and EEG. Insert oral airway and administer O_2 if necessary. Insert an IV catheter and draw venous blood for levels of anticonvulsants, glucose (check Dextrostik) electrolytes, calcium, BUN, CBC. Draw arterial antipyretics (acetaminophen). Perform frequent suction.
2	6–9 min	An IV line is placed with normal saline. Administer a bolus of 2 ml/kg 50% gluclose.
3	10–30 min	Initial treatment consists of an infusion of IV lorazepam given at a rate of 1–2 mg/min (0.1 mg/kg) to a maximum dose of 5 mg. This is followed by IV phenytoin, 18–20 mg/kg, infused at a rate not to exceed 1 mg/kg/min or 50 mg/min. Monitor ECG and blood pressure.
4	31–59 min	If seizures persist, administer a bolus infusion of phenobarbital at a rate not to exceed 50 mg/min until seizures stop or to a loading dose of 20 mg/kg.
5	60 min	If control is still not achieved, other options include: 1) Diazepam (50 mg) is diluted in a solution of 250 ml 0.9% NaCl or D_5W and run as a continuous infusion at 1 ml/kg/hr (2 mg/kg/hr) to achieve blood levels of 0.2–.8 mg/ml. The IV solution is changed every 6 hours as advised by certain authors, and short-length IV tubing is used. 2) Pentobarbital with an initial IV loading dose of 5 mg/kg with additional amounts given to produce a "burst suppression" pattern on EEG. Maintenance of pentobarbial anesthesia is continued for approximately 4 hours by an infusion of 1–3 mg/kg/hr. The patients are then checked for the reappearance of seizure activity by decreasing the infusion rate. If clinical seizures and/or generalized EEG discharges persist, the procedure is repeated; if not, the pentobarbital is tapered over 12–24 hours.
6	61–80 min	If seizures are still not controlled, call the anesthesia department to begin general anesthesia with halothane and neuromuscular blockage.

Continous EEG monitoring is recommended in the obtunded patient to assure that status elipticus has not recurred. In the management of intractable status, a neurologist who has expertise in status elipticus should be consulted and advice from a regional epilepsy center should be sought.

Lumbar puncture should be performed as soon as possible, especially in a febrile child or infant below 1 year.

For infants with a history of neonatal seizures, infantile spasms, or early onset seizures, pyridoxine, 100 mg IV, should be administered while EEG monitoring is being performed to diagnose and treat the rare patient with seizures with a vitamin B_6 deficiency.

kilogram, which is infused at a rate not to exceed 1 mg per kilogram per minute or a total of 50 mg per minute. ECG and blood pressure monitoring are recommended during phenytoin infusion.

If seizures persist, phenytoin therapy is followed by phenobarbital administration. Phenobarbital is administered at a rate not to exceed 50 mg per minute until the seizures stop or a loading dose of 20 mg per kilogram is given. This protocol is effective in stopping most cases of status epilepticus in children. In children seizures that are difficult to control and which do not respond to lorazepam, phenytoin, and phenobarbital require the same control as in adults. A diazepam drip followed by pentobarbital anesthesia is recommended. If seizures are still not controlled, general anesthesia is recommended.

Pyridoxine, 100 mg IV, is recommended for children or infants with a history of neonatal seizures, infantile spasms, or early onset seizures. The pyridoxine should be given while EEG monitoring is being performed. This allows the treatment and diagnosis of rare patients with seizures and a vitamin B_6 deficiency.

In our initial studies at the Medical College of Virginia, status epilepticus in children is a common problem, although it usually does not have as high a mortality rate as that of the adult population. Our findings also indicate that recurrent status epilepticus is more common in children. Further research needs to be developed to more definitively evaluate these observations.

As future research develops to define the risk management scale for mortality in status epilepticus in children and adults, the clinician will have a more definitive guideline for determining which patients need acute monitoring or follow-up. We recommend hospitalizing all patients who do not recover consciousness within 30 or 40 minutes after the cessation of status epilepticus in the neurologic intensive care unit. In this unit, the patients can have continuous EEG and vital sign monitoring. The patients who regain consciousness are hospitalized on the general neurology floor. Careful monitoring and follow-up of patients who do not recover rapidly from status epilepticus may often avoid complications that could be prevented by acute monitoring. This type of close observation may not be possible in all hospital settings, but it is recommended for patients who have prolonged seizures or significant associated medical complications.

SUGGESTED READING

Aminoff MJ, Simon RP. Status epilepticus: causes, clinical features and consequences in 98 patients. Am J Med 1980;69(5):657–666.
Delgado-Escueta AV, Waisterlain GC, Trieman DM, Porter RJ. Status epilepticus. New York: Raven Press, 1983.
Leppik IE, Derivan AT, Homan RW, et al. Double-blind study of lorazepam and diazepam in status epilepticus. JAMA 1983;249:1452–1454.
Rashkin MC, Youngs C, Penovich P. Pentobarbital treatment of refractory status epilepticus. Neurology 1987;37:500–502.
Wilder BJ, Ramsay E, Wilmore LJ, et al. Efficacy of intravenous phenytoin in the treatment of status epilepticus. Ann Neurol 1977;1:511–518.

PATIENT RESOURCES

Medical College of Virginia Epilepsy Center
Status Epilepticus Program Project
Robert J. DeLorenzo, M.D., Ph.D., M.P.H.
Department of Neurology
P.O. Box 599, MCV Station
Richmond, Virginia 23298

Epilepsy Foundation of American
4351 Garden City Drive
Landover, Maryland 20785

PAIN

PRINCIPLES OF PAIN MANAGEMENT

GREGORY W. ALBERS, M.D.
STEPHEN J. PEROUTKA, M.D., Ph.D.

The management of pain is one of the most common and difficult problems facing neurologists. Pain is a nonspecific symptom which may be a manifestation of a diverse array of pathologic conditions. Therefore, identification of the cause of pain is always the first objective of a patient evaluation. Once a tentative diagnosis has been established, a wide variety of treatment options may be considered. In general, the most common and effective mode of treatment for pain is pharmacologic. Surgical options are sometimes available for selected pain syndromes or for conditions refractory to standard treatment approaches. In some patients, therapeutic success may be achieved with alternative modalities such as physical therapy, biofeedback, and/or psychiatric intervention. A summary of the major options available to the physician is provided in Table 1.

DIAGNOSIS

The classification of pain syndromes is difficult, and pain terminology is often confusing. However, some simple generalizations are useful. Pain produced by activation of peripheral pain receptors (somatic or nociceptive pain) usually responds well to standard analgesics. Central pain (pain associated with central nervous system lesions) and neuropathic pain (pain associated with peripheral nerve damage) often respond best to atypical analgesics.

A second important diagnostic consideration concerns the differentiation of chronic pain disorders from acute pain disorders. Chronic pain differs from acute pain both symptomatically and pathophysiologically. For example, patients with chronic pain usually adapt to constant pain and therefore may appear to be quite comfortable. Unfortunately, this lack of apparent distress may lead the physician to question the validity of the patient's complaints. Generally, pharmacologic therapies aimed at treating patients with chronic pain must avoid the use of addicting substances such as narcotics.

PHARMACOLOGIC OPTIONS

The selection of an appropriate pharmacologic agent for the management of pain can seem quite difficult. Because the number of drugs used for pain may appear overwhelming, it is useful to classify these medications into four major categories: (1) prostaglandin inhibitors, (2) atypical analgesics, (3) narcotics, and (4) combination analgesics. Selection of an appropriate medication for pain relief requires knowledge of the pharmacologic properties and side effect profiles of each of these four drug groups.

Prostaglandin Inhibitors

Prostaglandin inhibitors are the drugs of choice for the management of mild to moderate pain. This group of agents includes aspirin, acetaminophen, and the nonsteroidal anti-inflammatory drugs

Table 1 Overview of Pain Management Options

Pharmacologic
    Prostaglandin inhibitors
    Atypical analgesics
    Narcotics
    Combination analgesics

Surgical
    Local anesthesia
    Epidural injections
    Nerve decompression
    Thalamotomy

Alternative options
    Psychological/psychiatric intervention
    Electrical stimulation (TENS)
    Biofeedback
    Physical therapy

(NSAIDs). Their mechanism of action involves the inhibition of prostaglandin synthesis primarily through the inhibition of the enzyme cyclooxygenase. These medications have principally analgesic, antipyretic and anti-inflammatory properties. However, it is important to note that the anti-inflammatory potency of acetaminophen is quite weak compared with that of aspirin and the NSAIDs.

Aspirin remains the prototypical prostaglandin inhibitor analgesic. It also remains the drug of choice for mild to moderate pain from headache, neuralgia, or myalgia. Nonetheless, the analgesic potency of aspirin tends to be underrated by most patients and physicians. In blinded studies, for example, 650 mg of aspirin is usually as effective as or more effective than 65 mg of codeine. The extremely low cost and effectiveness of aspirin make it an ideal analgesic for patients who can tolerate its gastrointestinal effects.

Acetaminophen is an excellent alternative for patients who are unable to tolerate aspirin. In general, acetaminophen appears to be equipotent to aspirin in its analgesic effects. However, because of its lack of significant anti-inflammatory actions, it is less effective for pain related to inflammation. Although acetaminophen has minimal gastrointestinal toxicity, it does carry the risk of hepatic necrosis, which may occur with chronic doses as low as 5 to 8 g per day or with an acute overdose of only 10 to 15 g.

NSAIDs offer several potential advantages over aspirin and acetaminophen. First, they have less gastrointestinal toxicity than aspirin. Second, because NSAIDs cause reversible inhibition of cyclooxygenase, their antiplatelet activity is of shorter duration. Third, their analgesic potency is often slightly better than that of aspirin or acetaminophen. Otherwise, NSAIDs have a mechanism of action and side effect profile similar to that of aspirin. Unfortunately, NSAIDs differ from aspirin and acetaminophen also in that they are considerably more expensive.

Although insufficient data are available to differentiate the various NSAIDs in terms of analgesic potency or risk of gastrointestinal hemorrhage, there are many significant differences among agents. For example, piroxicam (Feldene) has the longest half-life (approximately 45 hours), and this allows for once daily dosing. Diflunisal (Dolobid), sulindac (Clinoril), and naproxen (Naprosyn) can be administered in twice daily doses. Indomethacin (Indocin) has superior anti-inflammatory activity but appears to cause more frequent side effects than other NSAIDs. Meclofenamate (Meclomen) is asociated with incidence of diarrhea as high as 30 percent.

All NSAIDs carry a small risk of renal toxicity because of the role of prostaglandins in modulating renal blood flow. This risk is greatly accentuated in patients with pre-existing renal disease, congestive heart failure, or hepatic dysfunction. Several studies have suggested that sulindac (Clinoril) has minimal effects on renal prostaglandin synthesis and therefore appears to carry a relatively reduced risk of renal toxicity.

Since most NSAID side effects are dose-related, a low dose should be chosen initially and increased gradually as required. NSAIDs are highly bound to serum albumin (most are greater than 99 percent bound) and can potentially displace other highly protein-bound drugs such as coumarin anticoagulants, phenytoin, methotrexate, and oral hypoglycemics. Obviously, such interactions could potentially lead to toxicity.

Atypical Analgesics

Several drugs that were originally developed for other conditions such as depression or epilepsy have been found to be useful in pain management. These agents are primarily useful in treating chronic pain syndromes, particularly conditions involving central or neuropathic pain. For example, a substantial amount of data suggest that antidepressants can provide significant pain relief in both depressed and nondepressed patients. Although the exact mechanism remains unclear, effects on descending monoamine pathways involved in the modulation of pain transmission appear to be important.

Before pain therapy with antidepressant drugs is initiated, the rationale for using these agents for pain control, as opposed to depression, should be stressed to the patient. Patients with pain syndromes are often offended by the implication that they are depressed. Therefore, the physician should clearly state the reasons for using these agents for pain. Low doses should be used initially (Table 2). If pain relief is not obtained after 6 to 8 weeks of therapy, the dosage should be increased slowly to full antidepressant doses and continued for at least another 6 to 8 weeks. When a positive response is obtained, drug therapy should be continued for 3 to 6 months, after which a gradual withdrawal of the medication is attempted. If the pain recurs after medication withdrawal, treatment should be reinstituted.

As with the NSAIDs, there are insufficient data to rank the analgesic potency of the antidepressants. Many of the controlled trials have involved the use of agents associated with a high incidence of side effects, such as amitriptyline (Elavil) and imipramine (Tofranil). However, significant analgesic effects also occur with better-tolerated agents such as nortriptyline (Pamelor) and desipramine (Norpramin).

A second major class of atypical analgesics is that of the anticonvulsants. Carbamazepine (Tegretol), phenytoin (Dilantin), valproic acid (Depakene), and clonazepam (Klonopin) are the anticonvulsants

Table 2 Commonly Used Analgesics

Drug	Brand Name*	Typical Starting Dose
Prostaglandin inhibitors		
Aspirin		650 mg q4–6h
Acetaminophen	Tylenol	650 mg q4–6h
Ibuprofen	Motrin	400 mg q4–6h
Naproxen	Naprosyn	375 mg q12h
Sulindac	Clinoril	150 mg q12h
Diflunisal	Dolobid	500 mg q12h
Piroxicam	Feldene	20 mg q24h
Atypical analgesics		
Amitriptyline	Elavil	25 mg qhs
Nortriptyline	Pamelor	25 mg qhs
Carbamazepine	Tegretol	100 mg q12h
Narcotics		
Codeine		30 mg q4–6h
Pentazocine	Talwin Nx	1 tab q4–6h
Meperidine	Demerol	100 mg IM q4–6h
Combination analgesics		
Aspirin/ butalbital/ caffeine	Fiorinal	1 tab q4h
Aspirin/ butalbital	Axotal	1 tab q4h
Acetaminophen/ chlorzoxazone	Parafon Forte DSC	2 tabs q6h
Acetaminophen/ codeine	Tylenol #3	1 tab q4h
Acetaminophen/ hydrocodone	Vicodin	1 tab q6h
Aspirin/ oxycodone	Percodan	1 tab q6h

* Several brand names are available for some of these analgesics.

most frequently used for pain. These agents may be effective in the treatment of a variety of pain syndromes, including various neuropathies, neuralgias, and pain in multiple sclerosis or Guillain-Barré Syndrome. Carbamazepine (Tegretol) has proven to be the most effective agent for the treatment of trigeminal neuralgia. However, the data are limited on comparisons of the anticonvulsants in treating other painful conditions. Although the exact mechanism of action for pain control is unclear, a reduction of excitatory synaptic transmission within pain-modulating circuits has been postulated.

Several other medications such as anticholinergics, phenothiazines, and baclofen have been advocated for the management of various painful conditions. Unfortunately, very little data from controlled studies are available regarding the use of these drugs. The short-term use of anti-anxiety agents may also be helpful, particularly if pain is accompanied by significant anxiety.

Narcotic Analgesics

Although narcotics are the most effective analgesics available, we strongly believe that narcotic use should be restricted to the short-term relief of moderate to severe pain. We believe that narcotics should rarely be used for chronic pain control in neurologic patients. Quite simply, the problems encountered with long-term narcotic use (e.g., tolerance and addiction) far outweigh their benefits in patients with chronic pain disorders.

For the short-term relief of acute pain, codeine is usually the oral narcotic of choice. Its advantages include a relatively low dependence liability and good oral bioavailability. Unfortunately, like many narcotics, codeine has a short plasma half-life (only about 3.5 hours), necessitating frequent dosing. Codeine, as well as the other orally active narcotics, should generally be administered in combination with a prostaglandin inhibitor, as discussed in the following section of this chapter.

Propoxyphene (Darvon) is one of the least potent narcotics. In many studies it has proven to be less effective than aspirin or acetaminophen. We find that there is little use for this agent in treating neurologic patients. If more potent orally active narcotics are required, hydrocodone (Vicodin) or oxycodone (Percodan) may be considered. These agents are available only in combination with nonopioid analgesics. Of these, oxycodone is the more potent and appears to have higher abuse potential.

For parenteral use, meperidine (Demerol) is a recommended choice because of its relatively low incidence of gastrointestinal side effects. Meperidine hydrochloride (Demerol) can occasionally produce central nervous system side effects, including excitement and seizures, and should not be used for patients on monoamine oxidase inhibitors. Several mixed agonists-antagonists such as pentazocine (Talwin), butorphanol (Stadol), and nalbuphine (Nubain) appear to offer the advantage of less abuse potential than other potent narcotics. Their disadvantages, however, include the risk of precipitation of a withdrawal reaction in patients being treated with other opioids and occasional psychotomimetic effects.

Combination Analgesics

A variety of combination analgesics are available for use in moderate pain disorders. Aspirin or acetaminophen is frequently combined with caffeine and/or a barbiturate for the treatment of headaches (e.g., Excedrin, Fiorinal, Axotal) or with a muscle relaxant for acute musculoskeletal strain (e.g., Norgesic, Soma, Parafon Forte DSC). Certain analgesic combinations appear to offer synergistic effects greater than those obtained by doubling the dose of either individual agent. For example, the most successful combinations involve a prostaglandin inhibitor (usually aspirin or acetaminophen) coupled with an oral narcotic—for example, propoxyphene (Darvon compound), codeine (Tylenol with codeine), hydrocodone bitartrate (Vicodin), and oxycodone (Percodan, Tylox).

SURGICAL OPTIONS

A large variety of surgical or anesthetic procedures are available for specific pain syndromes. Focal neuropathies such as occipital neuralgia, painful neuromas, and carpal tunnel syndrome can be treated with local injections of anesthetic agents and corticosteroids. Occasionally, the pain relief that follows local infiltration is long lasting. Epidural or intrathecal injections may also provide pain relief for selected patients, and standard orthopedic and neurosurgical procedures such as laminectomy and peripheral nerve decompression are available for specific syndromes. For example, reflex sympathetic dystrophy often responds to sympathectomy and/or sympathetic blocking agents. More invasive procedures such as gangliolysis, posterior rhizotomy, cordotomy, or thalamotomy should be performed only in specialized centers.

ALTERNATIVE OPTIONS

A diverse variety of alternative (i.e., nonpharmacologic and nonsurgical) therapies is also available for patients with pain syndromes. In certain chronic pain patients, psychological factors may play a primary role in the pain syndrome and can severely complicate patient management. Fear and depression are also frequently associated with pain and sometimes need to be addressed specifically. For these individuals, psychological and/or psychiatric evaluations may be most appropriate.

Physical therapy and exercise are important options and may be particularly useful in treating pain syndromes related to muscle contraction or spasm. Other therapeutic options such as biofeedback, relaxation training, hypnosis, and transcutaneous nerve stimulation (i.e., TENS) are helpful for selected patients. Depending on the clinical situtation, multimodality therapy may be more successful than any single therapeutic option used alone. For instance, chronic headaches often respond well to a combination of drug therapy, cervical exercises, and psychological or psychiatric intervention.

SUGGESTED READING

Boynton CS, Dick CF, Mayor GH. NSAIDS: an overview. J Clin Pharmacol 1988, 28:512–517.
Beaver WT. Combination analgesics. Am J Med 1984, 77:38–53.
Hackett TP, Bouckoms A. The pain patient: evaluation and treatment. In Hackett TP, Cassem NH, eds. Massachusetts General Hospital handbook of general hospital psychiatry. 2nd ed. Littleton MA: PSG Publishing Co., Inc., 1987:42.
The International Association for the Study of Pain, Subcommittee on Taxonomy. Classification of chronic pain: descriptions of chronic pain syndromes and definitions of pain terms. Pain 1986; 3(suppl):S1–226.
Malone MD, Strube MJ. Meta-analysis of non-medical treatments for chronic pain. Pain 1988, 34:231–244.

PATIENT RESOURCES

International Association for the Study of Pain
909 N.E. 43rd Street, Suite 306
Seattle, Washington 98105
Telephone: (206) 547-6409

American Pain Society
1200 17th Street, N.W. Suite 400
Washington, DC 20036
Telephone: (202) 296-9200

ACUTE BACK PAIN AND DISC HERNIATION

RICHARD B. NORTH, M.D.

Low back pain is pandemic; a majority of adults experience a temporarily disabling episode. It is the most common cause of hospitalization, and its impact on the workplace is second only to that of upper respiratory infections, accounting for approximately one-quarter of lost work time. Associated health care and compensation costs, exclusive of lost productivity, are estimated to exceed $20 billion annually in the United States.

Degenerative lumbar disc disease is likewise ubiquitous, but it is only occasionally the cause of low back pain, and the need for surgical intervention is the exception rather than the rule. Even in patients with clear-cut disc herniation established clinically and by imaging studies, spontaneous recovery without surgery is common.

More than one-quarter million lumbar laminectomies and discectomies are performed annually in the United States, a rate which greatly exceeds that of other developed, industrialized countries. An estimated 30 to 40 percent of patients experience persistent pain after surgery; 25 percent are unable to return to their original occupations, and 10 to 15 percent undergo reoperation.

When the records and studies of patients with "failed back syndrome" (persistent, disabling pain occurring after one or more operations) are reviewed in detail, the original indications for surgery are commonly obscure. Secondary procedures are often necessary simply to correct the sequelae of primary procedures; in patients whose initial problem may have been a maladaptive or exaggerated response to minor pathology, the yield remains low.

Increasingly sophisticated imaging and other diagnostic tests are available for the evaluation of lumbosacral spine disease; however, clinical history and physical examination are of primary importance in the diagnosis and treatment of acute back pain, particularly during selection of patients for surgery. The sensitivity of modern diagnostic imaging (e.g., magnetic resonance imaging demonstration of disc degeneration) must be complemented by the specificity of a thorough clinical evaluation.

CLINICAL EVALUATION

Evaluation of the patient presenting with low back and/or lower extremity pain begins with a careful history. The patient's occupation, the circumstances under which symptoms developed (e.g., a lifting-related injury at work), and the effects of the condition on the patient's work and lifestyle should be recorded and considered. The relative magnitudes of low back and leg pain, the precise pattern of radiation, the quality of the pain, its aggravating and relieving factors, and associated neurologic symptoms should be noted. The latter include weakness, loss of sensation, abnormal sensations (e.g., paresthesias), changes in bladder or bowel habits or control, and changes in sexual function.

Pseudoradicular pain is a common manifestation of lumbosacral spine injury and degenerative disease. Experience with minor procedures involving paravertebral injections and radiofrequency denervations, with localization by electrical stimulation, shows that sciatica and other apparently radicular symptoms may occur in the absence of any nerve root compromise. On examination, referred pain syndromes of this sort are accompanied by mechanical signs, as opposed to neurologic or tension signs. Reproduction of pain by extension, for example, is a mechanical sign suggesting posterior element (facet joint) disease.

Although a detailed discussion of physical examination and differential diagnosis is beyond the scope of this chapter, some aspects of these deserve mention. The straight leg raising test, employed routinely in the physical examination, is often misinterpreted. If the patient complains only of low back pain with supine straight leg raising, this indicates a mechanical low back syndrome. A symptomatic disc herniation, on the other hand, should elicit complaints of ipsilateral (and sometimes contralateral) sciatica and should cause the patient to assume a protective position. When this occurs, the effects of simultaneous neck flexion and of dorsiflexion of the foot are noteworthy, as are the effects of popliteal and sciatic compression. Because of the variability between examiners in performing and interpreting these tests, recording the results as simply "positive" or "negative," as is done routinely, is of limited value. Explicit descriptions of these maneuvers and patient responses are much more informative.

Certain physical findings common in the "failed back" population predict a poor response to surgical treatment. As enumerated by Waddell, the most useful functional signs include the following:

1. Tenderness superficially (e.g., to gentle pinching of the skin of the low back) or in a nonanatomic pattern.
2. Simulated lumbosacral spine motion causing pain (e.g., axial loading at the vertex, trunk rotation).
3. Distraction (e.g., straight leg raising performed in the sitting position is well tolerated, but straight leg raising performed in the supine position is tolerated poorly).
4. Regional disturbances on neurologic examination (e.g., weakness or sensory loss that does not conform to a neuroanatomic pattern).
5. Overreaction to the examination, unexplained by cultural variability (e.g., pain behavior).

While it should be assumed that all patients complaining of low back pain have an organic basis for their complaint, individuals may vary greatly in their potential to respond to treatment for a given lesion. Patients with active workmen's compensation claims, personal injury litigation, or other issues of secondary gain are generally considered inferior candidates for surgery. Psychological tests have been developed or adapted for screening low back patients: the Minnesota Multiphasic Personality Inventory scales for depression, hypochondriasis, and hysteria, for example, are usually elevated in those who fail treatment. Personality disorders, somatization disorders, and other psychiatric diagnoses are common among patients with chronic low back pain or "failed back syndrome."

DIAGNOSTIC TESTS

Plain radiographs of the lumbosacral spine are the standard initial diagnostic study for patients with low back pain, although their yield and specificity are low. Findings of facet joint sclerosis, disc space narrowing or spurring, and other degenerative changes are of course ubiquitous even in asymptomatic patients, and should be interpreted accordingly. Not only the degenerative changes of spondylosis, but also those of spondylolysis and spondylolisthesis, are routinely assessed by plain films. Plain films also may disclose less common spinal conditions (e.g., infection or neoplasm) or extraspinal pathology (e.g., abdominal aortic aneurysm).

In patients presenting for initial evaluation, specialized diagnostic imaging such as magnetic resonance imaging (MRI), computed tomography (CT), and CT myelography should be reserved for those in whom there are specific indications that intervention may be required. As with plain radiographs, MRI, CT, and CT myelography commonly demonstrate signs of degenerative disease even in asymptomatic patients, but this does not contribute to the management of the acute low back syndrome. If, on the other hand, there are clinical indications of disc herniation or of another potential surgical problem, it is useful to obtain a definitive study early in the patient's management. If symptoms persist and are intractable, these studies are usually necessary to rule out significant pathology, even in the absence of a compelling clinical presentation.

As a noninvasive test that involves no exposure to ionizing radiation, MRI has obvious advantages over CT and CT myelography. Its ability to distinguish between soft tissues such as the thecal sac and the annulus and nucleus of the disc is a major advantage. It images cortical bone and calcifications poorly, however; CT provides a better demonstration of degenerative spurs, bony defects, and bony lateral recess and central stenosis of the spinal canal. While MRI is useful as a screening examination and may suffice as the sole imaging study (after plain films) for a clinically straightforward disc herniation, it has not replaced CT. With the addition of a small amount of water-soluble intrathecal contrast, CT remains the study of choice in demonstrating postsurgical arachnoid fibrosis.

Improvements in diagnostic imaging have reduced the need for ancillary electrophysiologic tests. Electromyography of lower extremity and paravertebral muscles remains useful, however, in confirming the diagnosis of radiculopathy (as opposed to pseudoradicular pain) in patients with equivocal clinical and imaging findings. Along with nerve conduction studies, it is useful in ruling out peripheral entrapment syndromes.

TREATMENT

Mechanical Low Back Syndrome

The patient presenting with acute onset of low back pain, with or without sciatica, with mechanical signs but without tension signs or neurologic symptoms or signs, may be diagnosed clinically as having an acute lumbosacral strain. Diagnostic evaluation may be limited to plain radiographs, and therapy to the traditional regimen of bedrest and analgesics. The duration of necessary bedrest is a matter of controversy; recent controlled studies suggest that restriction of activity is appropriate, but that the week or more of bedrest that has been prescribed routinely in the past is inferior to shorter periods.

If symptoms persist after the patient has undergone mobilization and low back education and exercise programs, further diagnostic study (CT or MRI) is indicated. In some patients with intractable mechanical low back pain, the lumbar facet joints are at fault. Facet joint syndrome may be defined empirically as mechanical low back pain that responds to medial branch posterior primary ramus blocks. Radiofrequency denervations are useful in this small subpopulation of patients.

Lumbar Disc Herniation

The patient presenting with radiculopathy—not only radiating pain, but tension signs and neurologic deficit—is a potential surgical candidate. However, even in patients with this condition, spontaneous recovery is common. Early diagnostic imaging is appropriate, to establish the diagnosis; but in the absence of a major neurologic deficit, conservative management is appropriate initially. As with acute lumbosacral strain injuries, even documented lumbar disc herniation will usually improve with conservative therapy and require no further intervention. Unlike the patient with acute lumbosacral strain, for whom prolonged bedrest and inactivity are not of proven benefit and may in fact be detrimental, the patient with acute lumbar disc herniation requires a more open-ended, individualized period of rest before mobilization.

The standard indication for surgical treatment of disc herniation is persistent, disabling pain despite an adequate trial of conservative care, with abnormal imaging studies sufficient to explain the patient's symptoms. The duration of an "adequate" trial is in general a matter of controversy and in each case a matter of clinical judgment. As spontaneous recovery is common, one might argue for extended conservative therapy. Another viewpoint, however, is that the results of surgery are less favorable after 6 to 9 weeks. Studies of these issues are difficult to interpret, particularly because of selection effects: Reported series of patients undergoing early surgery, for example, include some who might have improved spontaneously. On the other hand, those whose surgery has been delayed or postponed, whether by the physician or patient, would seem to be biased towards *a priori* inferior candidates for treatment. Prospective, randomized study data are scant; they suggest that there is short-term benefit for patients treated surgically, but little difference 1 year after presentation between those who have undergone operation and those who have not.

Lumbar disc herniation occasionally presents with a major neurologic deficit; this constitutes a neurosurgical emergency. Neurogenic bladder may occur with particularly large, central disc herniations, especially with pre-existing lumbar stenosis. Disabling weakness (e.g., foot drop) occurs more commonly. Although spontaneous recovery without surgery is possible, it is unpredictable; to maximize the chances of recovery, prompt surgical intervention is indicated.

Surgical Procedures

Although a detailed discussion of surgical techniques is beyond the scope of this chapter, some popular notions and procedures deserve discussion.

"Microsurgical" lumbar discectomy is common current terminology; it raises several technical issues: (1) the use of the operating microscope per se is considered less important than principles of microsurgical technique (i.e., gentle, meticulous dissection and hemostasis); (2) a small skin incision may permit adequate surgical exposure, but paravertebral muscle dissection should be of sufficient length to avoid traumatic focal retraction; and (3) if disc removal is limited to the herniated free fragment, the possibility of recurrent herniation may be greater, but if the surgeon must create a defect in the annulus to remove nuclear material, this may predispose to recurrence. Each side of these issues has its advocates and supporting case series; however, rigorous prospective study data are lacking.

In prospective studies, chymopapain chemonucleolysis has been found to compare favorably with placebo injections, although it compares unfavorably with traditional surgery in several respects. Its overall failure rate is higher, and the results of salvage surgery appear to be inferior to those of primary surgery—whether because of the effects of chemonucleolysis or because of the delay it introduces. It is occasionally complicated by catastrophic allergic reactions or toxic reactions to errant intrathecal injections. It may not be used for free fragment disc herniations that are sequestered and inaccessible to intradiscal injection. Percutaneous automated discectomy has been introduced recently as an alternative that may be used in the same subset of patients, but without the unique hazards of chymopapain.

Rehabilitation and Physical Therapy

Active participation in a daily exercise program is the most important aspect of rehabilitation after acute lumbosacral strain or postoperatively. The Williams flexion exercise program, which includes knee-chest stretching, pelvic tilts, and partial situps, is the best established and most widely applicable. The objective of any such program is strengthening deconditioned, strained paravertebral and abdominal muscles so as to provide necessary support and prevent further strain injury. After external bracing and prolonged disability and inactivity, exercises are a difficult undertaking for many patients, and a structured program is necessary to ensure compliance in many cases.

Education as to proper techniques for lifting and other activities of daily living is an important aspect of rehabilitation. Some patients with physically demanding jobs, despite compliance with these recommendations and with daily exercises, will continue to experience disabling lumbosacral strain injuries; for them, vocational rehabilitation may be appropriate.

SUGGESTED READING

King JS, Lagger R. Sciatica viewed as a referred pain symdrome. Surg Neurol 1976; 5:46–50.

Long DM, Filtzer DL, BenDebba M, Hendler NH. Clinical features of the failed-back syndrome, J Neurosurg 1988; 69: 61–71.

Spitzer WO, LeBlanc FE, Dupuis M, et al. Scientific approach to the assessment and management of activity-related spinal disorders: a monograph for clinicians. Report of the Quebec Task Force on spinal disorders. Spine 1987; (suppl): S1–S60.

Waddell G, McCulloch JA, Kummel E, et al. Nonorganic physical signs in low-back pain. Spine 1980; 5:117–125.

Weber H. Lumbar disc herniation: a controlled, prospective trial with ten years of observation. Spine 1983; 8:131–140.

PATIENT RESOURCES

Back Basics: Managing Spine and Disc Problems with Self Care. Krames Communications, 312 90th Street, Daly City, California 94015-1898.

Back Care. Medic Publishing Co., Drawer O, Issaquah, Washington 98027.

CHRONIC LOW BACK PAIN AND FAILED BACK SYNDROME

LARRY EMPTING-KOSCHORKE, M.D.

Low back pain should be assessed and treated as a pain syndrome. There are multiple possible pathophysiologies for this condition, and these may be compounded further in a patient who has already undergone one or more low back operations. Pain in one anatomic area can be from any local tissue or may be radiated or referred. The pathologic source of the pain may be malignant or benign and may or may not be amenable to surgical intervention. As physicians, we are concerned that dangerous pathology may be missed and, conversely, that surgery performed to treat this pathology may worsen the patient's condition. There is also a stunning difference in the degree of pathologic impairment and the extent of disability in different patients that is based primarily on their psychiatric profile. Pain has an incredibly potent effect on psychological defenses, mood, and ultimately, the degree of disability. We have all seen patients who have either minor pathology but major disability or rather impressive pathology with minimized complaints and minor disability. The problem is deciding for which patients and to what extent our increasingly expensive diagnostic technology is required. In this chapter, I delineate the anatomic, pathophysiologic, and psychiatric syndromal features of the various sources of low back pain and "failed back" as determined by the traditional assessments and newer technologies, and finally, clarify treatment interventions.

BASIC PRINCIPLES OF PAIN SYNDROMES

One should assume that there is some physiologic source for the pain that the patient complains of; purely psychogenic pain is rare. The pathology may be minor, however, and the patient's response may be one of inappropriate disability. The converse may be true in a stoic person.

A general medical history and examination are essential for determining systemic factors causing local pathology. The neurologic and orthopedic examination will best define the syndromal signs. The neurologic examination must be complete in its screening for clues of a more widespread process presenting focally (e.g., mononeuritis multiplex presenting as sciatic and low back pain).

The psychological effects that pain has on personality, mood, and interpersonal relationships should be noted early on; this allows ease of intervention if the pain proves primarily psychogenic.

Physiologic and psychiatric components should be assessed concurrently rather than sequentially since both are inevitably operative and management of both will be necessary for whatever somatic pathology is found.

A familiarity with the local anatomy, referral patterns, and syndromal features of the pathophysiologic diagnoses is also important. One should start with simple and less invasive diagnostic testing, although one should use whatever testing is necessary to be as definitive as possible, whether making a diagnosis of inclusion or exclusion. One should define the source of pain and determine whether the lesion is surgically approachable. If it is not, physical therapy and/or pharmacologic and psychiatric interventions are indicated.

ANATOMIC CONSIDERATIONS

In treating chronic low back pain, each specialist focuses on his or her own "anatomy of interest"; for example, neurologists focus on the neural elements of the condition, orthopedic surgeons on correctable spinal and/or bony abnormalities. However, nearly all tissues in the low back are capable of producing pain locally. With the exception of the nucleus pulposus, the spinal, ligamentous, and neural elements are innervated by multilevel somatic and sympathetic nociceptive afferents. Hence there is little value in attempting to localize pain to one or another vertebral level. Historic and reproducible radicular paresthesias to a specific dermatome and facet pain syndrome induced by extension with radiation to posterior thigh or hip, anterolateral thigh, or groin (but rarely below the knee) are actually the only two pain patterns that are routinely helpful.

Bony Anatomy

The vertebral column anteriorly and facet joints posterolaterally are the stabilizing and most stressed bony components of the spine and hence the most susceptible to degenerative arthritic changes. As a disc degenerates and shrinks in height, the anatomic relationship of the articular surfaces is further altered and painful spondylosis and mechanically induced low back pain are hastened. Activity worsens the pain, whereas rest alleviates it. The posterior location of the facets tends to cause pain when the patient extends. Connecting anterior and posterior elements, the most vulnerable component is the pars interarticularis, which when fractured (spondylolysis) can allow shift of one vertebra (forward or back) on another (spondylolisthesis). Spondylosis posteriorly and laterally on the vertebral body causes central bony canal stenosis and lateral recess stenosis, respectively. Stenosis centrally creates "spinal claudication" syndromes with walking-induced back pain, leg pain, weakness, and/or change in reflexes.

Lateral recess stenosis of course narrows the foramen that the nerve root must take out of the bony canal. Facet spondylitic changes further narrow or even obliterate that foraminal opening, often causing classical radicular/dermatomal symptoms.

Disc Anatomy

Flexion places dorsally directed force on the disc, causing herniation either centrally or laterally, and thereby causing canal stenosis or lateral stenosis, respectively, with symptoms similar to those associated with bony changes. Of course they are not mutually exclusive, and often herniation is also seen with spondylolisthesis. Forcing a fragment through richly innervated ligaments causes low back pain in itself, regardless of whether or not the herniated portion of the disc impinges on nerve roots per se. When dorsal column stimulators are implanted, stimulation over the coverings of the cord can cause paresthesias many levels up, which partially explains why ligamentous pain can radiate quite high in the spinal column. With pressure on roots at any level, nociceptive afferents within its coverings and vessels as well as the somatic and sympathetic axons themselves can elicit painful radiating paresthesias without segmental findings on examination or electromyography (EMG). With sympathetic nociceptive afferents, the pain also is localized poorly or even "mirrored" contralaterally. Injury along the course of the lumbosacral plexus or even in the sciatic nerve as low as the pyriformis has been shown to cause referred pain to the low back. Hence one must consider pathology anywhere along the dermatomal course, from cord to peripheral nerve, especially if the patient has radicular symptoms.

Musculoligamentous Anatomy

Muscle and ligamentous injury or strain (e.g., myofascial syndrome) cannot be imaged and must be measured on clinical examination only.

Because underlying and correctable pathologies can be primary and spasm and muscular trigger points can be secondary, one is obligated to work up chronic "myofascial" or "musculoskeletal" syndromes that do not respond well to conservative therapy.

Referred Pain

Pelvic retroperitoneal lesions and, to a lesser extent, abdominal lesions can cause referred pain to the low back. However, history and review of systems usually helps determine the source of this pain.

Anatomy of the Failed Back

Surgery has many effects on normal anatomy, sometimes even at sites distant from the site of surgery. A herniated disc fragment can certainly recur at the same level. Scarring caused by the primary pathology or occurring postsurgically is common in the lateral recesses along the course of the roots' egress. More extensive scarring of the multiple roots may occur with even a single level disc resection (i.e., arachnoiditis). These scarred elements are restricted in mobility, pull on one another, and often progress with compressive scar. Laminectomies can resect much of the lateral lamina or facets, leading to later fracturing of facets or spondylitic nonanatomic joints. "Fusions" may fail to fuse originally, reabsorb, form pseudoarthroses, and fail to incorporate the facet joints. The low back with a solid fusion must make up for that lack of motion either above or below the fusion causing "transitional" changes such as laxity of ligaments behond physiologic norms and accelerated spondylitic changes. Again, some of these are suited to surgical correction, while others are not.

DIAGNOSTIC ASSESSMENT

Always let your neurologic examination guide your diagnostic testing and imaging. The clinician has a tremendous advantage over the radiologist in that the history and examination can focus on specific anatomic details that may not otherwise standout.

Plain Films

Lateral flexion and extension films may be the only way to show a dynamic spondylolisthesis. Oblique views are necessary for facet and foraminal anatomy and pars interarticularis fractures (especially in trauma cases). Plain films also indicate the amount and location of spondylitic changes as well as decreased disc height suggesting degenerative changes.

Electromyography/Nerve Conduction Velocity (EMG/NCV)

In a patient who has not undergone prior surgeries, radicular findings can be useful in bolstering a clinical opinion, but lesions on imaging will determine if a surgeon should operate. The main limitation of EMG/NCV is that it can be negative for slowing or denervation even while a painful irritative process that could be relieved by surgery (e.g., a foramenal decompression) remains active. Also, once the resection of the first laminectomy has been performed, the paraspinous EMG is not helpful. EMG/NCV will, however, help rule out more distal or widespread processes confusing the clinical picture (e.g., mononeuritis multiplex with radicular involvement). Similar arguments hold for somatosensory evoked potentials, which for the most part are less useful.

Thermography

On the whole, thermography has not provided more information on low back pain than a good neurologic examination.

Magnetic Resonance Imaging

Magnetic resonance imaging (MRI) has proven exceptionally useful in illustrating soft tissue intrathecal processes and disc herniations. The quality varies tremendously, however, and MRI is poor at illustrating the bony anatomy so important in spine pathology. MRI is most useful in patients who have not undergone prior surgeries. New contrast agents are evolving (e.g., gadolinium) that are useful in delineating recurrent disc (avascular) with scar tissue (vascularized, enhancing, and with a much poorer outcome for reoperation). MRI has been the most useful tool in illustrating pelvic and retroperitoneal processes that can refer to the low back.

Myelography with Computed Tomography

The most definitive study, plain myelography with postmyelogram computed tomography (CT) illustrates the bony features best as well as their relation to the neural elements. This is particularly true in patients who have undergone back operations or who have had fusions. Three-dimensional reconstruction has proven especially useful in patients with fusions, pseudoarthroses, foraminal stenosis, and occult facet and pars fractures. The software varies significantly for three-dimensional studies, and the actual films represent a surface view only, so that quality and utility may vary significantly. Myelogram CT and MRI can be quite complementary in defining of complex cases.

Nerve Blocks

Diagnostic facet and selected root blocks may help confirm clinical and imaging suspicions in a functional manner and support an argument for radiofrequency facet denervation or foramenotomy. Although recent literature has illustrated generic epidural steroid "therapeutic" blocks that are not effective for low back pain, selected root or arachnoiditis cases have still shown some response to steroid root or intrathecal injections.

PSYCHIATRIC VARIABLES

Personality types and disorders as well as cognitive ability determine not only the repertoire and adaptability of patients in dealing with pain, but also the degree of disability. Personality disorders that are most problematic (and which are preexistent to the low back pain syndrome) include histrionism, dependence, passive-aggressiveness, and borderline and antisocial personalities. Limited cognitive resources also decrease coping strategies.

Mood abnormalities and disorders include lifelong dysthymia, adjustment disorder with depressed mood, and major affective (depressive) disorder. Almost all patients with pain syndromes have depressive features, many of them evolved to the point that the patients are responsive to antidepressant medications, which often have serendipitous peripheral benefit on pain mechanisms. Some psychiatric or psychological input is essential to treating these complex, distressed and distressing patients. They often require psychological and psychopharmacologic management while the structural/pathophysiologic aspects are addressed.

ASSESSMENT STRATEGIES

Assessment should be definitive, whether or not the source of the low back pain is surgically approachable or even if the pathology is relatively minor and incongruous with the degree of disability. This enables one to define realistically the surgical, pharmacologic, and psychiatric strategies.

Although each work-up is guided by clinical judgment, the following generalizations can be made:

1. In clinically suspicious cases, the combination of plain films and regular MRI gives excellent data about both bony and soft tissues, and thus may guide further work-up or answer any questions regarding a surgical lesion.
2. In patients with failed backs, plain films followed directly by three-dimensional CT myelogram are the best diagnostic tools. If there is a question of scar versus recurrent disc herniation, a gadolinium MRI may be helpful with blocks useful in facet/root pathologies.
3. The more complex the diagnostic process and the more psychologically disabled the patient, the more desirable it is to assess and treat the patient in a chronic pain diagnostic unit or "Pain Treatment Center."

4. Many patients with chronic low back pain or a failed back syndrome are already taking narcotics or other addicting medications (e.g., benzodiazepines) at the time of presentation. Maintaining them on these medications during the diagnostic work-up is reasonable. Then once the pathology has been defined, decisions can be made regarding surgery, permanent blocks, and pharmacologic intervention. For detoxification of high-dose narcotics and benzodiazepines and/or addicting medications used over a long period of time, it is often necessary to hospitalize patients in an Inpatient Pain Treatment Center with psychiatric expertise.
5. Tricyclics, especially the lesser anticholinergics (e.g., nortriptyline hydrochloride and desipramine hydrochloride), are useful for peripheral pain. These should be started at low doses and increased slowly. Although pain may be alleviated with low doses, the dosage may need to be increased to typical antidepressant serum levels. The nontricyclic antidepressants are less useful except for an affective component. Carbamazepine, clonazepam, and phenytoin are useful for neuritic and radicular symptoms.
6. Posterior column stimulators may be quite useful in the treatment of arachnoiditis and focal multilevel scarring. In some cases, morphine pumps are useful in moderating pain. Thalamic stimulators may be most useful in patients with "central pain" states. All of these should be used in the setting of a controlled protocol and multidisciplinary workup.

CERVICAL SPONDYLOSIS

ELLIOTT L. MANCALL, M.D.
MARK STACY, M.D.

Cervical spondylosis, an acquired disorder involving the intervertebral discs, the cervical vertebrae and processes themselves, and indirectly, the spinal roots and spinal cord, is a common degenerative disorder of midlife and old age. In this disorder, radiologic changes predominate in the fourth through seventh vertebral bodies; however, purely radiographic alterations, even when computed tomography (CT) scanning, magnetic resonance imaging (MRI), or myelography is used, often fail to explain fully the spectrum of clinical complaints. Pathologic examination may provide evidence of a complex assortment of changes, any or all of which may account for the symptomatology in a given patient. These include, *inter alia,* osteophyte formation, joint degeneration (spondyloarthropathy), central herniation of the intervertebral disc(s), and hypertrophy of the ligamentum flavum, all of which may narrow the spinal canal (and may potentially cause either direct cord compression or compromise of the spinal vascular network).

More laterally placed bony spurs involve the intervertebral foramina and compress the spinal roots; lateral extrusion of disc fragments may produce similar radicular affection. Osteophytic compromise of the vertebral foramina may also lead to compression of the vertebral artery, which is symptomatically manifest particularly with changes in position of the head and neck. Finally, entrapment of the greater occipital nerve may occur as a result of spasm of the cervical musculature. In such a complex setting, the patient's clinical symptoms and signs remain the most useful guide to the location, nature, and extent of the pathologic process.

From the therapeutic point of view, it is useful to divide the patients' complaints into several distinct groups, each reflecting a predominant, although not necessarily exclusive, constellation of clinical and pathologic alterations: headache, syncopal episodes, cervical radiculopathy, and cervical myelopathy. These may develop spontaneously in an insidious manner, or more acutely after trauma to the neck (e.g., a whiplash injury, the medicolegal implications of which should not be ignored in one's therapeutic approach).

HEADACHE

Spondolytic changes occurring superiorly at the cranio-cervical junction and within the upper cervical column may result in headache. In some patients, pain is lancinating in quality and radiates unilaterally or bilaterally from the neck or base of the skull to the vertex or forehead, sometimes into the orbit. Spontaneous pain may be reproduced by compression or percussion of the greater occipital nerve as it crosses the basiocciput. Spasm of the cervical musculature is almost invariably encountered; the pain in these instances of occipital neuralgia is likely caused by entrapment and compression of the occipital nerve as it traverses muscles of the posterior triangle of the neck.

More common is the aching or squeezing pain experienced at the occiput and radiating around the head in a band or vicelike manner, and again reflecting spasm of the cervical musculature as so-called insertional or muscle-contraction pain. It may be extremely difficult to distinguish this pain from that of the classical tension headache syndrome; in fact, the mechanism of headache in both conditions is probably similar if not identical.

Treatment of headache in patients with cervical spondylosis is basically symptomatic, and includes the use of massage, ultrasonography, regular applications of moist heat, suitable muscle relaxants—e.g., chlorzoxazone (parafon Forte DSC), 500 mg three times daily; cyclobenzaprine (Flexeril), 10 mg three times daily; or diazepam (Valium), 2 to 5 mg three times daily—and nonsteroidal anti-inflammatory agents. The use of narcotics should be avoided. Intermittent cervical traction may be helpful, particularly in patients with severe cervical spasm. In the face of neuralgic pain, agents such as amitriptyline hydrochloride (Elavil), 10 to 25 mg administered at bedtime, and/or carbamazepine (Tegretol), 800 mg per day or more as required, are helpful. In resistant cases of occipital neuralgia block of the greater occipital nerve, or as an extreme measure, avulsion of the nerve may be useful.

SYNCOPAL EPISODES

Syncope associated with head movements, particularly turning of the head with retroflexion, is associated with osteophyte formation with narrowing of the vertebral foramina, often with subluxation of the vertebral bodies. These changes result in compression—and sometimes frank occlusion—of the vertebral arteries. Symptoms are not confined to syncope alone; at times, a full-blown picture of vertebro-basilar insufficiency appears. Careful attention to the details of the patient's history should permit one to distinguish this osteophytic compromise of the vertebral arteries from the far more common transient ischemic attacks caused by atherosclerosis and stenosis of the posterior circulatory tree. If changes are demonstrated in the vertebral artery angiographically with changes in head posture, decompression of the vertebral canal may be beneficial.

CERVICAL RADICULOPATHY

Compression of the cervical roots, either by osteophyte formation within the intervertebral foramina or by traumatic lateral herniation of a disc fragment, results in cervical radiculopathy, characteristically presenting with severe lancinating pain that is generally referred in a dermatomal pattern to the shoulder, arm, or hand. Patients often complain of tingling paresthesias in the hand or arm. There may also be pain, particularly with a change in position of the neck or with coughing, sneezing, or other Valsalva maneuvers. Spasm of the cervical musculature with restriction of movement of the cervical spine is typically encountered, especially in acute cases of traumatic origin. Asymmetry or loss of the muscle stretch reflexes is common, and segmental weakness may be apparent. Sensory changes are more difficult to document, but in many cases, a dermatomal sensory loss is evident. Atrophy of muscle appropriate to the segmental level of the lesion may be noted.

The management of cervical radiculopathy is directed at relieving both pain and, ultimately, the nerve root compression itself. Cervical traction is useful, particularly in the face of cervical spasm and when supplemented by a cervical collar. Warm and/or cold compresses, massage, and ultrasonography are often beneficial. Muscle relaxants (see preceding section) may be helpful, and relief of pain with appropriate analgesics is especially important; one must bear in mind that the pain itself will induce cervical spasm, and one must break this unfortunate cycle of pain-spasm-pain if at all possible. Ibuprofen (Motrin), 600 mg every 6 hours, or other nonsteroidal anti-inflammatory agents may be helpful; narcotics should be used only with caution.

Other treatment modalities such as acupuncture or transcutaneous nerve stimulation (TNS) may be used in some patients but are not uniformly helpful. TNS is probably more useful in acute cases than chronic cases. If painful radiculopathy has been present for a long period of time, amitriptyline is of benefit, beginning with 25 mg administered at bedtime, increasing to 100 mg, as required.

If conservative measures fail to relieve symptoms, surgical correction (foraminotomy) with decompression of the compromised spinal root(s) is necessary. It should be emphasized that the vast majority of patients respond to conservative management, with surgery being required only as a last resort.

CERVICAL MYELOPATHY

Myelopathy is the most serious of the complications of cervical spondylosis. Compression of the cervical cord is generally insidious in onset and slowly progressive; a more rapid course may follow trauma. Among the more common symptoms are tingling paresthesia and sensory impairment of the hands, often radicular in distribution; weakness, clumsiness, or atrophy of the hands, at times with segmental fasciculations; and spasticity and weakness of the lower extremities. Urinary urgency and frequency and impotence are not uncommon. Radicular pain and spasm of the cervical musculature may appear. Cervical myelopathy results from either or both of two mechanisms: (1) direct compression of the spinal cord by osteophytic processes or disc degeneration with central protrusion of soft disc material often with cartilaginous overgrowth, in many cases associated with thickening of the ligamentum flavum or (2) compromise of the vasculature of the cord with a seondary ischemic myelopathy.

The management of cervical myelopathy caused by spondylosis is often unsatisfactory. First, one must be careful in making the diagnosis since in the absence of significant pain or sensory changes, it may be difficult to distinguish this myelopathy from amyotrophic lateral sclerosis. Tumor of the cervical cord, multiple sclerosis, primary lateral sclerosis, and subacute combined degeneration of the cord caused by B_{12} deficiency are among the disorders which must be excluded. Even when the diagnosis is clear, management is difficult. Cervical traction, a cervical collar, warm or cold compresses, massage, ultrasonography and muscle relaxants all play a role in the treatment of this condition. If such measures fail, however, patients may require laminectomy with posterior decompression of the cord. In appropriately selected cases, anterior discectomy with removal of centrally protruded disc material and fusion may be the surgical approach of choice.

SUGGESTED READING

Brain L, Wilkinson M. Cervical spondylosis and other disorders of the cervical spine. Philadelphia: WB Saunders, 1967.

Herkowitz HN. The surgical management of cervical spondylotic radiculopathy and myelopathy. Clin Orthop 1989; 239:94–108.

Larsson E-M, Holtås S, Cronqvist S, Brandt L. Comparison of myelography, CT myelography and magnetic resonance imaging in cervical spondylosis and disc herniation. Acta Radiol 1989; 30:233–239.

Lestini WF, Wiesel SW. The pathogenesis of cervical spondylosis. Clin Orthop 1989; 239, 69–93.

Teresi LM, Lufkin RB, et al. Asymptomatic degenerative disc disease and spondylosis of the cervical spine: MRI imaging. Radiology 1987; 164:83–88.

REFLEX SYMPATHETIC DYSTROPHY

ROBERT J. SCHWARTZMAN, M.D.

Reflex sympathetic dystrophy (RSD) comprises a group of related disorders that are similar manifestations of various inciting events. Recent research suggests that RSD is a form of reflex neurogenic inflammation that occurs after nerve injury and is initiated by sympathetic overactivity in the affected body part. It may involve sensory neuropeptides (substance P, calcitonin gene-related peptide, neuropeptide Y, somatostatin, and vasoactive intestinal peptide) in concert with inflammatory mediators such as histamine, bradykinin, and the prostaglandins. Sympathetic innervation has profound effects on muscle spindles, the reticular formation, glycolytic and aerobic muscle physiology, and peripheral nociceptive receptors.

Early in their illness, patients have sympathetic maintained pain, although after a variable period central mechanisms may be affected and the pain becomes sympathetically independent. At this point, there may be physiologic changes in the polymodal nociceptive neurons of Rexed Layer I of the spinal cord or in neurons projecting central pain. The best opportunity for curing the disease is during the period when the pain is sympathetically maintained. At some point in the illness, all patients manifest burning pain, vasomotor instability, and edema. If the syndrome does not abate spontaneously or with treatment, it progresses through defined stages and spreads proximally or in a mirror distribution to the opposite side of the body. Occasionally, the entire body may be affected. The syndrome may occur at any time from childhood through old age and affects women more frequently than men. Specific situations favor the development of RSD: (1) the casting of extremities after fracture, (2) partial nerve injuries, (3) soft tissue injuries such as sprains, (4) brachial plexus traction injuries, (5) disc disease, and (6) entrapment neuropathies. RSD also occasionally develops after myocardial infarction, stroke, or spinal cord injury. Almost invariably, the pain experienced is out of proportion to the initial injury. Stage I RSD encompasses all degrees of causalgia (burning pain) in association with varying degrees of vasomotor instability and edema. The pain may occur almost immediately after the injury is sustained or may be delayed for 7 to 10 days. During the early stages, the extremities are hyperemic, swollen, and hyperalgesic (overly sensitive to innocuous stimuli). Toward the end of Stage I disease (at 3 to 6 months), the nails may become brittle and hair growth is accelerated. Stage II of the illness is characterized by increased pain and dystrophic changes of hair, skin, nails, and subcutaneous tissue. Vasospasm, hyperhidrosis, and hyperpathia may predominate (the pain threshold is increased, but once it is exceeded, the pain progresses explosively and is appreciated after the stimulus is removed). During Stage III, the pain is lessened, but the extremity is atrophic, contracted, and ankylosed. Dystonia, difficulty in initiating movement, tremors, and a peculiar quivering of the affected muscles may be seen during any stage of the illness.

TREATMENT

Successful treatment depends on the following: (1) early diagnosis (during the first 2 weeks of the disease), (2) identification and treatment of the initiating cause, (3) effective sympathetic blockade, and (4) aggressive physical therapy. The severity of the initial symptoms is not a predictor of eventual outcome. If proper sympathetic blocks are performed within the first 2 weeks of the onset of Stage I RSD (at which time classic causalgia is first seen) in conjunction with intensive physical therapy, Stage II and Stage III disease may be prevented. Avulsion injuries of the brachial plexus are an exception and seem to respond only to dorsal root zone section (DREZ). Although Stage I disease has been reported to respond to treatment with corticosteroids, anticonvulsants, narcotic analgesics, calcium channel blockers, nonsteroidal anti-inflammatory agents, tricyclic antidepressants, and beta- and alpha-adrenergic blocking agents, all of these treatments have failed to effect a cure in my experience with more than 500 patients. My suspicion is that patients responded dramatically to these agents either because it was very early in the course of the disease or perhaps because they were destined for spontaneous resolution. I have not achieved sustained relief with any of these agents in any patient with Stage II or Stage III disease. During Stage I, on the other hand, all of these agents help afford some pain relief for varying periods of time.

Regardless of the stage of the disease, all patients with RSD suffer from spasms in the affected areas. Benzodiazepines (5 mg administered three times daily) and clonazepam (Klonopin, 0.5 mg administered three times daily) in increasing dosages are effective. In those patients with severe dystonia, baclofen (Lioresal, 90 to 120 mg per day) has been most effective.

Sympathetic Blocks

Sympathetic blockade of the superior cervical ganglia is used to relieve pain in the upper extremities, head, and trunk. Paravertebral sympathetic ganglia blockade from T12, L1–L2 has been most effective in the lower extremities. I recommend that the blocks be performed in series of five every other day (Fig. 1). Some patients may require as many as 20 blocks over a 3-month period in conjunction with intense physical therapy to attain relief of pain; Bupivacaine hydrochloride (0.25 percent), 5 ml, or mepivacaine hydrochloride (0.5 percent) is employed. A few patients have responded to 1 to 2 mg of labetalol (alpha- and beta-blocker) when other blocks have failed. The use of sufentanil blocks (5 μg), a morphine antagonist for both the stellate and the paravertebral ganglia, may provide a longer duration of action (12 to 48 hours) in some patients. If the blocks are only partially effective, it is worthwhile to block the opposite side since there may be cross-over of fibers at cervical levels and usually at L1–L2 in the lumbar area. My own suspicion is that if the RSD is diagnosed promptly and blocks nevertheless fail, the problem may be technical; either aberrant sympathetic tissue is in the nerve root foramina or there is extensive bilateral innervation. If at time of diagnosis there is bilateral RSD in the lower extremities, I use epidural sympathetic blockade for 48 hours first. In those patients with severe sympathetic dystonia of the upper extremities, axillary somatic blocks have been helpful. Several patients with dystonia have responded to high-dose Lioresal (80 to 120 mg) in conjunction with upper or lower extremity sympathetic blockade. Liver function must be monitored carefully in patients receiving these high doses. A good block of the superior cervical ganglia results in an immediate ipsilateral rise in skin temperature and a Horner's syndrome. Occasionally there is noncontinuity of the sympathetic chain and one may see an isolated Horner's syndrome without skin temperature changes. Immediately or up to 3 hours after the block, the patient may experience decreased pain and edema, increased skin temperature, and improved function of the extremity. The latter may be the result of blockade of the specific effects of sympathetic activity on the muscle itself or the muscle spindle, rather than of a lessening of pain. A significant portion of patients may have an excellent block but suffer a paradoxical increase in pain. Recent evidence suggests that as the extremity warms, heat sensitive nociceptive afferents are stimulated, increasing sympathetically maintained pain. It has been suggested that an increase in pain in response to either heat or cold stimuli may be used as a screening test for sympathetically maintained pain. The complications of sympathetic cervical superior ganglian blocks include the following: paralysis with vertebral artery dissection, recurrent laryngeal nerve block, pneumothorax, and bradycardia (following right superior cervical ganglia block).

During lumbar paravertebral blockade, there may be perforation of the vena cava, aorta, and kidney, as well as trauma to the genitofemoral or other somatic nerves. These complications are very rare in experienced hands. The techniques are well established, but the physician must be prepared to perform intubation and resuscitation. All of the blocks are performed in the surgical recovery room or in a specially equipped anesthesiology peripheral block area.

Sympathectomy

Patients who respond to sympathetic blockade and physical therapy but do not maintain this response over a 3-month trial period should be considered for sympathectomy. In my experience, complete cures have followed sympathectomy. I try to sympathetically denervate only one extremity; otherwise there is the potential for hyperthermia and hypotension (bilateral denervation below T_6). I have seen 21 patients with bilateral lower extremity and 16 with bilateral superior cervical ganglia sympathectomy with no complications. Approximately 30 to 40 percent of patients will suffer postsympathetic pain (sympathalgia). This may be treated with Tegretol at a dosage of up to 1,200 mg per day or with phenytoin (Dilantin), 300 to 400 mg per day. This complication usually abates spontaneously within 3 to 4 months. If pain recurs in the area of sympathetic denervation and the patient is still sweating in this area, chemical sympathectomy with 7 to 10 percent phenol may be accomplished. Ureteral stricture and infection have been seen after this procedure.

If the RSD is limited to the distal extremity, a series of guanethidine Bier blocks (10 to 20 mg) performed once per week for 4 weeks is often effective. These have been especially helpful after recurrence of pain after sympathectomy. There is evidence to support that primary intravenous regional sympathetic blockade (Bier blocks) may be used as a first

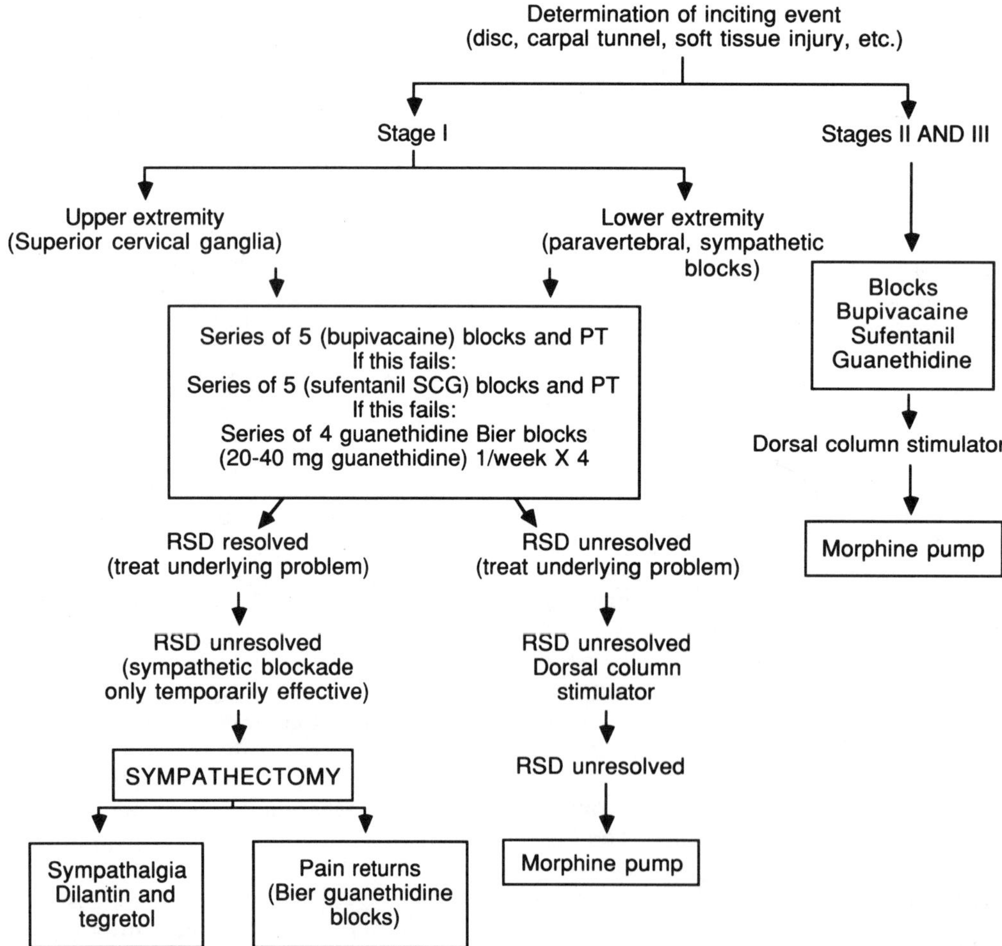

Figure 1   Approach to management of RSD. PT = physical therapy SCG = superior cervical ganglia.

method of sympathetic blockade. However, I have not found this to be as successful as SCG or paravertebral blocks. In my experience, bretylium Bier blockade has not been as effective as guanethidine Bier blocks.

Other Management

In general, once the RSD has been controlled, I attempt to correct the underlying problem. Such management includes disc and other back, neck, and spine surgery, carpal tunnel release, cryoneurolysis of neuromas, and the various approaches to brachial plexus decompression. Unfortunately, any surgery or intravenous placement in a patient already suffering from RSD may initiate a new flare-up of the disease. These exacerbations are sudden and usually local, but they may involve the entire sympathetic innervation of the affected side. These flare-ups can usually be successfully treated by regional intravenous sympathetic blockade.

Many patients with severe RSD are taking narcotics, calcium channel blockers, tricyclic antidepressants, nonsteroidal anti-inflammatory agents, and hypnotic sedatives. My practice is to prescribe these patients methadone hydrochloride, beginning at a dose of 5 mg administered twice daily and gradually increased to 20 to 40 mg per day until pain relief is achieved. Patients need their usual dose of narcotics for at least 4 days until the methadone becomes effective. The dose of methadone should be increased slowly to avoid nausea and vomiting. Fluoxetine (Prozac) at a dosage of 20 to 40 mg per day administered in the morning is helpful for depression. Nonsteroidal anti-inflammatories may be used during the day at 4- to 6-hour intervals.

If these therapies fail, I turn to dorsal column stimulation. These units can cover all parts of the body and be adjusted externally. One can expect significant pain relief in 50 percent of patients. I have found external transcutaneous electrical nerve stimulator units to be minimally effective.

In those patients with generalized RSD or whose life is ruined because of pain that is confined to one extremity, I implant morphine pumps. The pumps are associated with a high degree of success if the patient responds to doses of 10 mg of intrathecal morphine. Effective pain relief is usually attained with a dosage of 30 mg of intrathecal morphine per day. The success rate for this form of treatment is approximately 50 percent. If unsuccessful, the dorsal column stimulator system and the morphine pumps are removed. Clearly, treatment of RSD is currently frustrating and difficult, and it is successful in less than 50 percent of patients. All patients with RSD are severely incapacitated, depressed, and in need of general medical and psychiatric support.

SUGGESTED READING

Bonica JJ. Sympathetic nerve blocks for pain diagnosis and therapy. Vol 1. New York: Breon Laboratories, 1980:27–38.
Hannington-Kiff JG. Intravenous regional sympathetic block with guanethidine. Lancet 1974; 1:1019–1020.
Payne R. Neuropathic pain syndromes with special reference to causalgia and reflex sympathetic dystrophy. The Clinical Journal of Pain 1986; 2:59–73.
Rowlingson JD. The sympathetic dystrophies. Int Anesthesiol Clin 1983; 21:117–129.
Schwartzman RJ, McLellan TL. Reflex sympathetic dystrophy. Arch Neurol 1987; 44:555–561.

PATIENT RESOURCE

RSDS Association
PO Box 821
Haddonfield, New Jersey 08033
Telephone: (609) 428-6510
or
(609) 428-6980

HEADACHE AND FACIAL PAIN

MIGRAINE AND CLUSTER HEADACHE

DEWEY K. ZIEGLER, M.D.

A problem in reaching a consensus on the optimum treatment of migraine is the difficulty in establishing criteria for diagnosis. There is no verifying biologic test; each clinician must rely on his or her clinical judgment. A universally agreed on criterion, however, is recurrence of attacks, and there are therefore two treatment considerations: treatment of an acute attack and prophylactic treatment for prevention of recurrent symptoms.

The first treatment necessity is to rule out any underlying disease of which headache is a symptom. Headache is a common symptom of increased intracranial pressure, meningeal irritation, and vasculitis and can occur in association with any kind of encephalopathy (e.g., that caused by electrolyte derangement or anemia). For this reason, all patients with severe, constant, or recurrent headache must undergo a careful neurologic examination and some laboratory tests—a complete blood count, a measurement of the sedimentation rate, and a profile of blood chemistry values. Minor degress of abnormality on neurologic examination must be suitably evaluated. Although usually if there are abnormalities on neurological examination, patients have referable symptoms, occasionally such symptoms are absent. Minor degrees of impairment of fine finger movement, rapid gait, or ability to hop may be found. Reflex asymmetry, abnormality of visual fields on confrontation, or any degree of impairment of higher functions (e.g., memory, flow of speech) may also be important.

Once a presumptive diagnosis of migraine is made on the basis of the history and a negative examination, I present to the patient a brief summary of migraine as it relates to his or her case. This "mini-lecture" usually covers the following points:

1. Based on a review of the history and the negative neurologic examination, there is minimal possibility of brain disease (often a patient has the unspoken apprehension that he or she is harboring a brain tumor; not infrequently the physician discovers that a family member or close friend has had this illness).
2. Migraine is defined as an illness characterized by recurrence of severe headache and, often but not always, one-sided location and occurrence of nausea and vomiting.
3. There is no single cause for this condition; many kinds of biochemical abnormalities and physiologic abnormalities have been found in some patients.
4. In many patients, migraine is associated with a hereditary tendency—probably a susceptibility to headache brought on by various stimuli through mechanisms still unknown.
5. Because migraine is characteristically recurrent, prophylactic treatment is often effective for varying periods of time; it can be discontinued, but often later needs to be reinstituted.
6. Treatment of the acute attack and treatment to prevent recurrent attacks require different procedures.
7. Migraines are occasionally brought on by situations that can be avoided. Migraineurs should try not to skip meals since in some patients slight drops in blood sugar may precipitate attacks. Keeping regular sleeping hours is also important; some patients suffer attacks after missing sleep, others after particularly prolonged sleep (e.g., on weekends). Also to be avoided are excessive caffeine intake (contained in coffee and many soft drinks), chocolate, sharp cheeses, and red wine. In some individuals, a variety of other food substances have been reported to precipitate attacks.

TREATMENT OF ACUTE ATTACK

An urgent problem is the differentiation of an acute migraine attack from acute meningeal irritation caused by subarachnoid hemorrhage or bacterial meningitis. Distinguishing an acute attack from the latter is rarely a problem since infection is almost invariably characterized by fever and systemic signs of infection. Subarachnoid hemorrhage, however, presents more difficulties. Presence of any degree of nuchal rigidity, impairment of consciousness, or other abnormalities on neurologic examination mandates computed tomography (CT) scan of the head and a spinal fluid examination. The reason for the spinal fluid examination is that occasionally cases are seen before the blood is apparent on CT scan. Even without these clues, in a patient presenting with severe headache and no previous history of the same, these tests may be warranted—although clearly they cannot be made routine for each headache episode. I rely greatly on the previous history; if onset occurs at an early age, if attacks are fairly uniform, and particularly if the visual symptoms of classic migraine have occurred, I feel more confident that the attack is migraine. Positive family history also favors migraine to some degree.

I consider the treatment of the acute migraine attack to consist of five aspects: (1) avoidance of environmental stimuli, (2) antiemetics, (3) analgesics, (4) ergotamine, and (5) sedatives.

My first instruction to the patient with an acute attack is to initiate rest in a dark, quiet room. Most patients have discovered this treatment modality themselves, but some attempt to "tough it out"—go to work, often to a job that involves close visual work and causes "stress." Such an attempt invariably prolongs the headache.

The patient must decide when early symptoms herald a severe migraine attack and when they do not. Once migraine is diagnosed, administration of ergotamine is indicated (Fig. 1). Use of ergotamine early in the episode is far more effective than later. It can be given even during the aura of classical migraine. The caveat presented to the patient is that there is a danger of overuse of ergotamine; patients taking the drug when they are overly apprehensive may become psychologically dependent on larger amounts. The more psychologically unstable the patient, the greater the danger of such a dependence.

Often the severe migraine attack is accompanied by nausea and/or vomiting. These symptoms are

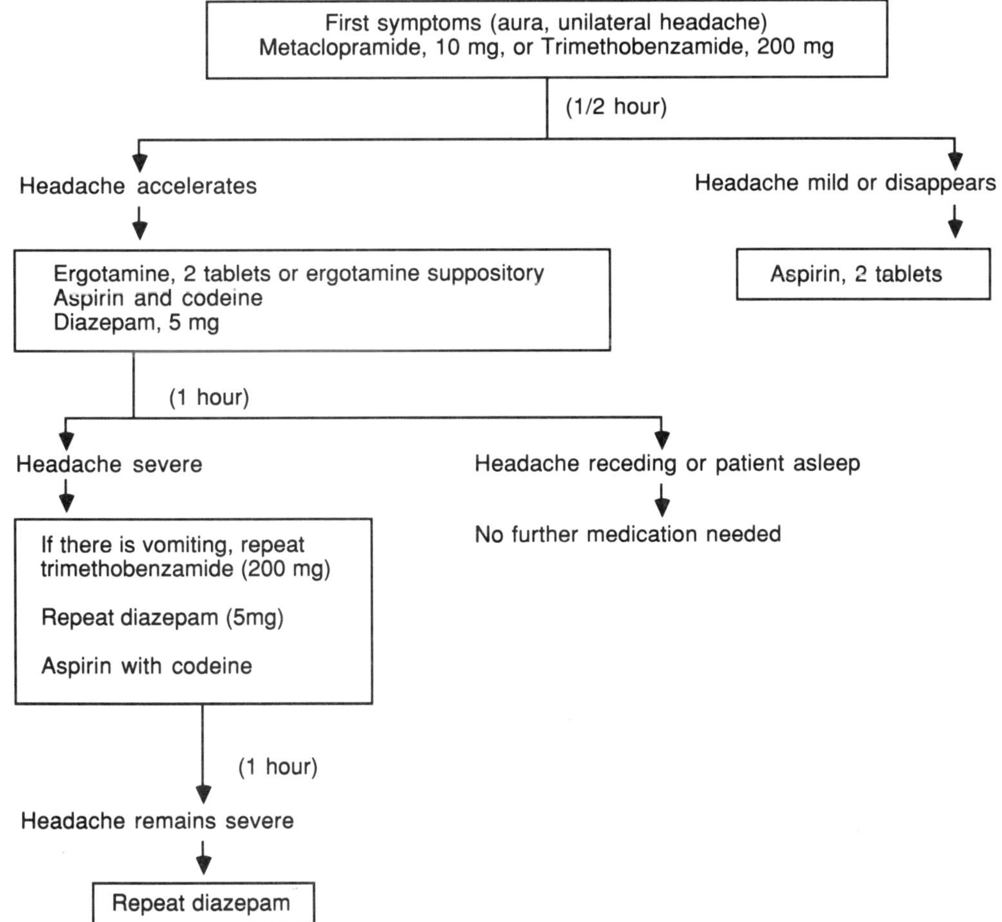

Figure 1   Treatment of acute migraine attack.

intensified, if not initiated by, ergotamine. If the patient has a history of nausea with attacks, I recommend initiation of treatment with an antiemetic before administering ergotamine. If nausea has begun, a trimethobenzamide hydrochloride suppository (200 mg) is useful, or if considerable agitation is present, a phenothiazine such as prochlorperazine may be preferable, likewise in the form of a suppository. If the patient can anticipate the nausea and therefore receive medication orally, I prescribe metaclopramide, 10 to 20 mg by mouth, as the first therapeutic agent.

I prescribe ergotamine to be taken 20 to 30 minutes after the acute antiemetic. If nausea is not present, ergotamine can be taken orally in the tablet form combined with caffeine or with caffeine plus a small amount of phenobarbital and belladonna. Since it is desirable for migraine patients to sleep, one must remember that these preparations do contain the stimulant caffeine. I recommend 2 mg of ergotamine taken orally, followed by three additional 1-mg doses at hourly intervals if needed. I do not recommend more than 5 mg ergotamine for any single attack. I have no real opinion as to the additional benefit conferred to the ergotamine-caffeine by the addition of phenobarbital-belladonna. I rarely use sublingual ergotamine since the degree of its absorption is questionable. Ergotamine may also be taken via nasal inhalation; absorption is excellent, but the preparation is costly and I have not used it.

For some patients, ergotamine must be taken in suppository form. Often patients awaken with a severe headache accompanied by nausea and therefore cannot take medication by mouth. Some find the onset of nausea so rapid that there is no time for oral medication to take effect. Absorption of the drug from rectal mucosa is more complete than from gastric mucosa; rarely does a patient require more than one suppository.

Because ergotamine is a vasoconstrictor, it should probably never be used in patients who have a history of any arterial disease and should be used only with great caution in the elderly. It is particularly important to warn patients of these vasoconstrictive actions and of the symptoms of dangerous vasoconstriction (e.g., chest pain, extremity pain). As a general rule, after discussing with the patient the side effects of any medication prescribed, I provide him or her with one of the excellent American Medical Association (AMA) printed sheets (if available) discussing that particular class of drug.

Patients can develop a psychological habituation to ergotamine. This is probably not a true addiction, but it is nevertheless an effect that occasionally requires hospitalization to undo. I warn patients that the weekly limit of ergotamine is 8 to 10 mg. Occasional patients benefit from the compound Midrin, which also contains a vasoconstrictor of much weaker potency.

Analgesics are of course needed for the acute attack; some patients may achieve adequate relief with aspirin, acetaminophen, or ibuprofen. Although these agents should be tried alone first, in my experience there is usually adequate evidence of some attacks of pain severe enough to justify the occasional use of more potent agents such as codeine (e.g., 30 mg), or codeine derivatives combined with aspirin or acetaminophen. Of also greater analgesic potency is propoxyphene. Occasional patients achieve superior relief when a sedative is compounded with analgesics (e.g., butalbital [Fiorinal]). Such agents should be used for limited periods of time only, and the patient should be informed that they contain a sedative which can well be habit forming if taken continually.

I try to evaluate more or less intuitively the degree of probability of drug abuse in each individual patient. In those in whom there are clues of emotional instability, prescriptions for more potent analgesics should be given in only small amounts. All patients, of course, should receive a limited number of such tablets, both per single attack and per week.

One of the major decisions is whether to recommend or permit potent opiates (e.g., meperidine hydrochloride) parenterally for patients with severe attacks. I strongly discourage such treatment because of the frequency of dependence on these drugs. If patients become used to the euphoria and analgesia produced by opiates, they are progressively more unwilling to tolerate any headache pain, and demands for injections usually accelerate. I tell patients that they can almost always avoid the necessity of parenteral opiates by instituting prompt oral therapy that includes enough sedation to put them to sleep. I therefore instruct them to take a strong sedative with analgesics and ergotamine. (For the average adult, I have been prescribing diazepam 10 mg.) The dose is to be repeated in 1 hour if the patient is not asleep by that time. (Patients in pain frequently require large amounts of this medication to induce sleep.) It must be made clear to the patient that the diazepam is to be used only in the event of acute attacks and to induce sleep and that it must not be used with great frequency.

PROPHYLACTIC TREATMENT

The decision of whether to administer medication on a daily basis for prophylaxis of headache is often a difficult one. Certainly in the patients with one or two episodes per year such treatment is not justified. Conversely, in patients with one or more attacks weekly, such treatment regimens should be tried. The patient should share in the decision in questionable cases, the possible benefits of treatment being weighed against possible drug side effects.

Although the prophylactic agents to be discussed are reported to be effective in treating migraine and not "muscle tension headache," I have been liberal in their trial. In many patients, episodic headache has some (although far from all) of the characteristics of migraine, and in many of these patients, one of the drugs will be effective. We do not yet know which, if any, specific combinations of variables predict response to one or the other drug.

Frequently patients have several questions before beginning a daily drug regimen. Such questions may include the following:

1. "Will I have to stay on this for the rest of my life?" The answer I give is that migraine is an intermittent problem and that, although we cannot surgically "remove" migraine, many persons go without attacks for months and even years. After a long interval during which headaches are few or rare, I instruct patients to taper medication.
2. "Are the drugs addicting?" The answer to this is "no" in the sense that withdrawal is usually not difficult.
3. "Will these drugs interfere with any other medication I am taking—for example for cardiac disease?" The answer to this question is also usually "no," although drug interactions should be investigated for each combination in question.

If the decision is made to use prophylactic treatment, I tell patients that there is currently medical literature supporting the trial of several different agents for this purpose, the most generally used being propranolol, amitriptyline, methysergide, naproxen, and verapamil. There is little medical literature providing guidance as to which patient characteristics might indicate the preferential trial of one of these drugs or whether combinations of two or more drugs might be superior to one drug alone.

I instruct patients that, as a general principle, dosage should be increased gradually until one of three end-points is reached: (1) good reduction in headache (as determined by the patient), (2) the occurrence of unacceptable side effects, or (3) a dose is reached at the upper range of that reported in the medical literature. Only after failure with trials with each of the single prophylactic agents do I move to polypharmacy (two drugs).

I frequently select propranolol for a first trial unless there is a specific contraindication, such as hypotension, asthma, or diabetes. It is wise to start with a low dose—for example, 20 mg twice daily with an increase in dosage at biweekly intervals. I have seldom achieved better results with any daily dosage of more than 160 mg, although much larger doses are used in patients with hypertension and have been used in some patients with migraine. Once the effective daily dose is established, I offer the patient the option of using the once-daily long-acting preparation, which can be supplemented, if necessary, by one or more short-acting doses. I point out to the patient the possibility of such side effects as orthostatic hypotension (which usually occurs only with large doses), the usual bradycardia, and the occasional fatiguelike state often described as a "loss of drive" rather than as sedation. However, this latter side effect may be a consideration in the choice of a drug; if a modest tranquilizing effect occurs with the use of propranolol, it is natural to select this drug for those individuals with manifest anxiety. Propranolol has been used as an agent in prophylaxis of anxiety attacks and is commonly used by entertainers just before a performance.

Several other beta-adrenergic-blocking agents have been used effectively for migraine prophylaxis; these are the compounds of the series which lack sympathomimetic effects. However there is no published evidence that any of these are superior to propranolol either in efficacy or diminution of side effects, and to date, only propranolol is FDA-approved for migraine. Nevertheless, if propranolol is ineffective and the patient seems a particularly good candidate for beta-adrenergic blocking therapy, I occasionally give a brief trial with metoprolol, 50 to 150 mg per day.

Patients taking beta-adrenergic blocking agents, particularly the elderly, should be warned not to discontinue use of the drug abruptly. Such abrupt action can produce hypertensive reactions, although this is rare with the comparatively small doses used to treat migraine.

Amitriptyline can be used as an one-dose nighttime medication, and I have found it particularly effective when insomnia complicates migraine. I always begin this drug with a small dose (10 to 25 mg nightly) since side effects disturb many patients and are lessened if dose is increased gradually. The therapeutic range is usually 50 to 100 mg nightly, although occasional patients benefit from a higher dose. Common side effects are sedation and dryness of the mouth caused by anticholinergic action. Since headache patients are frequently depressed, it is wise to bear in mind the caveat that this drug has been used effectively as a suicidal agent. There is little published experience with other antidepressants in the treatment of migraine, and there is no indication of the superiority of any of them to amitriptyline.

Methysergide (Sansert) was first discovered to be effective as a migraine prophylactic several decades ago. It seems that the more typical the migraine, the more likely this drug is to be effective as a prophylactic agent. Again, I begin with a dose of 2 mg twice daily—a dose that is usually below the therapeutic range. The dose is increased to 2 mg three times daily after a few weeks, and if results are still unsatisfactory, it is increased to 2 mg four times daily. Its limitations are its side effects. Even with small doses, some patients have unpleasant subjective sensations that they find difficult to describe but which have hallucinatory elements. Methysergide can also cause nausea and insomnia. The drug also has vasoconstrictor properties, and patients should be told to report any symptoms suggestive of cardiac or limb ischemia. The most dangerous side effect is growth of fibrous tissue into various sites (retroperitoneal space, lungs, cardiac valves), which occurs with prolonged use of methysergide. Patients must be warned to take a "vacation" from the drug for 1 month after 6 months' use.

The calcium entry channel blocker, verapamil, is another effective drug in the prophylaxis of migraine and has the advantage of carrying less potentially serious side effects than many of the others. As my experience with this drug increases, I tend to consider it among the best of the agents to be used for this condition. The usual drug dose is 320 mg daily. The common side effect is constipation, and flushing of the skin is not uncommon. In my experience, neither of these have been severe enough to necessitate withdrawal of the drug. Patients should probably take bulk stool softeners while receiving this drug.

The nonsteroidal anti-inflammatory drug naproxen is another choice for trial in prophylaxis of migraine. The usual dose is 375 to 500 mg 3 times daily. It has the advantage of some analgesic properties and is particularly valuable if patients have additional pain problems (e.g., arthritis). Several side effects must be remembered, the most troublesome being irritation of gastric mucosa and activation of peptic ulcer. It is wise to tell patients to take it with food or an antacid. In patients with some degree of pre-existing disease, the drug may also cause serious renal or hepatic dysfunction.

In many patients, headache frequency and severity diminish with nonpharmacological treatment. The most commonly used such treatments are instruction in general psychic relaxation, muscle relaxation, and biofeedback of neck or forehead muscle contraction (to demonstrate to the patient that such relaxation *has* occurred) or of hand skin temperature (to demonstrate that he or she has succeeded in raising skin temperature). There are reports of improvement in both migraine and nonmigrainous headache with this treatment, particularly with nonmigrainous headache. Currently it is not known whether any biofeedback demonstration to the patient with a recording device of some change in a physiologic variable is superior to instruction in muscle relaxation. My practice is to judge from the patient's history and "body language" during examination the degree to which the patient is "tense." If the degree appears to be high or if the patient himself links the attacks to stress, I give some simple instructions on relaxation. I recommend that the patient allot three or four 15-minute periods per day to retiring to a quiet, dark place (often an extremely difficult undertaking). The patient should then concentrate on relaxing each limb in turn and should repeat a series of semi-self-hypnotic phrases (Table 1). I have not used formal biofeedback with metering devices.

When migraine attacks recur with great frequency despite high doses of medication, I recommend hospitalization. During the hospital stay, the high doses of medication to which the patient has become habituated are withdrawn (gradually in the case of beta-adrenergic blocking drugs) and the patient is kept heavily sedated for a few days. This maneuver is particularly important if patients are taking large amounts of analgesics or ergotamine. These measures should be accompanied by a program of psychological counseling to enable the patient to avoid recurrence of migraine.

Table 1   Self-Administered Relaxation Phrases

I feel quite quiet . . . . I am beginning to feel quite relaxed . . . . My feet feel heavy and relaxed . . . . My solar plexus and the whole central portion of my body feel relaxed and quiet . . . . My hands, my arms, and my shoulders feel heavy, relaxed, and comfortable . . . . I feel all the tension in my neck letting go and relaxing . . . . My lower neck feels relaxed . . . . The upper neck at the base of my head is letting go . . . letting go . . . . My head feels free . . . . My jaws and my tongue are letting go . . . . The area around my eyes is letting go . . . . They feel relaxed . . . . I feel the areas around my mouth, my nose, and my forehead letting go and relaxing . . . . They feel comfortable and smooth . . . . My whole body feels quiet, heavy, comfortable, and relaxed.

I feel quite relaxed . . . . My arms and head are heavy and warm . . . . I feel quite quiet . . . . My whole body is relaxed and my hands are heavy and warm, relaxed and warm . . . . My hands are warm . . . . Warmth is flowing into my hands, they are warm . . . . I can feel the warmth flowing down my arms into my hands . . . . My hands are warm, relaxed and warm . . . . My forehead is relaxed . . . . I am relaxing every fiber . . . . The area around my eyes is soft, relaxed and letting go . . . . All the muscles in my face feel comfortable and smooth . . . .

My whole body feels quiet, heavy, comfortable, and relaxed . . . . My arms and hands are heavy and warm . . . . My forehead muscles are relaxed and smooth . . . . My mind is quiet . . . . I withdraw my thoughts from the surroundings and I feel serene and still . . . . My thoughts are turned inward and I am at ease . . . . Deep within my mind I am relaxed, comfortable, and still . . . . I am alert, but in an easy, quiet, inward-turned way . . . . My mind is calm and quiet . . . . I feel an inward quietness.

CLUSTER HEADACHE

In most patients, the syndrome of cluster headache is clearly distinguishable from migraine and responds to different therapeutic agents. The acute attacks are characterized by retro-orbital pain and are always unilateral, severe, and usually brief in duration (lasting 0.5 to 1 hour). Attacks are of great severity and characteristically repetitive during a short period of time. I have found few attacks to be responsive to treatment with ergotamine. Because the attacks are brief, oral analgesics do not have time to take effect. A further problem with the use of analgesics in patients with this condition is that the patients often take them in apprehension of the recurrent attacks. Occasional patients, however, do obtain relief from one of these agents, which must almost always be supplemented with codeine. I have found that inhalation of oxygen at 4 L/minute is effective in terminating attacks in most patients.

Patients with cluster headache should be warned to avoid alcohol; most of them have already discovered that even small amounts can precipitate attacks. Continuous prophylactic treatment is usually not needed since the "clusters" are separated by unpredictable intervals of time. Once the "bout" of headache attacks starts, I rely on adrenal steroid drugs to terminate the "cluster." I usually begin with 50 mg of prednisone administered daily and decrease the daily dose by 10 mg every week. When clusters are resistant to steroids or recur after only brief periods of relief, I have the patient begin taking lithium carbonate, beginning with one 300-mg tablet per day and rapidly increasing (over a period of 2 weeks) the dosage to 300 mg administered three times daily.

SUGGESTED READING

Jonsdottir BA, Meyer JS, Roger RL. Efficacy, side effects, and tolerance compared during headache treatment with three different calcium blockers. Headache 1987; 27:364–369.

Martin PR, Marie GV, Nathan PR. Behavioral research on headaches: a coded bibliography. Headache 1987; 27:555–570.

Tfelt-Hansen P. Efficacy of beta-blockers in migraine: a critical review. Cephalalgia 1986; 6 (suppl):15–24.

Ziegler DK, Ellis DJ. Naproxen in prophylaxis of migraine. Arch Neurol 1985; 42:582.

PATIENT RESOURCES

National Headache Foundation
5252 N. Western Avenue
Chicago, Illinois 60625

(There is a small membership fee. The organization provides up-to-date material concerning headache.)

Other sources of information:

Seymour Solomon, M.D.
Headache Clinic
Montefiore Hospital and Medical Center
111 East 210th St.
Bronx, New York 10467

Dewey K. Ziegler, M.D.
Headache Clinic
Department of Neurology
University of Kansas Medical Center
39th and Rainbow Blvd.
Kansas City, Kansas 66103

Neil Raskin, M.D.
Headache Clinic
Department of Neurology
University of California at San Francisco
505 Parnassus Avenue
San Francisco, California 94143

Joseph Sargent, M.D.
Menninger Headache Clinic
5800 West 6th Avenue
Topeka, Kansas 66604

Ninan Mathew, M.D.
Houston Headache Clinic
1213 Hermann Drive
Houston, Texas 77044

E.L. Speirings, M.D.
John R. Graham Headache Center
Faulkner Hospital
Allendale at Centre Street
Boston, Massachusetts 02130

Kenneth Welch, M.D.
Headache Clinic
Henry Ford Hospital
2799 West Grand Boulevard
Detroit, Michigan 48202

Seymour Diamond, M.D.
Diamond Headache Clinic
5252 N. Western Avenue
Chicago, Illinois, 66604

Joel Saper, M.D.
Michigan Headache and Neurological Institute
3120 Professional Drive
Ann Arbor, Michigan 48104

MIGRAINE IN CHILDHOOD

IAN J. BUTLER, M.B., F.R.A.C.P.

A physician training in pediatrics, family practice, or neurology may have little opportunity to confront a child with migraine. However, in clinical practices where children are evaluated, migraine in all its various forms is relatively common. Scandinavian studies estimate an incidence of 3 to 4.5 percent before puberty and increasing to 10 to 20 percent during the latter half of the second decade of life. The male:female ratio of incidence of migraine is approximately equal before puberty, whereas after puberty, females with migraine outnumber males 2:1.

Despite intensive study over the past 50 years, there is still a lack of consensus as to the pathogenesis of migraine. Initial studies indicated changes in the diameter and pulsations of external and internal cerebral vasculature as an explanation for the various prodromal, aura, and headache stages of the migraine attack. Later studies implicated serotonin and other bioactive amines. More recent studies have addressed the neural hypotheses implicating the brain (cortex and brain stem) and trigeminal nerve (substance P). The end result of the various hypotheses is a clinical syndrome of recurrent headaches in which, in an unfortunate few patients, involvement of the cerebral vasculature leads to transient or permanent ischemic changes to the brain and brain stem.

DIAGNOSIS

There appear to be several reasons for the failure of physicians to recognize migraine in children. In general, the medical profession and adult population, including parents, consider migraine to be a disorder of late adolescence and early adulthood that often improves during subsequent years. In the lay and medical community, there is also a strong misperception that most headaches in children are of psychogenic origin and are related to school phobias or other social stresses. In my experience, the majority of children with headache have migraine, with a minority having structural brain lesions (hydrocephalus, brain tumors, and abscess formation, benign intracranial hypertension, sinusitis, and psychogenic causes.

One of the major problems in recognizing migraine in childhood is the variety of forms of migraine in this age group. Paroxysmal disorders such as paroxysmal torticollis of infancy, recurrent abdominal pain syndrome, and benign paroxysmal vertigo of childhood may be the initial manifestations in a young migraineur. In an infant or child with a paroxysmal disorder, a family history of migraine often suggests that future migraine episodes will follow. In a young child presenting with migraine, I have frequently elicited a prior history of recurrent, periumbilical abdominal pain, sometimes sufficiently severe to necessitate hospitalization for vomiting.

Other difficulties in the diagnosis of childhood migraine relate to those children with initial onset of complicated migraine. For example, I have observed children with hemiplegia, aphasia, brain stem syndromes (ophthalmoplegic migraine), and disturbed mental states as the initial presentation of childhood migraine. Often there may be a history of vague recurrent headaches or of migraine in other first-degree family relatives. Basilar artery migraine presenting as an acute confusional state is frequently observed and may be a diagnostic dilemma until the child recovers, usually spontaneously over several hours. The onset of headache after head injury in childhood is common and on most occasions represents a postconcussive syndrome. However, I have observed many children with onset of migraine headache or even an acute confusional state shortly after a relatively mild head injury. Some children may have an episode of complicated migraine with visual phenomena (scintillations, scotomas, visual field defects), aphasia, or hemiparesis without an associated history of headache. Such episodes obviously present a difficult diagnostic dilemma until the natural history of recurrent headaches is revealed. Rarely have I diagnosed "ice-pick" headaches in children, and cluster headaches are also uncommon in this age group (however, approximately 1 percent of cluster headache sufferers present in childhood).

Although older children may have a history that typically indicates common migraine or classical migraine with hemicrania, visual phenomena, and hemiparesis or hemianesthesia, I have been impressed with the clinical distinctiveness of the natural history of migraine presenting during the first decade of life. This distinctiveness has been a source of diagnostic concern for physicians. During the first couple of years the headaches may be mild, may occur only intermittently, and may not require medical attention. There is frequently a crescendo leading up to the presentation, often with a mass lesion or psychogenesis being considered as causing the headaches. At this time, the headaches may occur daily or even several times daily. Often they are of brief duration (lasting only for several minutes) and are usually poorly defined to the top or front of the head. The headache may not be associated with nausea or vomiting. The frequency and severity of the headache at this point will often result in an emergency consultation with a negative computed tomography (CT) scan in hand and an alarmed referring physician and parents. This stage of the natural history of migraine may persist for several months (or less with treatment), and over the next several years, a more typical history of migraine, including frequency and duration of headaches, emerges.

Clearly the clinical history is the most important aspect in the management of these young children and adolescents. Questions should be directed at the child in addition to both parents. Often a history of the vivid visual hallucinations of the ''Alice in Wonderland'' syndrome (micropsia, macropsia) may be elicited only by gentle but persistent direct questioning of the child. (The child may be unwilling to admit to such strange and unnatural phenomena to the parents or pediatrician.) Occasionally there is a definite and repeated association of a migraine episode with a dietary source such as chocolate or oranges. Occasionally I have also observed a monthly periodicity of migraine episodes in prepubescent girls such that menstrual-related migraine may be predicted to occur in the future. Although a history of allergies are common in this age group, I am not convinced that migraine has an allergic basis.

A history of migraine in close family members should be sought vigorously and persistently. Frequently the headaches have been misdiagnosed as ''sinusitis'' or ''tension headaches'' and may be recognized as migraine only in the parent or parents at the time of the child's consultation. It has been stated, and I would agree, that if one parent is questioned, a family history of migraine is obtained in 80 percent of cases and in 90 percent if both parents are questioned.

A consistent aspect of the history in young migraineurs is the tendency to retire, often voluntarily, to a quiet, darkened room and the child's appreciation that sleep leads to relief of the symptoms of the migraine episode. Such a tendency often indicates that conservative management is possible. Furthermore, a parent with migraine, either as a youngster or persisting into adulthood, may be an excellent ''role model'' for the child, serving as an example of how one may successfully ''live with migraine.'' Obviously the reverse situation may apply and needs to be managed on an individual basis by appropriate psychological counselling.

TREATMENT

In general, the treatment of migraine in childhood should be highly conservative. The ritual of the consultation, examination, and explanation is frequently sufficient to allay the fears and expectations of the parents and child. Occasionally, in a very anxious family, neuroradiologic studies (usually a CT scan) may be necessary to convince other family members, friends, and referring physicians that a tumor or hydrocephalus is not present. Other studies, including measurement of cerebrospinal fluid pressure at lumbar puncture, are dictated by the examination and subsequent clinical course and are certainly not performed routinely. I rarely obtain an electroencephalogram unless there is a strong suspicion of an associated seizure disorder. Sometimes the history of basilar migraine may be difficult to distinguish from various types of seizures, such as complex partial seizures with absence or occipital epilepsy. Frequently after the consultation and recommendation of some simple remedies, there is apparent resolution of the emergent situation related to the headaches. I use analgesics such as aspirin, acetaminophen, or ibuprofen for the headache and I encourage the child to lie down in a quiet, darkened room to enable onset of sleep. Analgesic medications combined with a mild sedative can also be helpful in inducing sleep.

Dietary manipulations may be helpful in those children with headache episodes that are clearly linked temporarily to specific food or drug ingestion. In some older children and adolescents, a history of coffee drinking may indicate ''caffeine withdrawal'' headaches, and coffee drinking may need to be limited. Furthermore, I continue to recommend that oral contraceptive medications be discontinued or avoided in young female migraineurs and certainly in those patients with headache episodes that appear to have been initiated or exacerbated by such medication or who have a history of complicated migraine. Occasionally in a child with pernicious vomiting, medications may need to be administered parenterally or by suppository. Usually vomiting is a minor aspect of childhood migraine, and often the headache seems to be alleviated after vomiting. I have not used ergot alkaloid preparations in the acute treatment of childhood migraine.

During the initial evaluation, I also discuss with the parents and child the role of future migraine episode prophylaxis. Indications for migraine prevention usually include repeated school absences, a severe and continuing episode in which headaches occur every day (status migrainosus), headache episodes interfering with social or sporting activities, and severe, often prolonged headaches occurring more than once per month and usually weekly. Frequently parents do not want daily medications for their child and are willing to agree to a ''cooling-off period'' during which conservative management is used for several weeks or months.

Over the years, I have tried many types of daily medications for migraine prevention. During the last decade, I have used initially in children those anticonvulsants currently administered for seizure control. Phenytoin or phenobarbital and, more recently, carbamazepine are administered in small doses which are increased until headache prevention is achieved. The doses required are often less than what is required for seizure control, and suspected toxic manifestations can be readily monitored by anticonvulsant blood levels. The initiation of treatment with small doses and a simplified dosage schedule usually permits excellent patient compliance and successful decrease of the frequency and suppression of the severity of the headaches. If possible, I tend to avoid phenytoin treatment in young females because of the adverse cosmetic effects of this medication on skin and hair. Occasionally I use a combination tablet containing phenobarbital, ergotamine tartrate, and alkaloids of belladonna (Bellergal-S) in migraine prophylaxis. I suspect that phenobarbital is the active ingredient in this combination tablet.

In the minority of children who do not respond to this approach, I find it necessary to use propanolol in increasing doses. The long-acting form of propanolol may be helpful in avoiding the need to take medication during the school hours. I have not in the past found cyproheptadine (Periactin), clonidine (Catapres), or methysergide (Sansert) to be helpful in the prevention of childhood migraine. Rarely have I found it necessary to use an antidepressant or calcium-channel blocking agent for patients in this age group.

Medications used successfully in migraine prophylaxis are usually continued for 3 to 6 months or until the end of the current school year. During the summer vacation, I attempt to decrease or discontinue prophylactic medication. Should severe and frequent headaches recur, a further similar cycle of medication is advised. In school-age children, I attempt to use medications that require administration only once or twice daily since this avoids the adverse stigmata and the need for the child to take a midday dose at school. However, the school nurse does need to be involved since I frequently recommend that a headache episode beginning in the classroom be managed by the school nurse using analgesic administration. Frequently resolution of the headache follows a period of rest or sleep in the school infirmary. This approach avoids the necessity for parents to repeatedly remove the child from school, which can be especially inconvenient if both parents work. Furthermore, such an approach will decrease the stigmata attached to a chronically ill child who is repeatedly absent from school. A similar approach can be used at home such that the child learns to "live with migraine," completes homework assignments, and is able to compete successfully with his or her peers both socially and athletically.

SUGGESTED READING

Bickerstaff ER. Migraine variants and equivalents. In: Blau JN, ed. Migraine: clinical and research aspects. Baltimore: Johns Hopkins University Press, 1987:55.

Lance JW. Fifty years of migraine research. Aust NZ J Med 1988; 18:311–317.

Prensky AL. Migraine in children. In: Blau JN, ed. Migraine: clinical and research aspects. Baltimore: Johns Hopkins University Press, 1987:31.

Rothrock JF, Walicke P, Swenson MR et al. Migrainous stroke. Arch Neurol 1988; 45:63–67.

TRIGEMINAL AND GLOSSOPHARYNGEAL NEURALGIA

GERHARD H. FROMM, M.D.

Trigeminal neuralgia is a disorder of the sensory divisions of the trigeminal nerve consisting of brief paroxysms of electric shocklike or stabbing pain separated by pain-free intervals. The maxillary and mandibular divisions are more frequently affected than the ophthalmic division. The attacks are triggered by light tactile or vibratory stimulation of trigger points that are usually located periorally or intraorally. Trigeminal neuralgia is characterized by a tendency to exacerbations and remissions, with an overall progressive increase in the frequency, severity, and duration of the exacerbations.

Glossopharyngeal neuralgia is a similar disorder affecting the glossopharyngeal nerve, so that the pain is in the region of the ear, the base of the tongue, or the tonsillar fossa, or under the angle of the jaw, and is triggered by talking or swallowing. It is only about one-twentieth as common as trigeminal neuralgia. Glossopharyngeal neuralgia may be associated with syncope caused by severe bradycardia or asystole and for which the insertion of a cardiac pacemaker is required.

The diagnosis of trigeminal or glossopharyngeal neuralgia is made on the basis of a history of the characteristic attacks and a negative neurologic and dental examination. A magnetic resonance imaging (MRI) study should also be obtained to rule out a cerebellopontine angle mass lesion. The drugs that are effective in the treatment of trigeminal and glossopharyngeal neuralgia are not analgesics and are relatively specific for the painful paroxysms associated with these conditions. The surgical procedures currently available are similarly specific for these disorders. Successful medical or surgical management thus depends greatly on an accurate diagnosis.

MEDICAL MANAGEMENT

In view of its greater safety, I prefer to start treatment with baclofen (Fig. 1), even though it is not quite as effective as carbamazepine. The starting dose is 5 to 10 mg three times daily. This dose is increased by 10 mg per day every other day until the patient is pain-free or side effects occur. The usual maintenance dose is 50 to 60 mg per day. The biological half-life of baclofen varies considerably, but is usually approximately 3 to 4 hours. Patients with severe trigeminal or glossopharyngeal neuralgia therefore may need to take baclofen at 3- to 4-hour intervals.

The most common side effects of baclofen are drowsiness, dizziness, and gastrointestinal distress, and approximately 10 percent of patients are unable to tolerate the drug because of one or more of these symptoms. An acute confusional state that occurs shortly after initiation of baclofen therapy is a rare complication that clears up promptly after the drug is discontinued. The most important point to keep in mind when administering baclofen is that it should never be discontinued abruptly after long-term administration, as hallucinations and/or seizures may occur. Such withdrawal symptoms are treated by reinstituting the previous dose of baclofen and then gradually tapering it by 5 to 10 mg per day each week.

Since trigeminal neuralgia often exhibits spontaneous remissions, especially early in the course of the disease, I gradually taper the dose of baclofen after patients have been completely pain-free for several weeks. If the painful paroxysms do not recur, the patient does not require medication until the next exacerbation occurs. I advise patients to keep some tablets on hand so that they can restart the medication as soon as possible when the pains recur, without having to wait to get in touch with me, since recurrences usually do not happen during office hours.

As indicated in Figure 1, carbamazepine is the next drug of choice if baclofen is ineffective or causes unacceptable side effects. The starting dose of carbamazepine is 100 to 200 mg twice daily. This

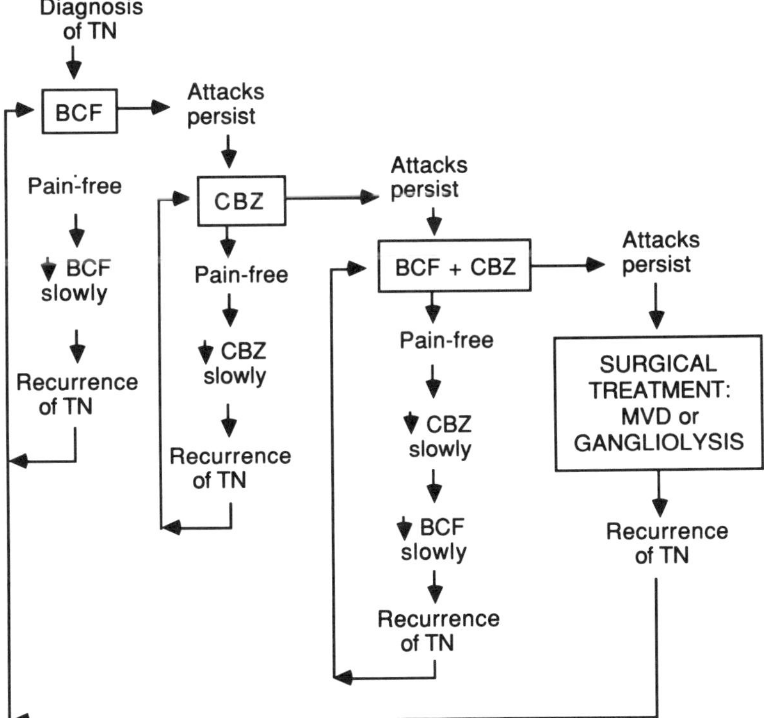

Figure 1 Steps in the management of trigeminal neuralgia. TN = trigeminal neuralgia; BCF = baclofen; CBZ = carbamazepine; MVD = microvascular decompression.
(Republished with permission from Fromm GH, ed. Medical and surgical management of trigeminal neuralgia. Mount Kisco, NY: Futura Publishing Co., 1987:67.)

dosage can be increased by 200 mg per day every other day until the patient is pain-free or side effects occur. The usual maintenance dosage is 600 to 1,200 mg per day, with serum levels of 5 to 12 μg per milliliter. Most patients will have to take this drug in at least three divided doses because, with chronic use, the half-life of carbamazepine is only 8 to 12 hours.

The most common side effects of carbamazepine are drowsiness, dizziness, unsteadiness, gastric distress, nausea, and anorexia. One or more of these signs and symptoms will occur initially in as many as 40 percent of patients. They usually subside within a few weeks, but in approximately 10 percent of patients, carbamazepine must be discontinued. The most serious potential side effect of carbamazepine therapy is aplastic anemia. Fortunately this occurs very rarely, but leukopenia, neutropenia, and/or thrombocytopenia do occur in approximately 2 percent of patients who take carbamazepine. Therefore, a complete blood count as well as hepatic and renal function tests should be obtained before starting treatment with carbamazepine. I then repeat the complete blood count every 2 weeks for the first 2 months, and quarterly thereafter. Carbamazepine should be discontinued if the leukocyte count drops below 3,000/μl or if the absolute neutrophil count drops below 1,500/μl. Patients should also be instructed to call their physician immediately if fever, sore throat, stomatitis, easy bruising, or petechiae should develop. Occasionally, carbamazepine induces imappropriate secretion of antidiuretic hormone. It is therefore useful to check serum electrolyte levels once per year in patients who need to take this drug chronically.

As with baclofen, the dose of carbamazepine should be gradually tapered after patients have been pain-free for several weeks, and can then be restarted when there is a recurrence of the trigeminal or glossopharyngeal neuralgia.

Because of the progressive increase in the severity of trigeminal and glossopharyngeal neuralgia, it is possible that neither baclofen nor carbamazepine alone will eventually succeed in controlling the painful paroxysms. When this happens, the combination of baclofen and carbamazepine will often relieve the attacks (see Fig. 1) because of the synergistic action of these two drugs. Baclofen in conjunction with phenytoin may be used in patients who cannot tolerate carbamazepine, as baclofen also has a synergistic action when used with phenytoin. Occasionally patients require a combination of all three drugs: baclofen, carbamazepine, and phenytoin.

Phenytoin is used primarily as an adjunctive drug to baclofen in patients who have become refractory to baclofen alone and who cannot tolerate carbamazepine. The usual dosage of phenytoin is 300 to 400 mg per day with serum levels of 15 to 25 μg per milliliter of total phenytoin or 1.5 to 2.5 μg per milliliter of free or unbound phenytoin. The latter measure is more accurate when there is impaired protein binding of phenytoin, such as in patients with hepatic or renal disease. The metabolism of phenytoin displays saturable kinetics, leading to large increases in serum levels with only small increments in the dose as saturation of the metabolizing enzymes in the liver is approached. The variation in absorption between different brands of phenytoin is therefore accentuated and may necessitate adjustments in the dose if patients switch from one brand to another. The most common side effects of phenytoin are drowsiness, dizziness, diplopia, and ataxia. Approximately 10 percent of patients cannot tolerate even low doses of phenytoin.

Phenytoin is also useful in the emergency treatment of patients who are having a prolonged flurry of very severe attacks of trigeminal or glossopharyngeal neuralgia and are therefore unable to take any medication orally. In such instances, a loading dose of 1,000 mg of phenytoin can be administered intravenously by slow infusion at a rate no greater than 25 mg per minute with continuous electrocardiogram (ECG) recording and frequent blood pressure determinations. The infusion must be terminated if arrhythmia or hypotension develop. The intravenous administration of phenytoin is contraindicated if there is sinus bradycardia, sinoatrial block, second- or third-degree atrioventricular block, or severe myocardial insufficiency.

SURGICAL MANAGEMENT

Patients who become refractory to all of these medications are candidates for surgical treatment. As indicated in Figure 1, microvascular decompression and radiofrequency or glycerol gangliolysis and rhizotomy are currently the procedures of choice for trigeminal neuralgia. For glossopharyngeal neuralgia the choices are sectioning the glossopharyngeal nerve or a radiofrequency lesion of the petrous ganglion.

Microvascular decompression attacks the presumed etiology of trigeminal neuralgia, preserves the nerve, and produces long-lasting relief in most patients. Radiofrequency or glycerol gangliolysis and rhizotomy avoid the risks of craniectomy, are associated with minimal morbidity and essentially no mortality, are much less expensive, and can be repeated easily. In younger, healthy patients, the chance of long-term pain relief with microvascular decompression is an important consideration, while the minor operative procedures are preferable in older patients and patients with significant medical problems. In the case of glossopharyngeal neuralgia, sectioning the nerve is the most commonly practiced surgical intervention, although there have been reports of successful radiofrequency gangliolysis and rhizotomy.

Unfortunately, none of the surgical procedures for trigeminal neuralgia is successful in all cases. Furthermore, there is a rather wide discrepancy between the success rate and the incidence of complications reported by various centers for each of these procedures, probably related to each center's own level of expertise and experience with a given operation. It is therefore important not only to decide which surgical approach is likely to be the best in each case, but also to be sure to refer the patient to a neurosurgeon who is skilled in that procedure and performs it regularly. In addition, it should be kept in mind that the painful attacks of trigeminal neuralgia can recur after any of these operations, including microvascular decompression, even if the patient becomes pain-free initially.

I have found that patients will often respond to another trial of medical therapy if their painful paroxysms recur after surgical intervention. Baclofen, carbamazepine, and phenytoin should therefore be tried once again at that time, as outlined in Figure 1.

SUGGESTED READING

Fromm GH, ed. Medical and surgical management of trigeminal neuralgia. Mount Kisko, NY: Futura Publishing Co., 1987.

DEVELOPMENTAL ABNORMALITIES

CONGENITAL HYDROCEPHALUS

PETER McL. BLACK, M.D., Ph.D.

Congenital hydrocephalus is a regularly encountered neurologic problem that may produce very little morbidity if appropriately managed. It is virtually always caused by obstruction to cerebrospinal fluid (CSF) flow absorption pathways and can be divided into two types: communicating and noncommunicating. In communicating hydrocephalus, the ventricles communicate with the subarachnoid space; in noncommunicating hydrocephalus, they do not, and lumbar puncture or other procedures that produce a CSF pressure gradient may produce foramen magnum herniation and death. The most common cause of neonatal communicating hydrocephalus is intraventricular hemorrhage associated with prematurity. Causes of noncommunicating hydrocephalus include posterior fossa cysts, tumors obstructing ventricular pathways, and congenital aqueductal stenosis. The hydrocephalus associated with myelodysplasia may be either communicating or noncommunicating.

The major clinical problems in childhood hydrocephalus are the initial diagnosis and management of hydrocephalus syndromes, recognition of shunt malfunction, and dealing with complications of shunting.

DIAGNOSIS

The diagnosis of hydrocephalus during the first few years of life is usually made by measuring an enlarging head circumference and obtaining confirmatory imaging studies. Computed tomography (CT), magnetic resonance imaging (MRI), or ultrasonography should be performed in any child with a head circumference that is at the 98th percentile at birth or that crosses percentile lines during early childhood. CT has the advantage of fast scan time but the disadvantages of irradiation and low sensitivity to tectal and intraventricular lesions that might be the cause of the hydrocephalus. In an infant, MRI usually necessitates sedation but provides superior visualization of the entire CSF pathway; it has been our policy to obtain an MRI in any child whose cause of hydrocephalus is not clear from history or CT. Untrasonography is particularly useful for following ventricular size in neonates with intraventricular hemorrhage; however, it requires an open fontanel and is not by itself adequate to establish precise ventricular anatomy. In these infants, CT or MRI imaging should be done at some point during the first few months of life.

HYDROCEPHALUS SYNDROMES

Hydrocephalus In Utero

Hydrocephalus is regularly diagnosed in utero by ultrasonography. It has been our policy to wait until delivery before proceeding with any further diagnosis or treatment. Although ultrasonography indicates ventricular enlargement, it does not provide a full evaluation of sites of obstruction or associated anomalies, and it is therefore necessary to obtain a CT or MRI scan to understand the anatomy satisfactorily. Head circumference may be monitored by sequential intrauterine ultrasonographic evaluations and delivery may be induced early or accomplished by cesarean section if there is a major increase in head size.

Hydrocephalus After Intraventricular Hemorrhage

Hydrocephalus that occurs after intraventricular hemorrhage requires special neurosurgical management because of the high protein content of CSF, which may obstruct a shunt valve. When possible, it is best to use sequential lumbar punctures or external ventricular drainage to keep the fontanel flat in the premature newborn for as long as possible. When a shunt is inserted, it may be inserted without a valve because of the problem of valve obstruction. This should be revised to a shunt with a valve approximately 1 month later as the CSF becomes normal in viscosity.

Hydrocephalus During the Neonatal Period

Modest ventricular enlargement without a tense fontanel or symptoms of increased pressure (vomiting, lethargy) may be initially observed with sequential head circumferences, as not all ventriculomegaly requires shunt placement. If the head circumference crosses percentile lines or if there is increasing ratio of ventricle:brain size on sequential CT scans, a shunt should be placed.

Symptomatic Hydrocephalus After Fontanel Closure

Until fontanel closure, increased intraventricular pressure is accompanied by enlarging head circumference. After the fontanel is closed, there will be ventricular enlargement at the price of parenchymal thinning. There are four syndromes of such progressive ventriculomegaly, depending on the rate of its development. In *acute* hydrocephalus, there is nausea, vomiting, headache, progressive obtundation, and death. Emergent ventricular decompression is necessary. In *chronic* hydrocephalus, persistent headache, inattention, memory loss, abducens palsies, papilledema, gait difficulty, and leg spasticity may be found, sometimes with endocrine abnormality. If symptoms are seen and imaging has been performed, a shunt should be placed; it is important to be as certain as possible about the cause of hydrocephalus in these patients, as MRI scans may reveal tectal tumors or other tumors where aqueductal stenosis seemed the cause. If hydrocephalus occurs more slowly, the patient may have *normal pressure* hydrocephalus, with delayed psychomotor development, clumsiness, a large head, and impaired learning. The syndrome of *arrested* hydrocephalus is sometimes difficult to distinguish from normal pressure hydrocephalus. Often a CT scan done for another reason than suspected hydrocephalus may show massive ventriculomegaly in a child with arrested hydrocephalus; the neurologic examination may be completely normal and there may be minimal symptoms or none at all. Shunting in such a case may be very hazardous because of the danger of subdural hematoma; whether it should be contemplated at all is a matter of experienced neurosurgical judgment. An antisiphon device may be a useful shunt component in these cases.

MANAGEMENT PROBLEMS IN SHUNTING

Shunt Types

Ventriculoperitoneal shunting is the procedure of choice for infants with hydrocephalus. A shunt has four components: (1) a ventricular catheter, which may be straight, J-shaped, or flanged, and which may be inserted frontally or parietally, (2) a valve, which may either be the slit valve type, opening when differential pressures across it are a certain magnitude, or the ball and spring type, (3) a tapping reservoir, which allows fluid removal and evaluation of shunt function, and (5) a distal catheter, usually placed in the peritoneal cavity.

Generally, a posterior parietal burr hole is used for the ventricular catheter situated just at the lambdoid suture and to the right of midline; the catheter is directed at the nasion and inserted so that its tip is beyond the coronal suture. The reservoir may be attached to the ventricular catheter, a position that allows direct access to the ventricular catheter, or it may be in line between ventricular catheter and valve. Valves may close at high (100 to 150 mm CSF), medium (50 to 110 mm CSF), or low (30 to 70 mm CSF) pressure. The peritoneal tubing may be blunt tipped or open at its tip. Twenty centimeters or more are usually inserted into the peritoneal cavity.

Optional components in a shunt are an on-off device, an antisiphon device, and a shunt filter. The on-off device allows one to turn the shunt off without invasive manipulation, although it may be problematic for that very reason. The antisiphon device stops the shunt flow at the level of the device when the patient sits upright. It may obstruct shunt function with time. A shunt filter keeps malignant cells from being spread to the peritoneum if a shunt is placed with a tumor; the filter will regularly obstruct if tumor cells flow through the shunt.

There may be distal runoff of a shunt to the peritoneal cavity (ventriculoperitoneal shunt), the pleura (ventriculopleural shunt), or the right atrium (ventriculo-atrial shunt). The peritoneum is much preferred, while the pleural cavity is a reasonable second choice in a young patient, and in an older child, the common facial vein may be cannulated for catheter insertion into the superior vena cava at its junction with the right atrium.

Assessing Shunt Function

When shunt malfunction is suspected, three tests are useful: a shunt series, CT or MRI, and a shunt tap. A shunt series consists of plain radiographs of the head, chest, and abdomen, and may demonstrate disconnection of tubing. CT may show enlarging ventricles. A shunt tap should be reserved for cases in which there is a serious likelihood of malfunction and should be performed by a neurosurgeon. With a shunt tap, there is a 1 percent chance of infecting the shunt. Tapping is done by inserting a needle into the reservoir after shaving and preparing the skin over the reservoir. If there is no flow from the shunt on tapping, ventricular catheter malfunction is likely; if there is good flow, the pressure can be measured to assess whether the shunt is maintaining the desired pressure.

Shunt Malfunction

Often the parents of the patient are the best judges of shunt malfunction. Sometimes diminished activity and appetite, clumsiness, and intermittent headache are the only signs. Severe headache, lethargy, and vomiting are more definite symptoms and should prompt urgent evaluation and, in most cases, shunt revision. When in doubt, it is best to seek neurosurgical consultation and evaluate possible shunt malfunction aggressively, as decompensation may occur within hours. At surgery, the head, chest, and abdomen are usually prepared to allow access to all shunt components.

Shunt Infection

Shunt infection may be insidious and subtle, presenting most often as peritoneal catheter obstruction. Rarely does it present with signs of sepsis. With ventriculo-atrial shunting, infection may present as glomerulonephritis or endocarditis. Its diagnosis is not easy to make; use of a shunt tap may enable one to make a correct diagnosis, but it also risks the possibility that skin contamination may be falsely interpreted as infection. The most common organisms are *Staphylococcus epidermidis* and skin diphtheroids. The most reliable samples are those taken from CSF at the time of shunt revision, avoiding skin penetration.

If cloudy CSF is encountered at shunt revision, a stat cell count and Gram stain should be done. If there are organisms or more than 10 WBC per cubic millimeter, the shunt should be externalized as if infected.

Shunt infection is best treated by removal of the shunt, replacement of the ventricular catheter to external ventricular drainage, and administration of intravenous antibiotics for 7 to 10 days until the CSF is sterile or until the white blood cell count in the CSF is less than 10 per cubic millimeter. Oxacillin or vancomycin are the best initial antibiotics, to be adjusted depending on the sensitivities of cultured organisms.

Slit Ventricle Syndrome

The slit ventricle syndrome is a peculiarity of hydrocephalus in children with shunts, usually in patients in whom a shunt was placed before fontanel closure. In this syndrome, the ventricles are very small and with shunt obstruction do not enlarge. The current theory is that the compliance of the brain is such that the ventricles cannot enlarge; high pressure is accompanied by persistent small ventricles.

This syndrome is difficult to manage. Although usually the ventricular catheter is obstructed and changing it relieves the syndrome, a higher pressure valve and antisiphon device may be added. Occasionally subtemporal decompression may be necessary.

Subdural Collections

Subdural collections may occur for unknown reasons in some patients who have had shunts placed for hydrocephalus. They may enlarge with time and are best treated by placing shunt catheters in them that are connected into the shunt system below the valve.

Trapped Fourth Ventricle

With a case of aqueductal stenosis and fourth ventricular outlet obstruction with a shunt in place, there may rarely be progressive enlargement of the fourth ventricle with symptoms of nausea, headache, and vomiting. This may require placement of a catheter directly into the fourth ventricle.

Prognosis of Shunting

The prognosis of shunting depends more on the underlying disease than on the shunt itself. Hydrocephalus corrected early without other abnormalities of the brain can be managed well by shunt placement, and patients may develop normally.

SUGGESTED READING

Dennis M, Fitz CR, Netley CT, et al. The intelligence of hydrocephalic children. Arch Neurol 1981; 38:607–615.
Milhorat TH. Hydrocephalus and the cerebrospinal fluid. Baltimore: Williams and Wilkins, 1972.
Milhorat TH. Hydrocephalus: historical notes, etiology, and clinical diagnosis. In: McLaurin RL, ed. Pediatric neurosurgery: surgery of the developing nervous system. San Diego: Grune & Stratton, 1982:197.
Nulsen FE, Rekate HL. Results of treatment for hydrocephalus as a guide to future management. In: McLaurin, RL, ed. Pediatric neurosurgery: surgery of the developing nervous system. San Diego: Grune & Stratton, 1982:229.
Portnoy HD. Treatment of hydrocephalus. In: McLaurin RL, ed. Pediatric neurosurgery: surgery of the developing nervous system. San Diego: Grune & Stratton, 1982:211.

PATIENT RESOURCE

National Hydrocephalus Foundation
Route 1
River Road, Box 210A
Joliet, Illinois 60436

MYELOMENINGOCELE

ROBERT W. MARION, M.D.
PAUL CHAMBERS, M.D.
LINDA F. SCHENDEL, P.N.P.

Myelomeningocele (MM), occurring in approximately one in 1,000 newborns in the United States, is the most common physically disabling birth defect in humans. Caused by failure of fusion of the caudal portion of the neural tube, the embryonic structure that gives rise to the central nervous system, MMs most often occur in the lumbar or sacral regions of the spine. Because of the neurologic deficit that occurs distal to the site of the MM, children affected with this congenital malformation often require intervention by many members of a diverse group of medical and surgical subspecialists, including neurosurgeons, orthopedic surgeons, urologists, rehabilitation and developmental medicine specialists, as well as general pediatricians. Because such a large number of physicians is necessary to deliver appropriate medical care to the child with MM, parents, who are attempting to deal with and accept the fact that their child has a problem that will require lifelong attention, are often bewildered and overwhelmed at a time when important decisions must be made. For this reason, it is essential that the specialists who care for children with MM be organized into a multidisciplinary team and that the team have a coordinator, an individual who can act as overseer of the medical care, advocate of the child and the family, and ombudsman between the patient, the family, and the rest of the team.

The purpose of this chapter is to describe the principles of management of patients with MM followed in the Spina Bifida Clinic at the Montefiore Medical Center/Albert Einstein College of Medicine. Both inpatient and outpatient care of infants, children, and adolescents will be considered.

MANAGEMENT OF THE NEWBORN WITH MYELOMENINGOCELE

Although through ultrasonography and amniotic fluid and maternal serum alpha-fetoprotein screening, prenatal diagnosis of MM is possible, in the majority of cases, the diagnosis of MM is made during the immediate neonatal period. At the time of birth, a sac is usually present in the midline of the affected child's lower back. The sac, which is covered by meninges, may contain cerebrospinal fluid (CSF) only or a combination of CSF and portions of the spinal cord and/or nerve roots. In the former case, the infant has a meningocele, which is usually associated with a normal neurologic examination and has a relatively good prognosis. In the latter case, the infant has a myelomeningocele, which is associated with neurologic deficits occurring below the level of the lesion; the severity of the deficit noted within the first few minutes of life is often predictive of that patient's long-term functional status. For this reason, a careful neurologic examination must be performed for any infant with a meningocele or a MM during the immediate neonatal period.

The protocol used for the management of newborns with MM at our center is detailed in Table 1. If the affected infant is born at a hospital distant from ours, arrangements for transfer to the Montefiore Medical Center are made as soon as the infant's cardiorespiratory status has been stabilized. If the diagnosis is made prenatally, attempts are made to transfer the mother to our center so that the baby can be delivered in a controlled manner, thus minimizing the risk of infection.

During the immediate neonatal period, the parents are as much patients as the infant. After expecting their child to be completely normal, these parents are faced with the realization that their baby has a serious congenital malformation, a defect that will cause permanent disabilities and require lifelong medical care. This must be addressed during the initial informing interview, which is usually attended by the team's neurosurgeon, genetic counselor, and pediatrician-coordinator. During this session, in addition to discussing the need for surgical repair of the defect, the possible need for ventriculoperitoneal shunting, and the long-term urologic and orthopedic sequelae caused by MM, the parents are informed that the coordinator is available to help in any way possible and to give them any information, advice, and support they may require. Often during the difficult days that follow the birth of a child with MM, this information can be extremely heartening.

After an initial work-up (see Table 1), the initial neurosurgical procedure to close the spine is most often performed at our center within the first 48 hours of life. Occasionally surgery will be delayed if the infant is physically unstable.

After surgery, the child is kept in a prone position, the surgical site is covered with a sterile drape to minimize the risk of infection, and the head circumference is monitored on a daily basis. If signs and symptoms of hydrocephalus, a complication that occurs in 70 percent of affected individuals, are present, ultrasonography or computed tomography (CT) scan of the head is repeated. If hydrocephalus is confirmed, a ventriculoperitoneal shunt (VPS) is placed. At our center, to minimize the risk of infection, placement of the shunt is never performed during the initial neurosurgical procedure, even when hydrocephalus is confirmed during the immediate neonatal period.

Table 1   Management Protocol for Newborns with Myelomeningocele

Preoperative
1. Keep infant prone at all times; minimize manipulation of the sac.
2. Keep sac covered with sterile gauze moistened with sterile saline.
3. Attempt to stabilize infant's cardiorespiratory status and inform neonatologist of record.
4. Alert the pediatric neurosurgeon, the pediatrician-coordinator of the Spina Bifida Clinic, and the genetic counselor.
5. If infant is born at a site distant from the medical center at which surgery is to be performed, make arrangements for transfer as soon as the patient is stable.
6. Generally all newborns with MM undergo operation within the first 48 hours of life. Occasionally, surgery is delayed for medical reasons. The decision of when to perform surgery is made by the attending staff.
7. Before surgery, obtain the following:
   CBC with platelets
   Type and cross for surgery
   Electrolytes, BUN, and creatinine levels
   Anteroposterior and lateral radiographs of the skull
   Urinalysis
   Urine for culture and sensitivity (obtained by catheterization)
   CT scan or sonogram of head
8. Obtain parental consent to perform the operation after the informing interview held with neurosurgeon, pediatrician-coordinator, and genetic counselor.

Postoperative
Neurosurgical
1. Keep infant prone and in Trendelenberg position until supine positioning has been approved by neurosurgery service.
2. Keep dressing clean and dry. All dressing changes must be done by neurosurgery service.
3. Check and chart infant's head circumference daily.
4. If head circumference is increasing, perform CT or sonogram.
5. If hydrocephalus is documented, schedule surgery for placement of VPS.
Urologic
1. Inform Spina Bifida urologist of infant's admission.
2. Obtain sonogram of kidneys and urinary tract to rule out hydronephrosis.
3. Note voiding pattern (e.g., voids spontaneously, dribbles).
4. Beginning at 4 days after surgery, catheterize the bladder after voiding for 2 days to check for the presence of residual urine.
5. Check initial urine culture report. If positive, begin appropriate antibiotic.
Orthopedic surgery
1. Inform Spina Bifida orthopedist of infant's admission.
2. Obtain radiographs of the hips in neutral and frog-leg lateral positions as soon as possible.

After a postoperative course during which the child's condition is carefully monitored, the infant is discharged from the hospital. In most cases, the initial inpatient stay lasts between 2 and 6 weeks. Longer stays, necessitated by complications of the initial surgical management such as localized infection, meningitis, sepsis, shunt malfunction, and Arnold-Chiari crisis, occur in 10 to 20 percent of our patients.

MANAGEMENT OF THE CHILD WITH MYELOMENINGOCELE

After the neonatal period, children with MM are followed in an outpatient clinic at the Blythedale Children's Hospital, a facility located a short distance from the Montefiore Medical Center. The clinic, which meets once a month, is designed to minimize the time and expense needed to provide children with MM the medical care necessary to ensure proper health and optimal functioning. The clinic is staffed by the neurosurgeon, urologist, orthopedic surgeon, rehabilitation medicine specialist, developmentalist, and psychiatrist, as well as the pediatrician-coordinator. In addition to these medical and surgical specialists, the following individuals are important members of our Spina Bifida team:

1. *Pediatric nurse practitioners,* who perform bladder catheterization on all arriving patients to evaluate postvoid residual urine volumes and obtain surveillance cultures. In addition, the nurses teach techniques of clean intermittent catheterization (which are reinforced through the use of simply worded instruction sheets) and previously taught concepts such as signs and symptoms of increased intracranial pressure, and help the pediatrician-coordinator in running the clinic.
2. *Social workers,* who help patients secure necessary health care benefits and needed equipment, serve as advocates for the patient and the family in their interfacing with social agencies and the public school system, run a parent and adolescent support group on a regular basis, and offer limited counseling services to patients who are having difficulty coping with the stresses caused by their disabilities.
3. The *orthotist,* who makes and fits orthotic devices to the specifications prescribed by the orthopedic surgeon and the physiatrist.
4. The *genetic counselor,* who prepares a complete family pedigree on all MM patients, explains the multifactorial inheritance pattern known to occur in families with a history of MM, counsels the parents regarding the 4 percent recurrence risk in future progeny, and arranges prenatal diagnostic services for couples who have already had one affected child.
5. *Laboratory personnel,* including an x-ray technician.
6. The *transportation coordinator,* whose responsibility it is to ensure that patients scheduled for clinic visits are aware of their appointment and are able to get to the hospital with all the necessary equipment.

The typical steps followed by patients during a

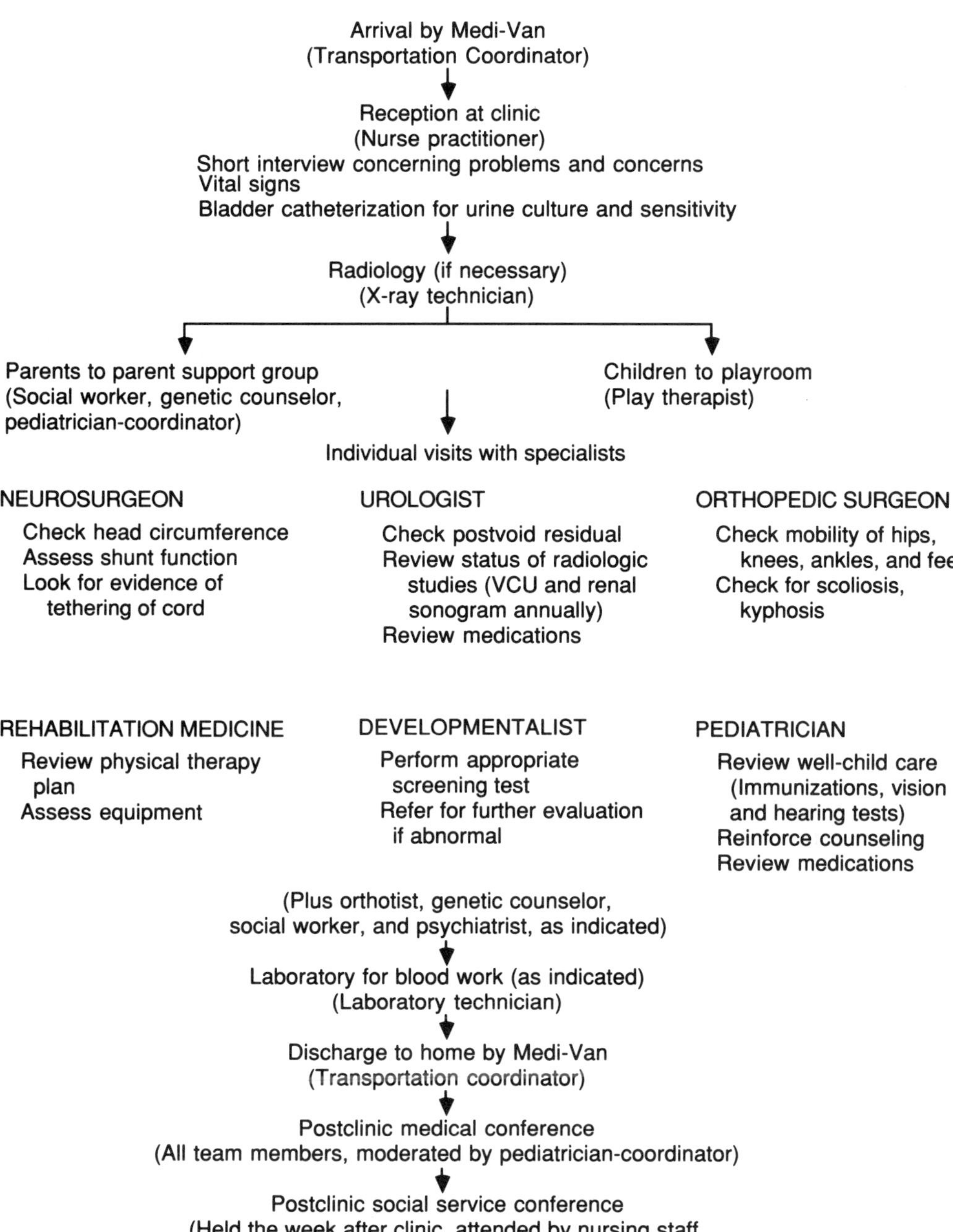

Figure 1 Management of patients with MM at Spina Bifida Clinic.

visit to our Spina Bifida Clinic are summarized in Figure 1.

Each physician involved in the care of patients with MM has developed his or her own protocol to assure that quality medical care is delivered. The principles of these protocols are as follows.

Neurosurgical Protocol

After the initial hospitalization, the neurosurgeon follows infants and children on a regular basis, looking for signs and symptoms of shunt malfunc-tion in those who have VPSs in place and for signs and symptoms of hydrocephalus in those who have not required shunts in the past. If evidence of these problems is found, the patient is rehospitalized, and replacement (or placement) of the VPS is performed. Additionally, the neurosurgeon vigilantly observes the patient for evidence of progressive neurologic dysfunction in bowel and bladder function and in lower extremity strength and mobility—signs and symptoms that may herald the onset of tethering of the spinal cord, an occasional complication of MM repair.

Urologic Protocol

In most patients with MM, urologic dysfunction is a serious, potentially lethal complication. For this reason, careful management by a urologist experienced in the care of children with neurogenic bladders is essential.

Children with neurogenic bladders fall into two categories: those with urinary retention and overflow, and those with total urinary incontinence. In patients with the former problem, increased sphincteric activity results in persistent retention of urine after voiding. Ultimately bladder thickening, upper urinary tract dilatation, vesiculoureteral reflux of urine, and recurrent urinary tract infections occur. In patients with high urinary residual volumes, clean intermittent bladder catheterization, coupled with frequent radiologic and urodynamic studies, is essential.

Patients with neurogenic bladders who demonstrate complete urinary incontinence are found by catheterization to have little or no retention of urine. These children, unlike those with urinary retention, are initially at no great risk. However, careful monitoring is essential, as infants who demonstrate total incontinence early in life often develop increased sphincteric tone later and ultimately retain urine.

During the neonatal period, as indicated in Table 1, the bladders of infants with MM should be catheterized after voiding, to assess the presence of residual volume. For those patients who demonstrate total incontinence, postvoid residual volumes must be carefully monitored during every visit to Spina Bifida Clinic.

Bowel incontinence is a disturbing problem for many patients with MM, a problem that becomes greater as the patient reaches adolescence. In our clinic, the urologist, in addition to managing bladder function, is responsible for bowel training. Working with the pediatric nurse practitioners, a bowel protocol is developed and prescribed for each patient who requests one.

Orthopedic Protocol

The goal of orthopedic management is to make the child with MM as functional as possible, based on the neurologic deficit caused by the lesion. Some children with MM will be able to walk without assistance; some will be able to ambulate with braces or other equipment; some will require walkers or parapodia for ambulation; some will never be able to ambulate but will be able to sit upright in a wheelchair. The orthopedic surgeon, working with the physiatrist and the orthotist, develops a plan for each child enrolled in the clinic. Early in life, children with MM commonly have one or more of the following problems: congenital dislocated hips, talipes equinovarus, and contractures of the hips, knees, and/or ankles. Later, scoliosis and/or kyphosis occur, abnormalities that are indirectly related to the initial defect in the spine. Surgical intervention must be carefully planned to correct each of these problems so that the quality of life can be improved.

Rehabilitation Medicine Protocol

The rehabilitation medicine specialist works with the orthopedic surgeon and the orthotist in developing a plan that allows the patient to be as functional as possible. This is accomplished through a carefully prescribed program of physical therapy tailored to the special needs of each individual and aided by the use of equipment such as braces, parapodia, walkers, and wheelchairs. The rehabilitation medicine specialist reassesses each patient on an annual basis, evaluating progress and revising the therapeutic plan accordingly.

Developmental Medicine Protocol

The mental development of children with MM covers a whole spectrum, from normal to severe mental retardation. The majority of patients in our clinic function in the normal or borderline range, but learning disability is very common in children with MM. Each child enrolled in the Spina Bifida Clinic therefore periodically receives a screening test appropriate for his or her age performed by a developmentalist. If a delay in development is documented, a complete evaluation is conducted, and intervention is offered in the form of referral to an infant stimulation program for infants and younger children or a recommendation regarding class placement for school-age children.

Psychiatric Protocol

Because reactions to the stress caused by chronic disorders such as MM are frequently manifested in the form of psychiatric disturbances, a child psychiatrist is part of the Spina Bifida Clinic team. Although not present during the monthly meetings of the clinic, the psychiatrist accepts referrals from other members of the clinic's staff who have identified possible disturbances in the patients and/or their families. A full psychiatric evaluation follows, and recommendations are made. Some clinic patients who have received a short course of psychotherapy have responded well; others receive on-going therapy on a weekly basis; and some have required administration of antipsychotic medication in addition to on-going therapy sessions.

Pediatrician-Coordinator Protocol

The pediatrician-coordinator must serve many roles. First and foremost, he must ensure that all of the above-mentioned forms of care are delivered to each patient enrolled in the Spina Bifida Clinic in a timely and efficient fashion. Next, he must be certain that the plan made by each of the other physicians is carefully explained to and understood by the child and his or her family. Additionally, he must ensure that each enrolled patient has a primary care provider and is receiving appropriate health care maintenance (the clinic is not equipped to deliver primary care to our patients) as well as any additional care that is not provided by the clinic. The pediatrician-coordinator must communicate with the patient's primary care provider after each visit to ensure that the provider is aware of the clinic physicians' management plans. Finally, he must serve as the clinic's physician-advocate, intervening on the child's behalf when necessary.

The pediatrician sees each patient for an in-depth intake visit before that patient's first full clinic appointment, and then for a short check-up on an annual basis. He runs the conference that convenes at the conclusion of each month and during which plans for each patient's future care are formulated. Additionally, he supervises the social service conference, held with the social workers, nurse practitioners, psychiatrist, and genetic counselor during the week after the monthly meeting of the Spina Bifida Clinic. At this conference, special problems between the child and his family, and the child and the environment, are discussed, and plans for specific interventions are made.

MANAGEMENT OF THE OLDER CHILD AND ADOLESCENT WITH MYELOMENINGOCELE

Adolescence is a particularly difficult period for individuals with chronic disorders, and MM is no exception. In addition to the problems common to all adolescents, patients with MM must begin to face adult life with the realization that the problems from which they have suffered since early childhood will not disappear in the future, and that previously unanticipated problems may develop. Problems of body image, urinary and bowel continence, and sexuality become important to the patient, often for the first time. For this reason, although adolescents with MM still attend the clinic and see the same panel of physicians, different issues are addressed. Two special programs for adolescents are detailed below.

Adolescent Peer Group

The adolescent group was assembled by a social worker and the psychiatrist for the specific purpose of giving teenage patients the opportunity to talk among themselves, to share experiences and coping mechanisms, and to "let off steam." The group, made up of patients between 13 and 20 years of age, meets on a monthly basis. The psychiatrist, vigilant for symptoms of dysfunctional behavior, evaluates patients noted to have particular difficulties in private sessions after the group meetings.

The group is viewed as a unique, extremely valuable opportunity by most of the adolescent patients, who discover for the first time that others are experiencing many of the same difficulties in their daily lives. These sessions are enthusiastically attended.

Urology

In addition to the duties with the younger patients, the urologist may assess sexual functioning in some of the adolescent males. Sexual dysfunction in men with MM include inability to produce an erection, sterility, and retrograde ejaculation. A careful evaluation of sexual function must be carried out in order to diagnose the problem correctly and offer therapeutic intervention.

Caring for the infant, child, and adolescent with MM is a challenge for the medical community. Although it is possible to care for the child with MM in a piecemeal fashion, a carefully planned, comprehensive multidisciplinary team approach is a much more favorable and cost-effective setting in which necessary care can be efficiently delivered.

SUGGESTED READING

Marion RW. Neural tube defects: meningomyelocoele and anencephaly. Current opinions in neurology and neurosurgery 1988; 1:353–357.
Shurtleff DB, ed. Myelodysplasias and exstrophies: significance, prevention, and treatment. New York: Grune and Stratton, 1986.

PATIENT RESOURCE

The Spina Bifida Association of America, National Office
1700 Rockville Pike, Suite 540
Rockville, Maryland 20852
Telephone: (301)770-7222

A national support group with local offices throughout the United States, the SBAA plays many important roles. It functions as an advocacy group for individuals with MM, as a family support group, and as a fund-raising organization that supports research and treatment. The organization publishes a bimonthly newsletter, "Insights into Spina Bifida," which is distributed free of charge to chapter members.

INTRACRANIAL HEMORRHAGE, PERIVENTRICULAR LEUKOMALACIA, AND HYPOXIC-ISCHEMIC ENCEPHALOPATHY IN THE NEONATE

MICHAEL V. JOHNSTON, M.D.

INTRAVENTRICULAR HEMORRHAGE IN THE PREMATURE INFANT

In premature infants, intraventricular hemorrhage with extension into the periventricular region of the brain is a common cause of later neurologic morbidity. Therapy begins with the identification of risk factors so that appropriate preventive measures can be taken. The most important factors contributing to intracranial hemorrhage in the premature infant appear to be rapid, wide fluctuations in intravascular and intracranial pressure, which overstress an immature capillary bed in the periventricular matrix. Hemorrhage extends into the adjacent brain, and ischemia within this area may further contribute to the damage. This pathophysiologic mechanism is worsened by hypoxia, hypercarbia, hypoglycemia, and sepsis. The incidence of each of these factors is markedly enhanced when the infant is born prematurely, and therefore the most effective treatment is to prevent prematurity.

Several actions appear to reduce the incidence and severity of hemorrhage when premature birth is inevitable. The mother should be transferred to a high-risk perinatal center before delivery, if possible, since special care in the delivery process may reduce the incidence of hemorrhage. Transport inside the uterus prevents environmental fluctuations, which increase the incidence of hemorrhage.

Although not yet standard therapy, several pharmacologic therapies have shown some ability to reduce the incidence of hemorrhage if administered before delivery. Giving the mother a loading dose of phenobarbital of 20 to 30 μg per milliliter 6 hours before delivery has been beneficial in some centers.

After delivery, the newborn at risk for intracranial hemorrhage should be treated in a manner to reduce the hemodynamic disturbances that appear to be risk factors. The infant's circulation should be supported with fluids or blood products to maintain adequate blood pressure and prevent hypotension, although overexpansion of the circulation should be avoided. Hypertonic solutions such as sodium bicarbonate should be avoided or administered slowly to avoid fluctuations in blood pressure. Special care should be taken to avoid periods of apnea, hypercarbia, or hypoxemia, which enhance circulatory instability. Protocols for minimizing stimulation of the infant by maneuvers such as suctioning may be helpful.

The premature infant should be studied serially with ultrasonography. Because small infants need to be transported out of the nursery, computed tomographic scanning is avoided in these neonates. Hemorrhage usually evolves within the first 24 hours after delivery. The severity of hemorrhage is graded according to the volume of the ventricular system that is filled with blood and according to the extent and location of echodensity within the periventricular parenchyma. Grade I hemorrhages occupy less than 10 percent of the ventricular area on several views, Grade II hemorrhages occupy 10 to 50 percent, and Grade III hemorrhages occupy more than 50 percent. Later neurologic outcome is closely correlated with the severity of the periventricular echodensity, which generally reflects areas of hemorrhagic infarction. Echodensity extending into the frontal, parietal, and occipital regions is associated with a high incidence of death and neurologic disability.

Specific treatments for preventing hemorrhage in the neonate show some promise. Neuromuscular paralysis in ventilated premature infants appears to be associated with a marked reduction in the incidence of intraventricular hemorrhage. This treatment has been shown to convert a widely fluctuating cerebral blood flow velocity pattern to a more stable one in infants with respiratory distress syndrome. The marked respiratory effort caused by respiratory distress syndrome is associated with dramatic changes in intracerebral hemodynamics. Pneumothorax is especially harmful because the sudden changes in intrathoracic pressure may alter cerebral hemodynamics. Other pharmacologic means for preventing intraventricular hemorrhage have received investigational interest but have not had proven value. These include the administration of phenobarbital, indomethacin, ethamsylate, and vitamin E. These agents may act to "stabilize" cerebral blood vessels and cerebral blood flow. Seizures occurring in the setting of intraventricular hemorrhage should be treated vigorously as described later in this chapter because they may help to extend injury.

In infants with enlarged ventricles secondary to posthemorrhagic communicating hydrocephalus, repeated lumbar punctures every other day are worth a trial over 1 to 2 weeks to prevent the need for a ventriculoperitoneal shunt. Cautious observation of head circumference and ventricular size through the use of ultrasonography is generally warranted. Morbidity appears to be more closely related to the area of ischemic infarction than to the degree of hydrocephalus. Ventriculomegaly related to hemorrhage may stabilize and become compensated. The availability of ultrasonography in the nursery makes it possible to observe this process frequently.

PERIVENTRICULAR LEUKOMALACIA IN THE PREMATURE INFANT

Periventricular leukomalacia (PVL) in premature infants is believed to represent symmetric areas of infarction in the frontal white matter surrounding the frontal horns of the ventricular system. The occurrence of these lesions in areas that represent a vascular watershed area is believed to reflect a combination of hypoxic ischemia and hypotension. Other factors such as gram-negative sepsis may contribute to the evolution of PVL. The evolution of the cystic lesions can be followed serially with ultrasonography. Echodensities appear in the periventricular zones before characteristic cystic areas evolve. PVL is associated with a form of cerebral palsy known as spastic diplegia involving all four extremities, the legs particularly. No effective preventive treatment or therapy has been proven to reduce the severity of PVL. As with intraventricular hemorrhage, efforts to prevent or treat hypotension and circulatory insufficiency, hypercarbia, hypoxemia, and acidosis are probably important for preventing this lesion and limiting its extension.

HYPOXIC-ISCHEMIC ENCEPHALOPATHY

Hypoxic-ischemic encephalopathy occurs in both full-term and premature infants. It is a syndrome affecting the brain as well as several other organs that evolves after an extended, severe episode of combined hypoxemia and ischemia.

Recognition of hypoxic-ischemic encephalopathy is important for instituting appropriate therapy and for accurate documentation in the medical record. Extensive epidemiologic data suggest that a documented postnatal episode of hypoxemia or ischemia or an event such as a difficult delivery does not produce permanent brain injury unless the infant develops the syndrome of hypoxic-ischemic encephalopathy within hours after the insult. Accurate recognition and documentation of hypoxic-ischemic encephalopathy in the infant's neonatal chart may be helpful retrospectively for clarifying the nature of later neurologic disability. Infants with severe encephalopathy lasting more than 48 hours generally have some permanent brain injury.

Brain dysfunction and behavioral changes in hypoxic-ischemic encephalopathy include lethargy, poor feeding, hypotonia, and seizures. Early in the episode, the infant may go through a period of hyperalertness. It is unusual for the brain to be injured by a hypoxic-ischemic episode if there are no associated complications in the cardiovascular, respiratory, hematopoietic, or renal systems. Hypoxic-ischemic encephalopathy is typically accompanied by evidence of renal dysfunction such as acute tubular necrosis or a period of decreased urinary output. Cellular elements of the kidney appear to be as sensitive as the brain to hypoxic injury. Involvement of other organs may worsen the hypoxic-ischemic encephalopathy, and these dysfunctions should be aggressively treated in the neonatal intensive care unit.

Behavioral abnormalities and seizures in infants with hypoxic-ischemic encephalopathy are produced by neuronal dysfunction. Although the brain injured by hypoxia-ischemia contains some neurons and other cellular elements that are destined to die, other populations may possibly be salvaged by appropriate therapy. At present, careful attention to cardiovascular and general supportive management are the primary focus of therapy, although more specific therapies that may improve salvage of damaged neurons may be developed in the future.

Measures should be taken to optimize cerebral blood flow and to match flow with metabolic demands. The circulation of the damaged brain appears to be more pressure-passive and has less autoregulatory control than the normal brain. Therefore the maintenance of optimal cardiac output and blood pressure is especially important. Unless absolutely necessary, severe fluid restriction to treat cerebral edema should be avoided because of the danger that hypovolemia will worsen ischemia. Hyperventilation may also be used to assist in reducing intracranial pressure, but a $P\text{co}_2$ of less than 20 should be avoided because it may reduce cerebral blood flow. Clinically useful measures for quantitating cerebral blood flow in infants should be developed.

In experimental settings, an elevated serum glucose may worsen asphyxial brain injury by elevating levels of lactic acid. The optimal blood sugar concentration for infants with hypoxia-ischemia is not known. A reasonable approach is to prevent or correct hypoglycemia while avoiding excessive infusion of glucose, which might produce high glucose levels. Elevated glucose levels may lead to rapid metabolic shifts, which could change cerebral circulation as well as contribute to excessive lactic acid accumulation.

Seizures are an important indicator of the severity of neuronal dysfunction in patients with hypoxic-ischemic encephalopathy. Seizures may also damage the brain directly in this setting both by allowing neurotransmitters and other substances released at synapses to reach toxic levels and by exhausting metabolic substrates. Frequent monitoring of electroencephalography in hypoxic-ischemic infants for detecting electrical evidence of seizure activity is desirable. It is not certain whether the severe injury associated with severe encephalopathy reflects hypoxic-ischemic neuronal injury or a contribution from seizures. My impression is that seizures in the context of hypoxic-ischemic encephalopathy should be treated aggressively because of their propensity to extend injury in the metabolically compromised brain.

Seizures should be anticipated and treated with anticonvulsants when they occur. Treatment should also include reassessment for metabolic causes of seizures such as hypoglycemia, hyponatremia, hypomagnesemia, and inborn errors of metabolism. Loading doses of 10 to 30 mg per kilogram of phenobarbital can be given safely if administered slowly. Serum concentrations as high as 50 μg per milliliter are usually well tolerated, but higher levels may compromise cardiac output. I usually recommend phenobarbital loading for any infant with evidence of hypoxic-ischemic encephalopathy even before seizures begin.

If seizures persist despite treatment with phenobarbital, phenytoin in a loading dose of 10 to 20 mg per kilogram is administered up to a serum level of 20 μg per milliliter. Phenytoin is difficult to use orally in newborns because of poor absorption and usually must be maintained with intravenous doses. Primidone in an oral loading dose of 15 to 25 mg per kilogram is sometimes useful as a third drug if seizures persist for more than several days. In individual cases, pyridoxine administration (50 or 100 mg IV or IM) should be considered in patients with refractory seizures to make certain that these seizures are not related to this treatable metabolic cause.

Cerebral edema in patients with hypoxic-ischemic encephalopathy is primarily related to neuronal and glial accumulation of water rather than to extravasation of edema from blood vessels. Measures useful for controlling edema in patients with hypoxic-ischemic encephalopathy include hyperventilation and fluid restriction. Steroids are not helpful in the treatment of hypoxic ischemia edema, and it seems unlikely that edema itself makes any significant contribution to the evolution of hypoxic-ischemic neuronal damage until it becomes quite severe. Excessively vigorous efforts to treat cerebral edema may be harmful, and primary efforts to control cerebral edema are not likely to alter the ultimate outcome of hypoxic-ischemic encephalopathy. Therefore the therapeutic focus should be on correcting cerebrovascular and metabolic abnormalities rather than on the edema itself.

SUGGESTED READING

Johnston MV, Silverstein FS. New insights into mechanisms of neuronal damage in the developing brain. Pediatr Neurosci 1986; 12:87–89.

Painter MJ, Pippenger C, MacDonald H, Pitlick W. Phenobarbital and diphenylhydantoin levels in neonates with seizures. J Pediatr 1978; 92:315.

Volpe JJ. Intraventricular hemorrhage in the premature infant: current concepts. Part 2. Ann Neurol 1989; 25:109–116.

CEREBRAL PALSY

ALAN I. ROSENBLATT, M.D.
FREDERICK B. PALMER, M.D.

Cerebral palsy (CP) has traditionally been defined as a disorder of movement and posture resulting from a static lesion of the developing brain.

Several points regarding this definition deserve special emphasis. First, in order to make a diagnosis of CP, the physician must be certain that the brain lesion is static. This may be clear from the medical history and neurologic examination, or it may require extensive laboratory or imaging studies to exclude possible progressive or neurodegenerative etiologies. Second, although the brain lesion in patients with CP is static, the neurologic symptoms may be expected to change with brain development. Thus the infant with prominent hypotonia may soon develop choreoathetosis and eventually become rigidly dystonic during adolescence. These changes in motor symptoms may require frequent changes in intervention strategies. Third, the child with a brain lesion resulting in motor deficits (CP) is almost certain to have other neurologic deficits in areas of cognition, language, sensory function, and behavior. Further, secondary nutritional, skeletal, and other medical deficits are extremely common. Often the associated deficits present the child with a far greater functional handicap than the motor impairment alone, and therefore become the major focus for treatment. Table 1 offers an abbreviated list of such deficits.

The overall goal of therapy is to provide the optimal setting for realizing the child's potential for development within the constraints of his or her organic deficits. It is generally accepted that a diagnosis of CP must include a characterization of the nature, topography, and severity of motor handicap. It must also include a complete (or as complete as possible) delineation of associated neurologic and

Table 1 Associated Dysfunctions

Cognitive
  Mental retardation
  Learning disability
Communication
  Speech disorders
  Language processing disorders (developmental dysphasia)
  Hearing loss
Visual
  Strabismus
  Refractive errors
  Field cuts
  Visual processing disorders
  Blindness (cortical, nerve)
Emotional/Behavioral
  Attention deficit hyperactivity disorder
  Self-injurious behavior
Sensory
  All modalities may be affected
Oral-Motor/Nutrition
  Inadequate intake
  Direct aspiration
  Gastroesophageal reflux
Seizures
  All types
  Infantile spasms
  Lennox-Gastaut
Pseudodegeneration
  Plateau
  Motor loss, cognitive loss

medical deficits and coexisting social or family problems. This is a prerequisite to rational treatment and is best coordinated by the managing physician. Individualized treatment plans usually involve several different disciplines and should be directed at the entire scope of the handicap rather than solely, or even primarily, at the motor aspect. Successful supervision of care enables the patient to avoid undesirable medical and surgical complications as much as possible and may enhance social conditions for the child such that he or she may participate in community life. Comprehensive diagnosis and management is a complicated process and generally requires an interdisciplinary team. Table 2 lists some of the indications and goals for involving nonphysician specialties in the evaluation and care of the child with CP and adds some clinically relevant comments regarding their utilization.

This chapter gives a capsule summary of the treatment approach used for children with CP at the Kennedy Institute for Handicapped Children. It is intended to reflect our experience, rather than be exhaustive. It is presented with the realization that little conclusive evidence is available to support the efficacy of individual interventions, but also with the recognition that careful, knowledgeable medical supervision of intervention is likely to be necessary for optimal outcome.

TREATMENT OF MOTOR ABNORMALITIES

A basic guideline for the management of the motor disorder in CP is presented in Figure 1. One of the key factors determining the aggressiveness of intervention necessary is the gross motor developmental quotient (MoQ). The MoQ is a ratio of the child's motor age, based on standardized milestones, divided by the child's chronologic age. For example, a child of 15 months whose best gross motor milestone is sitting with support (the best gross motor milestone of the average 6-month-old infant) would have a MoQ of 0.4 (6/15). Standardized milestones are available in most pediatric textbooks and in the Harriet Lane Handbook. In general, patients with a MoQ greater than 0.5 do not require vigorous motor intervention and may usually be monitored at regular intervals. Exceptions to this rule include infants with hemiplegia in whom only mild gross motor handicap is expected (although these infants have substantial fine motor abnormalities that traditionally require intervention).

Physical Therapy and Orthotics

Our approach to using physical therapy in the treatment of CP utilizes a modified version of the Bobath neurodevelopmental technique. In this method, manual guidance and repetition are employed to counteract abnormal patterns of movement and posture and facilitate more normal movement reactions. The use of proper positioning helps avoid interfering primitive reflexes, thereby enhancing function. For example, a child with increased trunk extension and shoulder retraction (tonic labyrinthine reflex) will have difficulty with visual-motor and adaptive skills such as finger feeding. Proper positioning in a modified seating device limits neck extension and subsequent reflexive retraction of the shoulders, thus allowing for more functional use of the upper extremities.

A combination of physical therapy and orthotic devices is used to prevent contractures, provide support, promote stability, and limit involuntary movement that might inhibit function. Passive stretching activities are intended to maintain maximum range of motion and are taught to family members. Leg braces and ankle-foot orthoses may permit weight bearing and better balance. Braces for the back, head, and neck may be manufactured to improve head control, thereby allowing for better visual fixation. Arm splints enable an athetoid child to control involuntary movements that thwart purposeful upper extremity activities. Sandbags and wedges are used for positioning of the child while in bed and may be adapted for use with seating devices.

Table 2 Use of Nonphysician Specialties in the Treatment of Children with CP

Specialty	Common Indications	Goals	Comments
Special Nutrition Services	Based on the weight for height curve, those patients at either the 5th percentile or the 95th percentile Based on the weight for height curve, those patients showing a marked weight loss over a short interval (even if they are not yet at the 5th percentile Other reason(s) for suspecting insufficient caloric intake (e.g., poor swallow, gastroesophageal reflux)	Estimation of present caloric intake based on the dietary history Estimation of caloric requirements based on ideal body weight Establishing desirable parameters for growth Establishing dietary recommendations for home and school, and monitoring progress	Nutritional problems in patients with CP often require extensive medical workups and may reveal significant gastroesophageal reflux, particularly in the more severely motor-handicapped patients. Oral feeding alone may be inadequate for meeting caloric requirements, and gavage or gastrostomy feeds may be necessary. Based on the weight for height curve, the ideal body weight for the child with CP is at the 10th percentile.

Occupational Therapy	Fine motor delay (DQ <0.5)*
	Presence of or risk of contractures in the upper extremities
	Based on the child's cognitive level, overdependence on others for activites of daily living
	Oromotor dysfunction, drooling, inadequate oral intake for meeting caloric needs, excessive time required for feeding
	Equipment needs
		Obtaining a profile of present skills:
		  upper extremity function, oromotor function, activities of daily living
		Establishing recommendations for intervention:
		  Therapeutic activities for school and home to facilitate upper extremity and oromotor skills and promote participation in activities of daily living
		  Avoiding undesirable movement patterns
		  Proper positioning and range-of-motion excercises
		Recommending or manufacturing orthotic devices:
		  Eating utensils and devices
		  Upper extremity splints (with orthopedics)
		  Seating and bathing devices; other adaptive devices for activities of daily living
			A cine-esophagram during feeding (using foods of different textures) will help evaluate swallowing and the potential for aspiration.
			The patient's ability to participate in activities of daily living is influenced by his or her cognitive level as well as by his or her motor capacity.

Physical Therapy	Gross motor delay (MoQ < 0.5)†
	Difficult or inefficient ambulation in the absence of prominent delay
	Persistence of primitive reflexes and abnormalities of tone interfering with function or management
	Presence of or risk of contractures in the lower extremities
	Transportation needs
		Obtaining a profile of present skills: gross motor function, locomotion, postural reactions
		Establishing recommendations for intervention:
		  Therapeutic activities for home and school that establish more favorable movement and postural patterns, avoiding abnormal primitive reflexes
		Recommending or manufacturing orthotic devices:
		  Braces and splints (with orthopedics)
		  Means of transportation (e.g., suitable wheelchair, walker, quad canes, single point canes)
		  Home equipment (ramps, rails, lifts, positioning devices)
			Videotaping the patient in conjuction with specific therapies (e.g., medications, physical therapy evaluation) is often helpful in qualitative assessments.
			It is helpful to have a physical therapist present for orthopedic evaluations.
			"One-time" consultations for children with an MoQ of 0.5–0.7 may provide parents with informal suggestions for appropriate motor activities and thereby allay anxieties.

Audiology	Hearing loss that may cause or confound disorders of language and communication	Determining whether hearing loss is conductive, sensorineural, central, or mixed
		Assessment or monitoring of:
		  Middle ear function
		  Peripheral auditory sensitivity to stimuli within speech frequencies
		  Brainstem auditory function
		Recommending and applying amplification, if indicated
			Because of the prevalence of hearing loss in patients with CP, initial evaluation is particularly useful.
			Office-based hearing screening is unreliable and insensitive.
			Brainstem auditory evoked responses (BAER's) are a nonspecific measure of hearing loss in high-risk premature infants during the newborn period. More specific results using BAER, behavioral audiometry, and acoustic impedance audiometry are obtained after the patient is 6 months old.
			Early treatment of hearing loss may significantly improve outcome.

Speech and Language	Global language delay
	Isolated expressive language delay
	Dysarthria
		Obtaining a language profile:
		  expressive language, receptive
		  language, articulation
		Establishing recommendations for
		  intervention:
		    Speech therapy in school and at home
		    Augmentative systems including communication
		      boards and electronic devices
		    Therapy for feeding problems
			Receptive language may be surprisingly better than expressive language and may be difficult to assess, especially in the choreoathetoid patient with oromotor and upper extremity involvement. Repeat evaluations may be necessary.
			Isolated articulation lessons are usually not rewarding.

Psychometric Testing	Mental retardation and/or learning disabilities Suspected plateau, degeneration, or difficulty in the assigned school setting	Obtaining a cognitive profile: IQ and patterns of strengths and weaknesses, achievement level in reading, math, and writing	Because the majority of children with CP are mentally retarded or have learning disabilities, it is helpful to have an assessment at the time of diagnosis and again before any anticipated change in educational placement. Re-evaluations are useful in patients with suspected plateau, degeneration, or difficulty in the assigned school setting. Achievement testing may be handled by Special Education. Parent and teacher input is crucial in assessing discrepancies between IQ and achievement Special testing instruments and methods may be necessary for children with severe motor or sensory impairment.
Special Education (Private or School-Based)	Child is entering first grade or change has been suggested Detailed testing is desired to delineate strengths and weaknesses (i.e., in developing an Individualized Education Plan)	Assessment of levels of current functioning across all academic areas Some assessment of the most and least successful modalities of academic performance (i.e., auditory vs. visual; time-restricted vs. unlimited time) Establishing recommendations for classroom placement and special adaptations necessary for teaching and grading the patient's work	Teacher input is invaluable. Special Education evaluation should take place in conjunction with psychometric testing. Special Education evaluation for a patient with an IQ of <55 may not be necessary.
Behavioral Psychology	Parent or teacher has difficulty managing the patient's behavioral problems Patient is prone to excessive physical punishment (risk for abuse).	Identification of target behaviors to be treated Establishing consistent behavior protocol for home and school Monitoring efficacy of protocol in all environments, and revising protocol as necessary	Behavior modification techniques may be enhanced by medication (e.g., methylphenidate). Teachers and other caretakers should be involved in program.
Social Work	Home environment and family dynamics are problematic The family's understanding of the patient's problems is insufficient Access to services and support networks are insufficient Additional sources of stress	Estimation of family's ability to meet patient's needs and adjust to child's disability Recommending and/or providing resources to family members for financial, emotional, interpersonal, and marital stresses Facilitation of family's understanding of diagnoses and recommendations	It is often impossible for the busy clinician to attend to the many details involved in this process without the aid of a knowledgeable social worker. Respite care services to ensure that primary caretakers are able to meet their own needs may be necessary to enhance the long-term outlook for family-provided care. Evaluation in cases of suspected child abuse is essential.

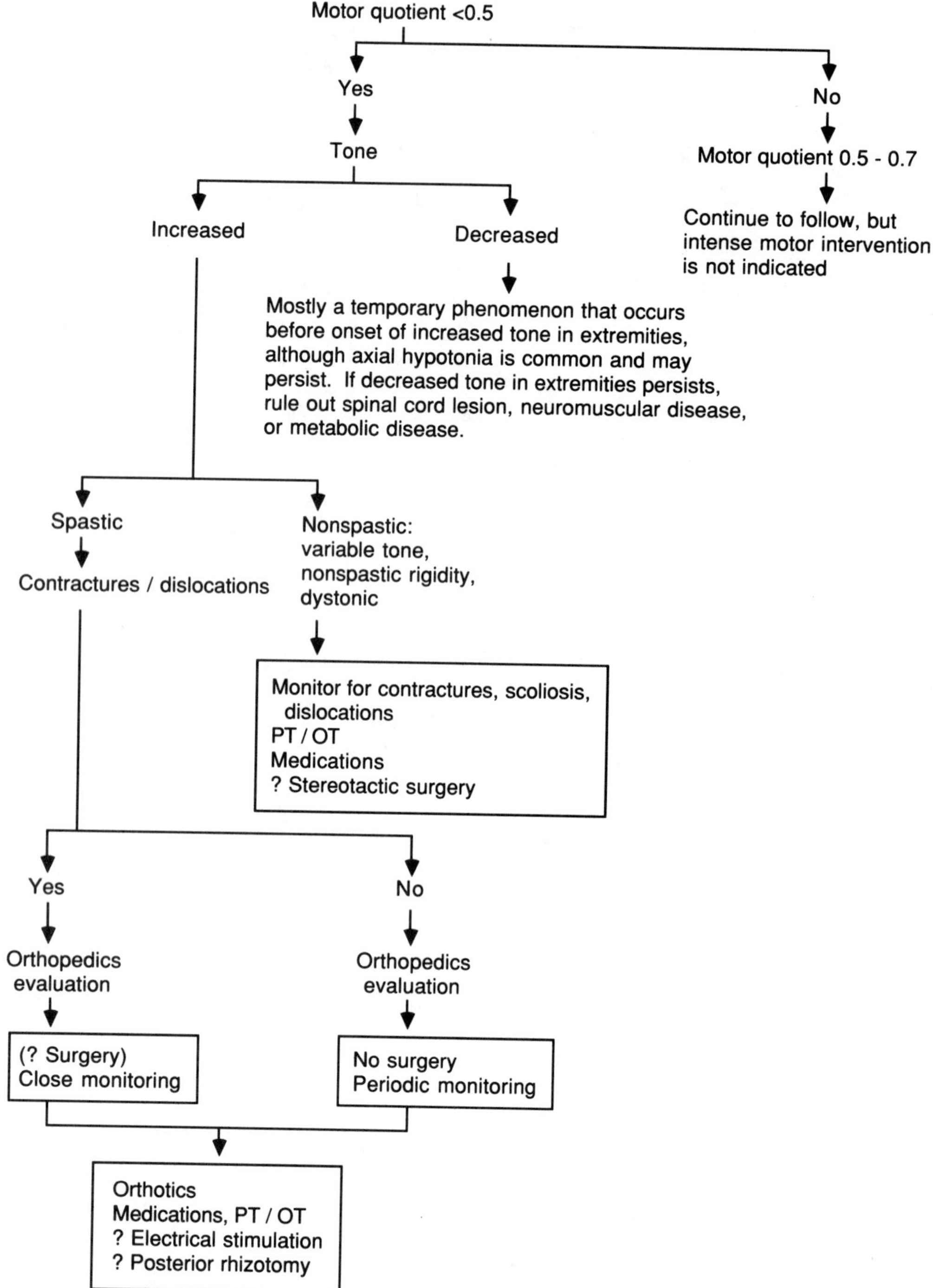

Figure 1 Management of cerebral palsy in the infant and preschool child.

Medications

The use of medication is primarily directed at reduction of hypertonus rather than at control of involuntary movements. The most commonly prescribed drug for this purpose is diazepam. It is used routinely in the patient who has undergone orthopedic surgery and who is at risk for pathologic fractures and may suffer pain from intense muscle spasms during the postoperative period. Diazepam may also be used as adjunctive therapy for control of muscle tone. Before prescribing this drug, one should define what effect of the medication is intended. One should aim to optimize both tone and function, in conjunction with the other modalities of treatment, producing a minimum of undesirable side effects. To determine its efficacy, drug therapy is generally coordinated with the reports of the child's caretakers and therapists.

Flexibility in dosage and in choice of medication is useful in developing a successful regimen. The dosage of diazepam for muscle relaxation usually ranges from 0.1 to 0.5 mg per kilogram per day, divided into oral doses administered three times daily or four times daily. For a child younger than 5 years of age, the usual dose is 1 to 2 mg. In older children, we seldom administer more than 5 mg per dose, although higher doses may be well tolerated. The dosage may need to be gradually increased over a period of several days or weeks to avoid excessive sedation. Other undesirable side effects include drooling and decreased oromotor function (to the point of interfering with feeding), ataxia, and excessive hypotonia. Abrupt cessation of diazepam may produce serious withdrawal symptoms.

Although they are seldom used in our center, baclofen and dantrolene sodium are alternatives to diazepam in adults and older children. Baclofen is given in a dose of 5 mg three times daily and increased by 5 mg per dose every 3 days until the desired effect is produced. The maximum daily dose is 80 mg. Side effects include drowsiness, nausea, and headache; sudden discontinuation of this agent may cause withdrawal symptoms or acute increase in spasticity. Dantrolene may not have a readily apparent effect, and therefore the dosage should not be increased more frequently than once per week. The initial dose is 0.5 mg per kilogram twice daily, then three times daily and four times daily, increased by 0.5 mg to 3 mg per kilogram four times daily, not to exceed 100 mg four times daily in children. It is contraindicated in patients with active hepatic disease, and liver function tests should be routinely monitored. Changes in sensorium, weakness, and diarrhea may be precipitated. Weakness which substantially reduces motor function is usually unacceptable even if spasticity is reduced.

Agents used to control movement disorders, such as benztropine, levodopa, carbidopa-levodopa, and trihexyphenidyl hydrochloride, generally have not been effective in our experience with cerebral palsy but do offer an option in the treatment of children with severe movement disorders.

Orthopedic Surgery

Candidates for orthopedic surgery include the following: (1) patients whose motor function is impaired by deformity, contracture, or muscle imbalance, (2) those with progressive spine deformity, and (3) those whose hips are dislocated or are at risk for dislocation. The goal of surgery is to maximize function, optimize posture and the ability to take part in the activities of daily living, relieve pain, and prevent further complications of untreated orthopedic deformities, such as compromised cardiopulmonary function in patients with severe scoliosis or chronic and/or recurrent pressure sores caused by hip dislocation. Procedures may involve (1) muscle releases, lengthenings, or transfers, (2) neurectomies, (3) osteotomies, and (4) instrumentation. Orthopedic surgeons are increasingly using gait analysis laboratories to identify problematic muscle groups more precisely, provide objective indications for surgery, and establish measures for assessing surgical outcome. We obtain a baseline orthopedic evaluation for patients with hypertonus and have physical therapists and sometimes occupational therapists present at the evaluation. It should be remembered that nonambulatory patients have decreased bone mineralization and may be prone to fractures from relatively minor injuries.

Neurologic Surgery

Despite reports in the literature of successful outcomes of various neurosurgical interventions, we do not recommend neurosurgical intervention except for patients with hydrocephalus or localized seizure foci that are refractory to pharmacologic treatment. Selective lumbar dorsal rhizotomy may offer a treatment option for lower extremity spasticity, but we do not believe that this technique is ready for widespread application until more objective long-term data have been collected.

Stereotactic thalamic and dentate lesions for the treatment of dystonia have also been reported, with disappointing results. Recent positive experience with Parkinson's disease incorporating microrecording and modern imaging techniques may eventually lead to useful neurosurgical approaches to CP.

Electrical Stimulation and Biofeedback

The use of transcutaneous, epidural, and cerebellar electrical stimulation has been described. To date, there are no convincing objective data in the literature to support the benefit of electrical stimulation, and the degree of invasiveness and discomfort associated with its use may be considerable.

Biofeedback training involves the use of behavioral techniques together with objective measurements of muscle tension (e.g., electromyography) to produce voluntary control of muscle activity to simulate normal patterns more closely. This method requires a great deal of motivation and cognitive capacity. Although the use of biofeedback is noninvasive, outcome results are most beneficial in children who have involvement of only a few muscle groups and have been reported for only a small number of patients. We have not relied on this technique to any significant extent in the routine therapy of our patients.

Special Equipment

A checklist of equipment for the motor-impaired child would consist of braces, splints, positioning devices (wedges, rolls, and sandbags), seating devices (car seat, high chair or wheelchair, and bathing seat), and mobility aids (stroller, wheelchair, canes, and walker).

Numerous devices are available to aid the child who has motor, sensory, and communicative disabilities: electric wheelchairs, remote-control toys and aids, communication devices with voice synthesizers, and computers that read, print, and operate various appliances. The National Institute on Disability and Rehabilitation Research in the United States Department of Education helps fund a national network of bioengineering and rehabilitation research centers to develop and apply advanced technology for the improvement of function and promotion of independence among the disabled. Appropriate application of this technology and the most suitable use of equipment must be individualized based on the needs and capabilities of each child.

Recreational Activities

Over the past several decades, strides have been made in society's general appreciation of the capacity of individuals with CP to participate in and enjoy physical exercise and sports. Young children with CP should be allowed to participate in physical activities similar to those of other children their age, provided that this poses no extensive risk to their health and as long as participation is carried out under appropriate guidance and supervision. The National Handicapped Sports and Recreation Association and a special committee of the United States Olympic Commission devoted to Sports and the Disabled Athlete promote training and competition on community levels as well as international levels. The Boy Scouts and Girl Scouts of America also have recreational activities for handicapped youngsters.

FAMILY MANAGEMENT

Successful treatment of the patient with CP requires that one consider the child's household and the needs of all of the family members. Extra stresses are inevitably placed on the family of any child with a disability, and there is generally a greater frequency of marital discord, separation, divorce, and perhaps a feeling of neglect among siblings of handicapped children. Many children come from single-parent homes, and the demands for care imposed by the disabled child may be excessive for a single caretaker. Feelings of guilt, depression, anger, and helplessness among other household members may not only compromise the quality of care, but may endanger the child and put him or her

at risk for abuse. These matters should be addressed in the ongoing care plans for each patient, and special counseling sessions may be necessary. Social workers, behavioral and clinical psychologists, and psychiatrists for the family may be crucial in the optimal management of the patient.

ACKNOWLEDGMENTS

Preparation of this chapter is supported in part by Project 917, Maternal and Child Health Service, U.S. Department of Health and Human Services.

SUGGESTED READING

Bleck EE. Orthopaedic management in cerebral palsy. Clinics in developmental medicine, Nos. 99/100. Philadelphia: JB Lippincott, 1987.

Crothers B, Paine RS. The natural history of cerebral palsy. Cambridge, MA: Harvard University Press, 1959.

Matthews DJ. Controversial therapies in the management of cerebral palsy. Pediatr Ann 1988; 17:762–764.

Rubin IL, Crocker AC, eds. Developmental disabilities: delivery of medical care for children and adults. Philadelphia: Lea & Febiger, 1989.

Scrutton D, ed. Management of the motor disorders of children with cerebral palsy. Clinics in developmental medicine, No. 90. Philadelphia: JB Lippincott, 1984.

Thompson GH, Rubin IL, Bilenker RM, eds. Comprehensive management of cerebral palsy. New York: Grune & Stratton, 1983.

PATIENT RESOURCES

Associations

American Academy for Cerebral Palsy and Developmental Medicine
1910 Byrd Avenue
Suite 118
PO Box 11086
Richmond, Virginia 23230
Telephone: (804) 282-0036

Council for Disability Rights
343 S. Dearborn #1503
Chicago, Illinois 60604
Telephone: (312) 922-1093

National Handicapped Sports and Recreation Association
1145 19th Street, NW
Suite 717
Washington, DC 20036
Telephone: (202) 393-7505

National Institute on Disabilities and Rehabilitation Research
U.S. Department of Education
400 Maryland Avenue, SW
Washington, DC 20202-2572
Telephone: (202) 732-1134

National Information Center for Handicapped Children and Youth
1555 Wilson Boulevard
Suite 700
Rosslyn, Virginia 22209
Telephone: (703) 893-6061

United Cerebral Palsy Association, Inc.
66 E. 34th Street
New York, New York 10016
Telephone: (212) 481-6300

Literature for Parents
An update to: a reader's guide for parents of children with mental, physical, or emotional disabilities. Baltimore: Maryland State Planning Counsel on Developmental Disabilities, 1983.

Batshaw ML, Perret YM. Children with handicaps: a medical primer. 2nd ed. Baltimore: Paul H. Brookes Publishing Co., 1986.

Finnie NR. Handling the young cerebral palsied child at home (Revised edition). New York: EP Dutton, 1975.

Fraser BA, Hensinger RN. Managing physical handicaps: a practical guide for parents, care providers, and educators. Baltimore: Paul H. Brookes Publishing Co., 1983.

Pueschel SM, Bernier JC, Weidenman LE, eds. The special child: a source book for parents of children with developmental disabilities. Baltimore: Paul H. Brookes Publishing Co., 1988.

The Exceptional Parent (magazine for parents of handicapped children).
1170 Commonwealth Avenue, Brighton, Massachusetts 02134
Telephone: (617) 730-5800

SYRINGOHYDROMYELIA

JOHN P. LAURENT, M.D.

In 1824, Olliver d'Angers described a cerebrospinal fluid–filled cavity in the spinal cord which may or may not communicate to an enlarged central canal. Such a cavity, the walls of which are largely composed of glial tissue, is classically called a syringomyelia. "Hydromyelia" is the term reserved for an enlarged central canal lined with ependymal tissue. Differentiation between hydromyelia and syringomyelia is clinically difficult, and theories of pathogenesis and treatment modalities are similar. I prefer to combine these two entities under a single name: syringohydromyelia. The syringohydromyelia syndrome is a chronic progressive myelopathy with well described neurologic findings. Asymptomatic patients will eventually lose some function.

The majority of patients with syringohydromyelia have probably had defective development of outflow tracts from the fourth ventricle with patency of the central canal by way of the obex. Hydrodynamic forces enlarge the canal (hydromyelia) and may cause diverticular formation (syringomyelia). Nonhydrodynamic pathologic factors causing cystic dilatation within the spinal cord include alar-basal laminae junction disorders, spinal trauma, arachnoiditis, and spinal cord tumors (these are not discussed in this chapter).

DIAGNOSIS

The diagnosis of syringohydromyelia should be suggested by both neurologic and electrophysiologic studies. Radiographic evaluation should include plain films of the skull and spine. Magnetic resonance imaging (MRI) of both brain and spinal cord aids in establishing the diagnosis and may show the central canal connecting to the fourth ventricle. Dilatation of the ventricles is present in approximately 10 percent of the cases. Although no CSF canal between the fourth ventricle and the central canal has been reported, the majority of our operative cases have demonstrated a large obex opening. The inability to visualize this connection on MRI does not preclude its presence; the diameter of the canal may be quite small.

TREATMENT

Traditional approaches for correction of cystic dilatation in the spinal cord have been directed primarily at the intramedullary cysts; bony decompression cyst aspiration, marsupialization, and other drainage techniques have been reported. Treatment techniques for syringohydromyelia not directed primarily at the intramedullary cysts have included Krayenbuhl's placement of a ventricular shunt in the presence of hydrocephalus, a procedure that successfully reduced progressive myelopathy in 50 percent of cases. Sectioning of the filum terminale has not been consistently effective.

In my experience, once nonhydrodynamic causes of the syringohydromyelia have been excluded, patients with hindbrain abnormalities have benefited from the surgical obstruction of the central canal at the obex (Fig. 1). Gardner directed attention to the cervical-medullary junction. His original procedure involved decompression of this area with a low suboccipital craniectomy extending into a C-1 to C-4 laminectomy. The dura was opened, the ectopic cerebellar tissue was separated, and an opening was made into the fourth ventricle through the inferior medullary velum.

I have performed a similar procedure, which includes the plugging of the central canal at the obex, in 14 children with syringohydromyelia and

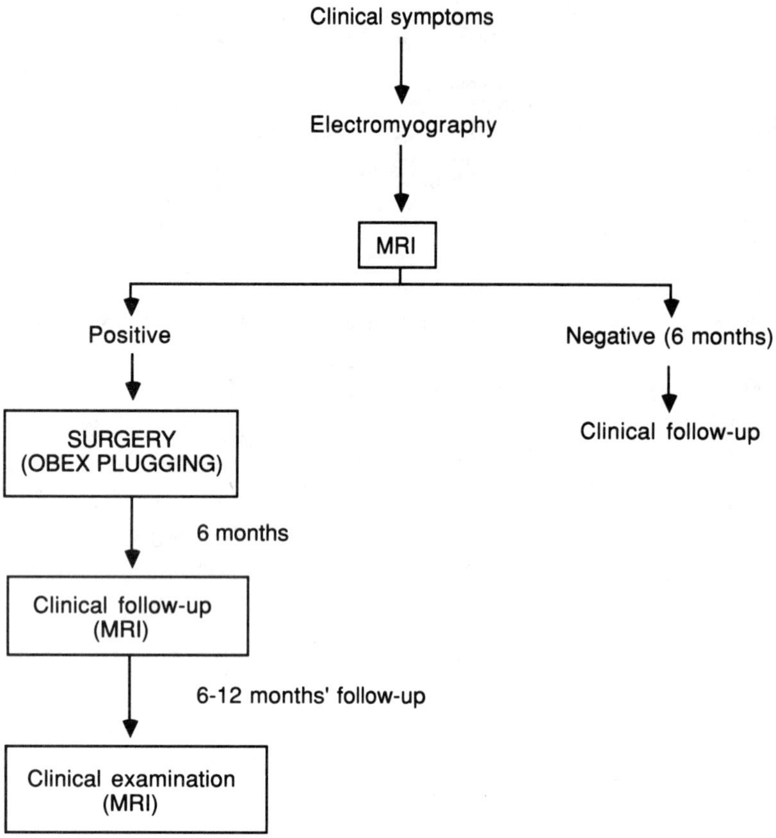

Figure 1 Clinical evaluation of syringohydromyelia.

have encountered very low morbidity and mortality rates. Neurologic function in each of these children has improved postoperatively with a decrease (as documented by MRI) in the size of the syringohydromyelic cavity.

My experience has led me to believe that plugging of the obex is the surgery of choice in children with hindbrain and cervical medullary abnormalities associated with syringohydromyelia.

SUGGESTED READING

Gardner WJ. Hydrodynamic mechanism of syringomyelia. J Neurol Neurosurg Psychiatry 1965; 28:247.

Krayenbuhl H. Evaluation of the different surgical approaches in treatment of syringomyelia. Clin Neurol Neurosurg 1974; 110.

Laurent JP. Syringomyelia and other cranial-cervical anomalies. Curr Opinion Neurol Neurosurg 1988; 1:361–363.

Peerless SJ, Durward QJ. Management of syringomyelia. Clin Neurosurg 1982; 30:531–576.

NEUROFIBROMATOSIS 2

ROSWELL ELDRIDGE, M.D.
ROBERT L. MARTUZA, M.D.
DILYS M. PARRY, Ph.D.

Neurofibromatosis 2 (NF2) or bilateral acoustic neurofibromatosis (previously termed central neurofibromatosis) is a heritable, autosomal dominant disorder distinct from neurofibromatosis 1 (NF1) or von Recklinghausen's disease. The clinical course of NF2 may be relatively benign. Contrary to prevailing opinion, the presence of acoustic neuromas does not lead inevitably to total deafness, diminished vision, or facial disfigurement. By contrast, surgical intervention may result in such changes quickly and with devastating effect. Thus it is imperative to distinguish the patient presenting with an acoustic neuroma of NF2 from the patient with a sporadic, unilateral acoustic neuroma. Diagnosis of and operation for the latter should never be performed in a young individual without first probing for a family history of hearing loss or brain tumors, examining the skin and scalp for changes of neurofibromatosis and the lens of the eye for posterior capsular opacities (which ordinarily are very rare), evaluating hearing in both ears, and excluding other brain or spinal tumors with gadolinium-enhanced high-resolution magnetic resonance imaging.

In this chapter we discuss the clinical and genetic distinctions among NF2, NF1, and sporadic, unilateral acoustic neuroma, and offer an approach to management of NF2 based on our experience with more than 100 patients (both those at risk for and those affected with NF2).

NF2: HISTORY AND CLINICAL FEATURES

More than 160 years ago, Wishart described a Scottish youth who had progressive hearing loss and imbalance that began during adolescence who probably had bilateral acoustic neuromas. He had several other brain tumors as well. Since then, multiple case reports of patients with bilateral acoustic neuromas have appeared, including many with meningiomas, schwannomas of other sensory cranial nerves, and low-grade astrocytomas.

During the 1930s, William James Gardner described a large family in which there were more than 30 individuals with bilateral acoustic neuromas. The trait was transmitted in an autosomal dominant fashion to approximately half of the offspring of an affected individual. Although relatively few had café au lait spots or neurofibromas, Gardner considered the trait to be an example of von Recklinghausen neurofibromatosis because of the pattern of inheritance and the bilaterality of the acoustic neuromas.

In 1970, our restudy of this family indicated more than 100 affected members in nine generations, with only one example of nonpenetrance, and that by history only. Onset of symptoms occurred typically at about 20 years of age but occurred a few years earlier in those who inherited the gene through the mother. The course was variable, with some individuals with acoustic neuromas surviving into their 60s and 70s, whereas others died while in their 20s of tumors or as a result of surgery. Several of those at risk for the disease were drowning victims. Because more than half of the affected individuals whom we examined had one or two prominent café au lait spots or peripheral neurofibromas (particularly over the scalp), or both café au lait spots and neurofibromas, we considered this trait to be a form of neurofibromatosis, albeit distinct from von Recklinghausen's disease because of the consistent presence of acoustic neuromas, which are absent in families with von Recklinghausen's disease. The designations of NF2 and NF1 for these conditions were proposed at a Consensus Development Conference on Neurofibromatosis held in 1987. In the course of screening those family members of the "Gardner kindred" who were at risk, it became clear that no single audiologic, vestibular, or imaging study available in 1970 was always abnormal in a newly diagnosed individual and that a battery of screening tests was required.

Several large families as well as many sporadic cases have been ascertained by several groups of investigators, suggesting that the disorder accounts for a sizable proportion of all patients with neurofibromatosis and for a considerable proportion of those with acoustic neuroma. However, no population-based epidemiologic study has yet been done to provide an estimate of the overall prevalence of NF2 or its contribution to NF1 and sporadic, unilateral acoustic neuroma.

During the early 1980s, our two groups independently confirmed a physical change of the lens of the eye consisting of opacities or actual cataracts in the posteriorly capsular portion of the lens. If present in a young individual at risk for NF2, such a change in the lens is highly suggestive of the disorder. If these opacities are large and dense, they can usually be detected by a clinician using a hand-held ophthalmoscope. One focuses first on the iris and then, without changing the setting, shifts to the lens where a black "cinder" indicates the opacity. The presence of small opacities and the important determination of their location just below the posterior capsule of the lens requires referral to an ophthalmologist for slit lamp evaluation.

Although brain tumors other than acoustic neuromas were not very common in the family Gardner studied, some affected individuals from other families who were studied subsequently have had five or more meningiomas of the brain in addition to multiple tumors of the spinal cord and its nerve roots. This suggested to one of us (RLM) that the gene for NF2 might be on chromosome 22, since this chromosome is frequently missing from or abnormal in cells from meningiomas. Studies of DNA from acoustic neuromas of NF2 were performed, demonstrating loss of genetic material only on chromosome 22. Later studies demonstrated loss of chromsome 22 in meningiomas and spinal neurofibromas of NF2 patients. It was therefore concluded that this chromosome was the site of a genetic alteration promoting transformation of Schwann cells to acoustic neuromas. Subsequently, genetic linkage analysis of one large family has shown that a single gene responsible for NF2 is linked to the site of a DNA polymorphism on the long arm of chromosome 22. Because variation exists in both the frequency and type of associated neural tumors among NF2 families, other genes may also be involved. Therefore similar linkage studies employing additional DNA polymorphisms in this region of chromosome 22 must be carried out in other families before one can conclude that the same gene causes all NF2.

One immediate and practical consequence of mapping the NF2 gene to chromosome 22 was to use this knowledge to distinguish this trait from that of von Recklinghausen neurofibromatosis or NF1. Investigators immediately examined NF1 families for evidence of linkage of the NF1 gene to chromosome 22. The results conclusively excluded linkage of NF1 to this chromosome. Soon thereafter, two independent laboratories produced convincing evidence in multiple families that the NF1 gene is on the proximal long arm of chromosome 17. These results confirmed our clinical impression that the two forms of NF are separate and distinct, with each having a different mutation, a different molecular defect, and probably a different mechanism of tumorigenesis (Table 1).

Distinguishing NF2 From NF1

One fundamental difference between NF1 and NF2 is the age of the patient at onset. NF1 is often diagnosed by examination of the skin at birth or

Table 1 Physical Features Found in Patients With NF1 and NF2 and Their Relative Frequency (Age Range When First Noted)

Organ System	*NF1*	*NF2*
Skin		
Café au lait spots	++++(0–10 yrs)	+ (youth)
Axillary and inguinal freckling	+++(10–20 yrs)	rare
Peripheral nerve		
Neurofibroma, dermal or plexiform	++++(0–20 yrs)	+(0–20 yrs)
Neurofibrosarcoma	+(0–70 yrs)	rare
Eye		
Lisch nodules of iris	++++(5–15 yrs)	0
Posterior capsular cataracts	0	+++(18–30 yrs)
Cranial nerves		
Optic glioma	+(infancy)	0
Optic meningioma	0	+(0–30 yrs)
Acoustic neuroma	0	++++(15–40 yrs)
Other schwannomas, neurofibromas of sensory nerves	+	++(<15 yrs)
Brain		
Meningioma, meningiomatosis	+	++(15–40 yrs)
Glioma	++(infancy)	++(20–40 yrs)
Macrocephaly	+++(childhood)	0
Mild cognitive impairment	++++(childhood)	0
Hamartoma, glioma, aqueductal dysplasia	++?	0
Spinal cord		
Schwannoma (sensory nerve root, intramedullary), neurofibromas	++(15–40 yrs)	++(15–40 yrs)
Meningioma	0(rare)	+(15–40 yrs)
Astrocytoma	0/+(rare)	++(15–40 yrs)
Ependymoma	+(rare)	++(15–40 yrs)
Syringomyelia	rare	rare
Lateral thoracic meningocele, dural ectasia	+(0–?)	
Skeleton		
Pseudoarthrosis of tibia	++(infancy)	0
Short stature, scoliosis	+++(youth)	0
Head circumference >97%	+++(0–70 yrs)	0
Endocrine		
Abdominal tumors (pheochromocytoma, carcinoid of ampulla of Vater), precocious puberty, renal artery stenosis, gastrointestinal neurofibroma	+	0

during infancy and almost always during the first decade of life. By contrast, NF2 generally does not become clinically evident until after the patient has reached puberty or is well into adulthood.

Because both forms of NF may involve skin, peripheral nerves, the eyes, brain, cranial nerves, and spinal cord (see Table 1), the terms "central NF" or "peripheral NF" have been discarded. Except in the spinal cord, there is often a qualitative as well as quantitative difference in the involvement. Thus in patients with NF1, axillary and inguinal freckling are common by puberty but are rare in patients with NF2. Both forms of NF are often accompanied by different, distinct eye changes that can be definitive in diagnosing each condition. Lisch nodules of the iris occur in more than 85 percent of postpubescent patients with NF1 but have not been seen in Caucasians with NF2. Posterior capsular opacities of the lens are seen in most patients with NF2 by age 30 but have not been described in patients with NF1. Acoustic neuroma, the hallmark of NF2, does not occur as part of NF1, while optic gliomas are not seen in patients with NF2.

By contrast, the spinal nerve roots may be involved with multiple Schwann's cell tumors in both conditions (see Table 1). In both forms of NF, tumors in this area, particularly when they involve the cervical cord and brain stem, are a major source of morbidity and death. In both forms of NF, there may also be glial tumors of the brain or spinal cord. In patients with NF1, optic gliomas are most common. In patients with NF2, spinal ependymomas and astrocytomas occur. However, developmental anomalies in the form of neuronal heterotopias, glial dysplasia, and hamartomatous formation, which are common in patients with NF1 and likely contribute to the macrocephaly, mild cognitive impairment, and subtle neurologic deficit frequently seen in patients with that disorder, are rare in patients with NF2. Because of these differences, a group of persons with NF1 would be found to differ clinically in many respects from a group of persons with NF2; however, when one is dealing *with an individual case,* making a precise distinction between NF1 and NF2 can be difficult. This is particularly true in those sporadic cases where patients present with very mild skin changes or with involvement of the spinal cord only. The minimal criteria necessary for the diagnosis of NF1 and NF2 are compared in Table 2. Theoretically, there should be no overlap between the two conditions; for instance, individuals with NF2 have fewer than six café au lait spots and no Lisch nodules, while in patients with NF1, these features are present in all but the elderly. In our practice, we have noted a few individuals (one of whom was black) who had bilateral tumors in the cerebellar pontine angle, at least one of which was a schwannoma of the facial nerve and posterior capsular lens opacities, six or seven café au lait spots, and

one or two Lisch nodules. It is important to note that the diagnostic criteria for NF1 and NF2 have been based on series consisting predominantly of Caucasians.

Distinguishing NF2 From Sporadic, Unilateral Acoustic Neuroma

It is even more critical to distinguish NF2 from the occurrence of sporadic, unilateral acoustic neuroma. Although the final molecular genetic events of tumorigenesis may be similar in these two conditions, the clinical consequences of each are different. Indeed, a major purpose of this chapter is to provide clinicians with the knowledge that will enable them to determine whether an individual in whom a single acoustic neuroma has been diagnosed has NF2 rather than a sporadic solitary acoustic neuroma. We continue to see young individuals, particularly women, who have had a presumed solitary, unilateral acoustic neuroma removed—usually with resulting unilateral deafness and some loss of facial expression—in whom the unexpected development of an acoustic neuroma on the contralateral auditory-vestibular nerve complex has been vexing to the patient and neurosurgeon alike. In many of these situations, had the involved physicians been aware of what to ask about and what to look for, the diagnosis of NF2 could have been made during the initial visit and the treatment plan might have been altered or appropriate counseling instituted earlier. At the very least, such an individual requires careful questioning regarding symptoms referable to the second ear, a family history of hearing loss, or balance difficulties; physical examinations for neurofibromata and café au lait spots; audiology and brain

---

Table 2 Criteria for Diagnosis of NF1 and NF2

NF1 may be diagnosed in Caucasians when two or more of the following are present:

  Six or more café au lait macules whose greatest diameter is more than 5 mm in prepubescent patients and more than 15 mm in postpubescent patients

  Two or more neurofibromas of any type, or one plexiform neurofibroma

  Freckling in the axillary or inguinal region

  Optic glioma

  Two or more Lisch nodules (iris hamartomas)

  A distinctive osseous lesion as sphenoid dysplasia or thinning of long-bone cortex, with or without pseudoarthrosis

  A parent, sibling, or child with NF1 on the basis of the above criteria

NF2 may be diagnosed when one of the following is present:

  Bilateral eighth-nerve masses seen by MRI with gadolinium

  A parent, sibling, or child with NF2 and either unilateral eighth-nerve mass *or* any two of the following:

    Neurofibroma, meningioma, glioma, schwannoma, juvenile capsular lenticular opacity, or abnormal asymmetrical audiologic or vestibular function without known cause.

---

stem auditory–evoked responses (BAERs) of both ears; magnetic resonance imaging (MRI) with gadolinium of the brain with emphasis on the posterior fossa; and ophthalmologic assessment of the lens by slit lamp with pupils dilated. In some series, NF2 is the cause of acoustic neuromas in as many as 20 percent of all patients and is most prevalent in those with early onset of symptoms. Differences that help distinguish NF2 from sporadic, unilateral acoustic neuroma are given in Table 3.

WHEN TO SUSPECT NF2

In what clinical settings should the diagnosis be considered? Figure 1 shows five groups of individuals at high risk for this condition.

Group 1 includes the identical twin or first-degree relative of a patient with NF2. An identical twin of an individual with NF2 is at a risk of nearly 100 percent for possessing the NF2 gene, while a fraternal twin, full sibling, parent, or child of an affected individual is at a risk of 50 percent. As an individual without signs or symptoms passes through the likely age of onset (which begins in the late teens) without signs or symptoms, this risk declines. By age 40, if all screening tests are negative, the risk is close to zero percent. As a corollary, once a physician has established the diagnosis of NF2, he

is obligated to see that all of the patient's siblings and children past puberty are screened. Both parents, regardless of their age, should be screened even if there is no family history of NF2, provided that their situations permit clinical evaluation. With this approach, we recently diagnosed NF2 in the 67-year-old father of an affected individual and made a presumptive diagnosis of NF2 in the paternal grandfather, who just months before at age 92 died with hearing loss and imbalance.

In our experience, the most important group (Group 2) in which to consider the diagnosis of NF2 are relatively young individuals with presumed sporadic, unilateral acoustic neuroma. Group 3 consists of youths and adults with only mild changes of NF, no positive family history, and no Lisch nodules, who therefore do not meet the diagnostic criteria for NF1. Group 4 includes children with one or two schwannomas or meningiomas. These children should be evaluated for NF2 since these tumors, regardless of site, are rare in children. Finally, when evaluating anyone with multiple brain tumors of unknown cause, one should consider the diagnosis of NF2.

SCREENING

When NF2 is suspected in a youth or adult, the following procedure should be followed. One should obtain a careful history stressing possible hearing loss, tinnitus and other noise in the head, and the occurrence of nighttime imbalance or difficulty sensing direction while swimming under water. One should also perform a physical examination stressing examination of the skin and scalp, evaluate the iris, lens, and fundus of the eye, and assess neurologic function (including the cranial nerves) and the spinal cord (see Fig. 1).

Symptoms of acoustic neuromas are usually referable to pressure on the vestibulocochlear and facial-nerve complex. In patients with NF2, symptoms usually begin during the teens or early 20s, but occasionally patients become symptomatic as early as during the first decade of life or as late as during the seventh decade of life. The first symptom is usually loss of hearing. This is generally unilateral and is often first noticed when the patient uses a telephone—one of the few daily activities that can be used to test unilateral auditory discrimination. With careful questioning, the patient may also describe a history of intermittent ringing or roaring in one or both ears or some unsteadiness, especially when walking at night on uneven ground. Other symptoms may include facial weakness, sensory change, headache, or a change in vision.

Patients may have features of NF as the first clinical sign. Café au lait spots and skin neurofibromas can be found in many affected persons on

Table 3 Distinguishing NF2 From Sporadic, Unilateral Acoustic Neuroma

	Sporadic Unilateral Acoustic Neuroma	Bilateral Hereditary Acoustic Neuroma (NF2)
Age at onset (yrs)	After 40	Before 40
Associated findings	None	Brain and spinal tumors, café au lait macules and neurofibromas, posterior capsular lens opacities
Means of diagnosis	Audiology and imaging of brain	Evaluation of skin, hearing, lenses of the eyes, imaging of brain and spinal cord
Management	1. Rule out NF2 2. Surgical tumor removal is usually curative; watchful waiting used only for the elderly or those medically unfit for surgery	*Individualize* Watchful waiting for stable patients; surgery for those with signs of deterioration

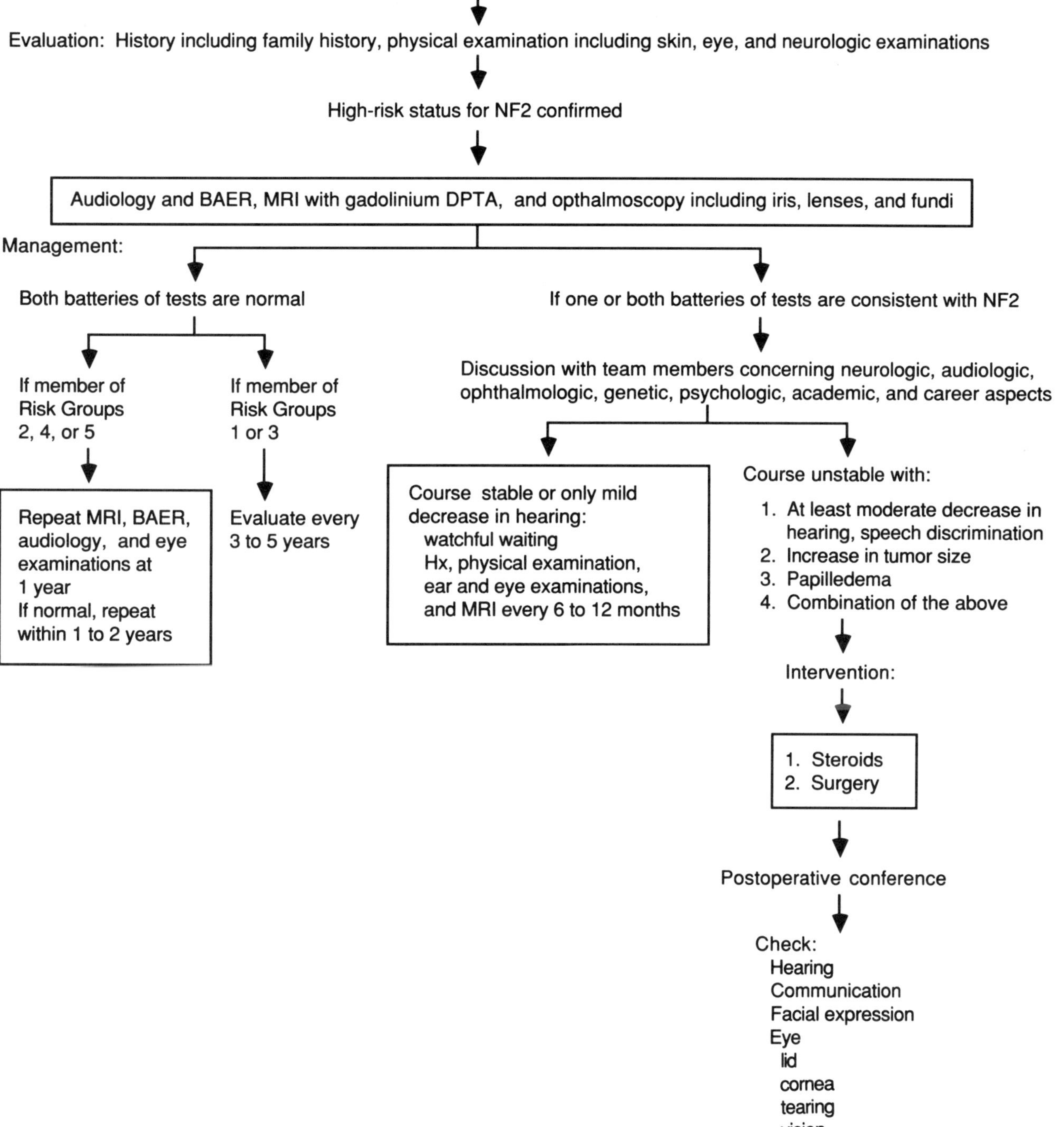

Figure 1 Management of NF2.

thorough examination. The macules themselves are not diagnostic of NF, but the presence of one or more of substantial size should raise the index of suspicion. Intertriginous freckling is uncommon in patients with NF2. Skin neurofibromas of NF2 are easy to overlook since they are usually less than 2 cm in diameter and are only minimally raised. Those occurring over the chest often have a roughened surface that may have more prominent hairs than the surrounding skin and are best seen when a light is shined on them from an oblique angle.

Other stigmata include visible or palpable masses, which may indicate plexiform NF on deeper nerves. Motor or sensory dysfunction suggests a nerve or spinal cord tumor. Ophthalmologic examination with emphasis on the lens and iris is necessary. Presenile lens opacities or actual capsular cataracts have been found in more than half of the patients examined and may precede the onset of symptoms of acoustic neuroma, allowing early identification of family members with the gene for NF2.

If the high-risk status of an individual is confirmed, the patient should be referred for audiologic assessment including evoked responses and for ophthalmologic evaluation including slit lamp examination of the lens with pupils dilated. At this point, we also obtain MRI of the brain before and after injection of gadolinium. Tests of vestibular function are also desirable since we have found them to be positive in a few individuals when all other tests were normal. The minimal criteria necessary for the diagnosis of NF2 are listed in Table 2.

EVALUATION OF THE PATIENT

If the initial screening studies are either diagnostic or suggestive of NF2, a complete evaluation at a center familiar with NF2 is in order to determine the extent of involvement in the following critical sites: the seventh and eighth cranial nerve complex and brain, the spinal cord and its nerve roots, and the lens of the eye.

COUNSELING AFTER DIAGNOSIS

Once a diagnosis of NF2 has been made, several issues must be addressed and a series of steps initiated. The diagnosis of NF2 does not mean that the patient's life is invariably altered. Many affected individuals have enjoyed a high-quality life for years. But the almost certain implications are that bilateral acoustic neuromas are inevitable, other nervous system tumors are probable, complete hearing loss and marked imbalance are distinct possibilities, and other family members are at high risk for the same. This information can be devastating, especially if it is delivered bluntly; therefore an ex-

perienced team and ample time for consultation and advice are required.

The extent of disease in the patient and the ramifications of the diagnosis should be addressed first. An experienced clinician should discuss the specific changes related to NF2 with the affected individual, together with his or her parents, spouse, or other close relative or friend. Thus, if one or both of the eighth cranial nerves are the site(s) of probable acoustic neuromas, their location, size, probable age (if known), and rate of growth should be discussed; if the patient wishes to see them, MRI may be used to clarify this information. The typical natural history as well as the extremes of behavior of this tumor together with some of the management options need to be mentioned. The importance of periodic monitoring of the tumors must be stressed. If useful hearing remains in one or both ears, the patient should be asked to test his or her hearing weekly by using the telephone. Because the vestibular portion of the eighth nerve may be involved early but go unrecognized until the patient attempts activities calling for precise balance or sense of direction, the patient should be told to exercise caution when engaging in activities such as swimming, diving, or climbing. Affected individuals should never swim underwater when alone. Stairs in the home should be well lit at night. If imbalance becomes a problem, the new field of "vestibular rehabilitation" should be explored. The importance of periodic monitoring with sensitive audiologic, ophthalmoscopic, and imaging techniques must be emphasized; such a program should be arranged and tailored to the individual patient's situation.

Consideration must be given to any other tumors found in the brain or in the spinal cord. Because tumors at any of these sites can undergo sudden change and because specialists at several centers may be involved in management discussions, we routinely provide affected individuals with copies of their critical audiologic, ophthalmologic, and imaging studies.

Some hearing loss is almost inevitable in those who have NF2; therefore an audiologist or some other appropriate specialist should discuss the potential benefits of sound amplification, lip reading, or sign language. To minimize the likelihood of loss of another important sense—vision—any involvement of the eyes, either directly by cataracts or indirectly by chronic papilledema resulting from one or more brain tumors or postoperatively by corneal ulceration or scarring resulting from faulty eyelid closure, reduced tearing, or diminished corneal sensitivity, should be carefully monitored. An eye specialist should discuss any changes noted in the lenses, optic discs, or cornea.

A practitioner familiar with NF2 should discuss with the patient important personal considerations, such as the effect of progression of NF2 on the patient's career. The patient and the patient's family should be informed of voluntary support organizations.

A counselor—whether geneticist, social worker, or nurse practitioner—is an essential member of the support team. Genetic counseling should be offered to the patient and the patient's family. Affected persons must be aware that there is a 50 percent risk of transmitting the gene for NF2 to any offspring and that, at present, no prenatal test is available. Their close relatives must be screened (see Fig. 1). A practical issue in family counseling concerns the probability that a person at risk who has no signs or symptoms of NF2 actually carries the gene and may therefore pass it on. A study of 18 such persons who later became affected provides useful information. The youngest patient was 15 years of age at the time of diagnosis, and half of the patients were younger than 25 years of age at the time of diagnosis. The diagnosis was made by age 45 in all but one patient. Newer diagnostic methods and routine ophthalmologic examinations for posterior capsular cataracts should now afford an even earlier diagnosis.

INTERVENTION

The growth patterns of acoustic neuromas in patients with NF2 is unpredictable. One or both tumors may progress relentlessly, leading to deafness, cerebellar symptoms, chronic headache, visual disturbances, paresis, and eventual death due to brain stem compression. More often, there may be only minimal growth for many years, so that the patient has few, if any, limitations. The typical course lies somewhere between these extremes but is impossible to predict. MRI with gadolinium has made it possible to follow the growth of individual tumors more accurately.

At present, surgical intervention is the usual procedure for attacking troublesome acoustic neuromas, as well as other brain and spinal cord tumors. In our experience, mortality from acoustic neuroma surgery is now rare, and, using expert intraoperative monitoring, morbidity related to facial nerve dysfunction can be avoided in the majority of patients. In some cases it has even been possible to preserve hearing. *However, no intervention is the initial appropriate choice for many patients.* Only two of the more than 20 NF2 patients we are following at the National Institutes of Health (NIH) have undergone surgery during the past 3 years. Watchful waiting is appropriate in the stable cases because there is little likelihood that intervention will improve the neurologic or audiologic status. Careful periodic clinical, audiologic, imaging, and ophthalmologic monitoring are essential.

The key question concerns the definition of a "troublesome" acoustic neuroma in patients with NF2. It is not the mere presence of a symptomatic acoustic neuroma since we now know that these tumors may grow slowly for as long as 40 or 50 years, causing hearing loss that is only mildly progressive over that time. In general, a "troublesome" acoustic neuroma in patients with NF2 is one associated with an unstable, deteriorating condition. Thus before one contemplates surgical intervention, there should be documented evidence of deterioration such as moderate to rapid hearing loss, decreasing speech discrimination, worsening BAER, or an increase in tumor size as determined by imaging. Complete surgical removal of an acoustic neuroma should be considered in those patients with small tumors or in whom one of the tumors is enlarging rapidly while there is useful and stable hearing in the opposite ear. In such patients, normal facial expression and useful hearing may be preserved with microsurgical removal of the acoustic neuroma by an experienced surgical team using intraoperative electrocochlear and BAER monitoring. When it is surgically feasible, tumors of any size should be removed when hearing is absent on the tumor-bearing side and the tumor causes neurologic dysfunction, or when a large acoustic neuroma in a young patient with a deaf ear could produce neurologic dysfunction with minimal additional growth. For patients with progressive hearing loss associated with an acoustic neuroma measuring 2 cm or more on the only hearing side, an attempt at complete tumor removal often results in total deafness. As a means of providing added years of useful hearing for such patients, partial tumor removal and internal auditory canal decompression are presently under investigation. Alternative methods of treatment such as focused stereotactic radiotherapy with a "gamma-knife" or with a proton beam are also being investigated. Although the results to date suggest that tumor growth may be slowed or arrested and seventh nerve function spared in some cases, long-term useful hearing has not been saved by the use of these alternative methods in most NF2 patients.

SUGGESTED READING

Kaiser-Kupfer MI, Freidlin V, Datiles MB, et al. The association of posterior lens opacities with bilateral acoustic neuromas in patients with neurofibromatosis type 2. Arch Ophthalmol 1989; 107:541–544.

Martuza RL, Eldridge R. Neurofibromatosis type 2. N Engl J Med 1988; 318:684–688.

Mulvihill J, Parry D, Sherman J, et al. Neurofibromatosis 1 (von Recklinghausen's disease) and neurofibromatosis 2 (bilateral acoustic neurofibromatosis)—1989 Update. Ann Int Med 1990 (in press).

Rouleau GA, Wertelecki W, Haines JL, et al. Genetic linkage analysis of bilateral acoustic neurofibromatosis to a DNA marker on chromosome 22. Nature 1987; 329:246–248.

Seizinger BR, Rouleau G, Ozelius L, et al. Common pathogenetic mechanism for three tumor types in bilateral acoustic neurofibromatosis. Science 1987; 236:317–319.

van Seters AP, van Dulken H, de Keizer RJW, Vielvoye GJ. Symptomatic relief of meningioma by buserelin maintenance therapy. Lancet 1989; 564–565.

PATIENT RESOURCES

The NF2 Sharing Network
10074 Cabachon Court
Ellicott City, Maryland 21043
Telephone: (301) 461-2245 (voice)
            (301) 461-5213 (TDD)

Acoustic Neuroma Association
P.O. Box 398
Carlisle, Pennsylvania 17013

Neurofibromatosis Inc.
3401 Woodridge Court
Mitchelville, Maryland 20721-8878

National Neurofibromatosis Foundation
Suite 7-S
141 Fifth Avenue
New York, New York 10010

Association of Late Deafened Adults
1027 Oakton
Evanston, Illinois 60202

TUBEROUS SCLEROSIS

WILLIAM GAILLARD, M.D.
GIHAN TENNEKOON, M.D.

DIAGNOSIS

Tuberous sclerosis, the second most common of the phakomatoses, is inherited as an autosomal dominant syndrome with variable penetrance; yet approximately 70 percent of cases are caused by new mutations. The criteria for making the diagnosis of TS are listed in Table 1 and the frequency with which a given sign occurs is presented in Table 2. The work-up of patients who satisfy the diagnostic criteria is presented in Table 3. The regularity with which these patients are followed depends on their clinical symptoms and signs.

TREATMENT

There is no specific therapy for TS. Management involves treatment of seizures, appropriate placement of children with mental retardation, and symptomatic management of CNS and other tumors.

Seizures

Seizures occur frequently in patients with TS, and their incidence correlates with the intelligence quotient of the patient. Seventy percent of those with average or above average intelligence have seizures, whereas all patients with mental retardation have seizures. The seizure types vary from complex partial to secondary generalized, and both forms are amenable to treatment with standard anticonvulsants. In addition, patients may have akinetic spells and infantile spasms.

Approximately 40 percent of patients have infantile spasms. The drug of choice is adrenocorticotropic hormone (ACTH) gel, 40 to 80 U per day administered intramuscularly, divided into two

Table 1   Criteria for Diagnosis

Any one of the following:
Adenoma sebaceum
Retinal phakoma
Radiologic findings of periventricular calcification, tubers, heterotopias
or
Any two of the following:
Ash leaf lesion
Shagreen patches
Infantile spasm
CNS calcification
Renal tumors
Cardiac rhabdomyoma
First-degree relative involved

Table 2   Frequency of signs in tuberous sclerosis

Clinical Signs	*Frequency*
Hypopigmented spot/ash leaf	70–85%
Adenoma sebaceum	85–95%
Shagreen patch	20–25%
Subungual fibroma	15–20%
Mental retardation	60–70%
Seizures	70–90%
Retinal phakoma	50%
Renal tumors/cysts	50–80%
Bone	50%
Pulmonary (usually in women)	20–40%
Cardiac	30%

Table 3 Work-up for TS Cases

Careful opthalmologic examination
Electrocardiography (for conduction defects)
Cardiac echo (to look for rhabdomyoma)
MRI (for heterotopias and cortical tubers, tumors)
CT scan (for periventricular calcification, tumors,
   hydrocephalus)
Renal sonography (for tumors and cysts)

equal doses. This therapy is continued until the electroencephalogram (EEG) pattern, hypsarrthymia, resolves and the seizures stop. The ACTH is then tapered; the total duration of therapy is approximately 6 to 8 weeks. A second trial of ACTH is recommended for clinical relapse, an all-too-frequent event in TS-related infantile spasms. In the patients who remain refractory to ACTH, prednisone (2 mg per kilogram per day) may prove efficacious. Alternative drugs include clonazepam (beginning with 0.05 mg per kilogram per day in two divided doses) and valproic acid (starting at 10 to 15 mg per kilogram per day and advancing to 60 mg per kilogram per day in divided doses, as necessary).

When steroids are administered, close follow-up is essential. Because of the immunosuppression caused by the steroids, infections are not well tolerated and patients may succumb to sepsis or opportunistic infection. Any fever or illness needs a thorough evaluation, while therapy aimed at the causative agent must be undertaken quickly. With the patient in such stressful states, steroid dosage may need to be increased. Blood pressure should also be monitored since hypertension may occur late in the treatment course and can be sufficiently severe to warrant decreasing the steroid dose. Potassium wasting may occur and may necessitate supplementation with oral potassium. Limiting food intake to avoid excessive weight gain is a constant and exasperating problem. Developmental regression is sometimes observed in patients who take steroids, although this phenomenon is reversible when therapy is discontinued. Other pharmacologic agents include clonazepam, which causes sedation, an increase in the amount of oral secretions, and an efficacy that may unfortunately be short lived. With valproic acid, another useful drug, there is a 1 in 500 chance of hepatic failure when administered to children younger than 2 years of age, and thus frequent monitoring of liver and bone marrow function is required.

If children with TS are treated early for infantile spasms, the long-term outcome with regard to mental retardation is better than that of patients with symptomatic infantile spasms. However, even if treated early, 60 percent of children with TS and infantile spasm continue to have seizures, 20 percent of whom develop a Lennox-Gastaut syndrome with a refractory mixed seizure disorder and associated mental retardation. In these children, the standard anticonvulsant drugs should be used first, but when the seizures are refractory, clonazepam, nitrazepam (mogadon, where available), lorazepam (Ativan), clorazepate (Tranxene), and a ketogenic diet should be considered. Should all medical therapies fail, surgical corpus callosotomy may be necessary. Of the 80 percent who do not develop Lennox-Gastaut syndrome, partial complex seizures are the most common and respond best to carbamazepine (10 to 15 mg per day) monotherapy. Generalized seizures should respond to treatment with standard anticonvulsants.

Mental Retardation

Of all TS patients, 34 percent have average or above average intelligence, while 38 percent are severely retarded, 14 percent moderately retarded, and 14 percent mildly retarded. Children who are severely retarded have seizures at an earlier age that are often more difficult to control. All mentally retarded children should be enrolled in an infant stimulation program; when these children are about 5 years old, they should undergo psychological testing to obtain a complete profile of their strengths and weaknesses. With this information, the physician, psychologist, and educator should design a program best suited to the child. The child's progress should be monitored at frequent intervals. Some of the severely retarded children have marked behavioral disturbances that may require additional therapy such as a behavior modification program.

CNS Tumors

Intracranial findings are cortical tubers, neuronal heterotopias, subependymal nodules, and giant cell astrocytomas (10 percent). Among patients with TS, the incidence of other intracranial tumors is similar to that in the general population.

Subependymal glial nodules often calcify and are demonstrated in more than 50 percent of plain skull radiographs when the patient reaches 5 years of age. CT is superior for imaging periventricular calcification, yet MRI provides better imaging of cortical tubers and heterotopias and is able to identify subependymal growths regardless of calcium content. Malignant degeneration is rare. However, as glial nodules commonly grow near the ventricular foramina, obstructive hydrocephalus may occur that may be life threatening. Surgical removal of the nodule or placement of a ventriculoperitoneal shunt is required in such cases. Head circumference and serial CT scans should be monitored in any patient with TS.

Non-Neural Manifestations

Skin.   Ash leaf lesions, which are often present at birth, do not require treatment. Adenoma sebacium, the most common and pathognomonic finding in TS, appears after the patient is two years of age and may not develop until age 5—well after the onset of seizures, mental retardation, or cardiac rhabdomyomas. Several reasons predicate removal of adenoma sebaceum. Some patients may have many angiofibromas that should be removed for cosmetic improvement. In patients with mental retardation, the angiofibromas are often traumatized and are a source of chronic infection and bleeding. The current approach is to remove angiofibromas by use of argon or carbon dioxide laser.

Retinal Lesions.   These phakomas require no special therapy.

Renal Lesions.   The most common tumor is an angiomyolipoma, a benign tumor that is often bilateral. These usually present with flank pain and hematuria, although in approximately 10 percent of patients there may be a massive hemorrhage. These tumors are detected by renal CT and ultrasonography. Lesions smaller than 4 cm are asymptomatic and should be followed at yearly intervals. Tumors larger than 4 cm require therapy with either angiography and embolization or surgery. Renal cysts are less common. These cysts may compress renal tissue and cause chronic renal failure, and therefore large cysts may require decompression or resection.

Cardiac Lesions.   Rhabdomyomas are common and may be present during the newborn period. Approximately 50 percent of patients with congenital rhabdomyomas have TS. They may present with congestive cardiac failure or arrhythmias. Although the tumor may be visualized by two-dimensional echocardiography, currently the best way to evaluate these children is by echo-gated MRI imaging. Treatment of patients with these tumors is primarily symptomatic: congestive cardiac failure should be treated by conventional means (digoxin and diuretics), and arrhythmias are treated with anti-arrhythmic drugs or a pacemaker. If there is obstruction to outflow, intracavitary tumors may be resected.

Pulmonary Involvement

Pulmonary cystic disease may develop in patients 20 to 30 years of age. It is more common in female patients, who generally have less severe neurologic involvement. Corpulmonale may develop, and recurrent and potentially life-threatening pneumothorax may occur.

Genetic Counseling

Genetic counseling is an integral part of the management of children with TS. In those families where several members are affected with TS, 50 percent of the offspring will have the disease. Unfortunately, there is no way of detecting affected children *in utero*. In those families with a strong family history, linkage has been detected to chromosome 9 in some cases and to chromosome 11 in others. When children present without a family history, both parents should be examined for stigmata of TS. The examination should include a complete physical examination, including a Wood's lamp examination of the skin and a fundus examination after pupillary dilation. CT scanning of the head to look for calcification should also be done. If no stigmata are found, TS is assumed to be the result of a new mutation.

SUGGESTED READING

Gomez MR, ed. Tuberous sclerosis. New York: Raven Press, 1988.

PATIENT RESOURCE

National Tuberous Sclerosis Association, Inc.
4351 Garden City Drive
Landover, Maryland 20785
Telephone: (301) 459-9888

VIRAL INFECTION

CONGENITAL VIRAL INFECTION

JAMES F. BALE, Jr., M.D.

Several different viruses can infect the fetus or newborn infant and damage the developing nervous system. Infections with certain pathogens, such as cytomegalovirus or rubella virus, typically occur in utero (i.e., congenital infections), whereas other agents, such as the herpes simplex viruses or enteroviruses, usually infect the newborn infant intrapartum (i.e., perinatal infections).

The presence of certain clinical features, such as rash, hepatomegaly, splenomegaly, jaundice, retinitis, cataracts, or microcephaly (features synonymous with the "torch" syndrome, a mnemonic referring to the principal causative agents, *Toxoplasma gondii,* *O*ther, *R*ubella, *C*ytomegalovirus, and *H*erpes simplex viruses) should suggest strongly the possibility of a congenital or perinatally acquired viral infection. Clinical signs in other infants, particularly those infants affected by the enteroviruses, may be difficult to distinguish from bacterial infection.

The immediate goals of the physician treating an infant with a suspected congenital or perinatal viral infection include (1) instituting isolation precautions that minimize exposure to other infants or susceptible hospital personnel, (2) completing a comprehensive diagnostic evaluation that should include serologic studies and virus cultures of urine, oral secretions (saliva or throat washings), stool (rectal swab), blood, and cerebrospinal fluid, and (3) initiating a treatment plan that should consist of general supportive measures and, possibly, specific antiviral chemotherapy.

Infants who survive congenital or perinatal viral infections are at high risk for cognitive, motor, visual, and auditory disabilities. Thus, such infants should receive periodic, comprehensive evaluation by a multidisciplinary team that includes physicians, speech and hearing specialists, physical therapists, and educational psychologists. Such evaluation is essential before the child's entry into an educational environment.

SPECIFIC VIRAL PATHOGENS

Rubella

Antiviral Therapy

Rubella virus infection cannot be effectively treated by postnatal antiviral therapy, but the congenital rubella syndrome can be prevented by immunization with the rubella virus vaccine (a component of the measles, mumps, rubella [MMR] vaccine), which was licensed in 1969. Immunization programs in the United States have reduced the incidence of congenital rubella syndrome by 96 percent.

Adjunctive Therapy

Congenital rubella virus produces a spectrum of clinical disease in infected newborns, a feature related to the timing of maternal infection. Infants with disseminated disease, characterized by low birth weight, jaundice, pneumonitis, encephalitis, cardiomyopathy, hepatitis, and rash, require intravenous hydration, phototherapy, and occasionally, mechanical ventilation. Anemia, thrombocytopenia, jaundice, and chemical hepatitis, common features of rubella infection, usually remit spontaneously.

Infants with congenital rubella syndrome often have a constellation of clinical features that includes eye lesions (cataracts, glaucoma, or pigmentary retinopathy), heart disease (cardiomyopathy, structural heart lesions such as a patent ductus arteriosus), and sensorineural hearing loss. Thus management of the infant with suspected congenital rubella syndrome should include (1) a thorough ophthalmologic examination, (2) an evaluation for heart disease (e.g., electrocardiography, chest radiography, cardiac ultrasonography), and (3) audiometry.

Infants with suspected or proven rubella infections require contact isolation (private room; masks, gowns, and gloves for persons having close patient contact). Rubella-infected infants should be considered contagious until 1 year of age (unless cultures of nasopharynx and urine are negative after 3 months of age). Serologic screening of all visitors and hospital personnel having close contact with such infants can determine their risk of infection. Seronegative, pregnant individuals must not care for infants with suspected or proven rubella virus infections.

Because survivors of congenital rubella syndrome may develop progressive sensorineural deafness, hearing should be evaluated periodically in order to institute appropriate remedial measures. In addition, children with congenital rubella syndrome require serial evaluation of growth and glucose tolerance because of an increased risk of diabetes mellitus (most commonly during the second and third decades of life), growth hormone deficiency, and hypothyroidism. Albeit rarely, children with congenital rubella syndrome may develop postrubella panencephalitis, a syndrome characterized by seizures, ataxia, and progressive loss of motor and intellectual skills.

Cytomegalovirus

Antiviral Therapy

Cytomegalovirus (CMV) infections in neonates can neither be prevented by vaccine nor treated effectively with specific antiviral chemotherapy. Consequently, CMV remains the most commonly identified cause of virus-induced mental retardation, affecting approximately 3,000 children annually in the United States. Certain antiviral agents, such as cytarabine, vidarabine, ribavirin, or interferons, inhibit CMV replication in vitro but have not been clinically useful. A recently developed 2-deoxyguanosine analogue, ganciclovir (9-[1,3-dihydroxy-2-propoxy)methyl]guanine), has been used to treat serious adult CMV infections such as pneumonia, retinitis, and gastroenteritis. No data are yet available regarding its efficacy in congenitally infected infants.

Adjunctive Therapy

Infants with congenital CMV infections display varied clinical signs at birth and therefore require individualized therapeutic strategies. Infants who exhibit microcephaly or retinitis only pose few therapeutic issues other than that the virologic diagnosis must be confirmed and appropriate neurodiagnostic studies initiated. By contrast, infants with disseminated infections, manifested by thrombocytopenia, anemia, jaundice, pneumonia, or hepatitis, require extensive supportive care that may include mechanical ventilation, transfusion therapy, phototherapy, or exchange transfusion for extreme hyperbilirubinemia.

All newborn infants with suspected or proven congenital CMV infections should receive (1) a thorough ophthalmologic examination to detect chorioretinitis, optic atrophy, or other CMV-induced ophthalmologic abnormalities, (2) a hearing screening to identify sensorineural hearing loss, a common complication of congenital CMV infection, and (3) a central nervous system (CNS) imaging study to identify CNS lesions. Although bedside cranial ultrasonography is useful as a screening test for periventricular abnormalities in unstable infants, I currently prefer cranial computed tomography (CT), a test that detects periventricular lesions (e.g., calcifications) and provides considerable data regarding cerebral parenchyma and cerebellar anatomy. Magnetic resonance imaging (MRI), a more expensive procedure, also effectively images the cerebral and cerebellar lesions associated with congenital CMV infections.

The majority of infants affected by CMV survive the neonatal period. Thrombocytopenia, petechiae, and chemical evidence of hepatitis may persist for several weeks but usually resolve spontaneously. Platelet transfusions are rarely required. Because progressive sensorineural hearing loss may develop postnatally, I recommend serial audiometry to be performed when the patient is 6 months, 1 year, and 2 years of age. Progressive ophthalmologic lesions have not been reported; however, a comprehensive ophthalmologic examination should be obtained when the child reaches school-age. Occasional infants require ventriculoperitoneal shunting because of progressive hydrocephalus.

Approximately 25 percent or more of the survivors have seizure disorders, consisting of infantile spasms, absence seizures, or generalized tonic-clonic seizures. Because there have been occasional reports of fatal, disseminated CMV infections during ACTH therapy for CMV-induced infantile spasms, valproic acid, administered at an initial dosage of 15 mg per kilogram per day, may be a safer alternative therapy in such infants. The pertussis immunization should be withheld from infants who have CMV-related seizure disorders.

Although CMV is not highly contagious, pregnant women should avoid direct "hands-on" contact with CMV-excreting newborns. Recent studies of day-care environments indicate that parents or adult caregivers who have direct contact with CMV-excreting children are at increased risk for acquiring CMV.

Herpes Simplex Virus Types 1 and 2

Antiviral Therapy

Neonatal herpes simplex virus (HSV) type 1 or type 2 infections are classified according to three modes of clinical presentation: (1) skin, eye, and mucous membrane involvement, (2) disease restricted to the CNS, or (3) disseminated infection, often without skin lesions. Although outcome correlates with the extent of organ involvement, all forms of suspected HSV disease require emergent evaluation and therapy. Virologic studies should include cultures of throat, skin vesicles, urine, cerebrospinal fluid, rectum, and eye (conjunctiva). Brain biopsy may be necessary in infants with suspected HSV encephalitis and negative surface and cerebrospinal fluid (CSF) cultures.

In contrast to the other congenital or perinatal viral infections, HSV infections can be treated with specific antiviral chemotherapy, using either vidarabine or acyclovir. Vidarabine, the first drug with proven clinical efficacy against HSV, can be given intravenously in a once-daily dose of 30 mg per kilogram over 12 to 18 hours for 10 to 14 days. Because vidarabine is relatively insoluble, large volumes of fluid are required for administration. Vidarabine distributes widely in body tissues and fluids and achieves CSF levels approximately 30 to 50 percent of those in serum.

Although rare in neonates, potential complications of vidarabine therapy include vomiting, diarrhea, tremor, myoclonus, and bone marrow suppression (thrombocytopenia, anemia, or leukopenia). Fluid overload during vidarabine administration can exacerbate volume-sensitive conditions such as cerebral edema. In the presence of renal failure, the vidarabine dose should be reduced by at least 25 percent.

Acyclovir, a 2-deoxyguanosine analogue, can be given intravenously at a dosage of 30 mg per kilogram per day in three divided doses for 10 to 14 days. Like vidarabine, acyclovir is phosphorylated intracellularly to a more active triphosphate form. However, because HSV-induced thymidine kinases phosphorylate acyclovir more efficiently than cellular kinases, acyclovir has a relatively specific action on virus-infected cells. As a result, the drug has few adverse side effects. Acyclovir also distributes widely in tissues and fluids, and the CSF level is approximately 50 percent of that in serum.

HSV keratoconjunctivitis may be treated topically with several different antiviral agents, including 1 percent trifluorothymidine or 3 percent vidarabine ointment administered five or six times daily for 14 to 21 days. Infants with intraocular involvement, such as uveitis, or any sign of systemic HSV disease require intravenous therapy with vidarabine or acyclovir.

At present, neither vidarabine or acyclovir can be judged superior for the treatment for neonatal HSV infections. All studies to date indicate that prompt initiation of specific antiviral therapy with either vidarabine or acyclovir is an important determinant of long-term outcome of HSV-infected infants. Updated information regarding the treatment of neonatal HSV infections can be obtained from investigators in the Department of Pediatrics, The University of Alabama, Birmingham.

Adjunctive Therapy

Because neonatal HSV infections frequently coexist with other medical conditions (e.g., prematurity), HSV-infected infants require treatment in an environment that can provide intensive neonatal care. The treating physician must carefully monitor fluid and electrolyte balance, respiratory functions, hepatic enzymes, clotting studies, and bilirubin levels. Transfusions of platelets and fresh frozen plasma may be necessary for infants with severe HSV infections accompanied by disseminated intravascular coagulation (DIC).

Seizures, a frequent occurrence in neonatal HSV encephalitis, may be treated with phenobarbital, administered in a loading dose of 15 to 20 mg per kilogram intravenously and a maintenance dosage of 5 to 7 mg per kilogram per day. Phenytoin, administered in a loading dose of 15 to 20 mg per kilogram, may be used if seizures persist despite adequate therapeutic levels of phenobarbital (25 μg per milliliter to as high as 40 μg per milliliter). Because CNS involvement or seizure activity is frequently subclinical in neonatal HSV encephalitis, electroencephalography has an important diagnostic role. CNS imaging studies, either CT or MRI, should also be obtained to determine the presence or extent of cerebral lesions.

Infants who survive neonatal HSV infections frequently have recurring herpetic skin lesions and should be excluded temporarily from day-care or center-based programs when lesions are active. If lesions involve a small surface area, they can be covered by clothes or dressings, allowing the child to resume normal activities. When lesions are not present or crusted, these infants pose no risk to other children or adult caretakers.

Enteroviruses

Antiviral Therapy

At present, neonatal enteroviral infections cannot be treated with specific antiviral chemotherapy.

Adjunctive Therapy

Infants with severe neonatal nonpolio enteroviral infections pose complex diagnostic and therapeutic dilemmas primarily because such infants can be difficult to distinguish from those with bacterial or disseminated HSV infections. Bacterial (blood, CSF, urine, and nasopharynx) and viral cultures (throat swab, rectal swab, and CSF) should be obtained, and antibiotics, such as ampicillin, cefotaxime, and/or an aminoglycoside, should be initiated as soon as possible. In addition, these infants may require initiation of anti-HSV agents, such as acyclovir, which should be continued until an etiologic diagnosis is established.

Infants with tachypnea, tachycardia, and liver enlargement, signs compatible with myocarditis associated with neonatal coxsackievirus B infections, require cautious fluid restriction, diuretics, and possibly, inotropic agents. Such infants should be carefully monitored for cardiac arrhythmias. Neonates with signs of DIC may require transfusions of platelets and fresh frozen plasma.

Varicella-Zoster Virus

Antiviral Therapy

Although acyclovir has not been extensively studied in neonates with perinatally acquired varicella-zoster virus (VZV) infections, it should be considered in those infants with severe infections, using the regimen outlined above for HSV infections. Varicella-zoster immune globulin (VZIG) prevents or modifies VZV infections in neonates exposed to VZV infection. VZIG should be administered as a one-time intramuscular dose of one vial (approximately 1.25 ml) administered at the following times: (1) as soon as possible after delivery if the mother had onset of varicella within 5 days before or 2 days after delivery, (2) within 96 hours of varicella exposure in hospitalized preterm infants younger than 28 weeks gestational age (due to poor placental transfer of antibody), or (3) within 96 hours of exposure in premature infants older than 28 weeks gestational age whose mothers deny having had prior chickenpox infections.

Adjunctive Therapy

Infants with fetal VZV syndrome, a rare disorder, typically have skin lesions as well as anomalies of the eye, CNS, and skeleton and thus require ophthalmologic examination and radiologic investigations, particularly CNS imaging studies. Perinatal VZV infections may be mild, requiring minimal therapy, or severe, resembling disseminated HSV infection. Intensive supportive care as well as therapy with acyclovir may be necessary.

Human Immunodeficiency Virus

The human immunodeficiency virus (HIV), the causative agent of the acquired immunodeficiency syndrome (AIDS), can be transmitted transplacentally, intrapartum, or via breast milk. Although most HIV-infected infants are asymptomatic at birth, failure to thrive or secondary infections may develop within the first 8 weeks of life. Because maternally derived antibodies may persist for many months, diagnosis relies on serial antibody assessment, detection of HIV antigen or nucleic acid, isolation of HIV, or the presence of secondary complications unique to AIDS. Management currently consists of treating secondary infectious complications, caused by such agents as CMV, *Pneumocystic carinii,* or *Toxoplasma gondii,* and initiating experimental anti-HIV therapy with drugs such as zidovudine.

Other

Other viruses, such as lymphocytic choriomeningitis virus or parvovirus B19, account for rare cases of congenital infection. Because specific antiviral medications are not currently available, therapy consists of supportive care and treatment of secondary complications.

SUGGESTED READING

American Academy of Pediatrics. The 1988 Red Book: Report of the Committee on Infectious Diseases. Elk Grove Village, Illinois: The American Academy of Pediatrics (AAP), 1988.

Andersen RD, Bale JF Jr., Blackman JA, Murph JR. Infections in children: a sourcebook for educators and childcare providers. Rockville MD: Aspen.

Bell WE, McCormick WF. Neurologic infections in children. Philadelphia: WB Saundners, 1981.

Johnson RT. Viral infections of the nervous system. New York: Raven Press, 1982.

Roberts RJ. Drug therapy in infants: pharmacologic principles and clinical experience. Philadelphia: WB Saunders, 1984.

PATIENT RESOURCES

The following groups may be of assistance to people seeking information or guidance with regard to congenital viral infections and their associated problems:

March of Dimes Birth Defects Foundation
1275 Mamaroneck Avenue
White Plains, New York 10605
Telephone: (914) 428-7100

National Foundation for Children's Hearing
  Education and Research
928 McLeon Avenue
Yonkers, New York 10704
Telephone: (914) 237-2676

Developmental Disabilities Center
  (formerly, Rubella Project)
St. Luke's—Roosevelt Hospital
428 West 59th Street
New York, New York 10019
Telephone: (212) 554-6565

Herpes Resource Center of the American
  Social Health Association
P.O. Box 100
Palo Alto, California 94302
Telephone: (415) 328-7710

VIRAL ENCEPHALITIS

LESLIE P. WEINER, M.D.

A patient presenting with an acute onset headache, fever, a change in mental status with or without obtundation, and a mononuclear cell pleocytosis should be considered as having a possible viral encephalitis. Such a presentation must be viewed as a medical emergency. Nonviral causes should be ruled out (Table 1) and attention turned to the differential diagnosis of viral encephalitis (Table 2). Of all the viral encephalidites, herpes simplex virus (HSV) encephalitis is the most important to identify; although only 10 percent of viral encephalidites are caused by HSV, more than half of deaths caused by viral encephalitis are attributed to it. An early etiologic diagnosis cannot easily be made even when sophisticated viral and serologic methodologies have been instituted.

EVALUATION

The diagnosis of viral encephalitis is dependent on epidemiologic, clinical, and laboratory data. A history of recent disease contacts at home, the workplace, or social gatherings, as well as documentation of recent travels can be of help. Risks such as contact with pets or other domestic animals, any wild animals, rodents, or ticks should be identified, particularly as they might suggest Lyme disease, lymphocytic choriomeningitis, or rabies. Regional virus activity is also important. Data may be obtained from the local health department suggesting an outbreak of St. Louis encephalitis or enteroviruses. In addition, seasonal activity provides further information. Late summer and early fall is associated with arbovirus and enterovirus infections, whereas spring is associated with mumps. An immunization history—particularly as it relates to poliovirus and mumps—may also be helpful.

The diagnosis of encephalitis may be aided by

Table 1 Disease That Simulate Viral Encephalitis

Infectious Diseases
  Bacterial processes
    Tuberculosis
    Mycoplasma pneumoniae
    Listeriosis
    Brucellosis
    Typhoid fever
    Syphilis
    Leptospirosis
    Lyme disease
  Bacteria-related
    Parameningeal infections
    Partially treated meningitis
    Brain abcess
    Mycotic aneurysms
  Fungi
    Cryptococcosis
    Candidiasis
    Coccidiodomycosis
    Histoplasmosis
    North American blastomycosis
  Parasites
    Toxoplasmosis
    Cysticercosis
    Echinococcosis
    Trypanosomiasis
    Plasmodium falciparum
    Amebiasis
    Trichinosis
    Schistosomiasis
    Toxocara
    Rickettsiae
    Typhus
    Rocky Mountain spotted fever
  Noninfectious disease
    Neoplasms
    Carcinomatosis meningitis
    Leukemic meningitis
    Diffuse gliomatosis
    Vasculitis
    Collagen vascular disease
    Granulomatous angiitis
  Others
    Sarcoidosis
    Behçet's syndrome

Table 2 Causes of Viral Encephalitis and Virus-Related Acute Encephalopathies

Viral encephalitis
  Sporadic
    Mumps
    Herpes simplex viruses
    Lymphocytic choriomeningitis virus
    Cytomegalovirus
    Epstein-Barr virus
    Adenovirus
    Rabies
  Epidemic
    Arboviruses (St. Louis, Eastern, Western, California, Venezuelan Equine, Colorado tick fever)
    Enteroviruses (coxsackievirus and echoviruses)
Postinfectious encephalomyelitis
  Measles
  Varicella
  Mumps
  Rubella
  Influenza
Viral infections in immunocompromised patients
  Cytomegalovirus
  Herpes simplex viruses
  Enteroviruses
  Adenoviruses
  Measles
  JC virus (Progressive multifocal leukoencephalopathy)
  Human immunodeficiency viruses (HIV)
Virus-associated encephalopathy
  Reye's syndrome

associated clinical signs. These include the following: (1) a rash that might indicate a childhood exanthem or an enterovirus infection, (2) oral thrush, which may be a sign of immunoincompetence, and (3) pneumonitis, which may suggest involvement with lymphocytic choriomeningitis, mycoplasma, or other bacterial infections. Pleurodynia and herpangina may be seen with different groups of coxsackievirus infections. Lymphadenopathy, splenomegaly, and hepatitis may be associated with cytomegalovirus, infectious mononucleosis, or human immunodeficiency virus infections.

It is important to make a correct diagnosis of encephalitis so that the patient may be spared therapies and diagnostic procedures that are potentially dangerous and expensive. An incorrect diagnosis of encephalitis may also prevent conditions other than encephalitis from being treated in a timely fashion and may thus result in a poor outcome. A definitive diagnosis may allow for the predictive course and outcome of the illness to guide the family and the patients in long-term care. Information which may be of public health importance may be obtained particularly as it relates to the need to control a vector. Finally, specific antiviral therapy such as antiherpes therapy may be administered.

Several conditions have clinical presentations that may mimic those of encephalitis. Table 1 lists the diseases that may simulate viral encephalitis. Some of these conditions may be difficult to diagnose because they are not ordinarily associated with an inflammatory process in the cerebrospinal fluid (CSF). On occasion, however, cryptic brain tumors, cerebrovascular accidents, and a subarachnoid hemorrhage associated with parenchymal damage may induce a CSF pleocytosis.

Another condition that may need to be differentiated from viral encephalitis is the syndrome of postinfectious encephalomyelitis. In this syndrome there is a history of a flu-like illness that occurs as early as 6 weeks before the sudden onset of neurologic deficits, fever, obtundation, and seizures. In most instances, the antecedent illness occurs 7 to 10 days before the onset of the encephalomyelitis. If the acute illness is associated with an identifiable childhood exanthem or systemic viral illness such as measles, the diagnosis is less difficult to make. In most instances, however, the acute syndrome is associated with an ill-defined and poorly documented flu-like process. It may not be possible to make the differentiation between a direct invasion by a virus and a perivenous immune-mediated demyelination on clinical grounds. An MRI, evoked potentials, or the presence of myelin basic protein in the CSF may be useful in suggesting a postinfectious demyelination; however, a biopsy may be required to differentiate these two entities in a patient whose condition continues to deteriorate.

HERPES SIMPLEX VIRUS ENCEPHALITIS

HSV encephalitis has no antecedent illness nor is there a seasonal variation. A history of or the presence of herpes labialis has no diagnostic value in implicating herpes simplex as the etiology of encephalitis. Typically, HSV type 1 encephalitis, the most important sporadic viral infection of the brain, is preceded by several days of fever, headache, and malaise. Behavioral abnormalities may be prominent during the early stages of the disease, prompting an inaccurate psychiatric diagnosis. The mental changes associated with this viral infection include withdrawal, agitation, hallucinations, and confusion. These may progress over hours or several days and gradually result in decreasing levels of consciousness. There may be an abrupt onset of major motor or focal seizures or a more slowly evolving aphasia, focal motor deficit, and sensory deficit. Localization to the medial temporal and orbital frontal regions of the brain is very suggestive of HSV type 1 encephalitis.

Routine laboratory studies including a complete blood count with a differential, an assessment of immune cells, blood chemistries including liver function studies, urine analysis, and chest x-ray examination may be useful in ruling out bacterial infections and the complications of an immunoincompetent state.

Examination of the CSF is the critical step in the differential diagnosis. Cerebral imaging should precede the CSF examination, and if there is no evidence of hydrocephalus, massive cerebral edema, or a shift of midline structures, a lumbar puncture should be performed. The computed tomography (CT) scan may be normal or show a low-density temporal lobe mass with edema. It may be that MRI may be a more sensitive early indicator of focal inflammatory disease than the CT scan; however, with regard to HSV type 1 encephalitis, the data are not yet available to support this.

The CSF may be under increased pressure. There is usually an increased number of mononuclear cells (7 to 500 cells per cubic millimeter). In as many as 5 percent of patients, however, there may be no increase in cells in the initial CSF. Although frequently there are red blood cells in the CSF, their presence is not considered diagnostic of HSV type 1 encephalitis. Protein is usually elevated but rarely exceeds 250 mg. The normal CSF sugar level is a critical value. In most instances, the ratio of CSF sugar to blood sugar is normal or very slightly depressed. Because the CSF sugar is normally two-thirds that of the blood sugar, it is essential that blood sugar be measured when the lumbar puncture is performed. If the initial spinal fluid examination is normal or if there is an unusual finding in the CSF such as polymorphonuclear cells, a repeat lumbar puncture should be performed within 24 hours.

In the absence of a focal temporal lobe lesion with brain imaging, electroencephalography (EEG) is perhaps the most sensitive test available. An emergency EEG, although not specific, may show unilateral or bilateral periodic epileptiform discharges over the temporal regions. Even in those instances where no periodic discharges are found, the presence of slow waves in the temporal area is suggestive of HSV encephalitis. Early in the course of the disease, radionucleotide scans may also be useful in demonstrating increased uptake in the temporal lobes when other methods have failed to demonstrate a focal lesion.

In those patients in whom focality has not been demonstrated within the first 24 hours, imaging and EEG should be repeated. If there is no evidence of focality or mass effect, the CSF should be re-examined to determine if there has been a change in the nature of the pleocytosis or the CSF sugar. Changes are most likely to occur in patients with partially treated meningitis. If the patient is deteriorating, a biopsy is indicated, even in the absence of focal signs.

TREATMENT OF SUSPECTED HSV TYPE 1 ENCEPHALITIS

In a patient who presents with personality changes, fever, focal seizures, and lateralizing signs of acute onset, the diagnosis of HSV type 1 encephalitis is strongly suggested. If the patient has a mass effect with a shift on CT scan or MRI, lumbar puncture is contraindicated and a biopsy of the temporal lobe should be performed as soon as possible. If the CSF can be evaluated, the indications for biopsy can be approached differently. The indications for brain biopsy in acutely ill patients do not so much confirm the diagnosis of HSV as help one diagnose a process for which a delay of treatment will result in a disasterous outcome. The best available information suggests that if the CSF sugar level is normal, there are few conditions that require an immediate change in therapy. In fact, although the estimated rate of complications such as hemorrhage and secondary infections (as reported in the literature) is probably less than 2 percent, it approaches the percentage of illnesses for which an immediate change in therapy is indicated. On the other hand, if there is a reduction in the CSF sugar, it is estimated that as many as 35 percent of patients presenting with focal neurologic signs will have a lesion for which treatment must not be delayed, or else the outcome will be poor. These conditions include bacterial cerebritis or abscess, tuberculoma, cryptococcal abscess, and an infectious vasculitis such as

syphilis. In summary, if the patient has focal temporal lobe mass and a CSF examination is contraindicated, a biopsy should be performed immediately. If the CSF can be examined and the sugar level is normal, I would not perform a biopsy; however, if the CSF sugar is reduced, a biopsy should be performed.

Treatment with acyclovir should be instituted as soon as the diagnosis is seriously considered. Important diagnostic information including viral isolation can be obtained up to 12 to 24 hours after the institution of acyclovir therapy. This antiviral agent should be administered at a dosage of 10 mg per kilogram every 8 hours for 10 days. This should be given intravenously in 100 ml of one-half normal saline over 1 hour. If a biopsy is being arranged, acyclovir treatment should be started while these preparations are being made.

The biopsy itself should be made in the area with the most disease. This should be carried out via craniotomy and not by CT- or MRI-assisted stereotactic biopsy. There are several reasons for performing craniotomy, the foremost of which is the low yield of diagnostic information from stereotactic biopsy. There have been approximately 2,000 stereotactic biopsies performed in my institution and although the accuracy with which brain tumors are diagnosed is greater than 90 percent, inflammatory lesions are diagnosed with an accuracy of perhaps 25 percent. Cultures are invariably negative, and 90 percent of patients in whom an inflammatory diagnosis is made have AIDS. The diagnoses in that group include toxoplasmosis, progressive multifocal leukoencephalopathy, and cryptococcosis. The open biopsy also allows the surgeon to have direct visualization of the area and at the same time serves to decompress an edematous temporal lobe.

The biopsy procedure in a particular institution should be guided by a formal protocol prepared by neurologists, the neurosurgeon, infectious disease specialists, and pathologists. The processing of the specimen should be prioritized. A portion of the specimen should be fixed in formalin for routine histologic examination. Tissue should be frozen for immunohistochemical staining using either fluorescent antibody or immunoperoxidase. Homogenates should be prepared to ensure proper culturing for aerobic and anaerobic organisms, fungi, and viruses. If possible, tissue should be prepared for electron microscopic examination.

In my experience, unless a specific alternative diagnosis has been made, acyclovir is continued for the full 10-day course even if the biopsy is negative. If the patient's condition continues to deteriorate and no obvious noninfectious complication such as a hemorrhage or ischemic lesion is evident, imaging and EEG are repeated. If the patient has not undergone biopsy and his condition continues to deteriorate, biopsy should be performed immediately. If the patient has a biopsy-proven HSV type 1, a rebiopsy may be necessary to determine if the HSV is persisting. If the HSV is persisting, a course of vidarabine, 15 mg per kilogram per day given continuously for 10 days, should be administered.

In my experience, few patients whose conditions deteriorate need to undergo biopsy or rebiopsy. Most deteriorate because of continued seizures, including electrical status, increased intracranial pressure, or complicating medical conditions such as fluid and electrolyte impairments and cardiorespiratory problems.

GENERAL SUPPORTIVE THERAPY

Several management decisions need to be addressed for a patient with suspected HSV type 1 encephalitis. Does the patient have an epidemic rather than sporadic encephalitis, and might the patient be contagious and require isolation? Should the patient be placed in an intensive care unit? Although strict isolation is not necessary, precautions should be taken in handling body fluids and waste material. Ideally the patient should be in an intensive care unit that has an isolation room, particularly if the patient has a viral exanthem. In any event, the patient must be in an area where close observation is possible.

Should the patient with HSV type 1 receive treatment with prophylactic anticonvulsants? Seizures are so frequent in patients with HSV that, even in the absence of clinical seizures, I routinely give patients a loading dose of 18 mg per kilogram of phenytoin if they have any focal activity on the EEG. Recurrent seizures are treated with intravenous benzodiazepine and phenobarbital. I do not administer anticonvulsants to patients who have no evidence of clinical seizures or lack focal signs or EEG changes. All patients who have undergone biopsy also receive anticonvulsants.

Does the patient have increased intracranial pressure? Does the patient's condition warrant endotracheal intubation? The use of an endotracheal tube to ensure proper oxygenation, to control ventilation rates, and to ensure against sudden respiratory failure from brain stem compression is indicated in patients with clinical or radiologic evidence of increased pressure. Tracheostomy is indicated in patients with prolonged coma. Treatment of increased intracranial pressure is difficult. Fluid restriction to one-half to two-thirds of the calculated daily requirement is useful. Controlled hyperventilation is important, with care taken to discontinue this treatment slowly as compensation takes place. Mannitol, 0.25 to 1 g per kilogram should be administered in small, repeated doses. Serum osmolarity should be maintained at approximately 310 mOsm per liter. Corticosteroids are indicated for the treatment of increased pressure in patients with HSV encephalitis. Dexamethasone is administered intravenously in a loading dose of 0.6 mg per kilogram followed by 0.2 mg per kilogram administered every 6 hours. There is no evidence that corticosteroids potentiates HSV encephalitis; however, prolonged use should be avoided if the diagnosis is in question.

Several other supportive measures are also necessary for proper management. These include daily assessment of electrolytes, blood glucose, and renal and pulmonary function. Inappropriate antidiuretic hormone secretion is a frequent complication of encephalitis. Urinary output should be carefully monitored, and in comatose patients, attention should be directed at maintaining proper nutrition. Finally, because viruses are thermolabile, fevers should not be treated too vigorously. A low-grade fever may be of some aid in the patient's recovery.

SUGGESTED READING

Nahmias AJ, Whitley RJ, Visentine AN, et al. Herpes simplex encephalitis: laboratory evaluations and their diagnostic significance. J Infect Dis 1982; 145:829–836.

Sawyer J, Ellner J, Ransohoff DF. To biopsy or not to biopsy in suspected herpes simplex encephalitis: a quantitative analysis. Med Decis Making 1988; 8:95–101.

Whitley RJ, Alford CA, Hirsch MS, et al. Vidarabine versus acyclovir therapy in herpes simplex encephalitis. N Engl J Med 1986; 314:1–149.

Whitley RJ, Soong S-J, Linnemann C, et al. Herpes simplex encephalitis: clinical assessment. J Am Med Assoc 1982; 247:317–320.

Wood M, Anderson M, eds. Neurologic infections. Philadelphia: WB Saunders, 1988:381–472.

HERPES ZOSTER

RICHARD T. JOHNSON, M.D.

Herpes zoster is as easy to diagnose as it is difficult to treat. Indeed, the patient usually makes the correct diagnosis of "shingles," and simple inspection without laboratory studies confirms the diagnosis.

The varicella-zoster virus causes almost universal infection in childhood with the clinical disease of chickenpox. During the course of that generalized blood-borne infection, the virus moves from skin lesions up sensory nerves and establishes latency in the sensory ganglion neurons. It remains latent for life. With activation, the virus spreads down the nerve, causing infection with vesicular eruption over the appropriate cutaneous dermatome. The virus may spread to immediately adjacent dermatomes, but in the immunocompetent patient, activated infection remains localized. Activation can occur at any time, but it is more frequent with increasing age or when a patient is immunosuppressed. It is estimated that by 80 years of age, 50 percent of all people will have had at least one episode of shingles. Lesions are most common over the trigeminal distribution and thoracic dermatomes, where the chickenpox blisters were most prevalent. Zoster is usually a benign, self-limited disease, but it may lead to persistent segmental motor paralysis. In two circumstances the disease is more severe. With increasing age, the acute disease is more painful and there is a greater likelihood of the development of postherpetic neuralgia. This is defined as severe, segmental pain persisting for more than 4 weeks after the onset of blisters. Disease is also more severe in patients who are immunosuppressed, where dissemination within the central nervous system (CNS) and visceral involvement may lead to severe and fatal disease.

TREATMENT OF UNCOMPLICATED ZOSTER

The rash begins as red papules, which become clear vesicles, and after approximately 3 days the fluid becomes turbid with the entry of inflammatory cells; the vesicles usually crust between 5 and 10 days. During this period, treatment should be symptomatic and should include the use of drying or soothing lotion such as calamine, trimming the fingernails to avoid excoriation and secondary infections, and the use of aspirin or acetaminophen. (Aspirin should never be used in children with chickenpox or zoster, however, because of the association of varicella with Reye's syndrome.) Once lesions have dried, capsaicin lotion may be used. Although this lotion contains the active ingredient of hot peppers and burns on application, it does over time cause cutaneous anesthesia. Ethyl chloride spray can similarly be used for transient relief of cutaneous dysesthesia.

Secondary infections of the lesions frequently occur. If localized, they can usually be treated with neomycin ointment. If cellulitis occurs with fever, cephalexin (500 mg four times per day) or dicloxacillin sodium (500 mg four times per day) should be given for 5 to 7 days.

Although herpes zoster is associated with Hodgkin's disease, cancer, and other diseases causing immunosuppression, it is not a first disease manifestation frequently enough to justify a costly search for underlying neoplasms or immunodeficiency diseases.

OPHTHALMIC ZOSTER

Involvement of the first division of the trigeminal nerve is second in frequency only to that of the thoracic lesions. With this involvement, there is often nuchal rigidity, obtundation, and greater severity of illness. A major complication of ophthalmic zoster is keratoconjunctivitis or iridocyclitis. One is forewarned of this complication if vesicles appear along the distribution of the nasociliary nerve on the lateral side and to the tip of the nose. Patients with first division ophthalmic zoster are also those at highest risk for developing cerebral vasculitis (see below).

In patients older than 60 years of age who have prodromal symptoms of greater duration and severe pain at onset, as well as in patients who are acutely ill with ophthalmic zoster (particularly with nasociliary branch involvement), oral acyclovir (800 mg five times per day) should be used. Lower doses of acyclovir given orally have been shown to be ineffective. It has been established that this dose shortens the healing time of lesions and decreases the duration and severity of acute pain, but its effectiveness in decreasing the incidence of postherpetic neuralgia has not been proven. In the uncomplicated cases of shingles, particularly in those patients younger than 60 years of age, the benefits do not justify the expense of oral acyclovir. Prednisone given during the acute phase of shingles has been claimed to decrease the frequency of postherpetic neuralgia, but the data supporting this are inconsistent. I do not believe that this uncertain effect justifies the slight increased risk of dissemination or immunosuppression associated with the use of corticosteroids.

THE IMMUNOCOMPROMISED PATIENT

Exposure of the immunocompromised patient to patients with varicella or zoster should be prevented, since immunocompromised patients can develop disseminated zoster after external exposure as well as after internal reactivation. Hospitalized patients with varicella or zoster should be placed under strict isolation; this is done not to protect the staff and the patient's family, but to protect other patients in the hospital who may be immunocompromised by disease or medical therapy. Zoster immune globulin protects immunocompromised children from contracting chickenpox after exposure to chickenpox or zoster, but it does not protect against zoster in children and adults with a past history of chickenpox.

If the patient is immunocompromised (e.g., patients who have undergone organ transplants) or if the lesions spread or show dissemination over more than three contiguous dermatomes, intravenous acyclovir should be instituted. If given within the first 72 hours, the agent is clearly effective. Doses of 10 mg per kilogram every 8 hours infused over a 1-hour period should be continued for 7 days. Because intravenous acyclovir is potentially nephrotoxic, the creatine should be followed carefully and adequate hydration should be maintained, even during the night. CNS toxicity also occurs, accompanied by tremor and disorientation. Dosage must be modified in patients with renal disease (e.g., organ transplant patients). If the rate of creatinine clearance is 25 to 50 ml per minute, the drug should be given every 12 hours instead of every 8 hours; if the rate is less than 25 ml per minute, infusion should be given every 24 hours; and if the rate is less than 10 ml per minute, only half of the single dosage should be given. The drug is removed by hemodialysis, and therefore the doses must be administered after dialysis.

VASCULITIS

On rare occasions, acute hemiparesis develops 2 to 10 weeks after the onset of ophthalmic zoster. Lumbar puncture may show some mild signs of inflammation, and angiography may show a localized vasculitis in the carotid artery near the trigeminal ganglion, or diffuse, bilateral vasculitis. The time of onset and the histologic features suggest that this granulomatous angiitis may be immune-mediated; on the other hand, some morphologic evidence suggests that virus may be present in the vascular lesions. Because of this uncertainty of pathogenetic mechanisms and the potential catastrophic effects of a generalized granulomatous angiitis, simultaneous treatment with both anti-inflammatory and antiviral drugs is justified. Large doses of steroids and full doses of intravenous acyclovir may be given.

POSTHERPETIC NEURALGIA

A pain persisting for more than 4 weeks occurs in only 9 percent of patients who suffer from shingles. Fifty percent of these patients have spontaneous resolution of pain by 8 weeks; less than 2 percent of patients with herpes zoster have postherpetic neuralgia lasting for 1 year or more. Postherpetic neuralgia is extremely rare in patients younger than 50 years of age. The greater the duration of the preherpetic symptoms, the more severe the lesions; the older the patient, the more likely there is to be severe and protracted postherpetic neuralgia.

The first step is to explain to the patient that this is generally a self-limited disease, although no guarantee can be issued since some patients have been described who have had postherpetic neuralgia for 10 years or more. Nonetheless, the statistics justify reassurance. Second, the use of narcotics should be avoided. In addition to having addictive properties, they are relatively ineffective for this form of pain. Local analgesic ointments or sprays provide only transient and usually trivial relief.

The drug of choice is amitriptyline, started at doses of 10 mg four times per day. In patients who feel too sedated by these spaced doses, it may be given as 50 mg at bedtime. The dose is increased until relief is achieved or until toxicity limits dosage. Doses of approximately 100 mg per day provide effective reduction of pain in most patients. When administered in conjunction with amitriptyline, carbamazepine, 150 mg per day increasing to 1,200 mg per day, may give greater relief, but the use of carbamazepine alone has not been evaluated in controlled studies. A recent double-blind cross-over study indicated that pimozide (4 to 12 mg daily) was more effective than carbamazepine in refractory patients; because of its side effects of tardive dyskinesias, memory impairment, and parkinsonism, it should not be the first option in the treatment of postherpetic neuralgia.

Although transcutaneous nerve stimulation has been reported to benefit some patients, it has been shown to be inferior to the medical treatment in controlled studies. In patients who have had prolonged disabling postherpetic neuralgia for several months and who are refractive to medical treatment, surgical intervention may be considered. Local root section and injection of nerve roots are ineffective since the neuralgia originates from the ganglion or proximal to the ganglia. Surgical interventions include lesions in the sensory ganglia, dorsal root entry zone, or spinothalamic tracts. The most effective surgical approach appears to be placement of thermal lesions in the dorsal root entry zone at the appropriate dermatome as well as at the dermatomes above and below the site of pain, yet even this destructive surgical approach has limited success. Therefore, medical treatment should be aggressive and prolonged, in the hope that the patient will experience spontaneous abatement of pain.

SUGGESTED READING

Balfour H, et al. Acyclovir halts progression of herpes zoster in immunocompromised patients. N Engl J Med 1983; 308:1448–1453.

Friedman AH, Nashold BS, Ovelmen-Levitt J. Dorsal root entry zone lesions for the treatment of post-herpetic neuralgia. J Neurosurg 1984; 60:1258–1262.

Huff JC, et al. Therapy of herpes zoster with oral acyclovir. Am J Med 1988; 85 (suppl 2A):85–89.

Lechin F, et al. Pimozide therapy for trigeminal neuralgia. Arch Neurol 1989; 46:960–963.

Max MB, et al. Amitriptyline, but not torazepam, relieves post-herpetic neuralgia. Neurology 1988; 38:1427–1432.

Wood MJ, et al. Efficacy of oral acyclovir treatment of acute herpes zoster. Am J Med 1988; 85 (suppl 2A):79–83.

RABIES

ALAN C. JACKSON, M.D., FRCPC

The rabies virus causes an acute infection of the central nervous system. With appropriate management, rabies can be prevented after an exposure (postexposure prophylaxis), and approximately 25,000 persons receive rabies prophylaxis every year in the United States. Although rabies is prevalent in wildlife in the United States, an average of only one to two human cases have occurred per year over the past 30 years.

PATHOGENESIS

The rabies virus is usually transmitted via the saliva of a biting animal. The virus is inoculated into muscles or subcutaneous tissues. There may be amplification of the virus in muscle at the site of exposure, accounting for the long incubation period in humans of a few days to a year or more (usually 30 to 90 days). The rabies virus attaches to muscle spindles and neuromuscular junctions and spreads within axons of peripheral nerves, reaching the spinal cord and brain. Subsequently, the virus spreads from the brain to the salivary glands, which is important for transmission of the virus in rabies vectors. The rabies virus may be present in an animal's saliva before the onset of signs of rabies.

CLINICAL FEATURES

Paresthesia or pain at the site of the wound may be an early symptom of rabies, and there may also be prodromal symptoms. Intermittent hyperactivity occurs in the classic form of disease. As many as half of affected patients have hydrophobia, which are associated with contractions of the diaphragm and other inspiratory muscles during attempts at drinking. Approximately 20 percent of patients develop a paralytic form of disease resembling the Guillain-Barré syndrome.

DIAGNOSTIC TESTS

Diagnostic tests for confirming rabies include the demonstration of the rabies virus antigen in corneal impression smears and in small nerves around hair follicles in skin biopsies taken from the nape of the neck (rich in hair follicles). The rabies virus can sometimes be isolated from saliva or cerebrospinal fluid (CSF). Serum-neutralizing antibodies do not usually appear until after the first week of clinical illness and are not useful in patients who have been immunized.

MANAGEMENT

Treatment of rabies is supportive since no antiviral therapy is effective. Survival has been reported in only three patients who were immunized before the onset of clinical disease. Intensive care is associated with prolonged survival of patients with rabies. Human-to-human transmission has never been documented except after corneal transplantation. Barrier techniques, including the use of gowns, gloves, and masks, should be practiced when one is caring for patients with suspected rabies because of the risk of transmission. Health care workers may require postexposure prophylaxis after high-risk contact with a patient with rabies.

Risk of Exposures

In a bite exposure, the animal's teeth breach the skin. In a nonbite exposure, saliva (or central nervous system tissue) contaminates an open wound, scratch, abrasion, or mucous membrane. Albeit rarely, rabies has been transmitted by an aerosol in bat-infested caves or in laboratory accidents. Approximately one-fifth of recent rabies patients in the United States have not given a history of an exposure.

When an exposure occurs, the likelihood of rabies transmission depends on whether rabies is known to exist or is suspected in the responsible species in the local area. For example, dog bites in New York City have not necessitated rabies prophylaxis for many years. Public health authorities are a valuable source of epidemiologic information. Most human exposures result from dog or cat bites. In the United States and Canada, the wildlife reservoir of rabies includes skunks, raccoons, foxes, and bats. In many developing countries, where most human cases of rabies occur, rabies is endemic in dogs, which are responsible for most exposures. Rodents (squirrels, chipmunks, hamsters, rats, and mice), rabbits, and hares rarely transmit rabies, and their bites do not usually necessitate rabies prophylaxis. Abnormal behavior of animals suggests the possibility of rabies, and the risk is greater with an unprovoked attack than with a provoked attack. A provoked attack may occur when a person attempts to feed or handle a healthy animal.

Management of Animals

After a bite or nonbite exposure from a dog or cat, the animal should be captured, confined, observed for a period of 10 days, and examined by a veterinarian before it may be released. However, if the dog or cat is a stray or unwanted, or if signs of rabies are present or develop during observation, the animal should be sacrificed immediately and the head transported under refrigeration for a laboratory examination. The brain should be examined for the presence of the rabies virus antigen, which is usually performed with the fluorescent antibody technique. Since the incubation period is uncertain for animals other than dogs and cats, these animals should be sacrificed immediately after an exposure and the head should be submitted for a brain examination. In high-risk exposures, rabies prophylaxis should be initiated before results from a laboratory examination are obtained. If the brain examination is negative, one may safely conclude that the saliva of an animal does not contain the rabies virus. If immunization has been initiated, it should be discontinued after a negative examination. If an animal escapes after an exposure, it should be considered rabid unless information from public health officials indicates that this is unlikely, and rabies prophylaxis should be initiated.

Postexposure Prophylaxis

After a decision has been made that postexposure prophylaxis is necessary, treatment includes local wound care and active and passive immunization. Treatment should be given as soon as possible. Initially, the wound should be thoroughly washed with soap and water. Devitalized tissues should be debrided, but primary closure of the wound should not be performed. Tetanus prophylaxis and measures to control bacterial infection should also be given when warranted.

Active Immunization

Human diploid cell vaccine (HDCV) is the best available vaccine for active immunization against rabies. Two hundred thousand courses of HDCV have been given over the last 12 years in North America and Europe, and there has not been a single case of rabies. A 1-ml dose should be administered intramuscularly in the deltoid area (in infants, in the anterolateral upper thigh) as soon as possible after exposure, but should be given regardless of the length of a delay. Four additional doses should be given on Days 3, 7, 14, and 28. Pregnancy is not a contraindication for immunization. Live vaccines should not be given for 1 month after immunization. Local reactions (pain, swelling, and itching) and mild systemic reactions (fever, myalgias, headache, and nausea) are quite common. Anti-inflammatory drugs and antipyretics may be used, but immunization should not be discontinued. Systemic allergic reactions are uncommon (11 per 10,000 people who have had vaccinations). Anaphylactic reactions should be treated with epinephrine and antihistamines. Corticosteroids may interfere with the development of active immunity. The risk of developing rabies should be carefully considered before discontinuing immunization because of an adverse reaction. A serum neutralizing antibody determination is necessary only after immunization of immunocompromised patients. In developing countries, alternative vaccines are commonly used that are less expensive. These vaccines, particularly ones derived from neural tissues, are associated with frequent systemic and neurologic reactions.

Passive Immunization

Human rabies immune globulin (RIG) should also be administered as passive immunization. RIG provides protection before the development of immunity from the vaccine. It should be administered at the same time as HDCV and should not be given later than 8 days after the vaccine. HDCV and RIG should never be administered at the same site or via the same syringe. The dose is 20 IU per kilogram; larger doses should not be given because the antibody has a dampening effect on the immune response. Immediately after the wound is washed, up to half of the dose (if anatomically feasible) should be infiltrated into the area of the wound and the rest should be given intramuscularly in the gluteal area.

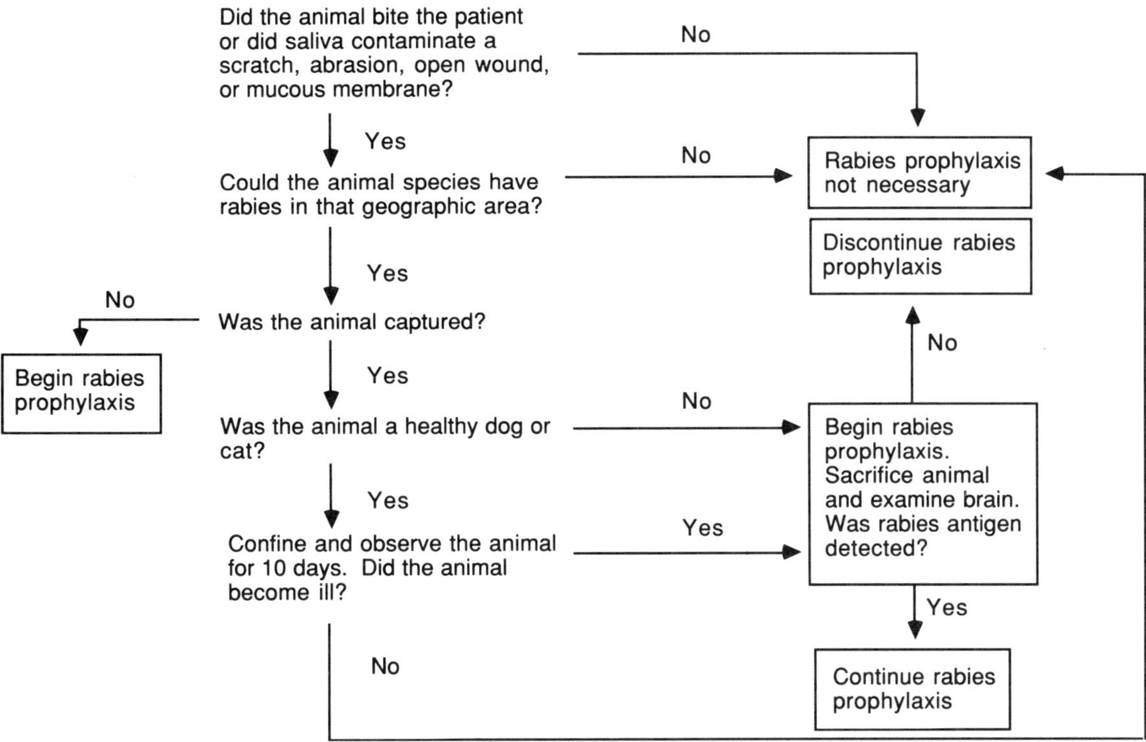

Figure 1 Algorithm for rabies postexposure prophylaxis. (Adapted with permission from Corey L. Rabies and other rhabdoviruses. In: Braunwald E et al, eds. Harrison's principles of internal medicine. 11th ed. New York: McGraw Hill, 1987: 714.)

In the case of an exposure involving a mucous membrane, the entire dose should be administered intramuscularly. Side effects of RIG include local pain and low-grade fever. If human RIG is unavailable, purified equine rabies immune globulin (ERIG) or equine antirabies serum (ARS) can be used in the same manner at a dose of 40 IU per kilogram. To assess hypersensitivity, intradermal testing with a 1/10 dilution should be performed before administration of ERIG or ARS. Anaphylactic reactions and serum sickness may occur, but the complication rate has been reduced in recent ERIG products.

Management decisions should be made quickly after a rabies exposure because delays in administering treatment will make it less likely to be effective. An algorithm for the management of patients after a possible exposure is shown in Figure 1. Physicians may need to seek advice from local, state, or federal public health officials for assistance in making decisions about postexposure prophylaxis.

Pre-Exposure Prophylaxis

Persons at risk for acquiring rabies, such as veterinarians, animal handlers, rabies laboratory workers, and certain international travelers, can be protected by immunization with three 1-ml doses of HDCV (pre-exposure prophylaxis) given on Days 0, 7, and 21 or 28. With special precautions, 0.1-ml doses of HDCV can be given intradermally for pre-exposure prophylaxis but not for postexposure prophylaxis. An adequate serum neutralizing titer should be demonstrated and repeated at intervals of 6 to 24 months, depending on the risk of exposure. Boosters should be given if the titer is inadequate. If a rabies exposure occurs in these individuals, local wound care and two doses of HDCV should be given. The first should be given immediately, and the second should be given 3 days later. Passive immunization (RIG) should not be administered to these patients.

SUGGESTED READING

Fishbein DB, Arcangeli S. Rabies prevention in primary care: a four-step approach. Postgrad Med 1987; 82:83–90, 93–95.
Kauffman FH, Goldmann BJ. Rabies. Am J Emerg Med 1986; 4:525–531.
Koprowski H, Plotkin SA, eds. World's debt to Pasteur. New York: Alan R. Liss, Inc., 1985.
Morrison AJ, Wenzel RP. Rabies: a review and current approach for the clinician. South Med J 1985; 78:1211–1218.
Immunization Practices Advisory Committee. Rabies Prevention: United States, 1984—recommendations of the ACIP. MMWR 1984; 33:393–402, 407–408.

NEUROLOGIC DISEASES ASSOCIATED WITH HIV-1 INFECTION

JUSTIN McARTHUR, M.B., B.S., M.P.H.

The nervous system is frequently involved during human immunodeficiency virus type 1 (HIV-1) infection, sometimes before advanced immune deficiency develops. Approximately 40 percent of patients with acquired immunodeficiency syndrome (AIDS) or AIDS-related complex (ARC) will develop one or more neurologic syndromes, and 10 percent of all patients will initially present with nervous system complaints. About half of the neurologic manifestations appear to be related to the direct or indirect effects of HIV-1, and the other half result from secondary complications of the immune deficiency induced by HIV-1. The HIV-1–related neurologic disorders are incompletely understood, and the full spectrum of nervous system involvement with HIV-1 infection remains unclear. However, treatment is available for most of the disorders, particularly if they are recognized at an early stage.

HIV-1–RELATED NEUROLOGIC DISORDERS

Some of these disorders occur early in the incubation period of HIV-1 infection, before any constitutional symptoms have developed. Others typically occur in patients with ARC or AIDS. The timing of these specific disorders, the differences in course, and the pathologic differences clearly suggest that different pathogenetic mechanisms underlie them.

HIV-1–Related Meningitis

One to two percent of recently infected individuals will develop acute aseptic meningitis with headache, meningismus, cranial neuropathies, and occasionally, transient encephalopathy. HIV-1–related meningitis appears to represent the initial response of the central nervous system (CNS) to viral invasion, and there is intrathecal synthesis of antibody to HIV-1. As many as 30 percent of HIV-1 carriers have a more indolent variant of HIV-1–related meningitis with chronic pleocytosis and headaches. Typically the acute symptoms of HIV-1–related meningitis are self-limited, require only symptomatic treatment with analgesics and antipyretics, and resolve within a few weeks. Serologic testing for HIV-1 (and probably human T-cell lymphotropic virus type 1 [HTLV-1]) should be part of the evaluation of patients with aseptic meningitis or chronic pleocytosis. It is uncertain whether the development of symptomatic meningitis or the detection of silent cerebrospinal fluid (CSF) abnormalities are predictive of subsequent progressive neurologic involvement.

HIV-1 Encephalopathy

Approximately 20 percent of patients with AIDS or ARC will show signs of a progressive subcortical dementia, and this syndrome has now been added to the list of AIDS-defining illnesses (Table 1). Also termed HIV-1–related dementia, AIDS dementia complex, and subacute encephalitis, the mental dulling, intellectual impairment, and memory loss can initially be mistaken for depression or other psychiatric syndromes. The disorder occurs in all groups at risk for HIV-1 infection, including children. The prevalence in *healthy* HIV-1 carriers is low. Based on current evidence, there is no justification for policies of employment disability based solely on HIV-1 serologic testing. Approximately 20 percent of patients with AIDS will develop a clinically significant dementia; however, during the early stages of dementia, the clinical features are nonspecific and stringent criteria should be used to avoid overdiagnosis of this condition (Table 2). Diagnostic precision is important not only for therapeutic reasons and because this disorder defines a case of AIDS, but also because the diagnosis carries serious prognostic and legal implications. Serial assessments of an individual are important in confirming progressive deterioration and excluding other potentially reversible causes of encephalopathy (see Table 2).

Although the pathogenesis of HIV-1 encephalopathy is unclear, zidovudine should be administered. The full dosage consists of 200 mg every 4 hours, and the drug should be administered in conjunction with the assistance of an internist or an infectious disease specialist because approximately 30 percent of recipients develop bone marrow sup-

Table 1 Major Neurologic Complications of HIV-1 Infection

HIV-1–Related	*Opportunistic Processes*
Acute aseptic meningitis	Cryptococcal meningitis*
Chronic pleocytosis	Toxoplasmosis*
HIV-1 encephalopathy*	CMV retinitis/encephalitis*
Vacuolar myelopathy	Other CNS opportunistic infections*
Predominantly sensory neuropathy	Herpes group radiculitis
Inflammatory demyelinating polyneuropathy	Progressive multifocal leukoencephalopathy*
Mononeuritis multiplex	Primary CNS lymphoma*
Myopathy	Systemic lymphoma*
	Neurosyphilis

* AIDS-defining condition.

Table 2 Criteria for Diagnosis of
HIV-1–Related Dementia

HIV-1 seropositivity (Western blot confirmation)
History of progressive cognitive/behavioral decline
Neurologic examination: nonfocal or diffuse CNS signs
Neuropsychological assessment: progressive deterioration on
   serial testing in at least two of the following areas: frontal
   lobe, motor speed, nonverbal memory
Absence of major affective disorder or active substance abuse
Absence of metabolic derangement (e.g., hypoxia, sepsis)
Absence of CNS opportunistic infections/neoplasms
   CT/MRI normal, atrophy, or white matter rarefaction
   CSF: negative VDRL and cryptococcal antigen

CT = computed tomography; MRI = magnetic resonance imaging.

pression necessitating blood transfusion and dose reduction. Other side effects include nausea, gastrointestinal upset, and during the first few weeks of treatment, headache. Patients with mild or moderate degrees of HIV-1 encephalopathy will often show improvement within a few weeks, particularly in memory and psychomotor speed. Several studies have demonstrated improvement in neuropsychologic test performance in both adults and children when zidovudine is used; however, the clinical benefits are usually limited to a few months and the disorder then continues to progress. Patients with far-advanced dementia rarely improve with zidovudine therapy. Symptomatic treatment is an important adjunct to antiviral treatment. Patients with mild or moderate dementia and marked apathy may respond to small doses of methylphenidate hydrochloride (Ritalin) starting with 5 mg twice daily. If marked depressive symptoms are present, tricyclic antidepressants may be attempted in a dose 25 to 50 percent of the usual dose. Patients with HIV-1 encephalopathy are extremely susceptible to the adverse effects of psychoactive drugs, and therefore hypnotics and anxiolytics should be avoided. Small doses of neuroleptics, such as haloperidol (Haldol) 0.5 mg administered as necessary, are useful in the agitated patient.

At an early stage before the dementia becomes too severe, one must discuss with patients with progressive dementia medicolegal issues such as arranging for power of attorney, completion of a living will, and arrangement of assets.

HIV-1–Associated Myelopathies

As many as 20 percent of patients with AIDS will be affected by a noninflammatory vacuolar myelopathy manifest by progressive spastic paraparesis and sensory ataxia and often accompanied by progressive dementia. As with HIV-1 encephalopathy, the pathogenetic mechanisms have not been elucidated, and toxic and metabolic factors may be important. The diagnostic approach should consider structural or compressive lesions and correctable nutritional deficiencies such as a vitamin B_{12} deficiency. A sensory level is unusual, so if one is present, particularly with back pain, magnetic resonance imaging of the spine or myelography should be performed to exclude extrinsic cord compression. Nonspecific CSF abnormalities are frequently present, but are not diagnostic. I have not found zidovudine to be useful in reversing the myelopathy, which usually progresses inexorably. Antispasticity agents such as baclofen (Lioresal) may relieve some of the spasticity.

Peripheral Nerve Disorders Associated with HIV-1

Predominantly Sensory Neuropathy

As many as 30 percent of patients with AIDS develop a neuropathy characterized by painful sensory symptoms in the feet. Most individuals develop this neuropathy late in the course of HIV-1 infection, usually in association with systemic opportunistic infections. This disorder can usually be recognized by characteristic complaints of dysesthesias and contact hypersensitivity in the feet with reduced or absent ankle reflexes and elevated sensory thresholds. Although electrophysiologic studies are helpful, they are not essential in the diagnosis and usually reveal a neuropathy affecting both sensory and motor fibers suggestive of a dying back axonopathy. Nerve biopsies are not usually helpful in the clinical setting. Consideration should be given to nutritional and toxic causes of sensory neuropathy, such as alcohol abuse, diabetes, pyridoxine excess, vitamin B_{12} deficiency, and the use of experimental neurotoxic antivirals, such as dideoxycytidine. Patients who develop predominantly sensory neuropathy are often already taking zidovudine because of their advanced immune deficiency. Although occasionally symptoms will stabilize with zidovudine treatment, more often there is no dramatic response, and symptomatic relief with pain-modifying agents such as amitriptyline hydrochloride (Elavil) or phenytoin (Dilantin) is more useful. Because of the potential for delirium, amitriptyline is started at a very small dose, 10 to 25 mg administered at every hour of sleep, and gradually increased to 50 to 100 mg.

Inflammatory Demyelinating Polyneuropathies

Several possibly immune-mediated phenomena have been described in association with HIV-1 infection, including inflammatory demyelinating polyneuropathy (IDP). In contrast to predominantly sensory neuropathy, IDP typically occurs at a relatively early stage of HIV-1 infection, before immunodeficiency develops. Typically there is profound motor weakness, sometimes developing acutely as

Guillain-Barré syndrome and associated with CSF pleocytosis. More often, IDP presents as a chronic, sometimes relapsing process. Because of this association between HIV-1 and IDP, a careful search for risk factors for HIV-1 infection and serologic testing should be carried out in any patient presenting with IDP. Plasmapheresis is the treatment of choice because it is less likely to cause additional immunosuppression than corticosteroids. In Guillain-Barré syndrome (GBS), a course of five plasma exchanges is given. With chronic inflammatory demyelinating polyneuropathy (CIDP), an induction course is followed by maintenance exchanges as needed. If plasmapheresis is impractical, short courses of corticosteroids are generally tolerated well without triggering opportunistic infections. For CIDP, I use a 4-day course of methylprednisolone, 15 mg per kilogram intravenously over 4 hours, followed by oral prednisone administered on the basis of an adjustable tapering schedule (60 mg administered over a period of as long as 2 months).

Myopathies

Polymyositis is an uncommon complication of HIV-1 infection that sometimes responds to treatment with immunosuppressive agents. Because of the potential for infectious complications, the use of these agents should be restricted to patients with severe weakness, greatly elevated serum creatine phosphokinase (CPK), and biopsy evidence of fiber necrosis and inflammatory infiltrates. A toxic myopathy can occur with the use of zidovudine, apparently after 6 to 12 months of full-dose treatment. The clinical features of toxic myopathy are not distinguishable from polymyositis. If a "drug holiday" of 2 to 4 weeks is accompanied by clinical improvement and a drop in CPK, I assume that the patient had a toxic myopathy and reduce the dose of zidovudine long-term.

OPPORTUNISTIC PROCESSES

Opportunistic infections and neoplasms of the CNS are common in the setting of HIV-1 infection, reflecting the underlying immune deficiency produced by infection and lysis of CD4 lymphocytes by HIV-1. Patients may have multiple concurrent opportunistic processes, or opportunistic processes may coexist with HIV-1–related neurologic disorders.

Intracranial Focal Lesions

A variety of disorders cause intracranial focal lesions, including toxoplasmosis, primary CNS lymphoma, progressive multifocal leukoencephalopathy, and other bacterial/fungal infections. Multiple concurrent opportunistic processes may coexist. Since specific treatment is available for many of these complications, early detection and accurate diagnosis is critical. A management approach based on empiric toxoplasmosis therapy has evolved (Fig. 1).

Cryptococcal Meningitis

Cryptococcus neoformans, a ubiquitous yeast, produces CNS infection in approximately 10 percent of patients with AIDS, and in some may be the first recognized opportunistic infection. The most common presentation is as meningitis with headache, meningismus, altered mentation, fever, and nausea. This constellation of symptoms mimics cerebral toxoplasmosis, other opportunistic processes, and when more indolent, HIV-1 encephalopathy. The CSF usually has *normal* cellular and protein constituents; however, uniformly cryptococcal antigen is detectable and fungal cultures are positive. A 6-week induction course with amphotericin B (0.6 mg per kilogram per day) is recommended. Flucytosine (Ancobon) is rarely tolerated by patients with AIDS because it causes diarrhea and myelosuppression. During successful treatment, both serum and CSF cryptococcal antigen titers can be expected to fall by at least four dilutions and fungal cultures will become negative. The CSF should be re-examined at the end of induction therapy or with recrudescence of symptoms. An end-of-therapy serum titer or CSF titer $\geq 1:8$ implies failure or relapse. Suppressive treatment with amphotericin B administered once or twice weekly via an indwelling Hickman catheter is necessary for lifelong maintenance. The median survival for patients diagnosed as having cryptococcal meningitis is about 9 months, and relapse occurs in approximately 60 percent. Alternative antifungal agents are being used more widely and include the agents fluconazole and itraconazole, which are still experimental. Fluconazole and itraconazole appear to be far less toxic than amphotericin B, are absorbed orally, and unlike ketoconazole, penetrate the blood brain barrier. They have shown promise both for primary therapy and as maintenance agents.

Cytomegalovirus Encephalitis/Retinitis

Cytomegalovirus (CMV) may cause infection of the retina, producing visual loss in as many as 20 percent of patients with AIDS. Less commonly, CMV produces an encephalitis that is clinically and radiologically indistinguishable from HIV-1 encephalopathy. An acyclovir analog, ganciclovir (Cytovene), is a useful suppressive agent, but frequently causes leukopenia and cannot be given in conjunction with zidovudine.

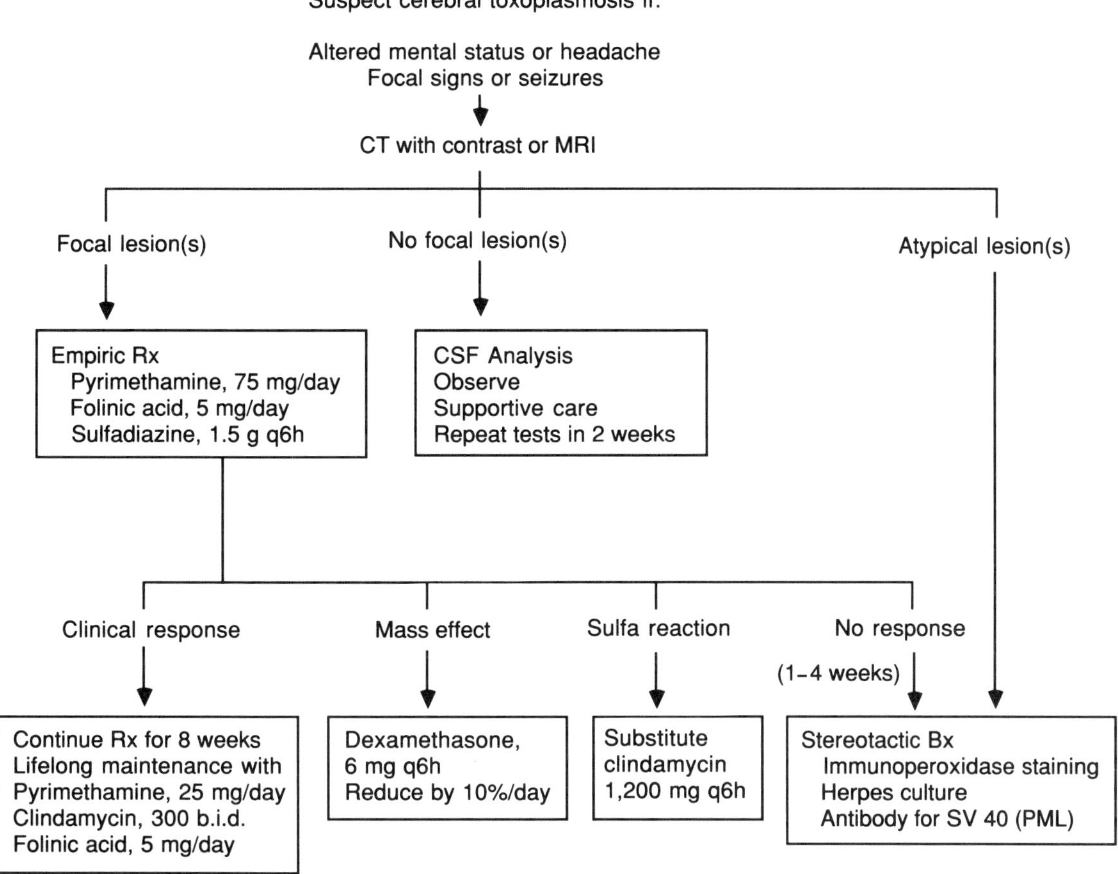

Figure 1 Management of intracranial focal lesions. CT = computed tomography; MRI = magnetic resonance imaging.

Cerebral Toxoplasmosis

Infection with *Toxoplasma gondii*, an obligate intracellular protozoan, causes necrotic and inflammatory abscesses that are often multifocal and scattered throughout the cerebral hemispheres with a predilection for the basal ganglia. Toxoplasmosis occurs in 5 to 10 percent of patients with AIDS, typically with fever, altered mentation, seizures, and focal neurologic signs developing over a few days. Imaging studies demonstrate multiple contrast-enhancing mass lesions; however, the radiologic appearances are not specific for toxoplasmosis and can be mimicked by lymphoma or other causes of abscess. Although serologic testing is not diagnostic, most patients with toxoplasmosis have detectable antitoxoplasma immunoglobin G (IgG), and a negative titer (<1:4) suggests an alternate diagnosis. Prompt initiation of antimicrobial therapy leads to clinical and radiologic improvement in approximately 80 percent of patients within 1 to 4 weeks. Corticosteroids should be restricted to patients with large lesions and mass effect. Lifelong suppressive therapy with two drugs, is necessary: pyrimethamine, 25 mg daily, and clindamycin (Cleocin), 300 mg twice daily. Relapse occurs in approximately 10 percent of patients.

Primary CNS Lymphoma

About 2 percent of patients with AIDS develop primary CNS lymphoma. The typical presentation is with slowly progressive neurologic deterioration leading to death within 3 months. Because the radiologic appearance cannot be distinguished from that of toxoplasmosis, biopsy is often necessary. CSF cytology is rarely diagnostic, and lumbar puncture may be contraindicated because of mass effect or the risk of herniation. The lymphoma is often multicentric and of B-cell origin, and it behaves aggressively. The response to whole-brain radiation or chemotherapy is poor, with a median survival of 2 months.

Progressive Multifocal Leukoencephalopathy

Progressive multifocal leukoencephalopathy (PML) develops in as many as 2 percent of patients with AIDS and typically presents with a progressive accumulation of focal neurologic deficits. Diagnosis is usually made from the typical clinical course, with imaging studies demonstrating multiple nonenhancing areas within the white matter without mass effect. Biopsy may be necessary to differentiate PML from cerebral toxoplasmosis, other opportunistic infections, or CNS lymphoma (see Fig. 1). Immunostaining with antibody to SV 40 or JC virus is necessary for definitive pathologic diagnosis. There is no effective treatment and the neurologic disorder usually progresses inexorably to death within weeks, or at most, a few months.

Herpes Group Radiculitis

Five to 10 percent of patients with HIV-1 infection develop herpes zoster radiculitis. Dermatomal herpes zoster does not require specific treatment unless cervical or lumbar dermatomes are involved. Here the potential exists for the development of severe myeloradiculitis with permanent motor deficits, and intravenous acyclovir (Zovirax) (30 mg per kilogram per day) should be used. The development of postherpetic neuralgia may necessitate the use of pain-modifying agents such as amitriptyline hydrochloride (Elavil) or carbamazepine (Tegretol). After the vesicles have completely healed, topical capsaicin (Zostrix) can reduce the neuralgic pains, but it must be used for at least 2 weeks. Recently cytomegalovirus has been identified as causing a progressive radiculopathy involving lumbar and sacral roots. Usually there is a polymorphonuclear pleocytosis and cytomegalovirus can often be isolated by culture from the CSF. An acyclovir analog, 9-(1,3-dihydroxy-2-propoxymethyl) guanine (DHPG) (ganciclovir [Cytovene]), has been tried.

Neurosyphilis

While not strictly an opportunistic infection, it has been suggested that the course of syphilis may be accelerated by the disturbance in cellular immunity accompanying HIV-1 infection. The clinical features of neurosyphilis may be modified and the time course from primary to tertiary syphilis shortened. There are reports of false-negative syphilis serology in individuals with biopsy-proven syphilis; however, in general, syphilis serology is reliable. Because of poor CSF penetration, benzathine penicillin should be avoided in patients with neurosyphilis. In a neurologically normal HIV-1 carrier with a history of *treated* syphilis who is sero-fast (rapid plasma reagin [RPR] $\leq$ 1:8 consistently), I do not

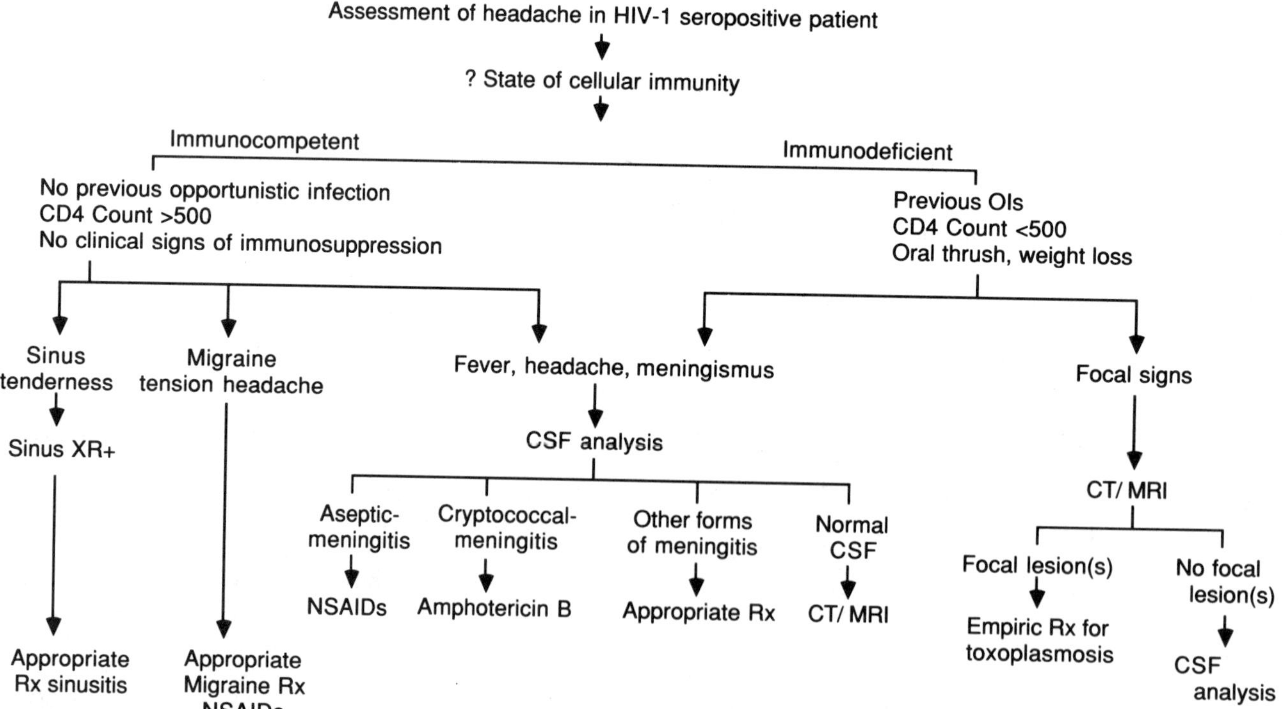

Figure 2 Assessment of headache in the HIV-1 seropositive patient. CT = computed tomography; MRI = magnetic resonance imaging; NSAIDs = nonsteroidal anti-inflammatory drugs; OIs = opportunistic infections.

advocate additional therapy or lumbar puncture. When neurologic symptoms are present, however, even if not typical of neurosyphilis, the CSF should be examined. If CSF Veneral Disease Reference Laboratory (VDRL) is positive or serum RPR is high (>1:16) and clinical features are suggestive of neurosyphilis, I favor treatment with intravenous penicillin, 24 mU for 10 days, or procaine penicillin, 2.4 mU with probenecid for 10 days, followed by re-examination of the CSF.

With an estimated 1.5 million Americans already infected with HIV-1, there is likely to be an increasing burden placed on neurologists for assessment of HIV-1 carriers with symptoms such as headache, memory loss, and neuropsychiatric symptoms. Usually knowledge of the systemic stage of HIV-1 disease and immune status is the most helpful information, and the approach shown in Figure 2 can be followed. One can usually reassure most HIV-1 carriers that serious neurologic complications are unusual at this stage of infection. Neurodiagnostic studies should be limited and lumbar puncture in particular is rarely useful at this stage because of the high frequency of silent HIV-1–related abnormalities.

SUGGESTED READING

AIDS Bibliography. Bethesda, MD: National Library of Medicine.

AIDS Experimental Treatment Directory. New York: American Foundation for AIDS Research (AMFAR).

Aronow HA, Brew BJ, Price RW. The management of the neurologic complications of HIV infection and AIDS. AIDS 2 1988; (suppl 1):S151–S159.

Cornblath DR. Treatment of the neuromuscular complications of human immunodeficiency virus infection. Ann Neurol 1988; 23 (suppl):S88–S91.

Haverkos H. Assessment of therapy for toxoplasma encephalitis. Am J Med 1987; 82:907–914.

McArthur JC. Neurologic manifestations of AIDS. Medicine 1987; 66:407–437.

Zuger A, Louie E, Holzman RS, et al. Cryptococcal disease in patients with the acquired immunodeficiency syndrome: diagnostic features and outcome of treatment. Ann Intern Med 1986; 104:234–240.

PATIENT RESOURCES

American Foundation for AIDS Research (AMFAR)
1515 Broadway 36th floor
New York, New York 10036
Telephone: (212) 333-3118

National Hemophilia Foundation
110 Greene St. Room 406
New York, New York 10012
Telephone: (212) 966-9247

AIDS Clinical Trials Information
Building 10 Room 11B09
Clinical Center NIH
Bethesda, Maryland 20892
Telephone: 1-800-TRIALS-A
    Monday–Friday, 9 AM–7 PM EDT

CDC AIDS Hotline
1-800-342-AIDS

Burroughs Wellcome (AZT [zidovudine] manufacturer)
Patient Temporary Assistance Program for Persons with AIDS
Telephone: 1-800-722-9292 (ext. 3633)

National AIDS Information Clearing House
P.O. Box 6003
Rockville, Maryland 20850

National Gay and Lesbian Task Force
Crisis Line
1-800-221-7044

Centers for Disease Control
1-404-639-3311

NONVIRAL INFECTIOUS DISEASE

BACTERIAL MENINGITIS

CHAD K. OH, M.D.
BURK JUBELT, M.D.

Meningitis is an inflammation of the meninges that is identified by an abnormal number of white blood cells in the cerebrospinal fluid (CSF). There is inflammation of the pia mater, the arachnoid, and the intervening CSF throughout the subarachnoid space of the brain and spinal cord (leptomeningits). The epenyma of the ventricles are also frequently inflamed (ventriculitis). Pyogenic meningitis is usually an acute infection caused by bacteria that evoke a polymorphonuclear (PMN) leukocyte response in the CSF. Much less frequent are subacute forms of bacterial meningitis (*Listeria monocytogenes, M. tuberculosis, T. pallidum*), which are characterized by a mononuclear cell response in the CSF. In a majority of cases, the meninges are infected by hematogenous seeding from a distant focus (i.e., septicemia or metastatic infection from the heart, lung, or other viscera). Direct extension of infection may occur from septic foci in surrounding tissues (sinusitis, otitis, osteomyelitis, brain abscess), fractures of the skull, nasal sinuses or mastoids, and neurosurgical procedures. While a diagnosis differentiating the type of meningitis may be difficult to make during the early stages of the disease, it is imperative that treatment be instituted as soon as possible since untreated bacterial meningitis is usually fatal.

DIAGNOSIS

The nervous system symptoms and signs, clinical course, and pathology of acute purulent meningitis are similar regardless of the causative organism. An acute onset of fever accompanied by generalized headache, and vomiting is the common mode of presentation. Signs of meningeal irritation ("stiff neck," Kernig's and Brudzinski's signs) are usually present except in infants, the elderly, or obtunded patients. A lumbar puncture (LP) should be performed and rapidly analyzed unless there is evidence of increased intracraninal pressure (papilledema, confusion, obtundation) or focality on neurologic examination. If these complications are present, a computed tomographic (CT) scan should precede the LP. The CSF should be analyzed with a cell count and differential, protein and glucose determinations, Gram stain, and culture. A simultaneous blood glucose determination should also be performed. A preponderance of PMN leukocytes and a low CSF glucose (<60 percent of the concomitant blood sugar) strongly suggest bacterial meningitis. Acid-fast and India ink stains should be performed when the gram stain is negative. When CSF examination is inconclusive, CSF should be sent for bacterial capsular polysaccaride antigens (available for pneumococcus, meningococcus, and *Haemophilus influenzae*), and the LP should be repeated within 12 to 24 hours. Throat and blood cultures should also be obtained as well as cultures from other extraneural sites, when appropriate. Antibiotic therapy should be initiated based on the statistical probability of which organism is commonly incriminated for that particular age group and those particular underlying conditions (Table 1).

GENERAL TREATMENT

General Supportive Measures

Once meningitis is suspected, it is essential to stabilize the patient. Intravenous access should be ensured. Assessment of vital signs with concomitant evaluation for shock, dehydration, electrolyte abnormalities, coagulopathies, and increased intracranial pressure must be performed rapidly.

Fluid Balance

The fluid and electrolyte balance must be carefully monitored. Dehydration and/or shock is common on presentation and must be corrected by blood volume expansion and/or vasopressors. Overhydration must be avoided, however, as it may worsen or precipitate cerebral edema. The syndrome of inappropriate secretion of antidiuretic hormone

Table 1 Common Etiologic Agents of Bacterial Meningitis by Patient Age and Predisposing Conditions

Age and Predisposing Conditions	Organism
Age	
Neonates	*E. coli*
	Group B streptococci
Infants and children	*H. influenzae*
	N. meningitidis
	S. pneumoniae
Adults	*S. pneumoniae*
	N. meningitidis
Predisposing Condition	
Neurosurgical procedure, head trauma, and intravenous drug abuse	Staphylococci
	Gram-negative bacilli
Diabetes mellitus	Gram-negative bacilli
	S. pneumoniae
	Staphylococci
Sickle cell anemia	*S. pneumoniae*
Alcoholism	*S. pneumococci*
Neoplastic disease, and immunosuppressed and immunocompromised patients	Gram-negative bacilli
	Listeria monocytogenes
	S. pneumoniae

(SIADH) is a common complication of meningitis requiring fluid restriction.

Cerebral Edema

Signs such as vomiting, lethargy, bulging fontanelle, hypertonicity, unequal or dilated pupils, bradycardia or apnea, impaired ocular movements, papilledema, and decorticate or decerebrate posturing may indicate advancing increased intracranial pressure and herniation. Controlled hyperventilation to a Pco_2 of 25 to 30 mm Hg rapidly lowers intracranial pressure through constriction of cerebral vessels. Osmotic agents should also be used for emergencies. A 20 percent solution of mannitol (0.5 to 1.5 g per kilogram) is infused intravenously over 30 minutes and repeated as needed. An indwelling urinary catheter should be placed. Fluid restriction is also advisable. Although there are no clinical studies specifically indicating that corticosteroids decrease cerebral edema because of bacterial meningitis, dexamethasone (0.6 mg per kilogram per day in four divided doses) should be added for moderate to severe edema.

Seizures

Seizures are a common complication of meningitis and usually occur during the first 24 to 48 hours of illness. Causes of seizures include bacterial toxins, cerebritis, infarction, fluid and electrolyte disturbances, and fever. Once seizures are noted, the airway should be ensured and appropriate anticonvulsants administered. If necessary, diazepam can be given initially to stop seizures, and thereafter longer-acting agents such as phenobarbital or phenytoin should be used to sustain seizure control. If there is only an isolated seizure, one may use phenobarbital or phenytoin for treatment without resorting to diazepam. Phenytoin does not generally depress the respiratory center like phenobarbital, but cardiac function must be monitored when phenytoin is given intravenously. After resolution of the meningitis, continuous anticonvulsant therapy is probably unnecessary unless persistent or focal seizures occur. Seizures are rare as a sequela of meningitis. Persistent or focal seizures imply an intracranial process (abscess, infarction) that should be reevaluated with CT scanning.

Complications

Coagulopathies

Disseminated intravascular coagulation (DIC) frequently occurs in patients with meningitis, particularly with meningococcal and other gram-negative bacteria. If DIC is confirmed by laboratory tests, treatment with heparin should be instituted with hematologic consultation. Mild forms of coagulation disorders, such as thrombocytopenia, may also be seen.

Subdural Effusions

This complication occurs primarily in infants younger than 1 year of age and occasionally in small children. It should be considered when worsening occurs during the 2nd week of therapy (recurrent fevers, headache, vomiting, irritability, lethargy, seizures, and fullness of the fontanelle). Subdural effusions are a collection of sterile fluid in the subdural space. If a CT scan reveals brain compression or displacement, treatment should be instituted with subdural taps. Surgical shunting or drainage should be considered only if repeated tapes are not successful or cannot be used as treatment.

Hydrocephalus

Hydrocephalus may complicate bacterial meningitis during the 1st or 2nd week of infection. The hydrocephalus may be noncommunicating because of obstruction of CSF flow at the aqueduct of Sylvius or at the outflow foramen of the fourth ventricle, or it may be communicating because meningeal inflammation blocks the arachnoid villi. Noncommunicating hydrocephalus is usually emergent, accompanied by papilledema, paralysis of upward gate, Babinski signs, and conditions ranging from lethargy to coma. Diagnosis can easily be made by

CT scanning and treatment instituted with ventricular drainage followed by shunting. Communicating hydrocephalus is not an emergency. Treatment involves resolving the meningitis, after which shunting is performed, if necessary.

Cortical Vein Thrombosis

Cortical vein thrombosis (thrombophlebitis) usually occurs during the 2nd week of the disease and results in fever, infarcts, and focal deficits. Because this late thrombosis suggests continuing infection, the choice of antibiotics should be re-evaluated and the CT scan and LP should be repeated.

Deafness

Bilateral sensorineural hearing loss is not an unusual complication of meningitis, especially in children. It does not correlate with the time of onset of treatment. Administration of corticosteroids (dexamethasone) during the first 4 days of illness may be preventative. Early evaluation (audiometry, auditory-evoked potentials) and treatment (speech therapy, hearing aids) are important in the management of this complication.

ANTIBIOTIC THERAPY

General Antibiotic Therapy

Antibiotic therapy should begin promptly after the LP has been completed. Since cultures and sensitivities will not be available for 24 to 48 hours, the choice of antibiotic will depend on the patient's age and predisposing condition (see Table 1), other clinical clues (e.g., rash, pneumonia), and the Gram stain. If the etiologic agent is unknown and is not seen on smear, treatment will consist of combined therapy with broad-spectrum antibiotics based on the most prevalent organisms for the patient's age group (see Table 1). In neonates, ampicillin with gentamicin or ampicillin with a third-generation cephalosporin (cefotaxime, ceftriaxone sodium) should be used. In children, because of the appearance of ampicillin-resistant strains of *H. influenzae*, initial therapy now often uses a third-generation cephalosporin (ceftriaxone sodium), although ampicillin with chloramphenicol is still an effective alternative. In adults, penicillin or ampicillin is the antibiotic of choice unless there is a predisposing condition suggesting staphylacocci or gram-negative bacilli. A specific antibiotic should be chosen as soon as cultures and sensitivities are available (Table 2). Antibiotics should be administered intravenously (or parenterally) throughout the treatment period. Therapy is continued for 10 to 14 days, depending on the response, and until the patient is afebrile for at least 5 to 7 days. The treatment of gram-negative bacillary meningitis is more prolonged (usually a minimum of 3 weeks), especially in patients with recent neurosurgical procedures.

Specific Antibiotic Therapy

Pneumococcal Meningitis

Meningitis caused by *Streptococcus pneumoniae* is often accompanied by acute otitis media, acute sinusitis, or pneumonia. Other predisposing factors for pneumococcal meningitis include head trauma with CSF leaks, sickle cell anemia, an altered host immune system, and alcoholism. The pneumococcus is a gram-positive diplococcus. Penicillin G is the drug of choice. Chloramphenicol or vancomycin are indicated for penicillin-allergic patients. Pneumococcal vaccine should be given after resolution of the meningitis.

Meningococcal Meningitis

The presence of petechiae, ecchymoses, or purpura in patients with meningeal findings implies a meningococcal infection, although rarely, similar lesions can be caused by *S. pneumoniae* and *H. influenzae*. Both sporadic and epidemic forms of the disease may occur. *Neisseria meningitidis* is a gram-negative diplococcus. Penicillin G is the antibiotic of choice in the treatment of pneumococcal meningitis. Contacts should be treated with rifampin. Vaccination is available to prevent epidemics.

H. Influenzal Meningitis

This type of meningitis is becoming more common in older children and teenagers. A third-generation cephalosporin (ceftriaxone sodium) or chloramphenicol should be used. Dexamethasone should be added because it appears to prevent complications (see the section on deafness earlier in this chapter). Contacts younger than 4 years of age should be treated with rifampin.

Staphylococcal Meningitis

Staphylococcal meningitis primarily occurs after neurosurgical procedures, after penetrating skull trauma, or with staphylococcal endocarditis (usually in intravenous drug abusers). Methicillin-resistant Staphylococcal meningitis is becoming a problem and vancomycin may be needed.

Gram-Negative Bacillary Meningitis

Even though this type of meningitis primarily occurs in neonates, it also occurs in adults with predisposing conditions. Gram-negative bacilli are a

Table 2 Antibiotic Therapy for Bacterial Meningitis With a Known Etiologic Agent

Organism	Antibiotic	Adult Dose Per 24 hrs*	Pediatric Dose Per 24 hrs*
Gram-positive			
Pneumococcus	Penicillin G	24 million U IV	300,000 U/kg IV
Penicillin allergy	Chloramphenicol	4 g IV	75–100 mg/kg IV
Multiply resistant	Vancomycin†	2 g IV	20–40 mg/kg IV
Streptococcus			
Groups A and B	Penicillin G	24 million U IV	300,000 U IV
Group D (enterococcus)	Penicillin G	24 million U IV	300,000 U IV
	+gentamicin	5 mg/kg IM or IV	3 mg/kg IM
Staphylococcus aureus	Nafcillin	12–14 g IV	200–300 mg/kg IV
Methicillin resistance	Vancomycin†	2 g IV	20–40 mg/kg IV
Listeria monocytogenes	Ampicillin	12 g IV	300–400 mg/kg IV
Gram-negative			
Haemophilus influenzae	Ceftriaxone sodium or	4 g IV	100 mg/kg IV
	chloramphenicol‡	4 g IV	75–100 mg/kg IV, IM
Meningococcus	Penicillin G	24 million U IV	300,000 U IV
Others§			
Escherichia coli,	Ceftriaxone sodium	4 g IV	100 mg/kg IV
Klebsiella, Proteus,	+gentamicin	5 mg/kg IM or IV	3 mg/kg IM
and similar organisms			
Pseudomonas	Ceftazidime or	6–8 g IV	20–50 mg/kg IV
	Ticarcillin	18 g IV	150–300 mg/kg IV or IM
	+ gentamicin	5 mg/kg IM or IV	3 mg/kg IM

* Antibiotics should be given in divided doses.
† Because of poor CSF penetration, intrathecal administration may be required.
‡ Unless organism is shown to be ampicillin-susceptible.
§ Other third-generation cephalosporins plus an aminoglycoside may be used as long as they have activity against the appropriate organism.

frequent cause of meningitis in patients with neoplastic disease, immunocompromised states, or following neurosurgical procedures or head trauma. A third-generation cephalosporin and an aminoglycoside are currently used for the treatment of gram-negative meningitides.

Modifying Circumstances

Neonatal Meningitis

In neonatal meningitis, meningeal signs are usually not present and septicemia is common. Thus, the diagnosis is not apparent by examination and LP is often indicated in the irritable or lethargic infant. Organisms that predominate are often from the mother's perineum. Initial therapy is as noted earlier in this chapter.

Shunt-Associated Meningitis

Meningitis with ventriculitis is a common shunt complication. *Staphylococcus epidermitis* is the major offending organism, although enterococci and gram-negative bacilli are also found. Blood, the surgical wound, both ends of the shunt, and CSF obtained from the shunt-valve reservoir should be cultured, in addition to the CSF obtained by LP. Treatment includes systemic and intraventricular antibiotics (probably vancomycin or third-generation cephalosporin) and, of course, shunt removal.

Recurrent Meningitis

Recurrence implies a CSF leak or a compromised immunologic system. A history of head trauma is much more frequent in patients with recurrent meningitis. The anatomic defect may produce a CSF leak (rhinorrhea, otorrhea). Rhinorrhea may be diagnosed by analyzing the fluid leaking from the nose for sugar content. Radioisotope techniques may be used to localize the leak. Tests for immune competence should also be performed (immunoglobulin levels, complement levels, T-cell levels, and T-cell functions such as skin testing).

Partially Tested Meningitis

Prior treatment may mask the diagnosis of meningitis by altering the CSF picture, or more often, by preventing isolation of the causative organism. Broad-spectrum antibiotics are indicated.

SUGGESTED READING

Committee on Infectious Diseases. Treatment of bacterial meningitis. Pediatrics 1988; 81:904–907.
Kaplan SL, Fishman MA. Supportive therapy for bacterial meningitis. Ped Infect Dis 1987; 6:670–677.
Lebel MH, Bishara JF, Syrogiannopoulas GA, et al. Dexamethasone therapy for bacterial meningitis: results of two double-blind, placebo-controlled trials. N Engl J Med 1988; 319:964–971.
Miller JR, Jubelt B. Bacterial infections. In: Rowland LP, ed. Merritt's textbook of neurology. 8th ed. Philadelphia: Lea and Febiger, 1989: 63.
Roos KL, Scheld WM. The management of fulminant meningitis in the intensive care unit. Crit Care Clin 1988; 4:375–392.

TUBERCULOUS MENINGITIS

PATRICK A. MURPHY, M.D.

The most difficult aspect of tuberculous meningitis is establishing the diagnosis. A classic case presents as a subacute illness lasting from a minimum of a few weeks to a maximum of a few months. The patient is usually a child who has a tuberculous relative or lives in a high-risk tuberculosis area. The usual history is of some weeks of nonspecific symptoms such as anorexia, irritability, and malaise, with low-grade fever. This is succeeded by a more definitely meningitic phase with progressively severe headache, vomiting, and drowsiness. The patient may develop ocular signs caused by palsies of the third, fourth, or sixth cranial nerves or parenchymatous lesions such as hemiplegia or cortical blindness. These lesions occur because of granulomatous inflammation around arteries, with subsequent thrombosis. Fever becomes more marked, and Kernig's and Brudzinski's signs are usually positive. The illness progresses by fits and starts, and sometimes a vasculitic lesion in a particular artery may be confidently diagnosed as the cause of a new symptom. The patient may apparently improve on several occasions, but the general course is progressively downhill, with accumulating focal deficits, increasing stupor, and multiple seizures.

Tuberculosis of the nervous system may present in unusual ways. Infants and the elderly may simply develop confusional states, with or without fever. A common diagnostic problem in urban hospitals is an elderly black person, usually a man, who is either known to be tuberculin-positive or clearly ought to be because he lived in the center of a large city 60 years ago when tuberculosis was common. When such a person develops fever and confusion, and a few cells are found in the cerebrospinal fluid (CSF), it is virtually impossible to either exclude or confirm the diagnosis of tuberculous meningitis. Many such patients are treated for tuberculosis, but most prove in the end to have some other condition such as multiple cerebral infarcts, central nervous system (CNS) syphilis, or carcinomatous meningitis. Occasionally, however, the CSF culture grows the tubercle bacillus, and the behavior is reinforced.

Tuberculous meningitis is always associated with the presence of multiple caseating granulomas in the CNS parenchyma. Sometimes these are large enough to act as mass lesions (tuberculomas) and may mimic a cerebral tumor. Rupture of a large caseous focus into the CSF may cause acute deterioration, which presents as an apparent bacterial meningitis.

The differential diagnosis is large and includes infections by viruses, spirochetes, brucella, fungi, and parasites, tumors such as leukemia, lymphoma, and carcinoma, and conditions of unknown etiology such as sarcoidosis. In particular patients it may be necessary to consider vasculitic processes such as a systemic lupus erythematosus or granulomatous cerebral angiitis.

To establish tuberculosis as the definite cause of a CNS illness is not easy. General examination of the patient, including chest x-ray examination, may fail to show a primary tuberculous lesion in more than half the cases. The tuberculin skin test is usually (although not always) positive in children or young adults and is often negative in infants and the elderly. Skin tests or a Ghon focus merely show that the patient *may* have tuberculous meningitis, and not that it actually exists.

LABORATORY TESTS

The CSF is virtually always abnormal in patients with tuberculous meningitis, with a typical pattern of increased cell count, lymphocytic preponderance, very low glucose levels, and raised protein levels. However, even the presence of a typical pattern does not prove that an illness is tuberculous, because exactly the same patterns are seen in fungal meningitis. Often the pattern is atypical in some way, and any or all of the above parameters may be normal. If the patient presents because of an acute deterioration, the cells may be mostly polymorphs, although subsequent specimens usually convert to a lymphocytic preponderance. About 30 percent of CSF smears are positive for tubercle bacilli, and about 50 percent of CSF cultures are eventually positive for tubercle bacilli. Even repeated examinations of multiple CSF specimens by highly skilled observers have yielded positive CSF smears 87 percent of the time and a positive culture 83 percent of the time. In approximately 15 percent of patients, confirmation of the diagnosis is impossible.

Since many of the entities that can be confused with tuberculous meningitis demand treatment in their own right, there is need for rapid diagnostic CSF tests that can establish the diagnosis early in the course of the disease. Many attempts have been made. They include detection of tuberculostearic acid, and detection of tuberculous antigens by enzyme-linked immunosorbent assay, latex particle agglutination, or radioimmunoassay. Assays for mycobacterial antigens in CSF are promising. A biotin-avidin radioimmunoassay was developed that detected antigen in all of 19 cases of tuberculous meningitis, and in none of 26 cases of viral meningitis. Two of 30 CSFs from patients with bacterial meningitis were positive for tuberculous antigen at a low level. The usefulness of this test clearly depends on the patient population to which it is applied. If tuberculous meningitis is common, it will be quite valuable. If tuberculous meningitis is rare, most of the positive results will be false-positives.

At present, the diagnosis of tuberculous meningitis is frequently made by intuition and by excluding other possibilities as far as possible. If the patient's condition is good, delayed treatment may be permissible while diagnostic studies continue. If the patient improves while receiving ordinary antibiotics such as penicillin, this strongly suggests that the diagnosis is not tuberculous meningitis, and spontaneous improvement in patients not taking any antibiotics would strongly suggest viral meningitis. However, if the patient is severely ill or if his or her condition deteriorates while under observation, antituberculous therapy should be started without delay. Attempts to demonstrate tubercle bacilli by smear and culture should continue. Frequently one must be satisfied with indirect evidence such as suggestive symptoms, residence in a high-risk area for tuberculosis, tuberculosis in a close relative, a positive skin test, or abnormal chest x-ray examination. These indications, plus slow improvement in the patient receiving antituberculous therapy, must suffice for the diagnosis of tuberculous meningitis. During the 1930s, meningeal biopsy was the definitive method for establishing the diagnosis of tuberculous meningitis, and this procedure may still be considered in a difficult case.

Other etiologies of subacute meningitis should be excluded as far as possible. Serologic tests for syphilis should be done. Where relevant (in certain regions of the world) one should consider brucellosis, leptospirosis, relapsing fever, and Lyme disease. The most common cause of fungal meningitis worldwide is cryptococcosis, but it is relatively easily excluded by the latex agglutination test for cryptococcal antigen. Culture of CSF for fungi is notoriously difficult; large volumes and repeated specimens are required. Serologic tests for fungi by themselves are not of great value. However, if antifungal antibody can be demonstrated in the CSF in a titer higher than would be expected from the CSF globulin content, there has probably been fungal replication within the nervous system. As with tuberculous infection, fungal meningitis is often diagnosed indirectly by showing a chronic progressive meningitis in the presence of active fungal disease in some other part of the body.

The diagnosis of parasitic infection of the brain by toxoplasma, *Strongyloides,* or cysticerci is difficult to make. The most direct method is to biopsy a lesion demonstrable on CT scan. However, the demonstration of antibody to the organism in the CSF in a higher titer than that expected from the CSF globulin content is frequently used. In fact, the same logic can be used to support the diagnosis of CNS infection with any organism, whether it be parasite, fungus, mycobacterium, spirochete, bacterium, or virus.

Chronic viral meningitis caused by human T-cell lymphotropic virus (HTLV-1) or human immunodeficiency virus (HIV) infection has become quite common in some areas, and may be associated with parenchymatous involvement. Chronic meningitis due to herpes simplex virus (HSV)-2 is seen in some normal people, and other herpes viruses such as Varicella-zoster may cause meningitis in the immunosuppressed.

Tumors involving the meninges may be demonstrable by cytology of the CSF. The diagnosis should be supported by histologic evidence of tumor elsewhere in the body, or by meningeal biopsy.

DRUG THERAPY

The antimicrobial treatment of tuberculous meningitis has been varied. Because treatment has to be continued for months or years, it is difficult to know whether relapses are caused by antibiotic failure or poor patient compliance. In addition, the disease is uncommon in developed countries, so that most academic physicians have little personal experience with it. The published evidence at the moment would support that 9 months of isoniazid and rifampin, without additional drugs, is adequate treatment for all forms of tuberculosis, including tuberculous meningitis. However, many people think that because tuberculous meningitis is a highly severe form of tuberculosis, virtually always fatal if untreated, somehow more drugs are required. There is no reasonable basis for this belief and no support for it in published data on the treatment of tuberculous meningitis.

If more than 2 drugs are to be used, published evidence would suggest the use of 4 drugs for the first 2 months of therapy, followed by isoniazid and rifampin for another 4 months. One thus gains by shortening treatment, at the expense of some increase in toxicity. The 2 additional drugs during the first 2 months should be any two of streptomycin, pyrazinamide, and ethambutol hydrochloride. The precise selection made may be influenced by patient considerations. One might eschew pyrazinamide in an alcoholic, or streptomycin in a deaf, elderly man or a pregnant woman.

More than 2 drugs are used in a patient or in a part of the world where resistance of the tubercle bacillus to isoniazid or rifampin is likely. However, this situation is not common; there is no evidence of it in several large series of patients treated with just isoniazid and rifampin. Nevertheless, one can imagine patients to whom this treatment would apply.

The outcome is strongly influenced by the state of the patient at the start of treatment. Virtually all patients with no focal deficits and only minor lethargy recover, most without sequelae. Comatose patients have a mortality of 50 percent and a high incidence of residual disability. Steroids are frequently added to the regimen in seriously ill patients, especially if there is evidence of spinal block, hydrocephalus, or cerebral edema. The hope is that by suppressing the inflammatory response temporarily, one may avoid permanent damage resulting from arteritic lesions, cranial nerve palsies, or obstruction of the CSF circulation. Even when the diagnosis of tuberculosis is correct, the usefulness of corticosteroid treatment is disputable. The effects of steroids on other CNS infections misdiagnosed as tuberculosis may well be disastrous. It is therefore customary to insist that the diagnosis of tuberculous meningitis be firmly established before steroids are given.

In some parts of the world, tuberculoma accounts for as much as one quarter of all intracranial mass lesions. The diagnosis may require surgical exploration, but once it is established, most cases can be treated medically. The only exception is where the lesion is large and situated where it may cause death by mass effect. This usually means a posterior fossa tuberculoma, which is treated by complete or partial excision under an umbrella of antituberculous chemotherapy.

SUGGESTED READING

Daniel TM. New approaches to the rapid diagnosis of tuberculous meningitis. J Infect Dis 1987; 155:599–602.

Kadivel GV, Samuel AM, Telisforo BM, et al. Radioimmunoassay for detecting *Mycobacterium tuberculosis* antigen in cerebrospinal fluids of patients with tuberculosis meningitis. J Infect Dis 1987; 155:608–611.

Kennedy DG, Fallon RJ. Tuberculous meningitis. JAMA 1979; 41:264–268.

BRAIN ABSCESS AND PARAMENINGEAL INFECTION

JOHN E. GREENLEE, M.D.

Brain abscess and parameningeal infections—epidural abscess and subdural empyema—are potentially fatal neurologic conditions whose onset may be so insidious as to obscure their serious nature or whose presentation may be so fulminant as to leave little room for diagnostic delay or therapeutic error. Patient survival and prevention of permanent neurologic sequelae are dependent on prompt diagnosis and the institution of appropriate medical and surgical therapy. The first three sections of this chapter deal with therapy of brain abscess, intracranial parameningeal infections, and spinal parameningeal infections. The final section discusses treatment of complications of brain abscess and parameningeal infection. It must be stressed that all of the conditions discussed in this chapter may produce headache, neck or back pain, nuchal rigidity, and alteration of mental status, all of which suggest meningitis. If meningitis is suspected in a patient with possible brain abscess or parameningeal infection, antibiotic therapy for meningitis should be instituted immediately, followed by emergent magnetic resonance imaging (MRI) or computed tomography (CT) of the head or spine, as appropriate. Lumbar puncture should be carried out if these radiologic studies do not reveal a space-occupying lesion. Under no circumstances should initiation of antibiotic therapy in patients with suspected meningitis be delayed until brain abscess or parameningeal infection has been ruled out by neuroradiologic studies.

BRAIN ABSCESS

Brain abscesses are most frequently consequences of hematogenous dissemination of organisms from pulmonary infections, infective endocarditis, or venous spread of organisms from sinusitis, otitis, or mastoiditis. Abscesses may also be associated with penetrating trauma, neurosurgical procedures, or facial or dental sepsis. Single or multiple abscesses may be present. Brain abscess begins with the formation of microscopic focus of sepsis, usually within white matter or at the gray-white junction. Growth of bacteria within this focus results in a localized encephalitis or "cerebritis," which undergoes necrosis and liquefaction as the abscess forms. Host response to the abscess includes dense infiltration by inflammatory cells, alteration in microvascular integrity with localized, frequently intense cerebral edema, and a gliotic and fibrotic response that results in the development of a capsule. The abscess capsule develops slowly and is thickest on its cortical surface and thinnest medially. Abscesses tend to expand toward and to rupture into the ventricular system rather than into the subarachnoid space. The enlarging abscess and its surrounding cerebral edema form a mass lesion that may produce death from uncal or tonsillar herniation. Abrupt clinical deterioration and death may also follow rupture of the abscess into the ventricular system.

Etiologic Agents

Aerobic, microaerophilic, and anaerobic streptococci, including agents of the *Streptococcus intermedius* group (*Streptococcus anginosus* and *Streptococcus milleri*), are found in 60 to 70 percent of brain abscesses. Anaerobic and microaerophilic streptococci are common in abscesses arising from sinusitis or dental infections. *Bacteroides* species and enteric bacteria including *Escherichia coli*, *Proteus* species, and *Pseudomonas* species are present in 20 to 40 percent of patients. *Staphylococcus aureus* is found in 10 to 15 percent of patients and is the most common isolate from brain abscesses associated with penetrating trauma or neurosurgical procedures. Abscesses—in particular those associated with sinusitis or otitis—frequently contain mixed flora. *S. aureus* may be present in pure culture in cases associated with trauma or endocarditis.

Isolates from brain abscesses in immunologically impaired patients may differ from those recovered from abscesses in immunologically intact individuals. Fungi including *Candida, Mucor,* and *Aspergillus* species may be associated with brain abscess in diabetics and immunocompromised patients, or in patients abusing intravenous drugs. The most common cause of focal intracranial infection in patients with the acquired immunodeficiency syndrome (AIDS) is *Toxoplasma gondii,* followed by *Cryptococcus neoformans* and *Mycobacterium tuberculosis.*

Clinical Presentation

Brain abscess most commonly presents as a rapidly or subacutely developing space-occupying lesion, often without findings to suggest an infectious process. Duration of symptoms is 2 weeks or less in 75 percent of patients. Development of clinical signs, however, may be much more indolent or may occur so rapidly as to suggest cerebral infarction or acute meningitis. Headache occurs in approximately 75 percent of patients. Nausea and vomiting occur in about 50 percent. Approximately one-third of patients present with focal or generalized seizures. Nuchal rigidity is present in approximately 25 percent. Localizing neurologic signs, although suggestive of brain abscess, may be extremely subtle and are absent in as many as 50 percent. Papilledema is present in only 25 percent and is frequently absent in rapidly developing abscesses.

Diagnosis

Brain abscess should be considered in any patient presenting with new, severe headache and symptoms or signs of a rapidly developing space-occupying intracranial process or with the new onset of focal or generalized seizures. A history of systemic or pericranial infection, carious teeth, drug abuse, or activities constituting risk factors for AIDS should increase suspicion that an abscess may be present. Sinusitis or other pericranial infection may be silent, however, and the patient may deny a history of drug abuse or homosexual activity. Fever is present in only about 50 percent of patients, and even when present, may be 38°C or less. The peripheral white blood cell count is often normal and is elevated to more than 20,000 cells per cubic millimeter in less than 10 percent of patients.

The diagnostic study of choice in patients with suspected brain abscess is MRI, with use of gadolinium enhancement if initial images are negative. MRI may detect abscesses at the stage of cerebritis not seen on CT. Contrast-enhanced CT should be used if MRI is not available. The sensitivity of contrast-enhanced CT may be increased if the scan is repeated 30 to 60 minutes after contrast infusion. Both MRI and CT will delineate the edema surrounding the abscess and may detect silent sinusitis or otitis. With close physician monitoring for respiratory depression or other signs of neurologic deterioration, sedation should be used if required to prevent motion artifact in delirious or severely agitated patients. Where sedation is required, we use midazolam hydrochloride (Versed), titrated in 0.5-mg increments until the desired level of sedation is reached, usually not to exceed 5 mg. Lumbar puncture is contraindicated in the treatment of brain abscess; spinal fluid abnormalities are usually nonspecific, and the procedure itself is accompanied by a 10 to 18 percent risk of brain herniation and death. Evaluation of patients with suspected brain abscess should include rapid, thorough examination for remote sources of infection with appropriate cultures of blood and other fluids such as sputum, pus from sinuses, or material obtained during myringotomy.

Therapy

Therapy of brain abscess involves prompt administration of appropriate antibiotics, surgical drainage or removal where indicated, and control of cerebral edema. Abscesses at the stage of cerebritis may respond to antibiotics alone. Surgery may be deferred if the abscess is still at the stage of cerebritis or if its size is less than 3 cm in diameter and the patient is neurologically stable. Liquefaction of the abscess center, however, may permit organisms to survive within pus despite levels of antibiotic that would be bactericidal in vitro. For this reason, encapsulated abscesses should be surgically drained or

excised, as should any abscess which enlarges despite antibiotic therapy.

Recommended antibiotics for brain abscess are listed in Table 1, and suggested dosages are given in Table 2. Antibiotics used for brain abscess fall into four major groups:

1. Antibiotics specific for *Streptococci* and other gram-positive organisms: penicillin G; chloramphenicol in patients allergic to penicillin.
2. Antibiotics specific for penicillinase-producing strains of *Staphylococcus aureus:* oxacillin or nafcillin (oxacillin is less likely to produce thrombophlebitis); vancomycin in patients allergic to penicillins or in whom nafcillin resistance is suspected.
3. Antibiotics with activity against gram-negative organisms: cefotaxime sodium, ceftazidime, or ceftriaxone sodium.
4. Antibiotics with activity *Bacteroides* species: metronidazole or chloramphenicol.

In choosing antibiotics, one must remember that a mixed culture of organisms may be present. In pa-

Table 1   Provisional Antibiotic Treatment of Brain Abscess and Intracranial Parameningeal Infection*

Cause of Initial Infection	*Probable Organism(s)*	*Recommended Initial Therapy*
Unknown	Aerobic and anaerobic streptococci *S. aureus* *Enterobacteriaceae* *Bacteroides* *Haemophilus*	Nafcillin, oxacillin,† or vancomycin‡ Plus metronidazole or chloramphenicol Plus cefotaxime§ or ceftriaxone[4] sodium§
Frontal, ethmoidal, or sphenoidal sinusitis	*S. aureus* *Enterobacteriaceae* *Bacteroides* *Haemophilus*	As above
Dental sepsis	Mixed *Fusobacterium, Bacteroides,* and streptococci	Penicillin‡ plus metronidazole or chloramphenicol
Penetrating trauma or surgery	*S. aureus* Streptococci *Enterobacteriaceae* *Clostridium*	Nafcillin or vancomycin Cefotaxime or ceftriaxone
Congenital heart disease	*S. intermedius,* other anaerobic, and microaerophilic streptococci *Haemophilus*	Penicillin‡ and chloramphenicol or cefotaxime or ceftriaxone sodium
Pulmonary infections (lung abscess, pulmonary empyema, bronchiectasis	*Fusobacterium* *Actinomyces* *Bacteroides* Streptococci	Penicillin‡ and mentronidazole or chloramphenicol Chloramphenicol (if penicillin allergy is present)
Bacterial endocarditis	*S. aureus* Streptococci	Nafcillin or vancomycin
AIDS (brain abscess only)	*T. gondii*	Sulfadiazine and pyrimethamine (with folinic acid)

* Drugs listed represent recommended provisional therapy and should be modified as culture results and sensitivities become known. Doses for provisional therapy are given in Table 2. Renal or hepatic insufficiency may require adjustment in dosage amount and interval.

† Oxacillin is less likely to produce thrombophlebitis than is nafcillin.

‡ If *S. aureus* is suspected as an infectious agent, penicillin should be replaced by oxacillin or nafcillin. Vancomycin should be used if penicillin allergy is present or if nafcillin resistance is suspected.

§ Data concerning penetration of third-generation cephalosporins into brain abscess or parameningeal infections is limited. The above recommendations concerning cephalosporins are based on their use in meningitis. Addition of gentamicin should be considered in epidural abscess or subdural empyema where Gram-negative organisms are strongly suspected, or as therapy for systemic Gram-negative infection.

Table 2 Dosages of Antibiotics Used in the Treatment of Brain Abscess and Parameningeal Infections

Antibiotic	Sensitive Organisms	Total Dose Per 24-hour Period (Dosage Interval)*
For initial use		
Penicillin	*S. pneumoniae* *N. meningitidis* Group B Streptococci	Infants <1 week of age: 150,000 U/kg/24 hrs IV (q6–8h) Infants 1 week–2 mos. of age: 150,000–200,000 U/kg/24 hrs IV (q6–8h) Children <50 kg: 250,000 U/kg/24 hrs IV (q4h) Adults: 20,000,000 U/24 hrs IV (q4h)
Ampicillin	*H. influenzae* (most but not all strains) Organisms sensitive to Penicillin G	Infants <1 week of age: 100 mg/kg/24 hrs IV (q6h) Infants 1 week–2 mos. of age: 150–200 mg/kg/24 hrs IV (q6h) Children <50 kg: 200–400 mg/kg/24 hrs IV (q4h) Adults 4 g/24 hrs IV (q4h)
Nafcillin	*S. aureus*	Infants <2 mos. of age: 100 mg/kg/24 hrs IV (q6–8h) Children <50 kg: 200 mg/kg/24 hrs IV (q4h) Adults: 12 g/24 hrs IV (q4h)
Oxacillin	*S. aureus*	Infants <2 mos. of age: 100 mg/kg/24 hrs IV (q6–8h) Children <50 kg: 300 mg/kg/24 hrs IV (q4h) Adults: 12 g/24 hrs IV (q4h)
Vancomycin	*S. aureus*§ *S. epidermidis*	Children <50 kg: 40–60 mg/kg/24 hrs IV (q6h) Adults: 2–3 g/24 hrs IV (q6–8h)
Chloramphenicol	*H. influenzae* *S. pneumoniae* *N. meningitidis* *Bacteroides* *Salmonella*	Premature and full-term infants <7 days of age: 25 mg/kg/24 hrs IV (q12h)† Full-term infants 7–30 days of age: 50 mg/kg/24 hrs IV (q8h) Full-term infants, 1–2 mos. of age: 50–100 mg/kg/24 hrs IV (q6h) Children <50 kg: 75–100 mg/kg/24 hrs IV (q6h) Adults: 3–4 g (50 mg/kg)24 hrs IV (q4h)
Metronidazole	*Bacteroides*	Children <50 kg: 15 mg/kg over 1hr; thereafter 30–40 mg/kg/24 hrs (q6–8h) Adults: 15 mg/kg over 1 hr; thereafter 30 mg/kg/24 hrs IV (q6h)
Cefotaxine sodium‡	*S. pneumoniae* *N. meningitidis* *H. influenzae* Gram-negative bacilli	Infants <1 week of age: 100 mg/kg/24 hrs IV (q12h) Infants 1 week–2 mos. of age: 150 mg/kg/24 hrs IV (q6h) Children <50 kg: 150 mg/kg/24 hrs IV (q6h) Adults: 6 g IV (q4h)
Ceftazidime‡	Gram-negative bacilli *H. influenzae*	Infants <1 mo. of age: 60 mg/kg/24 hrs IV (q12h) Children <50 kg: 100 mg/kg/24 hrs IV (q8h) (to a total of 6 g/24 hrs) Adults: 6 g IV (q8h)
Ceftriaxone sodium‡	*S. pneumoniae* *N. meningitidis* *H. influenzae* Gram-negative bacilli	Infants and children: 75 mg/kg IV; thereafter 50 mg/kg IV over 10 min (q12h) Adults: 4 g (q12h)
For brain abscess or subdural empyema associated with meningitis (in infants) or for adjunctive use in intracranial parameningeal infections		
Gentamicin§ or Tobramycin§	Gram-negative bacilli *Pseudomonas aeruginosa* (most strains)	Infants <1 week of age: 5 mg/kg/24 hrs IM or IV (q12h) Infants <2 mos. of age: 7.5 mg/kg/24 hrs IM or IV (q8h) Adults: 5 mg/kg/24 hrs IM or IV (q8h)
Pseudomonas Infections Carbenicillin	*P. aeruginosa*	Infants: 300 mg/kg/24 hrs IV over 1–2 hrs (q6–8h) Children <50 kg: 400–600 mg/kg/24 hrs IV over 1–2 hrs (q4h) Adults: 30–40 g/24 hrs over 1–2 hrs (q4h)
Ticarcillin	*P. aeruginosa*	Infants: 200–300 mg per kg per 24 hrs IV over 1–2 hrs (q6–8h) Children and adults: 200–300 mg per kg per 24 hrs IV over 1–2 hrs (q4h)
For brain abscess in AIDS patients		
Sulfadiazine	*T. gondii*	Adults: 4 g (q6h)
Pyrimethamine	*T. gondii*	Adults: 75 mg (q8h)

 * Drugs and dosages listed represent provisional therapy and should be modified as culture results and sensitivities become known. Side effects for each agent, including volumes of fluid required for IV drug administration should be reviewed. Renal or hepatic insufficiency may require adjustment of dosage amount and interval.

 † Neonates and young infants do not metabolize or excrete chloramphenicol effectively, and the use of excessive doses may cause fatal toxicity ("gray syndrome"). Neonates and infants treated with chloramphenicol should be observed carefully throughout the period of therapy, and the drug should be discontinued if the child develops poor feeding, vomiting, abdominal distention, tachypnea, or cyanosis.

 ‡ Experience with third-generation cephalosporins including cefotaxime and ceftriaxone is limited, as is knowledge of their ability to penetrate brain abscesses. Dosages recommended are those used in the treatment of bacterial meningitis.

 § Aminoglycosides do not reach adequate concentrations in brain abscesses in adults. Their use in neonates is directed primarily against the accompanying meningitis. The ability of these agents to reach therapeutic levels in epidural abscess or subdural empyema are uncertain, but adjunctive use in combination with a third-generation cephalosporin or penicillin should be considered.

tients who do not have penicillin allergy, initial therapy should include oxacillin or nafcillin, cefotaxime, and either chloramphenicol or metronidazole. Vancomycin and chloramphenicol should be used in patients known to be allergic to penicillin. The antibiotic regimen should be revised as data become available from cultured abscess material. The length of therapy is determined by patient course and follow-up MRI or CT. In general, antibiotics should be continued for at least 8 weeks if surgery is not undertaken or for 4 weeks if the abscess is drained or excised.

Surgical therapy of brain abscess may involve aspiration or excision. Aspiration, particularly under stereotactic CT guidance, is less traumatic to the central nervous system (CNS) than is excision, effectively reduces intracranial pressure in most cases, and removes the purulent center of the abscess, rendering the abscess more amenable to antibiotic therapy. Recurrence of the abscess may require repeat aspiration. Excision should be considered in patients with surgically approachable abscesses if ventricular rupture is considered imminent or in patients with large or multiloculated abscesses, abscesses located in the posterior fossa, or abscesses that do not respond to aspiration. *The response of a given abscess to antibiotic therapy or aspiration cannot be predicted with certainty from the initial CT or MRI. Frequent follow-up imaging is thus essential if a decision is made to defer surgery or if aspiration is used.* A follow-up MRI or CT should be obtained within 24 to 48 hours after initial therapy. Intervals between subsequent neuroradiologic examinations depend on the patient's status but during the first 2 weeks should not be greater than 3 to 5 days. MRI and CT may remain abnormal for many weeks despite apparent clinical recovery. (The therapy for coexisting cerebral edema and other complications of brain abscess is discussed later in this chapter.)

In patients with brain abscess who are fully alert at presentation, the survival rate approaches 100 percent, but falls to 41 percent in patients responsive only to pain, and to 18 percent (82 percent mortality rate) in patients who are comatose. Prognosis is poor if diagnosis is delayed, if the abscess is large, multiloculated, or within the posterior fossa, or if intraventricular rupture has occurred. Neurologic deficits secondary to the abscess itself and to surgical intervention are found in 30 to 55 percent of surviving patients and may be incapacitating in 17 percent of patients. Seizures occur in approximately 35 percent of patients. Onset of seizures may be delayed for as long as 12 months after surgery.

The major cause of focal CNS infections in patients with AIDS is *T. gondii.* Initial therapy of localized infection should be sulfadiazine and pyrimethamine. Because pyrimethamine is a folic acid antagonist, folinic acid should be administered orally or intramuscularly at a dosage of 2 to 10 mg per day, and complete blood counts, including platelets, should be followed. If the lesion shrinks in size, the etiologic agent should be presumed to be *T. gondii,* and therapy should be continued indefinitely. Diagnostic aspiration or drainage should be employed if the abscess enlarges while the patient is receiving therapy for toxoplasmosis.

INTRACRANIAL PARAMENINGEAL INFECTIONS

Intracranial epidural abscess represents localized infection between the skull and the outermost layer of the meninges, the cranial dura. Subdural empyema represents infection between the dura and arachnoid. Both most frequently represent complications of sinusitis, otitis, or mastoiditis. Organisms may also reach the subdural space in the course of bacteremia, sometimes by seeding of a pre-existing subdural hematoma. Epidural abscesses form by stripping tightly adherent periosteum from bone and are usually sharply circumscribed. Subdural empyemas, on the other hand, represent infection in a potential space and may rapidly spread over the lateral and medial surfaces of an entire cerebral hemisphere or a large portion of the posterior fossa. Extension of epidural infection into the subdural space, which occurs in more than 75 percent of patients, may produce subdural empyema and rapid clinical deterioration.

Etiologic Agents

The causative agents of intracranial epidural abscess and subdural empyema are similar. Aerobic streptococci are present in approximately 35 percent of patients and *S. aureus* in 17 percent. *Streptococcus pneumoniae, Haemophilus influenzae,* and gram-negative organisms are found in 14 percent. Anaerobic and microaerophilic streptococci, *Bacteroides fragilis,* and other anaerobic organisms are found in 33 to 100 percent of cases in which careful anaerobic culturing techniques are employed. Polymicrobial infections are common. Rarely, epidural abscess may be associated with rhinocerebral mucormycosis.

Clinical Presentation

Epidural abscess and subdural empyema may occur at any age, but they are more common in the young and more likely to occur in males than in females. Initial clinical features of both conditions include localized cranial pain, focal or generalized headache, and subsequent development of focal neurologic signs followed by evidence of increased intracranial pressure. Alteration in mental status is common in both disorders, as are focal or generalized seizures. An epidural abscess at the tip of the petrous bone may involve cranial nerves V and VI, producing unilateral facial pain and lateral rectus weakness (Gradenigo's syndrome). Findings in patients with epidural abscess tend to remain sharply localized. By contrast, neurologic signs of subdural empyema usually progress over hours to days, indicating involvement of an entire cerebral hemisphere, with hemiparesis and hemisensory deficit, or suggesting extensive involvement of posterior fossa structures with ataxia and brainstem findings. Onset of symptoms may be insidious in cases that develop after neurosurgical procedures. Nuchal rigidity is common in both epidural abscess and subdural empyema but is not invariable. Papilledema is frequently absent early in the course of the illness. In patients with subdural empyema, progression may occur so rapidly that death occurs before optic disc swelling becomes clinically evident. Meningitis, brain abscess, or septic intracranial venous thrombosis occurs in 14 to 38 percent of patients.

Diagnosis

The diagnostic procedure of choice in patients with intracranial parameningeal infections is MRI. CT with contrast is less reliable, although it should be employed if MRI is not available and may be required in addition to MRI if there is need to image bone. Patient sedation with careful monitoring of vital signs (as discussed earlier in this chapter for brain abscess diagnosis) may be essential to achieve an adequate study. Coronal views should be included to exclude subdural empyema at the base of the brain or in the posterior fossa. Films should also be studied for the presence of sinusitis, otitic infection, cerebral edema, and (particularly when MRI is used) evidence of cortical vein or venous sinus thrombosis.

Therapy

Epidural abscesses too small to be drained may be treated with antibiotics and close radiologic monitoring to confirm resolution and exclude subdural extension. Larger epidural abscesses should be drained. Subdural empyema, on the other hand, represents one of the most urgent of all neurosurgical emergencies. Early cases of subdural empyema may respond to drainage with burr holes followed by irrigation of the subdural space. Drainage by craniotomy is the procedure of choice for large, multiloculated, or posterior fossa empyemas. During surgery, the possibility of basilar or parafalcine extension of the empyema must be kept in mind. Pus obtained at the time of surgery for epidural abscess or subdural empyema should be meticulously collected for anaerobic as well as aerobic culture. Initial antibiotic therapy of intracranial parameningeal infections should be directed against *S. aureus,* aerobic and anaerobic streptococci, *H. influenzae,* and other anaerobic organisms, and should include nafcillin or oxacillin, a third-generation cephalosporin such as cefotaxime and chloramphenicol or metronidazole (see Tables 1 and 2). Adjunctive use of gentamicin should be considered, although its ability to penetrate the subdural space is not known. Antibiotic therapy should be continued for at least 3 weeks. Extensive cerebral edema is commonly present beneath the empyema. (The therapy of coexisting cerebral edema and other complications of epidural abscess and subdural empyema is discussed later in this chapter.) The prognosis for intracranial parameningeal infections, like that for brain abscess, varies greatly with the patient's neurologic status at the time of admission. Late seizures occur in as many as 42 percent of patients.

Intracranial Subdural Empyema in Infants and Children Younger Than 5 Years of Age

Intracranial subdural empyema in infants and young children is almost invariably the consequence of bacterial meningitis, and the organisms associated with the empyema are those which cause meningitis. In infants, subdural empyema is most frequently associated with gram-negative organisms and Group B streptococci. In older infants and small children, the organism is usually *H. influenzae* or, less frequently, *S. pneumoniae* or *Neisseria meningitidis.* Therapy is aimed at the associated meningitis (see Tables 1 and 2); cefotaxime or, alternatively, ampicillin combined with gentamicin should be used in infants younger than 8 weeks of age. Ampicillin and chloramphenicol, ceftriaxone, or cefotaxime should be used in children older than 8 weeks of age.

SPINAL PARAMENINGEAL INFECTIONS

The spinal dura, unlike the cranial dura, is separated from the overlying vertebral bodies by a fat-filled epidural space that provides little resistance to the spread of infection. Spinal epidural abscess usually occupies one to five vertebral segments and may extend the length of the cord. The spinal subdural space, like its intracranial counterpart, also permits rapid, extensive spread of infection. Spinal epidural abscess may arise as a complication of bacteremia by direct spread from vertebral osteomyelitis or by lymphatic spread from infections within the retropharyngeal space, posterior mediastinum, or retroperitoneal space. Spinal subdural empyema is a much less common disorder and is almost invariably the result of metastatic infection.

Etiologic Agents

S. aureus is the causative agent in 60 to 90 percent of epidural abscesses and is also the most common agent in spinal subdural empyema. Other organisms include aerobic and anaerobic streptococci, gram-negative agents, and *Staphylococcus epidermidis*. *M. tuberculosis* may be associated with chronic epidural abscess.

Clinical Presentation

Both spinal epidural abscess and subdural empyema most commonly involve the thoracic and lumbar spine and are usually posterior to the cord. Epidural abscess may be located anterior to the cord in the cervical region or in cases caused by *M. tuberculosis*. Although the temporal course of spinal epidural abscess is highly variable, most cases present within 1 to 3 weeks of onset. Clinical signs typically progress from localized, frequently severe pain to radicular symptoms, followed by signs of spinal cord compression. More chronic abscesses may mimic an extrinsic spinal cord neoplasm. Signs of systemic infection including fever and leukocytosis are common in acute spinal epidural abscess but are often absent if the infection is chronic. Spinal subdural empyemas characteristically present with rapidly progressive signs of spinal cord compression and with radicular signs at multiple levels. Rapid longitudinal spread of infection in either condition can result in cord necrosis extending over multiple vertebral segments.

Diagnosis

Because of its ability to visualize the cord over its entire length, MRI is the diagnostic procedure of choice in patients with spinal parameningeal infections. Myelography supplemented by CT should be employed if MRI is not available. Care should be taken during myelography to introduce the contrast medium at a level distant from that believed to be occupied by the abscess or empyema (e.g., by lateral cervical puncture if lumbar infection is suspected) in order to avoid seeding the subarachnoid space with organisms from the abscess or empyema.

Therapy

Spinal epidural abscess and subdural empyema require urgent surgery in almost all cases. If the causative agent is unknown, initial antibiotic therapy should be directed against *S. aureus* and the streptococci and should include oxacillin or nafcillin (Tables 2 and 3). Vancomycin should be used if there is a history of penicillin allergy or if a nafcillin-resistant organism is strongly suspected. Cefotaxime and gentamicin should be used as provisional therapy if a gram-negative paraspinous infection is identified. Final selection of antibiotics is based on isolation of organisms from abscess material and determination of antibiotic sensitivity. The prognosis for neurologic recovery is excellent for patients with epidural abscess if treatment is given before signs of cord compression occur. The prognosis for spinal subdural empyema is poor unless therapy is begun early in the course of the illness.

ADDITIONAL THERAPEUTIC CONCERNS IN BRAIN ABSCESS AND PARAMENINGEAL INFECTIONS

Cerebral edema is invariably present in brain abscess and intracranial parameningeal infections. Hyperventilation to a P_{CO_2} of less than 28 torr and mannitol are most rapidly effective in reducing intracranial pressure. Mannitol is administered as a 20 percent solution in an initial dose of 1 to 1.5 g per kilogram over a 10-minute period to a total amount of 2.5 to 3 g per kilogram over a period of 1 to 1.5 hours. The patient should be catheterized before mannitol is begun, and careful attention must be given to serum electrolytes and osmolality. Dexamethasone, although of uncertain use in the treatment of intracranial infections, is effective in reduc-

Table 3 Provisional Antibiotic Treatment of Spinal Parameningeal Infection

Cause of Initial Infection	Probable Organism(s)	Recommended Initial Therapy*
Unknown or suspected gram-positive organism	*S. aureus* Streptococci	Oxacillin,† nafcillin,† or vancomycin‡
Unknown—gram-negative organism suspected	*Enterobacteriaceae* *Pseudomonas aeruginosa*	Cefotaxime sodium plus gentamicin Ticarcillin plus gentamicin

* Drugs listed represent recommended provisional therapy and should be modified as culture results and sensitivities become known. Doses for provisional therapy are given in Table 2. Renal or hepatic insufficiency may require adjustment in dosage amount and interval.

† Oxacillin is less likely to produce thrombophlebitis than is nafcillin.

‡ Vancomycin should be used if penicillin allergy is present or if nafcillin resistance is suspected.

§ Data concerning penetration of third-generation cephalosporins into spinal parameningeal infections are limited. The above recommendations concerning cephalosporins are based on their use in meningitis. Gentamicin should be added in epidural abscess or subdural empyema where gram-negative organisms are strongly suspected.

ing vasogenic edema, and a short course of 10 mg IV initially followed by 4 mg IV every 4 to 6 hours should be considered if control of intracranial pressure is of greater concern than time. The placement of a transcranial device to monitor intracranial pressure is frequently invaluable in guiding therapy. If there is inappropriate secretion of antidiuretic hormone or development of diabetes insipidus, one may need to pay strict attention to fluid and electrolyte balance. Administering 5 percent dextrose in water without other electrolytes may lead to profound hyponatremia.

Treatment of seizures should begin with diazepam, 10 mg IV, or 4 mg of lorazepam given over a 2-minute period and repeated after 15 minutes if seizures persist. This initial therapy should be followed by a loading dose of intravenous phenytoin, 10 to 15 mg per kilogram, given in normal saline at a rate no faster than 50 mg per minute (1 mg per kilogram per minute in neonates). The electrocardiogram and blood pressure should be monitored during phenytoin administration. Maintenance therapy with phenytoin should be continued if seizures are controlled. Phenobarbital or other agents should be used if generalized seizures persist.

Adjacent or remote sources of infection are commonly present in brain abscess and parameningeal infections. These must also be sought and treated. Major pericranial sites of concern in intracranial space-occupying infections are the sinuses, middle ear, mastoid, and teeth. Sites of possible primary infection in spinal parameningeal infections include abscesses within psoas muscles, perinephric tissues, posterior mediastinum, or retropharyngeal space. Intracranial infections and spinal epidural abscess may be accompanied by cranial or vertebral osteomyelitis.

Care of the patient after recovery from brain abscess or parameningeal infection must be determined on an individual basis. Low-dose subcutaneous heparin should be considered in patients for whom extended periods of bed rest are necessary. Anticonvulsants may need to be maintained or adjusted, and the late appearance of seizures may require initiation of therapy with phenytoin or other agents weeks to months after recovery from the infection itself. Careful withdrawal of anticonvulsant drugs should be considered after 2 years in those patients who have seizures early in the course of their disease but who remain seizure-free and without focal neurologic deficits or electroencephalographic abnormalities.

Recovery from the neurologic deficits that follow brain abscess or intracranial or intraspinal parameningeal infections may occur slowly and incompletely. Physical and occupational therapy should begin as early as possible, and the program of rehabilitation should be modified over time as the patient improves. The acute illness and its sequelae are frequently physically, psychologically, and financially devastating to the patient and his or her family. The gradual nature of neurologic recovery should be stressed from the outset, and as the extent of neurologic injury becomes more certain, the patient and family should be assisted in developing long-term plans for dealing with the illness and its effects on their lives.

SUGGESTED READING

Chun CH, Johnson JD, Hofstetter M, Raff MJ. Brain abscess: a study of 45 consecutive cases. Medicine 1986; 65:415–431.
Greenlee JE. Anatomical considerations in central nervous system infections. In: Mandell GL, Douglas RG Jr, Bennett JE, eds. Principles and practice of infectious diseases. 3rd ed. New York: John Wiley and Sons, 1989:732.
Harris LF, Haws FP, Tripplett JN, MacCubbin DA. Subdural empyema and epidural abscess: recent experience in a community hospital. South Med J 1987; 80:1254–1258.
Hodges J, Anslow PI, Gillett G. Subdural empyema: continuing diagnostic problems in the CT scan era. Q J Med 1986; 59:387–393.
Lasker BR. Cervical epidural abscess. Neurology 1987; 37:1747–1753.
Wispelwey B, Scheld WM. Brain abscess. Clin. Neuropharmacol 1987; 10:483–510.

NEUROSYPHILIS

JOSEPH R. BERGER, M.D.

Syphilis is the result of infection with *Treponema pallidum,* a spirochete that is highly sensitive to penicillin. The combination of the ready availability of penicillin and the sensitivity of the organism to this antibiotic has led to the widely held belief that syphilis in contemporary times is rare. Although the annual incidence of syphilis in the United States declined eighteen-fold, from a peak of 72 cases per 100,000 individuals in 1943 to four per 100,000 in 1956, the current incidence is approximately 12 per 100,000. In some areas of the country, the incidence may be substantially higher than the national average. For instance, in Florida the incidence is 37.6 cases per 100,000 individuals, which is three times the national average. Groups that have experienced increased rates of syphilis—chiefly, homosexual and bisexual men and female prostitutes—are also those groups with an increased incidence of human immunodeficiency virus (HIV) infection, resulting in an increasingly frequent recognition of concomitant infection.

Infection with *T. pallidum* is divided into several stages. The initial manifestation of infection, primary syphilis, is an ulcerated, painless lesion with firm borders referred to as a chancre that develops at the site of epidermal or mucous membrane inoculation and is accompanied by regional adenopathy. This lesion occurs approximately 3 weeks after infection, although the time to development ranges from 3 to 90 days, depending on the size of the inoculum. Although the lesion is a local manifestation, the spirochetes, even at this early stage, have disseminated systemically. Early systemic dissemination is substantiated by the ability to transmit syphilis by blood donation from incubating seronegative donors. Other evidence for early systemic dissemination includes the detection of abnormalities in the cerebrospinal fluid (CSF) and the ability to culture *T. pallidum* from the CSF. Nine to thirty-five percent of newly infected patients display abnormal CSF parameters before the development of the rash of secondary syphilis, and *T. pallidum* was recently isolated from two of seven of patients (29 percent) with primary syphilis.

Within 2 to 8 weeks of the appearance of the chancre, the features of secondary syphilis appear. These features are largely attributed to a bacteremic phase of the illness and include a macular, maculopapular, or pustular rash that often involves the palms and soles, mucous patches, and alopecia. The skin manifestations may be accompanied by constitutional signs, diffuse adenopathy, iridocyclitis, hepatitis, periostitis, and arthritis. A brisk immune response is observed and immune complex deposition may lead to nephrotic syndrome. In this stage of syphilis, an aseptic meningitis occurs in 1 to 2 percent of patients. In my experience, the incidence of symptomatic syphilitic meningitis appears to be inordinately high in individuals with concomitant HIV infection. Syphilitic meningitis is characterized by fever, headache, nausea, vomiting, photophobia, and meningismus. On occasion, seizures, cranial neuropathies (most commonly cranial nerves VII, VIII, VI, and II) and other focal neurologic findings may be observed. Although clinical features of meningitis ordinarily occur in a small percentage of patients, CSF analyses indicate that more than 30 percent of patients with secondary syphilis have an aseptic meningitis, and 80 percent of patients with the rash of secondary syphilis have some CSF abnormality. In a recent study, *T. pallidum* was recoverable from the CSF of ten of 33 patients (30 percent) with secondary syphilis. Furthermore, in the absence of an abnormal CSF pleocytosis, abnormal protein level, or positive Veneral Disease Research Laboratory (VDRL) test, spirochetes have been recovered from the CSF of individuals with secondary syphilis.

The latent stage of syphilis is regarded as a quiescent phase of syphilis that precedes the development of tertiary complications. It is divided into two stages, early (within 2 years of infection) and late (greater than 2 years), to reflect the probability of recurrence of secondary syphilitic manifestations. Nonspecifically abnormal CSF results are not uncommon in patients with latent syphilis, with frequencies as high as 50 percent being reported. These abnormalities are more commonly observed in early latent syphilis, and in some patients the CSF abnormalities may resolve over time. A diagnosis of asymptomatic neurosyphilis is predicated on abnormalities detected in the CSF.

The clinically apparent central nervous system manifestations that result from tertiary syphilis affect less than 10 percent of untreated patients. These manifestations were documented to occur in 4 percent of untreated American black men in the Tuskegee study and 6.5 percent of Scandinavians in the Oslo study. A classification of neurosyphilis is provided in Table 1. Some of these forms of neurosyphilis may overlap with one another. An atypical form of neurosyphilis referred to as "modified neurosyphilis" has been attributed to the use of antibiotics for conditions other than syphilis in patients with unrecognized syphilis. This illness is characterized by a negative CSF VDRL and clinical features that are outside the spectrum of classically described features of neurosyphilis. However, the contention that these manifestations are syphilitic in origin has been debated. My own belief is that although "modified neurosyphilis" is a real entity, its frequency has been greatly exaggerated.

Table 1 Classification of Neurosyphilis

Asymptomatic neurosyphilis

Syphilitic meningitis

Cerebral forms of neurosyphilis
  Meningovascular syphilis
    Cerebromeningeal syphilis
    Cerebrovascular syphilis
  General paresis
  Cerebral gumma

Spinal forms of neurosyphilis
  Tabes dorsalis
  Spinal meningomyelitis
  Syphilitic spinal pachymeningitis
    Syphilitic hypertrophic pachymeningitis
    Spinal cord gumma
  Spinal vascular disease

Optic atrophy

Syphilitic otitis

Spinal and cranial syphilitic osteitis

DIAGNOSIS

In the absence of a readily applicable "gold standard," the diagnosis of neurosyphilis is established clinically. Unfortunately, no consensus exists regarding diagnostic criteria. At one end of the spectrum, a diagnosis of neurosyphilis has been recommended in patients with serologic evidence of syphilis and one or more of the following abnormalities in their CSF: a pleocytosis, an elevated protein level, a decreased glucose concentration, or a positive VDRL. However, neurosyphilis is undoubtedly overdiagnosed using these criteria. For instance, in the presence of concomitant HIV infection, a CSF pleocytosis and an elevated CSF protein level are frequently observed. Furthermore, other markers of neurosyphilis, such as an elevated CSF immunoglobulin level or CSF oligoclonal bands, are not useful in patients with HIV infection. At the other extreme, diagnostic criteria for neurosyphilis include a reactive CSF with increased cell count and protein level *and* a positive CSF VDRL. The dogmatic reliance on a positive CSF VDRL for establishing a diagnosis of neurosyphilis is unsuitable because of the insensitivity of this test. The VDRL is neither consistently positive in the serum of patients with syphilis nor consistently positive in the CSF of patients with neurosyphilis. The serum VDRL is positive in 72 percent of patients with primary syphilis, in nearly 100 percent of those with secondary syphilis, in 73 percent of those with latent syphilis, and in 77 percent of those with tertiary syphilis. Therefore, approximately one-fourth of patients with neurosyphilis have a negative serum VDRL. In the presence of concomitant HIV infection, the likelihood of a false-negative serum VDRL may be even greater. One recently described HIV-seropositive patient with secondary syphilis and negative serologic studies for syphilis required darkfield examination of a skin biopsy to establish the diagnosis. However, my own experience indicates that the serologic response for syphilis is preserved in most HIV-seropositive patients.

The CSF VDRL is positive in approximately 75 to 80 percent of patients with symptomatic neurosyphilis. Its frequency appears to vary with the clinical form of neurosyphilis, and in patients with asymptomatic neurosyphilis, it may occur considerably less often than in those with symptomatic disease. Clearly, the CSF VDRL is too insensitive to be relied on to exclude the diagnosis of neurosyphilis. I and others have observed pathologically confirmed neurosyphilis in patients with nonreactive CSF VDRLs. Also, a recent study in which CSF was cultured in rabbit testicles isolated *T. pallidum* from the CSF of 12 of 40 patients (30 percent) with primary and secondary syphilis. The CSF VDRL was positive in only four of the 12 patients (33 percent) from whom CSF treponemes were isolated. Therefore, to establish the diagnosis of neurosyphilis, measures other than a positive CSF VDRL must be relied on. The CSF fluorescent treponemal antibody absorption test (FTA-ABS) has been suggested as a sensitive screening test for detecting neurosyphilis. I believe that the CSF FTA-ABS is a highly nonspecific test and that its use as a screening modality still remains to be established. A reliable CSF test that exhibits both a high degree of sensitivity and specificity for neurosyphilis would be ideal. The currently available treponemal tests are of dubious value in this regard, and the physician must refrain from adhering rigidly to narrow guidelines in making this diagnosis. Perhaps the development of newer tests for syphilis, such as polymerase chain reaction or monoclonal antibodies directed against *T. pallidum* antigens, may solve this dilemma.

TREATMENT

Since the clinical recognition of syphilis during the late fifteenth century, many treatment modalities, such as the use of heavy metals (mercury, bismuth, arsenic) and fever therapy, have been advocated for the treatment of this disease. In 1943, the treatment of syphilis was rewritten when Mahoney convincingly demonstrated the efficacy of penicillin. Perhaps no other disease has been as dramatically affected by the discovery of penicillin as syphilis. However, the adequacy of currently recommended treatment regimens remains in question. In fact, there have been no controlled, randomized, prospective studies as to the optimal dose or duration of therapy for the treatment of neurosyphilis. The treponemicidal level of penicillin is 0.03 μg per milliliter. Although the organism has been demonstrated to be capable of acquiring plasmids that produce penicillinase, there is no evidence that penicillin has lost its efficacy in the treatment of *T. pallidum*. If penicillin levels become subtherapeutic, the spirochetes begin regenerating within 18 to 24 hours. The Center for Disease Control (CDC) recommends administering 2.4 million U of benzathine penicillin intramuscularly at weekly intervals for 3 weeks in the treatment of neurosyphilis, but the recordable penicillin levels in the CSF during treatment fail to reach treponemicidal levels. The concentration of penicillin in the CSF is typically unmeasurable, probably not exceeding 0.0005 μg per milliliter, which is 1 to 2 percent of the serum levels. Furthermore, viable treponemes have been recovered from the CSF at the completion of therapy. Another "recommended" regimen is procaine penicillin, 600,000 U IM daily for 15 days. This regimen, too, may fail to achieve treponemicidal levels of penicillin in the CSF. Ideally, treatment of neurosyphilis should consist of administering crystalline aqueous penicillin, 12 to 24 million U IV daily (2 to 4 million U every

4 hours) for 10 to 14 days. This regimen generally necessitates hospitalization. Because of the expense of treatment, I have occasionally resorted to the placement of an indwelling catheter and prescribing self-administered or visiting nurse–assisted infusions to be performed at home, provided that the patient is reliable and well motivated. The penicillin should be administered no less frequently than at 4-hour intervals to maintain the penicillin levels consistently at or above treponemicidal values, avoiding subtherapeutic troughs that occur when the drug is administered at less frequent intervals. An alternative approach to the use of parenteral penicillin is the daily oral administration of amoxicillin (3 g) and probenecid (1 g) for 14 days. This regimen achieves treponemicidal levels of amoxicillin in the CSF. An alternative regimen employs ceftriaxone, 1 g intramuscularly daily for 14 days.

In patients who are penicillin allergic, treatment with erythromycin, 500 mg four times daily, or tetracycline, 500 mg four times daily, for 30 days has been recommended. Erythromycin does not diffuse readily into the brain and CSF, nor has its efficacy been demonstrated in the treatment of neurosyphilis. Similarly, oral therapy with tetracycline yields very low CSF tetracycline concentrations, and it, too, has unproven efficacy in the treatment of neurosyphilis. Ideally, in the penicillin-allergic patient with unequivocally established, clinically manifest neurosyphilis, the prudent course is hospitalization, desensitization to penicillin, and subsequent high-dose aqueous penicillin treatment. In those penicillin-allergic patients with asymptomatic neurosyphilis or in those for whom the diagnosis is less firmly established, a trial of oral doxycycline, 200 mg administered twice daily, followed by close follow-up of their clinical course and CSF parameters may be cautiously employed.

Determining the adequacy of therapy depends on careful follow-up of the patient. Conversion of the serum VDRL or RPR (rapid plasma reagin) from a reactive titer to a nonreactive titer should occur within 1 year after treatment of primary syphilis, within 2 years after treatment of secondary syphilis, and within 5 years after treatment of latent syphilis. This delay to reversion from a seropositive status reflects the duration and severity of the illness. The presence of persistently positive serum VDRL or RPR suggests either persistent infection, reinfection, or a biological false-positive test.

In the treatment of neurosyphilis, fixed neurologic deficits may not improve with treatment and some abnormalities, such as tabes dorsalis and optic atrophy, may worsen despite adequate therapy. The best determinant for the adequacy of treatment is resolution of the CSF abnormalities. Examination of the CSF within several days of the institution of treatment with penicillin may be confusing since the CSF cell count may rise initially, particularly if accompanied by a Jarisch-Herxheimer reaction. However, the CSF should be examined at the termination of treatment to document a decrease in cell count, and thereafter should be examined at 3- to 6-month intervals for 2 to 3 years. The cell count should return to normal within 1 year after treatment (usually 6 months), and the protein level should return to normal within 2 years. The disappearance of the CSF VDRL typically parallels its resolution in the serum. The long hiatus before its eventual clearing makes it less useful for determining the adequacy of treatment than the CSF cell count or protein tests. With effective therapy, however, the CSF VDRL titers should not increase over time. An approach to the management of neurosyphilis is outlined in Figure 1.

Because neurosyphilis has been documented to occur in patients who have been treated for primary and secondary syphilis with CDC-recommended doses of penicillin, all patients with a history of prior treatment of primary, secondary, or latent syphilis should undergo CSF analysis. Examination of the CSF is particularly important in patients with concomitant HIV infection in whom currently recommended treatment regimens, at least in some instances, appear to be inadequate.

CONCOMITANT HIV INFECTION

Concomitant HIV infection may significantly alter the natural history of neurosyphilis. When it occurs in association with HIV infection, syphilis appears to be not only more aggressive, but also more difficult to treat. These observations suggest that the host's immune response is critical in controlling syphilis. The inability of the HIV-infected patient to establish delayed hypersensitivity to *T. pallidum* may prevent secondary syphilis from evolving to latency or may cause a spontaneous relapse from a latent state. This impairment of delayed hypersensitivity may account for a more rapid progression of neurosyphilis in HIV-infected individuals than would otherwise be expected. *T. pallidum* can be isolated from the CSF of HIV-seropositive patients with primary, secondary, or latent syphilis after currently recommended CDC penicillin therapy has been administered. The impracticality of culturing the organism and the frequency with which CSF abnormalities are detected in patients with HIV infection suggests that aggressive high-dose amoxicillin and probenicid or parenteral penicillin administration is a prudent course of management in HIV-seropositive individuals during the early stages of syphilis. Careful CSF follow-up analysis is required for those individuals who initially display abnormal results. Other than reversion of a positive CSF VDRL in those cases where it was initially present, a decline in the CSF pleocytosis

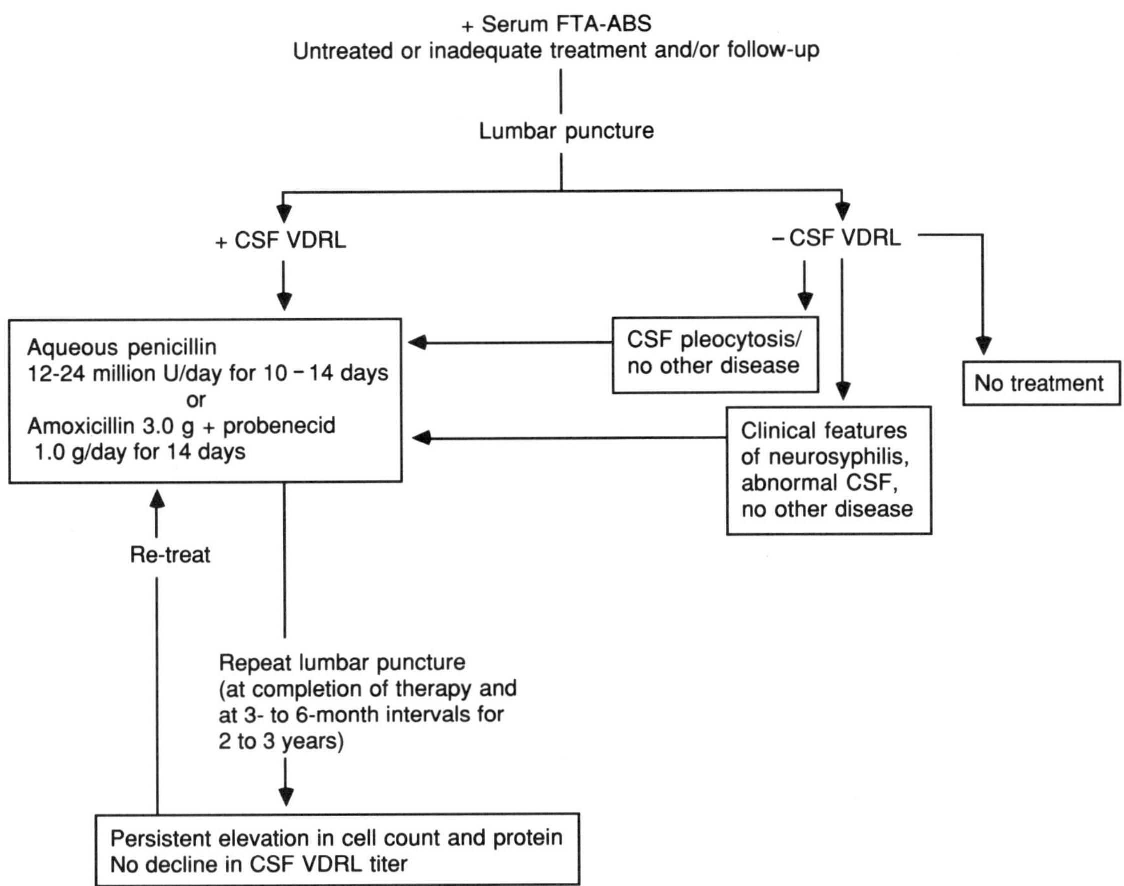

Figure 1   Treatment of neurosyphilis.

may be of greatest value in monitoring the success of therapy. I have seen syphilis recrudescence in rare HIV-seropositive patients treated with high-dose parenteral penicillin. This observation suggests the potential need for secondary prophylaxis in treating syphilis in the HIV-infected patient, as is employed in the management of CNS toxoplasmosis and cryptococcal meningitis, but further studies are warranted before it can be broadly recommended.

OTHER CONDITIONS

Certain ophthalmologic manifestations of syphilis may result in neurologic consultation. Although the characteristic ophthalmologic abnormality is the Argyll Robertson pupil, other conditions that may result from *T. pallidum* infection include interstitial keratitis, chorioretinitis, and optic atrophy. As recommended for the treatment of neurosyphilis, high-dose parenteral penicillin is required. Syphilitic optic atrophy, which is commonly unilateral and may occur with or without an associated basilar meningitis, is notoriously difficult to treat effectively. Progression is observed in as many as 50

percent of patients. For these patients, a trial of oral corticosteroids (prednisone 60 mg daily for 2 to 4 weeks) along with careful observation is suggested.

Syphilitic hearing loss, either acute or gradually progressive in nature, may occur in association with cochlear end-organ damage. Vertigo may also be a feature of this illness. Although syphilitic eighth nerve dysfunction is largely recognized as a late manifestation of congenital syphilis, it is also observed in acquired illness. This form of syphilis is relatively refractory to treatment regimens. Parenteral therapy with 12 to 24 million U of aqueous crystalline penicillin administered daily or oral therapy with 3.5 g of amoxicillin with 1 g of probenecid daily for 6 weeks to 3 months is recommended. Prednisone, 30 to 60 mg daily, in combination with the antibiotic regimen for this disorder is also recommended.

SUGGESTED READING

Clark EG, Danbold N. The Oslo study of the natural course of untreated syphilis: an epidemiologic investigation based on re-study of the Boeck-Bruusgard material. Med Clin North Am 1964; 48:613–624.

Hook EW III, Baker-Zander SA, Moskovitz BL, et al. Ceftriaxone therapy for asymptomatic neurosyphilis: case report and Western blot analysis of serum and cerebrospinal fluid IgG response to therapy. Sex Transm Dis 1986; 13:185–188.

Lukehart SA, Hook EW III, Baker-Zander SA, et al. Invasion of the central nervous system by *Treponema pallidum:* implications for diagnosis and treatment. Ann Intern Med 1988; 109:855–862.

Merritt HH, Adams RD, Solomon HC. Neurosyphilis. New York: Oxford University Press, 1946.

Rockwell DH, Yobs AR, Moore MB Jr. The Tuskegee study of untreated syphilis: the 30th year of observation. Arch Intern Med 1964; 114:92–798.

Swartz MN. Neurosyphilis. In: Holmes KK, Mardh P-A, Sparling PF, et al, eds. Sexually transmitted diseases. 2nd ed. New York: McGraw-Hill, 1990: 231.

Yim CW, Flynn MN, Fitzgerald FT. Penetration of oral doxycycline into the cerebrospinal fluid of patients with latent or neurosyphilis. Antimicrob Agents Chemother 1985; 28:347–348.

LYME DISEASE

LOUIS REIK, Jr., M.D.

Lyme disease is a multisystem inflammatory disease of worldwide distribution caused by a tick-transmitted spirochete, *Borrelia burgdorferi*. Although other ticks and biting insects may transmit the spirochete, the usual vectors are small, hard-bodied ixodid ticks.

The skin, heart, nervous system, and joints are the organ systems most often involved, frequently in sequence, and the illness is said to have three stages. Stage I begins 3 days to 1 month after the tick bite has been sustained with a characteristic skin lesion (erythema chronicum migrans [ECM]) accompanied by systemic symptoms and resolves spontaneously within 3 or 4 weeks. Stage II begins either while the skin lesion is still present or 1 to 6 months after it has resolved, and is characterized by neurologic abnormalities, cardiac involvement, and another skin lesion, borrelial lymphocytoma. Stage III, the chronic stage of Lyme disease, begins months to years after the initial tick bite and is characterized by Lyme arthritis, acrodermatitis chronica atrophicans (ACA), the third-stage skin lesion, and tertiary neurologic abnormalities (Table 1).

DIAGNOSIS OF NEUROLOGIC ABNORMALITIES OF LYME DISEASE

Lyme disease should be suspected in any patient with compatible neurologic abnormalities (Table 2). When these abnormalities follow ECM, accompany or occur after the development of Lyme arthritis, or accompany borrelial lymphocytoma or ACA, the diagnosis is straightforward. However, nervous system involvement in Lyme disease may occur alone. In such cases, a history of tick bite, onset during the summer, or travel and residence in an endemic area are clues.

Once the disease is suspected on clinical grounds, the diagnosis can usually be confirmed by detection of antibody to *B. burgdorferi*. By the time neurologic abnormalities develop, most patients have elevated levels of immunoglobin G (IgG) antibodies, whereas immunoglobin M (IgM) antibodies may or may not be present. False-positive tests do occur, especially in patients with syphilis and relapsing fever. Once these are ruled out, however, a positive test in a patient with compatible neurologic abnormalities is strong evidence for the diagnosis. When there is doubt, tests for antibody using the Western blot technique may help, as they are both more sensitive and more specific.

In some cases, particularly when neurologic abnormalities first develop, serologic tests may be negative. Testing of the cerebrospinal fluid (CSF) should then be done, as specific antibody often appears in the CSF before the serum in Stage 2 meningopolyneuritis. In cases of very short duration, both serologic and CSF tests may be negative initially, and treatment may have to be prescribed before laboratory confirmation of the diagnosis is obtained.

Similarly, early treatment with oral antibiotics sometimes abrogates the antibody response to *B.*

Table 1 Major Clinical Features of Lyme Disease

Stage	General Features	Neurologic Involvement
I	ECM and systemic symptoms	Headache and neck stiffness without pleocytosis
II	Borrelial lymphocytoma carditis	Lymphocytic meningitis Encephalitis Myelitis Cranial neuritis Radiculoneuritis/plexitis Mononeuritis Guillain-Barré syndrome
III	Lyme arthritis ACA	Progressive encephalomyelitis Encephalopathy with magnetic resonance imaging abnormalities Latent CNS borreliosis Others (?)

Table 2 Neurologic Abnormalities That May be Caused by Lyme Disease

Aseptic meningitis
Chronic lymphocytic meningitis
Acute meningoencephalitis
Focal encephalitis
Brainstem encephalitis
Demyelinating encephalitis
Chronic progressive encephalomyelitis
Cerebral vasculitis
Encephalopathy with MRI
  abnormalities
Acute transverse myelitis
Cranial neuritis (Bell's palsy)
Mononeuritis simplex or multiplex
Radiculoneuritis
Lumbar or brachial plexitis
Distal axonal neuropathy
Demyelinating polyneuritis
Carpal tunnel syndrome
Focal myositis

burgdorferi without eliminating the organism from the nervous system. In this case, late Lyme disease may develop in a seronegative patient. In some cases, but not others, immunoblots are positive, and treatment may again have to be prescribed on the basis of clinical features alone.

Moreover, the full spectrum of nervous system abnormalities occurring later in Lyme disease is probably not yet known, and it is not yet clear what is the best method for diagnosing late nervous system borreliosis. A positive serologic test indicates exposure rather than infection, and in some areas, the ratio of symptomatic to asymptomatic infection is probably 1:1. Because of this, and because antibody can persist in high titer for years after apparently successful treatment, a positive serum antibody test may not be sufficient for diagnosis. Measurement of specific antibody in the CSF may provide one clue, but it is not clear that the reactivity of the CSF is the best measure of activity in late disease.

With these uncertainties in mind, and because I practice in an endemic area, I perform serologic tests for Lyme disease in all patients with compatible neurologic abnormalities. All patients with a positive serologic test have a lumbar puncture with measurement of CSF anti-*B. burgdorferi* antibody. I prescribe antibiotic therapy for all those with pleocytosis, an elevated protein level, or locally synthesized anti-*Borrelia* antibodies. I treat patients with late polyneuropathy with antibiotics regardless of CSF reactivity, since such patients often have normal CSF. I also prescribe the same antibiotic treatment for patients with compatible neurologic abnormalities, a positive serum antibody test, and a normal CSF who have no explanation for their symptoms other than Lyme disease, especially if the symptoms are progressive. In addition, I routinely obtain a serum immunoblot and examine the CSF of seronegative patients with neurologic abnormalities of unknown cause who have a history of ECM or of a well-documented tick bite in an area endemic for Lyme disease; however, I generally treat these patients with antibiotics regardless of the result.

TREATMENT

The aims of treatment of Lyme disease are threefold: (1) to stop ECM and its associated symptoms; (2) to prevent the development of late skin, joint, heart, and nervous system abnormalities; and (3) to arrest and reverse those late abnormalities that do develop. It is not clear, however, which are the best antibiotic regimens for accomplishing these aims.

B. burgdorferi is sensitive to several antibiotics. *In vitro*, it is most sensitive to ceftriaxone sodium, cefotaxime sodium, and erythromycin; it is also sensitive, although less so, to amoxicillin, tetracycline, doxycycline, minocycline, lincomycin, imipenem, and ciprofloxacin. In vivo sensitivities in infected laboratory animals generally parallel those in vitro except in the case of erythromycin, which is much less active in vivo. The organism is only moderately sensitive to penicillin, both in vivo and in vitro.

Early Lyme Disease

Treatment with several of these antibiotics does shorten the course of ECM and its associated symptoms and also prevents the subsequent development of joint, heart, and nervous system abnormalities. Early treatment regimens using oral tetracycline and penicillin speeded the resolution of ECM, but treatment with erythromycin did not. All three antibiotics, however, seemed to prevent the occurrence of serious late complications in most cases. Yet some patients did develop late complications in spite of oral antibiotic therapy, particularly those patients with more severe systemic symptoms or multiple secondary skin lesions, and many others continued to have minor symptoms for weeks or months after apparently adequate treatment. Late nervous system involvement in patients treated with oral antibiotics early in the course of the disease seems particularly common, possibly because of inadequate penetration into the CNS.

B. burgdorferi is more sensitive to amoxicillin than penicillin V, and amoxicillin when given in conjunction with probenecid can achieve treponemicidal levels in the CSF. Consequently, I now treat patients with Stage I disease with amoxicillin 500 mg plus probenecid 500 mg four times daily, for 2 weeks in mild cases and for 4 weeks in severe cases (Table 3). Because doxycycline achieves higher tissue levels than tetracycline hydrochloride, I prescribe dox-

Table 3 Antibiotic Treatment of Lyme Disease

Stage	Abnormality	Treatment
I	ECM and systemic symptoms	Amoxicillin 500 mg q.i.d. plus probenecid 500 mg q.i.d. or Doxycycline 100 mg b.i.d. for 2 to 4 weeks
II	Isolated facial palsy	Amoxicillin or doxycycline as for Stage I disease
	Meningitis, CNS disease, neuritis	Ceftriaxone 2 g daily for 14 days or Aqueous penicillin G 20 million U IV for 10 days or Chloramphenicol 1 g IV q.i.d. for 14 days
III	Progressive encephalomyelitis	Ceftriaxone or aqueous penicillin G as for Stage II disease
	Distal axonopathy, encephalopathy	Ceftriaxone 2 g daily for 2 to 4 weeks or Doxycycline 100 mg b.i.d. for 30 days or Chloramphenicol 1 g q.i.d. for 2 weeks

ycycline 100 mg twice daily over a similar time period to penicillin-allergic patients with Stage I disease. Minor symptoms, particularly arthralgias, fatigue, and musculoskeletal pain, may continue for a few weeks or even 1 to 2 months despite adequate treatment. I find it helpful to warn the patients of this possibility in advance in order to allay any anxiety that may develop later. Although I do not believe that continued minor symptoms are an indication for re-treatment, unless they persist for more than 1 to 2 months without improvement, treated patients with continuing symptoms should be followed carefully. I have not found follow-up serologic tests helpful in assessing the response to treatment.

Neurologic Involvement in Late Lyme Disease

Once neurologic abnormalities have developed, treatment with oral antibiotics is probably no longer adequate and parenteral treatment is necessary in most cases.

Stage II

Treatment with high-dose (20 million U daily for 10 days) intravenous penicillin is effective in eradicating infection in patients with Stage II meningopolyneuritis. When intravenous penicillin is given to patients with Stage II disease, pain and fever may worsen temporarily during the first 18 hours, but

severe Herxheimer reactions have not been described. Once treatment is instituted, meningeal and systemic symptoms begin to improve within days, while radicular pains decrease over weeks and motor deficits improve over several weeks. Some patients continue to have headaches for weeks, however, and others continue to have frequent arthralgias, musculoskeletal pain, and fatigue. Stage II CNS abnormalities are arrested by treatment and may improve slowly, but some residual deficit is common in severe cases. CSF cell counts are usually lower by the end of treatment but may not return to normal for several months. Similarly, the CSF protein content is usually lower by the end of treatment, but it may remain elevated for a year or more. Failure of meningeal symptoms to improve during treatment or of the CSF cell count to decrease by the time a repeated lumbar puncture is performed at the end of treatment should prompt consideration of alternative antibiotic treatments.

Intravenous doxycycline (200 mg on Day 1, followed by 100 mg daily for 10 days) has been used to treat Stage II meningitis and some patients, although not all, have responded to this treatment. Others who have failed penicillin therapy have responded to intravenous cefotaxime (2 g three times daily for 10 days), ceftriaxone sodium (2 g once or twice daily for 14 days), or chloramphenicol (1 g four times daily for 2 weeks).

However, not all patients with Stage II neurologic disease need parenteral antibiotic therapy. Facial palsy in particular may occur without CSF pleocytosis and can be treated adequately with oral antibiotics. I examine the CSF of all patients with Lyme disease and facial palsy, and if there is no pleocytosis or intrathecal antibody synthesis and no other extracutaneous disease, I prescribe oral amoxicillin and probenecid or doxycycline as for Stage I disease.

Stage III

Progressive borrelia encephalomyelitis also responds to high-dose intravenous penicillin. With this treatment, most patients are stabilized, some improve partially, and a few become clinically normal. Pleocytosis resolves within approximately 3 months and CSF protein content usually decreases by then also, but specific antibody can persist in the CSF for a year or more.

Other Stage III neurologic abnormalities respond less well to intravenous penicillin. In many of the patients with these abnormalities, intravenous ceftriaxone (2 g once daily for 2 weeks) appears to be much more effective. Both patients with distal axonopathy of late Lyme disease and those with late mental changes improve when given ceftriaxone, but often they do not respond when treated with penicillin. However, improvement with ceftriaxone treatment is slow. Little change is apparent during the course of treatment; improvement develops over ensuing weeks and may not be complete until 6 months have elapsed. Not all patients respond to intravenous ceftriaxone, and some seem to improve initially and then relapse. I have treated several such patients with a longer, 1-month course of ceftriaxone (2 g once daily) with good response.

SUGGESTED READING

Berger BW. Treatment of erythema chronicum migrans of Lyme disease. Ann NY Acad Sci 1988; 539:346–351.

Dattwyler RJ, Halperin JJ, Volkman DJ, Luft BJ. Treatment of late Lyme borreliosis: randomised comparison of ceftriaxone and penicillin. Lancet 1988; 1:1191–1194.

Neu HC. A perspective on therapy of Lyme infection. Ann NY Acad Sci 1988; 539:314–316.

Skoldenberg B, Stiernstedt G, Karlsson M, et al. Treatment of Lyme borreliosis with emphasis on neurological disease. Ann NY Acad Sci 1988; 539:317–323.

Steere AC, Pachner AR, Malawista SE. Neurologic abnormalities of Lyme disease: successful treatment with high-dose intravenous penicillin. Ann Intern Med 1983; 99:767–772.

PATIENT RESOURCE

The Lyme Borreliosis Foundation, Inc. has organized patient support groups throughout the country, has literature available depicting some of the common features of Lyme disease, and will refer both patients and physicians needing advice to clinicians expert in diagnosing and treating Lyme disease:

The Lyme Borreliosis Foundation, Inc.
Box 462
Tolland, CT   06084
Telephone: (203) 871-2900

NEUROCYSTICERCOSIS

LARRY E. DAVIS, M.D., F.A.C.P.

For optimal treatment of neurocysticercosis, one needs an accurate diagnosis and classification of the disease. Patients may present with a variety of signs including seizures, increased intracranial pressure with headache and papilledema, altered mental status, or focal neurologic findings. This variety of clinical signs occurs because the cysts may develop in the brain, spinal cord, ventricles, or meninges. Furthermore, the larvae in cysts may be alive, but they are quiescent, degenerating and causing inflammation or dead and calcified.

DIAGNOSIS

The diagnosis of neurocysticercosis is most often made by computed tomography (CT). CT often demonstrates one or more parenchymal cysts 5 to 20 mm in diameter that may or may not show contrast enhancement of the cyst ring. Intraventricular and subarachnoid cysts are isodense with cerebral spinal fluid (CSF) and are difficult to recognize by CT. Hydrocephalus may be present, but nonionic contrast CT ventriculography may be needed to outline the ventricular cysts. Magnetic resonance imaging (MRI) imaging in active disease may demonstrate both parenchymal and ventricular cysticerci as cysts with MRI signal properties paralleling CSF. Degenerating cysts may be surrounded by a high intensity rim of tissue edema.

Until recently, serologic tests for cysticercosis were seldom helpful because they had poor sensitivity and specificity. An improvement occurred with the cysticercosis enzyme-linked immunoabsorbent assay (ELISA). A new cysticercosis immunoblot test detects both immunoglobulin M and immunoglobulin G antibodies to cysticerci antigens. This test is reported to have a specificity of virtually 100 percent and a sensitivity of approximately 98 percent in both serum and CSF. Presently, serum and CSF samples can be sent via state health departments to the Parasitic Disease Branch of the Centers for Disease Control (CDC). For tests that should be rapidly performed, it is recommended that one telephone the CDC Parasitic Disease Laboratory directly (404-488-4054). These newer serologic tests are helpful in the evaluation of unexplained chronic meningitis, a large cystic lesion, or a cyst that appears atypical.

Because the treatment varies (Table 1), the disease should be classified once the diagnosis is made. Although several classification systems exist, most separate neurocysticercosis into active and inactive disease. In active disease, the cysticerci in the CNS are alive or actively degenerating. In inactive disease, the cysticerci are dead with collapse of the cyst walls, which may be calcified.

TREATMENT

Active cysticercosis is usually treated with praziquantel. This drug has few side effects—mainly mild gastrointestinal symptoms, headache, vertigo, and a decreased sense of well being. The usual dosage is 50 mg per kilogram per day administered in three divided doses, taken by mouth for 15 days.

Table 1 Treatment of Neurocysticercosis

Disease	Treatment
Active disease	
Parenchymal cysts, small	Praziquantel
Parenchymal cysts, large and symptomatic	Praziquantel or surgical removal
Meningitis/arachnoiditis without hydrocephalus	Praziquantel + careful monitoring of patients for development of hydrocephalus
Meningitis/arachnoiditis with hydrocephalus	Ventricular shunt and praziquantel
Intraventricular cyst	Surgical removal or praziquantel Ventricular shunt may be needed if hydrocephalus is present
Spinal cord cyst	Praziquantel or surgical removal
Inactive disease	
Calcified granulomas	Symptomatic (e.g., anticonvulsants)

The drug is well absorbed from the gastrointestinal tract and has a plasma half-life of 1 to 1.5 hours. There is a wide variation in plasma levels of praziquantel after the patient has taken a standard dose. Some of this variation appears to result from extensive primary hepatic metabolism of praziquantel during its first passage through the liver. In blood, most praziquantel is bound to plasma albumin. Free praziquantel readily crosses the blood-brain barrier, usually achieving therapeutic concentrations in the CSF and brain. It also appears to penetrate cysticerci fairly rapidly. The exact mechanism of action of this agent is unknown.

Patients with multiple cystic lesions in the subarachnoid space or ventricles may develop increased CNS symptoms shortly after praziquantel treatment is initiated. This appears to result from death of cysticerci, release of cysticerci antigen into the surrounding brain, and stimulation of reactive inflammation. If symptoms worsen with praziquantel treatment, dexamethasone (12 to 24 mg per day) or prednisone (40 to 60 mg per day), frequently is given. Ocular cysticercosis probably should not be treated with praziquantel at all.

Some controversy exists as to whether it is necessary to give praziquantel to patients with mild symptoms or without symptoms in whom one or two small intraparenchymal brain cysts are seen on CT. In my experience, these patients generally have a good prognosis regardless of treatment.

Patients with ventricular or subarachnoid space cysts are more difficult to treat and manage because the cysts may not be killed by praziquantel. Intraventricular cysts also frequently dislodge or shift, causing obstruction of CSF outflow. Therefore, the cyst is frequently surgically removed. If hydrocephalus develops, ventriculoperitoneal shunting is indicated. Unfortunately, CSF cellular debris from the chronic inflammation may make it difficult to maintain shunt patency.

Occasionally, large parenchymal cysts that cause localized pressure effects are surgically removed. Similarly, spinal cord cysts that do not respond to praziquantel may be surgically removed.

Another drug, albendazole, is used in the treatment of neurocysticercosis in Mexico and other South American countries. This drug appears to have the same efficacy as praziquantel but is less expensive (a 2-week treatment with praziquantel costs between $500 and $700). The dosage of albendazole is 15 mg per kilogram per day divided into three doses, taken by mouth for 1 to 4 weeks. The drug is well tolerated and has few side effects. It has not yet received Food and Drug Administration (FDA) approval in the United States.

One-year follow-up studies of patients who received praziquantel treatment for neurocysticercosis in Mexico have reported permanent cures or marked improvement in approximately 90 percent of patients with parenchymal cysts but only in about 50 percent of patients with arachnoiditis. In patients who fail to show evidence of improvement on CT scan or clinically, retreatment with praziquantel or albendazole is recommended.

Patients with inactive disease do not respond to praziquantel because the cysticerci are already dead. Generally, these patients should be treated symptomatically with anticonvulsants for seizures. Occasionally, obstructive hydrocephalus may develop in these patients, necessitating ventriculoperitoneal shunting.

PREVENTION

Stools of the patient and members of his or her immediate family should be examined for ova and proglottids to *Taenia solium*. Approximately 10 percent of patients or their family will have an intestinal tapeworm. If these are identified, the individual should be treated with praziquantel (a single dose of 20 mg per kilogram, taken by mouth) or niclosamide (a single dose of 2 g for adults, taken by mouth) to eradicate the tapeworm and decrease the risk of autoinfection or community spread of the disease. When one is traveling in endemic areas, the risk of developing neurocysticercosis can be minimized by avoiding eating ova-contaminated food such as raw vegetables (these may be contaminated with human ova-containing stool). If pork is thoroughly cooked or frozen to ⁻20°C for several days, cysticerci is inactivated and intestinal tapeworm is prevented.

SUGGESTED READING

Earnest MP, Reller LB, Filley CM, Grek AJ. Neurocysticercosis in the United States: 35 cases and a review. Rev Infect Dis 1987; 9:961–979.

King CH, Mahmoud AAF. Drugs five years later: praziquantel. Ann Intern Med 1989; 110:290–296.

Sotelo J, Escobedo F, Rodriguez-Carbajal J, et al. Therapy of parenchymal brain cysticercosis with praziquantel. New Engl J Med 1984; 310:1001–1007.

Sotelo J, Penagos P, Escobedo F, Del Brutto OH. Short course of albendazole therapy for neurocysticercosis. Arch Neurol 1988; 45:1130–1133.

Sotelo J, Torres B, Rubio-Donnadieu F, et al. Praziquantel in the treatment of neurocysticercosis: long-term follow-up. Neurology 1985; 35:752–755.

OTHER INFLAMMATORY AND DEMYELINATING DISEASES

NEUROSARCOIDOSIS

ROBERT P. LISAK, M.D.

Sarcoidosis is an inflammatory granulomatous disease of unknown etiology. The extent of this disease ranges from asymptomatic involvement of perihilar nodes detected incidently on routine chest x-ray examination to widely disseminated disease involving liver, spleen, pulmonary parenchyma, heart, skin, joints, the muscle, and the eyes, as well as the central and peripheral nervous systems. The disease may be clinically evident in several organs, or involvement of one or two organ systems may predominate, but histologic or other studies may demonstrate the true extent of the disease in the individual patient. Sarcoid may present in an acute or subacute manner or may be slowly progressive. Patients may switch from one course to another. Therefore, while it is the general impression that the acute form tends to respond better to therapy and/or eventually subside when compared with a more progressive course, even when involving the same organ systems, there are clearly exceptions to this rule. Thus in the absence of controlled studies, proof of therapeutic efficacy of any treatment and especially its long-term benefit is lacking.

The diagnosis of nervous system sarcoidosis, which occurs in approximately 5 percent of patients with sarcoidosis, is not difficult to make when a clinical syndrome characteristic of neurosarcoidosis such as a seventh nerve palsy develops in a patient with known sarcoidosis. It is somewhat more difficult when a similar syndrome (Table 1) develops in a patient not previously known to have sarcoid (as many as 40 to 50 percent of those 5 percent who develop neurosarcoidosis). Such syndromes are clearly not specific for neurosarcoidosis. When a patient with one or more of these clinical neurologic syndromes appears without another unequivocal etiologic explanation, it is necessary to conduct an extensive search for evidence of sarcoid in other organ systems. This frequently requires obtaining tissue from another organ after laboratory and imag-

Table 1 Neurologic Manifestations of Sarcoidosis

Cranial neuropathies (II; III, IV, and VI; V; VII; VIII are the most frequent)
Aseptic meningitis
Hydrocephalus
Central nervous system parenchymal disease (hypothalamic, other hemispheric, spinal cord)
Vasculopathy-vasculitis/encephalopathy
Peripheral neuropathy (distal symmetric sensory motor, mononeuritis)
Myopathy
Nerve root implants

ing studies are performed to increase the yield of the procedure. I find an opthalmologic evaluation useful, as well. In a few patients (1 to 5 percent) the neurologic symptoms and signs may be the only evidence of sarcoid despite an extensive investigation, and biopsy of the appropriate area of the nervous system (meninges, intracerebral mass, muscle, peripheral nerve) without attempting complete surgical removal may be necessary. In addition, on rare occasions I have found it necessary to biopsy involved tissue to distinguish a neurologic complication of therapy for sarcoid from a newly appearing neurosarcoidosis syndrome (muscle biopsy to distinguish steroid myopathy from sarcoid of the muscle; biopsy of a mass lesion to distinguish focal infection from sarcoid within the nervous system if the distinction cannot be made based on clinical, laboratory, or imaging criteria).

CORTICOSTEROID THERAPY

In patients with cranial nerve involvement, aseptic meningitis, parenchymous disease, encephalopathy (not secondary to a metabolic cause such as hypercalcemia), vasculitis, or clinically significant myopathy or neuropathy, therapy should be begun with prednisone, 40 to 60 mg per day (or an equivalent dose of another oral corticosteroid such as methylprednisilone or dexamethasone). I administer this dose to the patient for 6 to 8 weeks, and if there is a good therapeutic response, I gradually taper the dose by 5 mg per day each week until I reach a level of 20 to 25 mg per day. If there is no deterioration, reduce the dose by 5 mg per day every 3 weeks. If there is a flare of disease activity, I return to the last dose at which the disease was suppressed, and after another 6 to 8 weeks, attempt to taper the dose again. Some patients will respond but will need long-term, low-dose suppression of 10 to 20 mg per day. The many complications of corticosteroids, both short- and long-term, are covered elsewhere in this volume.

Some patients neither improve nor worsen while receiving corticosteroid therapy, and it is difficult to decide what should be done under these circumstances. If the patient worsens, however, I generally try to give a higher dosage of steroids (80 to 120 mg per day) for several weeks and then once again try to taper the dose. Pulse therapy with intravenous methylprednisilone has also been reported to be helpful under these circumstances. I would try 500 mg given over 4 hours twice daily to four times daily, and then return the patient to the prior oral dose of corticosteroids.

OTHER THERAPIES

In the case of mass lesions of the brain and spinal cord, radiation has been reported to be of help in corticosteroid-resistant patients, and I have personally observed both successful and unsuccessful attempts at such treatment. Hydrocephalus, either caused by obstruction or an absorptive defect, may require ventriculoatrial or ventriculoperitoneal shunt. The more chronic intraparenchymous-presenting lesions may not respond well to any therapy or may require long-term corticosteroid therapy.

Therapy involving various cytotoxic and other immunosuppressive therapies, for patients resistant to corticosteroid and radiation therapy have been suggested for non-neurosarcoidosis cases, and even more recently, for patients with neurosarcoidosis. These therapies include cyclophosphamide, azathioprine, chlorambucil, and more recently, the more helper T-cell selective agent cyclosporin A. I have had no personal experience with any of these agents in the treatment of neurosarcoidosis, and would simply suggest that, given the uncontrolled nature of therapeutic studies and the unpredictable nature of this disease, one needs to exercise great caution in choosing to use these in patients with neurosarcoidosis.

SUGGESTED READING

Bejar JM, Kerby GR, Zeigler DK, Festoff BW. Treatment of central nervous system sarcoidosis with radiotherapy. Ann Neurol 1985; 18:258–260.

Grizzanti JN, Knapp AB, Schetcter AJ, Williams MH Jr. Treatment of sarcoid meningitis with radiotherapy. Am J Med 1982; 73:605–608.

Lisak RP. Neurologic manifestations of systemic inflammatory-autoimmune diseases. Curr Opin Neurol Neurosurg 1989; 2:169–173.

Luke RA, Stern BJ, Krumholz A, Johns CJ. Neurosarcoidosis: the long-term clinical course. Neurology 1987; 37:461–463.

Stern BJ, Krumholz A, Johns C, et al. Sarcoidosis and its neurologic manifestations. Arch Neurol 1985; 42:909–917.

PATIENT RESOURCE

Sarcoidosis Family Aid and Research Foundation
760 Clinton Avenue
Newark, New Jersey 07108
Telephone: (201) 676-7901

POSTINFECTIOUS AND ACUTE TRANSVERSE MYELITIS

BRUCE A. COHEN, M.D.
HOWARD L. LIPTON, M.D.

Acute transverse myelitis is an inflammatory condition of the spinal cord, usually involving multiple segments, which may be static or ascend progressively. The precise clinical manifestations in a given case are determined by the level of involvement and the extent of white and gray matter injury. Characteristically, the neurologic examination reveals elements of motor weakness, often initially with flaccidity but later with spasticity, sensory loss with a discrete level of demarcation, and bowel and bladder dysfunction. Symptoms develop rapidly, usually progressing over a period of days, and constitute a syndrome requiring immediate diagnostic evaluation.

The most urgent concern is to exclude a mass lesion producing a compressive myelopathy. Intrinsic lesions may be vascular, neoplastic, or inflammatory, and careful history with judicious use of clinical testing must be applied to this sometimes difficult problem of differential diagnosis (Table 1). Diagnostic modalities include imaging procedures, cerebrospinal fluid (CSF) and serum analyses, and in some cases, electrophysiologic studies. Figure 1 indicates the evaluation process we pursue. When

Table 1 Etiologies of Acute Transverse Myelopathy

Extramedullary compression
  Neoplastic
    Malignant (e.g., metastatic tumors)
    Benign (e.g., metastatic tumors)
  Infection
    Epidural abscess
  Mechanical
    Disc protrusion
    Spinal deformities
Intramedullary processes
  Neoplastic
    Ependymoma, glioma
  Vascular
    Spinal cord infarction, AVM
  Infectious
    Syphilis, HSV, VZV, CMV, enteroviruses, HIV-1,
      HTLV-1
  Postinfectious and postvaccinial
    Varicella, measles, mycoplasma, legionella
  Inflammatory (other)
    Systemic, lupus, Sjögren's syndrome, sarcoidosis
    Multiple sclerosis
  Toxic-metabolic
    Substance abuse

AVM = arteriovenous malformation; CMV = cytomegalovirus; HIV-1 = human immunodeficiency virus type 1; HSV = herpes simplex virus; HTLV-1 = human T-cell lymphotropic virus; VZV = varicella-zoster virus.

magnetic resonance imaging (MRI) is used, it is important to obtain strongly T2-weighted images. We also recommend routinely freezing an aliquot of CSF in case further serologic or immunologic studies become important.

Once a diagnosis of acute transverse myelitis is made, therapy is divided into two general categories: direct treatment focused on the presumed inflammatory mechanisms and attendant edema, and supportive measures to prevent secondary complications and enhance the recovery process.

DIRECT THERAPY

It is our practice to treat patients seen within the first 10 days with corticosteroids. Although no controlled studies have established the value of these agents, we have been impressed anecdotally by the dramatic response in some patients. We prefer to use intravenous methylprednisolone in a dose of 1 g in 500 ml of normal saline administered in the morning over a period of 2 to 4 hours, for 3 to 5 days. We then switch the patient to prednisone, starting with 60 to 80 mg taken orally and tapering the dose by 10-mg increments every 3 days. There is no established laboratory parameter for following response to therapy other than clinical status.

Alternatively, corticosteroid therapy can be initiated with prednisone at a dose of 1 to 1.5 mg per kilogram taken orally daily for 7 to 14 days followed by tapering doses as above. Some physicians prefer to administer adrenocorticotropic hormone (ACTH), 40 to 50 U twice daily for 7 days, and then to taper doses over a 2-week period. None of these regimens has been established by controlled trials to be superior.

SIDE EFFECTS OF CORTICOSTEROID THERAPY

Regardless of the regimen employed, several potential side effects of steroid therapy need to be anticipated. Fluid retention and transient weight gain are to be expected, and hypertension may be precipitated. We check blood pressures four times daily and weigh patients every other day. If diuretic therapy is required, a potassium-sparing agent should be used. We monitor electrolytes twice weekly.

We routinely administer antacids 1 hour after meals and at bedtime for prophylaxis against ulceration. Histamine receptor (H_2) receptor antagonists may also be used, and we employ them when treating a patient with a history of peptic ulcer or gastritis. Because these drugs are a potential cause of toxic delirium, we prefer to use antacids when treating asymptomatic individuals. Stools should be checked daily for occult blood.

Some patients develop alterations of mood, behavior, or mentation while receiving steroid therapy, sometimes with marked fluctuations. These side effects can be treated with benzodiazepines, such as alprazolam, 0.25 to 0.5 mg three times daily, or diazepam, 2 to 5 mg three times daily. If these agents are ineffective, lithium carbonate, 300 mg three to four times daily, may be used on a short-term basis.

Patients should be monitored for hyperglycemia and increased intraocular pressure. Wound healing may be impaired, acneform skin lesions may erupt, and cutaneous ecchymoses may occur. For patients receiving steroid therapy for less than 3 to 4 weeks, we do not routinely delay initiation of treatment for tuberculosis skin testing. When treatment is anticipated for a longer period, as in the setting of known collagen-vascular disease, a tuberculin skin test and anergy battery should be applied, and a slit lamp examination for cataracts and measurement of intraocular pressure should be performed. If the skin test is positive or the chest radiograph shows a Ghon complex, the use of isoniazid (INH) 300 mg daily and pyridoxine hydrochloride 50 mg daily should be considered.

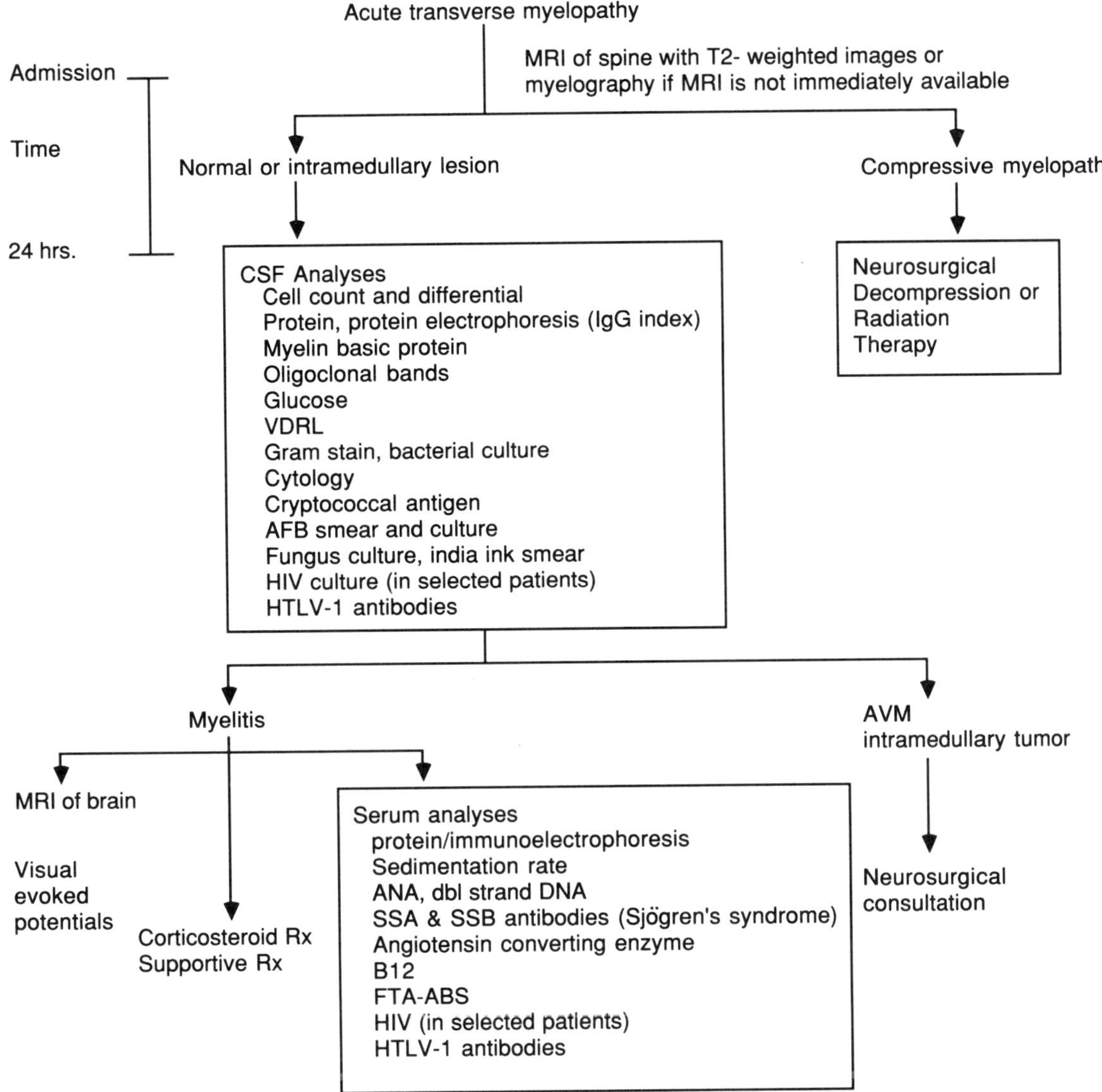

Figure 1 Diagnosis of acute transverse myelopathy. AFB = acid-fast bacilli; ANA = antinuclear antibodies; FTA-ABS = fluorescent treponemal antibody absorption test; SSA = Sjögren's syndrome A; SSB = Sjögren's syndrome B; VDRL = venereal disease research laboratory.

SUPPORTIVE CARE

Bladder disturbances are commonly encountered in these patients. Urinary retention with bladder distention is often present initially. In patients with a hypotonic bladder, manual voiding using the Credés maneuver at regular intervals may be attempted, but residual volumes should be maintained at less than 100 ml. If this fails, intermittent catheterization is preferred. This should be done often enough to prevent bladder overdistention (>400 ml), usually every 4 hours. If accurate input and output measurements are required or if intermittent catheterization is required more frequently than every 4 hours or cannot be performed, it may be necessary to use an indwelling catheter. In such cases, irrigation and antibiotic prophylaxis with trimethoprim-sulfamethoxazole double strength daily may be used, although some physicians prefer not to use prophylactic antibiotics to prevent selective colonization. The indwelling catheter should be removed as soon as possible.

If an uninhibited neurogenic bladder results in urinary incontinence, anticholinergic agents such as propantheline bromide, 15 to 30 mg at bedtime nightly and 7.5 to 15 mg three times daily, oxybutynin chloride, 5 mg three times daily, or imipramine hydrochloride, 25 to 75 mg daily, may be used. Care should be exercised to limit postvoid residual volumes to 100 ml or less.

When bladder dysfunction persists beyond the acute phase of illness, urodynamic investigation to assess for detrusor-sphincter dyssynergia should be performed. Prolonged catheterization may lead to stone formation, and occasionally, anatomic abnormalities of the bladder may be present, complicating management.

Constipation commonly accompanies immobilization in acute transverse myelitis. We routinely give patients bulk-forming agents such as psyllium and add docusate sodium, 50 to 100 mg daily, if needed. Mild laxatives may be used, and in the patients who fail to respond, enemas should be performed once or twice weekly. On occasion, manual extraction is necessary. The use of a bowel program in which glycerine or bisacodyl suppositories are used every other day as needed to maintain continence may prevent fecal impaction.

Careful attention to maintenance of skin integrity is essential in the treatment of any immobilized patient, and we use "egg crate" mattresses and elbow and heel pads to protect pressure points. Frequent turning of the patient at 2-hour intervals and daily inspection for early signs of decubitus formation are routine. Care is taken to prevent contact of desensitized skin with hot, abrasive, or moistened surfaces. If no necrosis is present, Duoderm dressings can be applied to affected areas every 4 to 7 days. When minor local skin necrosis appears, saline-wet to dry dressings can be used. If deep ulcerations occur, surgical consultation should be obtained.

Pain is not an uncommon problem in these patients. For dysesthetic pain, we prefer to administer carbamazepine, 100 to 200 mg three to four times daily, or phenytoin, 100 mg three to four times daily. Tricyclic agents such as amitryptyline (50 to 100 mg daily) may also be used, although their sedative and anticholinergic effects may interact with other medications or complicate urinary management. For muscular pains, we administer agents such as methocarbamol, 500 to 1,000 mg three to four times daily.

We prefer air compression boots as prophylaxis for deep vein thrombophlebitis until mobility is restored. Heparin may also be used, either subcutaneously at a dosage of 5,000 U twice daily or intravenously, titrating the intravenous dose so that a partial thromboplastin time of one and a half times the control is obtained. The use of heparin entails potential risks of hemorrhage and thrombocytopenia, and these must be watched for.

When patients develop painful or functionally limiting spasticity, we administer baclofen, 5 to 10 mg three times daily initially, increasing this dos-

age to a maximum of 80 mg daily. If an additional agent is required, we prefer diazepam, 2 to 5 mg three to four times daily. Dantrolene sodium (25 mg per day initially, with the dosage gradually increased in increments of 25 mg every 4 to 7 days) can also be used, but liver enzymes should be monitored serially and the drug discontinued if no benefit occurs within 45 days.

In patients with cervical myelitis, respiratory function should be monitored with forced vital capacity measurements taken twice daily. When patients require ventilatory assistance, negative inspiratory force, forced vital capacities, and arterial blood gases are used to assess respiratory capability and decide when the patient can be safely extubated once neurologic progression has stabilized. Adequate suctioning and, when required, chest physical therapy and postural drainage should be employed to prevent complicating pneumonias.

Nutritional management should not be overlooked. We prescribe low-sodium diets with adequate fluid replacement and caloric intake, ensuring 125 to 150 g of protein with supplements as needed. If the patient is unable to take oral feedings, parenteral alimentation may be required.

We start physical and occupational therapy as soon as feasible with splinting to prevent contracture formation and institution of passive range of motion of affected limbs at the bedside. The patient progresses to active resistance exercises, transfer, activities of daily living, and gait training as his or her condition permits. Appliances such as ankle-foot orthoses or leg braces, and walkers or multipoint canes may facilitate early ambulation.

Most patients improve, but some do not recover sufficiently to resume their previous occupational or daily activities. Social service, psychological support, and vocational retraining may be required and should be initiated as soon as prolonged or permanent limitation is anticipated. Adjustments in the home environment, such as support railings or special equipment, and training of family members or home health aides may be required and should be initiated early enough to allow the patient to have a smooth transition from the hospital to home.

SUGGESTED READING

Altrocchi P. Acute transverse myelopathy. Arch Neurol 1963; 9:21–29.

Dowling PC, Bosch VV, Cook SD. Possible beneficial effect of high-dose intravenous steroid therapy in acute demyelinating disease and transverse myelitis. Neurology 1980; 30:33–36.

Lipton H, Teasdall RD. Acute transverse myelopathy in adults. Arch Neurol 1973; 28:252–257.

Ropper AH, Poskanzer DC. The prognosis of acute and subacute transverse myelopathy based on early signs and symptoms. Ann Neurol 1978; 4:51–59.

MULTIPLE SCLEROSIS

ROBERT M. HERNDON, M.D.

DIAGNOSIS

Treatment of multiple sclerosis (MS) begins with diagnosis and classification. Approximately 10 percent of referrals to MS clinics are misdiagnosed. Although the spectrum of misdiagnosis has changed with the advent of magnetic resonance imaging (MRI), the rate of misdiagnosis has changed little. Misread and overinterpreted MRIs have become a common cause of misdiagnosis. *The diagnosis of MS remains a clinical diagnosis.* It is based on evidence of dissemination in time and clinical or paraclinical, *objective,* evidence of dissemination in location. It is important to realize that other disease processes can produce syndromes that meet formal diagnostic criteria for multiple sclerosis. Thus, atypical features such as absence of visual or oculomotor signs, normal cerebrospinal fluid, absence of bladder involvement, strictly posterior fossa signs, or a normal MRI should alert the physician to the possibility of misdiagnosis. Accurate diagnosis is especially important when more aggressive therapies are being considered, but it is also important in general, since many of the disorders that may be mistaken for MS can be effectively treated.

Classification

Once the diagnosis is clearly established, treatment depends on the type of disease and the severity of the process. Treatment can be divided into two categories; (1) treatment directed at the basic disease process and (2) symptomatic therapy. Treatment of the disease process is either immunosuppressive or immunomodulatory, and treatment selection is based on severity and classification (Fig. 1). In general, younger people with the disease are more likely to have an exacerbating remitting or exacerbating progressive course with relatively acute episodes of demyelination followed by periods of improvement or relative stability. In many of these cases, significant progression of the disease between attacks may be largely masked by the superimposed exacerbations and remissions. Improvement in one area after an acute attack will mask other symptoms that are continuing to progress, so that the patient may be improving in some areas and progressing in others simultaneously. In older patients, generally those older than 40 years of age, acute attacks are increasingly uncommon and the disease manifests itself primarily as a progressive loss of function without acute exacerbations or periods of remission.

THERAPY DIRECTED AT THE DISEASE PROCESS

Diet

Numerous claims have been made regarding the therapeutic efficacy of a host of different diets, vitamin supplements, and mineral supplements. To date, the only credible evidence of the efficacy of diet in treating MS is that a dietary supplement of linoleic acid achieved with two tablespoons of sunflower seed oil daily produces a slight reduction in the frequency and/or severity of acute attacks. The effect is not great, but it has been seen in more than one properly controlled study. Aside from this, however, there are no convincing studies demonstrating that special diets have any beneficial effect on the course of the disease.

Caution should be taken in the use of mineral supplements since there is evidence suggesting that zinc can enhance immune responses, and also epidemiologic evidence suggesting that zinc might have an adverse effect on MS.

Rest

Bedrest, a time-honored treatment for MS, is frequently recommended. In the case of acute at-

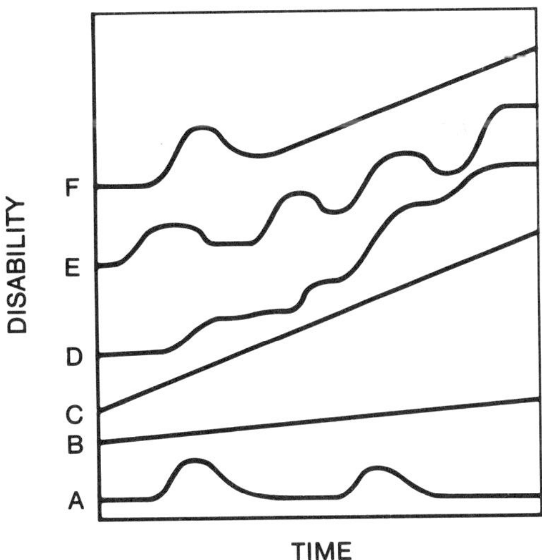

Figure 1 The varied course of multiple sclerosis. A = benign course; B = slowly progressive course; C = more rapid, steadily progressive course; D = intermittently progressive course; E = combined course with acute attacks, incomplete recovery, and a progressive component largely obscured by attacks and incomplete remissions; F = single acute attack followed by steady progression.

tacks in a person who is not severely handicapped, bedrest may provide some modest benefit in terms of reduced stress and anxiety. There is no evidence that it improves the rate of recovery. Bedrest is not recommended for individuals with progressive disease and especially for those with spastic paraparesis that has become chronic. Even 2 or 3 days in bed may be enough to convert an ambulatory patient with spastic paraparesis into a wheelchair-bound patient. Loss of muscle strength and tone occurs rapidly in paretic patients, and it is extremely difficult to make up lost ground.

Prevention of Acute Attacks

No treatment thus far reported is known to prevent acute attacks. Although there is preliminary evidence that beta-interferon and copolymer-1 (COP-1) reduce the number of acute attacks, these agents are still in the experimental stages. Therapeutic trials currently in progress may establish the place of these agents in the therapeutic armamentarium, but to date, they do not appear to be of much value in the treatment of progressive disease.

Azathioprine (Imuran) has been used to reduce the number of acute attacks of patients with MS, but controlled clinical trials have failed to demonstrate that it has a clear effect on exacerbation.

The Acute Attack

The acute attack of MS may be very mild with little impairment of important functions. In this case, and if the symptoms of the acute attack do not interfere with the patient's normal activities and are not uncomfortable for the patient, no treatment is necessary. There is no evidence that treatment of the acute attack improves the ultimate level of functional recovery. Although steroids will hasten the recovery process at the cost of side effects of varying severity, the ultimate level of recovery is probably not affected. The use of steroids in patients with optic neuritis may be an exception, however, because the optic nerve may become swollen and, since it passes through the restrictive optic canal, can be damaged by pressure and ischemia. Thus I believe that significant optic neuritis should be treated with steroids routinely, pending the outcome of the current multicenter optic neuritis treatment trial.

Severe acute attacks that interfere with the patient's livelihood or daily activities or that produce significant discomfort may be treated with adrenocorticotropic hormone (ACTH) or prednisone. Although many neurologists express a strong preference for one or the other, there is little evidence to support that one is significantly superior to the other. There is good evidence that ACTH shortens the duration of acute attacks, and the experience of most clinicians is that prednisone is equally efficacious. The two are by no means identical, and if one does not work, the other may. Individuals who have not been treated previously will often respond rapidly to prednisone in a dose of 60 mg daily, but with repeated courses, higher doses of as much as 100 mg daily or more may be required. Prednisone is best given as a single morning dose. I usually give the initial dose for 5 days, then taper. Recrudescence of symptoms is a common problem when the drug is tapered rapidly. When this happens, I find that resumption of full doses is usually required to regain the lost ground, and even then, the initial level of improvement may not be regained. Recrudescence during the taper can be minimized by using a slow taper (Table 1).

Acute attacks may also be treated with ACTH gel in a dosage of 40 to 80 U per day. In this case, the full dose is maintained for approximately 5 days, then decreased by 20 U every 3 days until the patient has discontinued the medication, or in some patients, may be completed with the patient receiving 20 U per day for 3 days followed by three alternate-day doses of 20 U each.

Steroid Dependence

Steroid dependence occurs when the steroid dose cannot be decreased without a significant recrudescence of symptoms. This is unusual and occurs in no more than 1 to 3 percent of patients. If three successive attempts to taper the steroids result in recurrence of significant, disabling symptoms, the patient should be considered steroid dependent. When this is the case, I have found that a slow taper to 30 mg of prednisone daily and a slow taper to 30 mg every other day can usually be achieved without a flair in the symptoms. Levels of 20 to 30 mg of prednisone administered on an alternate-day schedule can be maintained for long periods of time with minimal side effects. My experience has been that these patients remain remarkably free of acute attacks on the alternate-day schedule. I do not advocate continuous therapy for patients who can

Table 1 Treatment with Prednisone

Day	Dose (mg)
1–4	100
5–7	80
8–10	60
11–13	40
14–16	30
17–20	20
21–23	15
24–26	10
27–29	5
30	0

be withdrawn from steroids without recurrence of symptoms. In addition, I usually try to reduce the alternate-day dose to the minimum that will keep the patient free of recurrence of the symptoms. After 1 year of the alternate-day schedule, I usually reattempt to decrease the dose, although my success rate in withdrawing these individuals from steroids without a recurrence of symptoms has been low.

Progressive Disease

Steroids and ACTH

The use of steroids and ACTH in the treatment of progressive MS has been disappointing. Transient improvement often occurs but usually disappears within a few days or weeks after treatment is discontinued. One can delay the onset of wheelchair dependence for several months by administering steroids continuously, but because of the high rate of complications and particularly of osteoporosis, I do not recommend this approach.

In patients with severe spastic paraparesis, high-dose methylprednisolone will significantly reduce spasticity for a substantial period. The drug is given in a dose of 1 g daily for 3 days by intravenous infusion. I prefer to administer this dose as 0.5 g twice daily for 3 days. Although the dose is usually well tolerated, complications have been seen. In particular, immobile patients with deep vein thrombosis are liable to develop pulmonary emboli if they begin to move their legs more freely. Such emboli are dangerous and can be fatal. If one is in doubt regarding the possibility of deep vein thrombosis, appropriate studies and/or anticoagulation should precede treatment. Aseptic necrosis of the head of the femur is also seen as an uncommon complication.

Immunosuppressive Therapy

Cyclophosphamide in combination with ACTH or a synthetic steroid has been reported to be useful in treating progressive MS. My experience suggests that, in a carefully selected group of patients, the treatment does have substantial benefit. It also carries significant risks, however, and deaths have occurred, particularly with the shorter, more intensive, 8-day course that some have advocated. I have not included a treatment protocol in this discussion because I do not recommend that this treatment be undertaken by clinicians not familiar with chemotherapy or by those who are treating only a small number of patients. It should be undertaken only after a thorough study of the literature on the subject, and preferably only after discussion with someone who has used this form of therapy. For patients in whom this approach is indicated, we recommend referral to a center that has an active treatment program.

Selection of appropriate patients to be referred for chemotherapy involves consideration of the following factors.

Age. Younger patients respond much better than older patients. We rarely use chemotherapy in patients older than 55 years of age. Younger patients are much more likely to show significant improvement than older patients. The few exceptions to this have been older patients with an unusually rapid course, which is rare in this age group.

Rate of Progression. The more rapidly the disease is progressing, the more effective immunosuppressive therapy is likely to be and the greater the probability of significant clinical improvement. In patients with an indolent or slowly progressive course, improvement is significantly less likely and, because of the slow rate at which the patient is changing, arrest of progression is difficult to observe.

Disability. The response to therapy is less and the complication rate much higher in severely disabled patients. I do not treat patients who are wheelchair-bound unless they have been using a wheelchair for only a short time and can still stand (bear weight) and self transfer. Patients who are effectively paraplegic usually have significant impairment of respiratory function and are at risk for pulmonary infection as well as for bladder infection.

Reproductive Status. Because cyclophosphamide therapy may cause sterility and may also damage DNA, it should not be used in individuals who plan to have children and should never be used in someone who is pregnant.

Complicating Medical Disorders. Patients with significant medical illness in addition to MS must be evaluated individually. Diabetes in particular presents a problem since steroids add to the difficulties in controlling the diabetes and because these patients are much more susceptible to infection, particularly if the diabetes is severe. In general, I prefer not to treat insulin-dependent diabetics. Other disorders such as malignancies and heart disease should be evaluated on a case-by-case basis.

Side Effects. To be selected for chemotherapy, patients should be able to accept side effects including hair loss, nausea, and vomiting, and other risks inherent in the treatment.

Azathioprine

Azathioprine (Imuran) has been widely used over the past two decades despite a paucity of studies demonstrating its effectiveness. Studies to date suggest that, in doses of approximately 100 mg per day, it is fairly well tolerated for long periods. The drug appears to have little effect on the exacerbation rate, but it appears to have some effect on the overall rate of progression. Although the effects of this drug on progression are not great, they may be sufficient to warrant its use in some patients. Further clinical trials are needed to better define its place in the therapeutic armamentarium.

Cyclosporin

Cyclosporin has been used in a recently completed clinical trial and appears to have some beneficial effect on the disease process; however, renal toxicity and hypertension appear to be a substantial problem when the doses that are used are high enough to be effective. Because of this, I do not recommend its use at this time.

Plasmapheresis

The role of plasmapheresis in the treatment of MS remains uncertain. Good results have been reported in at least one controlled study; however, other studies have shown much less clear-cut results. A large controlled trial is currently in progress and should help define the proper role of plasmapheresis in the treatment of MS. Until further research results become available, I do not recommend this expensive and unproven approach.

Several other therapies including hyperbaric oxygen and transfer factor have been recommended by some, but these have not proven useful when properly tested.

SYMPTOMATIC TREATMENT

Spasticity

Spasticity is very common and troublesome in patients with MS, but in patients with pyramidal weakness, it also plays a role in maintaining the ability to stand and walk. In patients with spastic paraparesis, the spasticity may provide the extensor strength for bearing weight. Thus effective drug therapy for spasticity often increases weakness and a balance must be found between the two.

Effective treatment of spasticity begins with physical therapy. Stretching is essential to prevent contractures and also reduces spasticity. Active exercise will help maintain strength and mobility. I regard physical therapy as the mainstay of therapy for spasticity.

Baclofen (Lioresal) has proven to be the most effective and useful drug for the treatment of spasticity. The proper dose is "enough but not too much." Some patients receive considerable relief from as little as 5 mg taken once or twice daily and become weak when taking 10 mg per dose, while others require much higher doses and do well with doses of as much as 200 mg (although the maximum recommended dose according to the manufacturer is

80 mg per day). Baclofen should be started in a dose of about 10 mg administered twice daily and increased by 10 mg per day until the spasticity is adequately relieved or weakness occurs. When weakness develops, the dose should be decreased to a point below that at which weakness occurs. If this does not produce significant reduction in spasticity, there is little point in continuing therapy unless the patient is willing to tolerate some weakness in return for reduced spasticity.

Diazepam (Valium) is another effective muscle relaxant and may be used when results with baclofen are unsatisfactory. It is usually started at a dosage of 5 mg twice daily and increased gradually. It is considerably more sedative than baclofen, is habituating, and may interfere with cognitive function. I reserve it for patients who cannot tolerate baclofen or, in some instances, as an adjunct to baclofen therapy, particularly in patients who have a high level of anxiety in addition to their spasticity.

Dantrolene has not proven useful in the therapy of spasticity in MS patients in my experience. It appears to be much less effective than baclofen or diazepam and carries a greater risk of toxicity, particularly liver toxicity.

More drastic measures may be needed for patients with spasticity that is refractory to drug treatment. I reserve such measures for patients with essentially complete paraplegia. These include chemical neurolysis by injection of phenol either into motor nerves (using electromyographic guidance) or into the motor point. Alternatively, ethanol can be injected intrathecally to block the lumbar nerve roots. Although this usually produces relief that lasts for at least 6 months and can be repeated if necessary, it should be reserved for patients who have lost bladder and bowel control. More permanent relief can be achieved with neurosurgical intervention either via dorsal rhizotomy or by Bischoff's myelotomy. These drastic procedures result in a flaccid paralysis that is permanent. Such procedures are rarely needed but may be used in patients with long-standing sensory loss, urinary retention, and flexor spasms or spasticity that is refractory and seriously interferes with patient care. Considerable attention to the prevention of decubitus ulcers is needed in patients with impaired sensation that is either a direct result of MS or a result of destructive treatment aimed at relieving spasticity.

Bladder Dysfunction

Frequently, both small spastic bladders with urgency and incontinence and large flaccid bladders with overflow incontinence are a problem in patients with MS. Management of both types of neurogenic bladder is discussed elsewhere in this book.

Bowel Dysfunction

Constipation is a regular occurrence in patients with MS. Bowel motility is decreased, presumably because of altered autonomic function. This is aggravated in many patients by a low fluid intake, which is a common response in patients with urinary urgency, frequency, and incontinence. It is normally best to manage the bowel with stool softeners such as docusate sodium (Colace) in a dose of 50 to 200 mg per day and bulk laxatives such as bran. Increased fluid intake is also helpful. If these measures prove inadequate, bisacodyl (Dulcolax) may be useful. Bisacodyl tablets will usually work overnight and the suppositories within 1 to 2 hours. Severe constipation should not be ignored since obstipation with rupture of the bowel has been known to occur in patients with MS.

Cognitive and Emotional Aspects

While many MS patients have little clinically evident emotional or cognitive disturbance, most patients with well-established disease do have measurable changes in their cognitive abilities and many have disturbances in the emotional sphere. There are several relatively simple measures that can help in the management of these problems, although little can be done to help those few patients with serious cognitive impairment.

Depression, Euphoria, and Pathologic Laughing and Weeping

Depression. This is a common problem in patients with MS, and mania is also fairly common, particularly in patients receiving steroids. These affective disorders must be distinguished from the problems of exaggerated or perverted affective display described below. There is evidence of an increased incidence of true *bipolar disease* in MS patients and in relatives of MS patients, although the reason for this is unknown. These disorders usually respond to traditional treatment with lithium carbonate or with carbamazepine (Tegretol). Hypomanic episodes occurring during steroid treatment may usually be managed with Tegretol in a dose of 300 to 400 mg daily. This works more rapidly than lithium and can be easily introduced if sleeplessness and other signs of mania occur. If Tegretol does not work satisfactorily or cannot be used because of toxic side effects, lithium carbonate will usually prove effective.

Most depression associated with MS is probably situational, but endogenous depressions are also common. Tricyclic antidepressants are usually effective in the management of this disorder. The required dose is often much less than that traditionally used in the treatment of depression. I have found doses of amitriptyline hydrochloride of as little as 10 mg per day to be effective in some instances, and a dose of 25 to 50 mg at bedtime is typically adequate. The much higher doses traditionally used to treat depression are rarely required.

Pathologic Laughing and Weeping. Pathologic laughing and weeping are extreme examples of lability of affective display. In these extreme examples, the affective display (i.e., the laughter or crying) may bear little relationship to the feelings of the patient. The patient is unable to modulate affective expression, so that even relatively mild emotional stimuli bring on an affective display that is exaggerated in intensity and that may be inappropriate in relation to the patient's feelings or internal affective state. In milder cases, an exaggeration of the appropriate affective display is all that is seen.

These disorders of affective display, often described somewhat inaccurately as "emotional lability," are socially disabling and particularly prone to disrupt personal relationships since the patient's emotional displays are invariably interpreted as reflecting his or her feelings rather than recognized as an exaggerated and perhaps perverted expression of those feelings. It is extremely hard for the spouse, or indeed the physician, to recognize depression in someone who is laughing. We are taught from infancy to believe facial expression, and if the facial expression does not accurately reflect what the person is saying, we believe the expression. Thus emotional communication is disrupted for these patients, sometimes with devastating effects on interpersonal relations.

Both pathologic laughing and weeping and lability of affective display are responsive to treatment in the majority of cases. Amitriptyline hydrochloride in a dose of 10 to 50 mg daily, usually administered as a single bedtime dose, is effective in reducing lability of affective display in 80 to 90 percent of patients. The effect of this agent in treating these disorders is more rapid than in the treatment of depression. The result is a reduction in the extreme emotional expression so that the affective display is more consonant with the internal affective state. The use of L-dihydroxyphenylalanine(L-DOPA) has been recommended for pathologic laughing and weeping in patients with cerebrovascular disease, but its use in treating MS has not been reported.

Inability to Focus Attention

Many MS patients can do only one thing at a time. For example, many cannot walk and have a conversation at the same time because they need to concentrate on their walking. Such patients have a great deal of difficulty with concentration in a distracting environment. They are able to function reasonably well in a quiet, nondistracting environment but are unable to filter out distracting stimuli. This problem frequently leads to irritability and can significantly interfere with work performance. Such patients are extremely intolerant of typical family life in which children are running in and out, the television is often on, and multiple simultaneous conversations are taking place. The simple expedient of removing as much of the distraction as possible or of providing a quiet room where the patient can do one thing at a time without distraction will often greatly improve temper and allow him or her to cope with the frustrations of the disease much better. Similarly, removing distractions from the workplace may result in improved job performance.

SUGGESTED READING

McDonald WI, Silberberg DH. The diagnosis of multiple sclerosis. In: McDonald WI, Silberberg DH, eds. Multiple sclerosis. Boston: Butterworth Publishers, 1986:1.
Rudick RA, Schiffer RB, Schwetz K, Herndon RM. Multiple sclerosis: the problem of misdiagnosis. Arch Neurol 1986; 43:578–593.
Ellison GW, Myers LW, eds. Rationale for immunomodulating therapies of multiple sclerosis. Neurology 1988; 38 (suppl): 89.
Ellison GW. Treatment aimed at modifying the course of multiple sclerosis. In: McDonald WI, Silberberg DH, eds. Multiple sclerosis. Boston: Butterworth Publishers, 1986:153.
Sibley WA. Therapeutic claims in multiple sclerosis. New York: Demos Publications, 1988.
Schiffer RB, Rudick RA, Herndon RM. Pathological laughing and weeping: treatment with amitriptyline. N Engl J Med 1985; 312:1480–1482.

PATIENT RESOURCES

Literature

Scheinberg LS. Multiple sclerosis: a guide for patients and their families. New York: Raven Press, 1983.
Therapeutic claims in multiple sclerosis. Published by the International Federation of Multiple Sclerosis Societies (IFMSS). Available from the National Multiple Sclerosis Society (see address below, under "Associations").
Wolf JK, ed. Mastering multiple sclerosis: a handbook for MSers and families. Chicago: Academy Books, 1984.

Associations
National Multiple Sclerosis Society
205 East 42nd Street
New York, New York 10017
Telephone: (212) 986-3240

(Local chapters throughout the United States are listed in telephone directories.

URINARY PROBLEMS IN MULTIPLE SCLEROSIS AND OTHER SPINAL DISEASES

JACEK L. MOSTWIN, M.D., D. Phil.

THE NORMAL BLADDER CYCLE

Periodic filling and emptying of the bladder takes place in a cyclical manner. At the beginning of each cycle, the empty bladder begins to fill. Intravesical pressure is minimal and equivalent to surrounding intra-abdominal pressure. As the bladder slowly fills to its normal capacity of 350 to 450 ml, the pressure in the bladder does not rise, but the normal individual does become aware of gradual distention leading to a sensation of fullness and eventual urgency. Sensation of filling is transmitted by stretch receptors in the bladder wall and routed by way of long latency fibers along the dorsal spinal cord to the pons. (In tabes dorsalis, these fibers are damaged, resulting in gradual, painless low-pressure dilatation of the bladder.) From here they are represented in consciousness to the cortex. Although bladder pressure does not rise during filling, external sphincter activity progressively increases in a "guarding reflex" along with awareness of filling. The external sphincter responsible for this guarding reflex consists of fibers of striated muscle from the levator ani, innervated by pudendal nerve somatic afferents and efferents. Pudendal nerve activation is associated with reflex inhibition of parasympathetic activation of bladder contraction, a reflex mediated by pathways in the sacral spinal cord. In the normal individual, voiding can be postponed indefinitely, even until pain is induced. Bladder contractions occurring when the bladder is filled nearly to capacity can be inhibited by voluntary contraction of the external sphincter. When voiding is allowed to commence, the first event observed is relaxation of pelvic floor musculature associated with a drop in pressure at the bladder neck and in the proximal urethra. Radiographically this is evident as funneling of the bladder neck and posterior descent of the bladder base. Electromyography of periurethral striated muscles at this point will show complete cessation of activity. Synchronized release of acetylcholine to muscarinic receptors throughout the bladder muscle then causes a sustained contraction of the smooth muscle of the bladder resulting in total evacuation of its contents at a reasonable level of intravesical pressure unassisted by abdominal straining. The normal subject can feel this occurring and will know when the bladder is empty. The cycle can then begin again.

Animal experiments have shown that the micturition center is located in the rostral pons. As long as the spinal cord is intact to this level, cyclic filling and emptying, although unconscious, occurs with sphincteric coordination. Thus the demented or brain-damaged patient who is incontinent because of unawareness of bladder cycling usually shows no urinary tract damage. When the spinal cord is partially or completely severed or involved in disease, several abnormalities may result, the most serious being loss of bladder compliance and bladder instability with a dyssynergic external sphincter. Functional abnormalities may present as partial or complete retention, incontinence, or irritative syndromes combining frequency, nocturia, and urgency which may progress to urinary urge incontinence. Pain is rarely a feature in these abnormalities. Advanced complications may sometimes present, overshadowing the underlying functional abnormality; these include stones, chronic infection, bacteriuria, or sepsis, vesicoureteral reflux, hydronephrosis, or renal insufficiency (Table 1).

CLINICAL EVALUATION OF THE VOIDING CYCLE

For a patient with a neurologic disease or injury and any of the symptoms listed in Table 1, a cystometrogram is nearly always indicated. The various symptoms may be combined in any given patient in many different ways, and rational management will depend on a thorough functional evaluation, supplemented when necessary by cystoscopy, estimations of renal function, or imaging studies such as excretory urography, voiding cystourethrography, or renal or prostatic ultrasonography. Because catheterization is required, prophylactic antibiotics should be administered to patients requiring endocarditis prophylaxis as well as to those with a history of infection or with known residual urine, and to those suspected of voiding at high pressure against obstruction. A cystometrogram performed under the direction of a urologist familiar with normal and abnormal voiding events provides good approximation of all the events associated with the patient's voiding cycle (Table 2). The study measures the intravesical and intra-abdominal pressures during filling and emptying, the conscious responses to these events, and the coordination of the sphincters. The pressure and flow rate during voiding and the contribution of intra-abdominal pressure are measured. Residual urine is also measured. Even if voiding is abnormal, the method by which urine escapes the bladder can be characterized. Electromyography of the external sphincter is frequently utilized. Simultaneous fluoroscopy is occasionally used for difficult diagnoses.

GENERAL FEATURES OF BLADDER DYSFUNCTION ASSOCIATED WITH SPINAL DISEASE

Bladder Instability

Demyelinating disease such as multiple sclerosis or suprasacral spinal injuries that have stabilized after spinal shock commonly results in unstable (involuntary) bladder contractions occurring at low volumes of filling. These are often associated with simultaneous contractions of the external sphincter, referred to as "detrusor-external sphincter dyssynergia." The high pressures associated with the development of this dysfunction may become injurious to the upper tracts, with reflux and hydronephrosis resulting. The associated symptoms are urgency and urinary incontinence, difficulty initiating a voluntary stream, and hesitant or intermittent stream. Various degrees of retention may be found. Patients with multiple sclerosis who desire some degree of mobility find these symptoms particularly distressing; 10 percent of patients with multiple sclerosis present with urinary symptoms at the onset of multiple sclerosis, and 90 percent have symptoms of

Table 1 Symptoms of Bladder Dysfunction

Dysfunctional voiding
  Retention
  Incontinence
  Irritation
    Urgency
    Frequency
    Nocturia

Advanced complications
  Infection
  Stone
  Reflux
  Hydronephrosis
  Uremia

Table 2 Significant Variables Tested by Urodynamics

Sensation
Stability
Compliance
Capacity
End-filling pressure
Mechanism of voiding (Intrinsic contraction vs. abdominal straining)
Flow rate/voiding pressure
Sphincteric coordination
Completeness of emptying

bladder instability during the final stages of the disease.

Loss of Bladder Compliance

After a period of spinal shock, sacral or pelvic crush injury or tumor in which the motor nerves to the bladder are destroyed eventually produce a progressively stiffer, noncompliant bladder that fills until the fixed resistance of the internal (bladder neck) and external sphincters is passively overcome. Because of the associated pudendal nerve damage, the external sphincter may not respond to changes in bladder filling, and thus pressure may be low. In such a case, "pseudovoluntary" voiding can be achieved by applying external pressure to the bladder, either in the form of abdominal straining (Valsalva's maneuver) or direct suprapubic pressure (Credé's method). The bladder undergoes hypertrophy, and cellules and diverticula develop. The bladder neck is involved in this process and the pressures required for emptying the bladder increase until hydronephrosis and reflux develop. "Overflow incontinence" is found in this setting.

Sensory Denervation

The type of bladder once described as "flaccid" or "atonic" is found only in patients with purely sensory deficits such as tabes dorsalis, diabetes mellitus, or pernicious anemia. The result is a thin, compliant bladder that continues to stretch and empty to progressively lesser degrees.

COMPREHENSIVE MANAGEMENT OF BLADDER DYSFUNCTION

The goals of management are to provide continent storage of urine at low pressures for tolerable intervals and to provide complete low-pressure evacuation in the absence of stones and infection. The use of indwelling catheters may usually be avoided. Renal function and the integrity of the upper tracts must always be considered. The tools at the clinician's disposal include drugs, catheters, and occasionally, surgery. A complete functional diagnosis must be established before a treatment regimen is instituted, regardless of the type of neurologic injury or illness the patient may have. Even though certain patterns of bladder dysfunction can be anticipated by knowing the neurologic diagnosis, balancing the bladder by the combined use of drugs, catheters, and surgery requires detailed knowledge of the individual's bladder cycle.

Bladder Instability

Bladder instability (uninhibited bladder contractions) is usually experienced as urinary urgency and frequency. If the patient has easy access to a toilet, urgency may merely be a nuisance that limits or interferes with his or her lifestyle. Urinary incontinence will result if the instability persists, if voiding is deferred even momentarily, or if the patient (particularly those with limited mobility) does not have easy access to a toilet or a commode. Urinary incontinence also results if the patient is unable to prevent bladder contraction by pudendal nerve activation, or if the pressure generated by the instability is high. Patients with multiple sclerosis commonly present with urgency and urinary incontinence. Oxybutynin hydrochloride (Ditropan), an antimuscarinic drug with direct smooth muscle spasmolytic properties, in a dose of 2.5 mg twice daily to 5 mg three times daily taken orally on an empty stomach, has become the most effective drug used in the United States for the management of instability in patients with multiple sclerosis. In most patients with multiple sclerosis, a dose of 2.5 mg three times daily reduces the symptoms of urgency and urinary incontinence and avoids the antimuscarinic side effects of mouth dryness, blurred vision, and constipation that can occur when full doses are taken. Instability, however, may still be found on cystometry. In the presence of glaucoma, the medication should not be used without ophthalmologic consultation. If a dose of 5 mg three times daily does not control the instability, patients may be taught to dissolve a 5-mg Ditropan tablet in sterile saline and instill the drug directly into the bladder twice daily by catheter. This may be combined with oral administration as long as side effects are tolerated. A commercial preparation of Ditropan for intravesical use is not currently available, but production is being considered. Terbutaline sulfate is used extensively in Europe but has just become available for use in the United States. A tricyclic antidepressant such as imipramine hydrochloride produces antimuscarinic bladder blockade at doses of 10 to 75 mg per day, which is much less than the dosage range used for antipsychotic medication. Propantheline bromide (Pro-Banthine) in doses beginning at 7.5 to 15 mg four times daily is less effective than Ditropan, but is still useful. Spasmolytics such as flavoxate hydrochloride or topical analgesics such as phenazopyridine hydrochloride (Pyridium) are rarely helpful in the presence of neurologic disease but avoid the risk of confusion or central nervous system (CNS) side effects that develop with the use of antimuscarinic drugs.

Clean Intermittent Self-Catheterization

Patients with multiple sclerosis who are receiving antimuscarinic medication, especially if they already have some degree of detrusor-external sphincter dyssynergia, often develop urinary retention after beginning antimuscarinic medication. For this reason they may require catheter drainage. At my institution, we prefer the technique of clean intermittent self-catheterization, both for these patients and any other patients who may have urinary retention caused by sensory or motor failure, or who have temporary retention after abdominal, cranial, or spinal surgery. Rather than allow the various nursing units in the hospital to teach patients intermittent technique, we allow one urodynamic nurse specialist to teach all patients. This standardizes the approach and assures quality of care. We use Mentor 14-Fr clear polyvinyl catheters, 6 inches for women and 14 inches for men, and smaller as needed for boys and girls. These catheters are made available by Mentor Corporation of Minneapolis, Minnesota. We give written and illustrated instructions to the patients and follow them on a regular outpatient basis. We teach patients to perform catheterization on arising in the morning, before retiring at night, and every 4 hours during the rest of the day (Table 3). Waking at night to catheterize is unnecessary. Patients wash their hands with soap and water and rinse the catheter with soapy water. The urethral meatus is cleansed with soapy water or with an obstetrical toilette containing benzalkonium chloride. Men should lubricate the catheter with a sterile, water-soluble lubricant. We teach patients to catheterize in the sitting position (preferably while seated on a toilet or commode) so that urine can run out by gravity. Frequency of catheterization rather than aseptic technique is the most important factor in preventing infection. Bacteriuria will be found in as many as 40 percent of patients who perform clean intermittent catheterization. There is debate over which patients should be treated for bacteriuria, since studies have shown that this will clear spontaneously in most patients, whether they are treated or not. At my institution, we prefer to reserve antibiotic treatment for patients with infections whose symptoms include fever, pain, hematuria, or increased bladder dysfunction. We do not administer prophylactic antibiotics since this may lead to the emergence of resistant organisms. We do not advise our patients to boil catheters or soak them in alcohol- or iodine-containing solutions, as these techniques have not been shown to be beneficial.

We prefer to limit the technique of clean intermittent catheterization to patients who can perform

Table 3   Technique of Clean Intermittent Self-Catheterization

Technique is performed on arising in the morning, immediately before retiring at night, and q4h in between
Hands and catheter are washed with soap and water
Catheters should not be cleaned with alcohol, iodine, or by boiling
Antibiotics are usually not needed
Good hand function is required
Sterile technique is used for inpatients

it themselves. This means that they must have adequate hand function and coordination. Once these are learned, the urethral meatus may often be found by touch alone, so that good vision is not a prerequisite. We have not encouraged the spouses or families of adult patients to perform the catheterization, since we feel that this is an excessive imposition on an already burdened support system, and families can rarely adhere to the four-hourly schedule necessary for good technique. In this situation, or if hand function is inadequate or leg spasticity is severe (in women), we place an indwelling urethral silicone-coated Foley catheter that can be changed every 4 to 6 weeks during an outpatient visit or by a visiting nurse. These catheters may require periodic irrigation to clear precipitated phosphate debris from the bladder, which often clogs the catheter prematurely. Chronic bacteriuria is an unavoidable consequence of permanent indwelling catheters, and we do not attempt to eradicate it by using prophylactic antibiotics. We reserve suprapubic catheters for selected cases in which urethral catheters cannot be tolerated.

For hospitalized patients, we allow the unit nurses to perform sterile intermittent catheterization every 6 hours. This has helped prevent nosocomial infections with multiple drug-resistant organisms. In the setting of acute illness, intensive care, or the postoperative or immediate post-traumatic period, we favor the use of an indwelling catheter for simplicity of management. Intermittent catheterization can be begun when the patient is transferred to a regular unit.

Credé's Method and Suprapubic Percussion

These techniques are relics of the post-World War II rehabilitation era, but patients who use them may still be encountered, and they may return to favor someday in the future. The Credé technique of firm suprapubic pressure over the bladder is effective in patients with cauda equina or sacral or pelvic crush injury in which motor roots to *both* the bladder and the external sphincter have been damaged. The low outflow resistance allows externally applied bladder pressure to overcome the sphincteric resistance. Some overflow incontinence will be associated with the regimen. It is presently believed that high pressures applied to the bladder are damaging to both the bladder and the upper tracts, but there are adult patients who have used this technique for as long as 20 years without upper tract deterioration or infection.

Suprapubic percussion or stroking has been used by patients with high spinal injury to initiate a bladder contraction at regular intervals to allow emptying. If sphincter dyssynergia is present, these patients are at high risk for upper tract deterioration and an alternative regimen should be considered.

Surgical Options Including Augmentation and Reconstruction

If obstruction is present in the form of a spastic external sphincter or a hypertrophied bladder neck and catheterization is not feasible or desirable, transurethral electroresection of these structures in men can be performed to allow low-pressure drainage. This may be especially necessary in patients with high spinal cord injury, where autonomic dysreflexia results from bladder contraction against a closed external sphincter. An external condom catheter or similar device is usually required after such a procedure. Because a similarly effective device is not available for women, sphincterotomy is not performed in female patients. In ambulatory patients or those who have good hand function, an artificial urinary sphincter (manufactured by American Medical Systems) may be used to restore continence in suitable low-pressure compliant bladders with no resistance to outflow. These devices may, however, necessitate reoperation for mechanical malfunction or erosion into the urethra within a 5-year period.

Newer surgical techniques have made it possible to augment severely contracted or spastic bladders that cannot be controlled by medication and catheterization with segments of large and small intestine. Several techniques have been developed for the construction of continent internal urinary reservoirs fashioned from bowel which can store large volumes of urine at low pressure and require emptying by periodic regular intermittent catheterization. The operations are a major undertaking for both patient and surgeon and should be performed only after very careful consideration. The interested reader is advised to consult the references.

Present methods of precise urodynamic evaluation, pharmacologic control, catheterization and surgical reconstruction have extended the traditional options available for patients with bladder dysfunction from spinal disease, expanding possibilities for rehabilitation. The choices for management of incontinence or retention are no longer limited to indwelling catheter and urinary diversion alone. The urologist interested and familiar with these problems can be a valuable asset to the neurological and neurosurgical service caring for such patients.

SUGGESTED READING

Barrett DM, Wein AJ. Voiding function and dysfunction. Chicago: Year Book Medical Publishers, 1988.
Bors E, Comarr AE. Neurological urology. Baltimore: University Park Press, 1971.
Guttman L. Spinal cord injuries: comprehensive management and research. 2nd ed. Oxford: Blackwell Scientific Publications, 1976.
King LR, Stone AR, Webster GD. Bladder reconstruction and continent urinary diversion. Chicago: Year Book Medical Publishers, 1987.
McGuire EJ. Clinical evaluation and treatment of neurogenic vesical dysfunction. Baltimore: Williams and Wilkins, 1984.
Yalla SV, McGuire EJ, Elbadawi A, Blaivas JG. Neurourology and urodynamics: principles and practice. New York: MacMillan, 1988.

PATIENT RESOURCES

Help for Incontinent People (HIP)
P.O. Box 544
Union, South Carolina 29739

National Multiple Sclerosis Society
205 East 42nd Street
New York, New York 10017
Telephone: (212) 986-3240

Eastern Paralyzed Veterans
432 Park Avenue South
New York, New York 10016

SEXUAL PROBLEMS IN SPINAL CORD DISEASE

PETER J. FAGAN, Ph.D.
THOMAS N. WISE, M.D.
CHESTER W. SCHMIDT, Jr., M.D.

The sexual function of patients with spinal cord disease is often an important factor of their quality of life. Whether the sexual problem is a dysfunction (e.g., impotence) secondary to a chronic, progressive disease such as multiple sclerosis, or the result of an acute injury associated with issues of mobility, self-care, and bowel and bladder function, patients will, when medically stable, ultimately focus on their sexual function. Furthermore, many patients with diseases of the spinal column are young adults in the procreative stage of their life and for whom sexuality is a major issue. Thus the evaluation and treatment of sexual problems is an important aspect of the care and management of patients with spinal cord disorders.

While most neurologically impaired patients have obvious biogenic factors causing sexual dysfunctions, they must also be thoroughly evaluated for psychogenic factors that may contribute to their sexual problems. Treatment will then consist of interventions that address both the medical and psychological aspects in order to maximize the sexual function and subjective satisfaction of the patient.

THE NEUROLOGIC EVALUATION

Lesions of the cord between T-12 and L-4 may compromise the sympathetic input for (psychogenic) erection and vaginal lubrication, the emission phase of ejaculation, and the closure of the sphincter muscle to the bladder during ejaculation. Lesions of the S-2 to S-4 parasympathetic region may compromise (reflexogenic) erection and vaginal lubrication as well as the contractions during ejaculation and orgasm. Impairments of bowel or bladder function should alert the clinician to probable sexual dysfunction. Therefore patients who present with urinary tract infections secondary to spastic bladder should be presumed to have arousal disorders for which they should be evaluated.

Patients with spinal cord disease who can be sexually aroused may report absent orgasm. Since orgasm is generally believed to be a cerebral event with peripheral correlates, the diminution or lack of orgasmic sensation in neurologic patients presumably results from lesions in the S-3 to S-4 levels that receive input from the genital sensory nerves. However, because it is a cerebral event, higher lesions (i.e., of the cord or central nervous system) should also be sought.

Male patients who experience orgasm with no ejaculate or diminished ejaculate may be suffering from a disorder of emission or a disorder of retrograde ejaculation. The differential diagnosis of these two disorders is especially important for couples who wish to conceive. Emission takes place through a smooth-muscle reflex controlled by the autonomic nervous system involving nerves originating at T-10 to L-3. In severe cases, when no emission occurs, sperm is not available. If the patient wishes to conceive, referral should be made to a fertility specialist. Ephedrine sulfate, a drug that stimulates the sympathetic nerves that control emission, has been successfully used to compensate for impaired transmission from spinal cord centers and sympathetic ganglia. Because its effectiveness is compromised with continued use, it is usually administered to assist in erections only during times of likely conception.

Retrograde ejaculation or "dry orgasm," however, is a neurologic defect that prevents closure of the bladder neck during emission, thus depositing sperm in the bladder rather than in the posterior urethra. The conditions can be differentiated by examining the urine for sperm and fructose after orgasm.

NOCTURNAL PENILE TUMESCENCE STUDIES

Nocturnal penile tumescence (NPT) studies are useful for developing objective evidence of the contribution of organic factors in erectile dysfunction. The procedure records the frequency, duration, and when a "buckling" challenge is performed, the rigidity of penile tumescence episodes. Additional data include correlation of tumescence and rapid eye movement (REM) stages of sleep, penile blood flow and bulbocavernosus and ischiocavernosus muscle activity. These latter data are especially important for the evaluation of neurologically impaired men.

Current research has raised some questions about the ability of NPT studies to differentiate biogenic from pschogenic erectile dysfunction with absolute certainty. With the exceptions of hyperprolactinemia and the vascular steal syndrome, a normal NPT generally indicates adequate neurologic and vascular competency for an erection sufficient for coitus. However, abnormal NPT studies have been recorded in older males who are sexually functional in intercourse (confirmed by partners) and in patients with erectile disorders and with major mood disorders. In the latter case, a careful mental status examination must be done to rule out the presence of a depressive state which in itself can result in an abnormal NPT study.

THE PSYCHOSEXUAL EVALUATION

An essential component of the psychosexual history is the premorbid (baseline) level of sexual function the patient formerly enjoyed. Once a decrement in function has been established, the patient is usually cognitively and emotionally prepared to review with the clinician the data relevant to a sexual history. Table 1 provides an outline for a sexual history which the clinician can modify according to the needs and circumstance of the patient.

THE PRESENT-STATE SEXUAL EVALUATION

This part of the evaluation is based on conceptualizing the four phases of the human sexual response cycle: desire, arousal, orgasm, and resolution. Using this cycle as a framework, the patient is asked to describe his or her general level of sexual interest or libido (indicated by frequency of sexual fantasies or thoughts, masturbation, desire for sexual activity) and most recent attempt at engaging in sexual activity. A detailed review of the most recent or typical sexual activity allows the clinician to identify which dysfunction is present, or if there appears to be more than one, which dysfunction is primary. It is important to ascertain quantitative data—for example, the nature of and duration of foreplay, at

Table 1 Outline for a Sexual History

Childhood
  Source of sexual knowledge
  Parental attitudes about sex
  Sexual abuse or incest
  Sex play with siblings or peers
  Expressed affection in home
Puberty
  Age at the time of menarche/first ejaculation and patient's
    reaction to the experience
  Reaction to development of secondary sex characteristics
  General body image during puberty
  Masturbatory practices and fantasies
  Homoerotic fantasies and behaviors
  Dating experiences
  Age at which patient first engaged in sexual intercourse and
    his or her reaction to the experience
Young adulthood
  Sexual activities with others
  Paraphiliac behavior
  Venereal diseases
  Extended or live-in sexual relationships
  Previous marriage(s)
    Courtship
    Sexual practices (dysfunction?)
    Reason for termination of the relationship
Adulthood
  Homosexual activity
  Possible exposure to acquired immunodeficiency syndrome
    (AIDS)
  Extramarital relations
  Present primary sexual relationship
    Courtship
    Nonsexual problems (e.g., money, alcohol abuse)
    Children (problems?)
    Infertility/contraceptive practices
    Masturbation practices and frequency
    Variety of sexual behaviors with partner
    Frequency of sexual intercourse throughout relationship
    Previous sexual dysfunction in either partner
    Patient's assessment of stability of relationship
  Onset and history of present problem

what point erection is lost, or whether there is adequate lubrication.

After the patient has provided a clear description of his or her typical sexual functioning, the clinician should inquire about the patient's subjective reaction to the dysfunction and his or her perception of the partner's reaction to the problem. In many cases, the partner's reaction may be an important prognostic factor. A partner who is understanding and does not see the dysfunction as a personal rejection is more likely to be helpful and participate in the recommended treatment program.

To complement the psychosexual examination, the clinician must also recognize that other psychiatric disorders in either the patient or the spouse may affect sexual enjoyment and function. Thus an examination of the patient's mental state is a necessary part of the evaluation and includes an assessment of the patient's general appearance, behavior, and manner of speech. Does the patient have any unusual idiosyncratic ideas—i.e., does he or she view the illness as a punishment for past behavior? What is the patient's mood? Is he or she significantly depressed, or does he or she have problems with sleep that are unrelated to the physical disorder? Finally, what is the patient's cognitive capacity? Patients with multiple sclerosis may have a dementing process that can foster hyposexuality or, as a result of frontal lobe inhibition, increase sexual drive. Any indication that the patient has a major psychiatric disorder must be considered in conjunction with other elements of the evaluation.

If, at the conclusion of the psychological evaluation, the clinician judges the sexual dysfunction to have significant psychogenic components (Table 2), the patient should be referred to a physician or psychologist who specializes in the treatment of sexual dysfunctions associated with medical disorders. Patients whose dysfunction is caused by inadequate information or by mild anxiety may be helped by specific suggestions (e.g., that there should be more direct penile stimulation before the patient attempts penetration) and by reassurance that such problems are not uncommon and can be of short duration. Should recurrent urinary tract infection be associated with the patient's disease, as in women with multiple sclerosis, the clinician should advise that cunnilingus be avoided and that coitus might be related to infection.

MEDICAL TREATMENT

Many classes of medication, especially antihypertensives, antidepressants, anxiolytics, and the newer antacids have been reported to cause adverse sexual side effects. Therefore the patient's drug regimen should be reviewed for those agents that may impair sexual functioning (Table 3). When a medication is suspected of impairing sexual function, it can be discontinued or decreased, or a substitute may be considered. Having the patient take a "drug holiday" is one means of determining the effect of a medication on sexual function.

Table 2 Indicators of Psychogenic Sexual Dysfunction

History of sexual trauma or abnormal sexual development
Restrictive religious or moral sexual attitudes
Dysfunction (even episodically) existed premorbidly
Dysfunction is situational or partner-specific
Evidence of morning or masturbatory full tumescence (in men)
Evidence of masturbatory arousal and orgasm (in women)
Sexual dysfunction secondary to psychiatric disorder (e.g.,
  depression)

Table 3 Drugs That May Impair Sexual Functioning in Patients With Spinal Cord Disease

Drug	Dysfunction
Diuretics	
Chlorothiazide	Impotence
Spironolactone	Impotence, decreased libido
Adrenergic inhibitors	
Propranolol	Impotence
Clonidine	Impotence, decreased libido
Aldomet	Impotence, ejaculatory failure
Guanethidine	Impotence, ejaculatory failure
Reserpine	Decreased libido
Phenoxybenzamine	Ejaculatory failure
Tricyclic antidepressants	Erectile failure, anorgasmia
Trazodone	Priapism
Thoridazine	Ejaculatory failure
Digoxin	Erectile failure, decreased libido
Cimetidine	Erectile failure, decreased libido

CONDITIONS THAT LIMIT SEXUAL FUNCTION

Patients whose gross body movements are impaired may require assistance by another (usually the partner) to position them for sexual interaction. Under these conditions, it is helpful to learn from the patient how his or her body should be situated relative to the partner for sexual activity. Varied positions and the use of pillows for hip support and positioning can be tested out by the patient and partner. Consultation with a physical therapist skilled in treating disabled patients with sexual problems is helpful in designing sexual routines for severely disabled patients.

Spasticity of the lower extremities, especially adductor spasms in women, may increase with sexual arousal and may be managed with benzodiazepines (taken as necessary) or baclofen. However, since benzodiazepines may decrease sexual desire, dosage will require monitoring.

Patients who experience bowel or bladder incontinence during intercourse should be instructed to evacuate their bowel and/or bladder before engaging in sexual activity. Indwelling Foley catheters need not prevent intercourse. Men may fold the catheter along the side of the penis and then secure it with a condom; women may empty the bag before engaging in sexual activity and tape the catheter to their leg.

A excellent source on specific suggestions for impaired patients (e.g., physical movement, use of sexual aids such as vibrators) is the book *Not Made of Stone: The Sexual Problems of Handicapped People,* which is cited among the patient resources given at the end of this chapter.

SPECIFIC PHASE DISORDERS

Disorders of Desire

Hypoactive sexual desire secondary to illness-related fatigue and malaise should be recognized as such, and the patient should be encouraged to conserve energy and plan for sexual activity. Although estrogen replacement after hysterectomy and oophorectomy does not appear to affect libido and sexual drive directly, it often improves the patient's general sense of well-being, which in turn may increase desire for sex. Topical estrogen and systemic estrogen reduce the occurrence of dyspareunia secondary to inadequate lubrication and vaginal atrophy in postmenopausal women.

Exogenous testosterone (testosterone cypionate, 200 mg IM every other week) will restore sexual desire in men with low plasma levels of testosterone if the hypogonadism is not caused by pituitary or hypothalamic disease. Exogenous testosterone will not affect sexual drive or cure erectile dysfunction in men with normal plasma levels. Testosterone appears to enhance sexual fantasies, but not actual erectile functioning if neurologic damage is the cause of the erectile failure. Supplementation may actually enhance the distress of a patient who experiences increased sexual drive but continues to have limited erectile functioning. Bromocriptine (1.25 mg daily to 2.5 mg twice daily) will restore both sexual desire and arousal in male patients with hyperprolactinemia secondary to microadenomas of the pituitary.

Recent clinical trials of centrally acting agents to increase sexual desire and resolve dysfunctions have been inclusive. Interest has focused on aphrodisiacal effects of serotonin antagonists and dopamine agonists. Yohimbine, an alpha-adrenergic blocker, at a dosage of 2 mg orally three times daily has been reported to improve sexual desire and arousal. Diminished sexual desire is usually associated with depressive disorder. In such cases, the mood disorder should be treated first with both psychological and pharmacologic strategies before one attempts to treat the sexual dysfunction.

Disorders of Arousal

A common cause of insufficient arousal in women is painful intercourse (dyspareunia) caused by inadequate lubrication. Nonpetroleum vaginal lubricants are helpful in those situations when lubrication deficiency is secondary to organic factors. It should not be used as a substitute for adequate foreplay, and patients prone to infection should be advised against using jellies. Carbamazepine has been reported to diminish dyspareunia caused by clitoral hypersensitivity.

With demonstrated adequate vascular competency (a penile-brachial index >0.65), men with neurogenic impotence can experience pharmacologically induced erections with intracavernosal injections of vasodilating drugs. Goldstein and colleagues reported the successful treatment of 22 men with neurogenic impotence over a 15-month period using test doses of 0.42 to 0.83 mg of phentolamine mesylate and 12.5 to 25 mg of papaverine hydrochloride in a total volume of 0.5 to 1 ml. Hypersensitivity to the drugs is managed by titrating the dosage accordingly.

Pharmacologically assisted erection sufficient for penetration usually occurs with physical stimulation within 15 minutes after injection. Injection sites should be alternated on the sides of the penis and injections should not be administered more than two times per week. Palpable fibrosis has been reported after 1 year of usage. The erection should not last for more than 2 hours. If priapism occurs, it can be relieved with corporal epinephrine irrigation.

Because some penile prostheses require normal digital dexterity, patients with dexterity limitations should be offered only those implants that are mechanically simple (e.g., silastic rods). When either a prosthesis or the use of intracavernosal injections is selected as treatment, patient satisfaction (which includes the satisfaction of the patient's sexual partner) is facilitated by preprocedure and postprocedure education concerning the nature of the treatment and by counseling with both partners.

Special Circumstances

Patients without sexual partners, elderly patients, and homosexual patients present special challenges for the clinician. The patient without a sexual partner must rely on auto-arousal techniques for sexual gratification. The elderly, disabled patient without a partner may experience a global waning of sexual interest that is more pervasive than that of healthy counterparts. The clinician must be sufficiently comfortable with human sexuality to explore these issues in an unbiased manner.

The homosexual patient who is in a stable relationship with a single partner should be managed in a manner identical to that of a heterosexual patient. Single patients with multiple partners require counseling about safe sexual techniques and monitoring for sexually transmitted diseases.

SUGGESTED READING

Barrett M. Sexuality and multiple sclerosis. New York: National Multiple Sclerosis Society, 1982.
Sexuality and Disability: a journal devoted to the study of sex in physical and mental illness. (Published by Human Sciences Press, 233 Spring Street, New York, New York 10013-1578.)
Shover LR, Thomas AJ, Lakin MM, et al. Orgasm phase dysfunction in multiple sclerosis. J Sex Research 1988; 25:548–554.
Shover LR, Jensen S. Sexuality and chronic illness. New York: Guilford, 1988.

PATIENT RESOURCES

Heslinga K. Not made of stone: the sexual problems of handicapped people. Springfield, IL: Charles C Thomas, 1974.

CEREBROVASCULAR DISEASE

TRANSIENT ISCHEMIC ATTACK

JOSÉ BILLER, M.D.
HAROLD P. ADAMS, Jr., M.D.

A transient ischemic attack (TIA) is an important predictor of the subsequent development of a stroke. If no therapy is instituted, cerebral infarction develops in one-third of patients with TIAs. The interval since the most recent TIA appears to be the single most important factor in forecasting the risk of cerebral infarction. Of those patients who will have a cerebral infarction, half do so within 1 year after a transient ischemic attack and approximately one-fifth during the first few months of follow-up. The rate of recurrence of TIAs or the risk of stroke during the first few days after a TIA is not clearly established, but appears to be greatest during this time. Because the risk of stroke cannot be predicted by the number of TIAs, the duration of symptoms, or the type of TIA, all patients are considered at risk, and those with recent onset (within the last 10 days) should be evaluated on an urgent basis. Likewise, although it is clear that TIAs are strong predictors of stroke, several studies have shown that myocardial infarction is the most common cause of death in these patients, accounting for a mortality rate of 5 percent per year.

DIAGNOSIS

The diagnosis of TIA is made on the basis of the history obtained from the patient or any observer. A TIA is characterized by a short-lived episode of focal, nonconvulsive loss of function caused by the reversible interference of the blood supply to an area of the retina or brain. Onset is abrupt and usually unprovoked, reaching maximal intensity almost immediately. A TIA usually persists for 2 to 20 minutes and only rarely for as long as 24 hours. An episode that lasts a few seconds is probably not a TIA. The 24-hour time frame that differentiates a TIA from an infarction is imprecise and does not reflect the mechanisms responsible for the development of transient focal brain ischemia. A TIA is part of the spectrum of ischemic stroke that includes events that produce neurologic signs that persist for more than 24 hours but resolve within 3 weeks: "reversible ischemic neurologic deficit" (RIND) and partial, nondisabling infarction. These conditions should be viewed as different expressions of the same dynamic process with probably similar underlying pathophysiology, and therefore investigations and treatment for each condition are essentially alike.

The symptoms of a TIA are outlined in Table 1. Because there is a differential diagnosis for TIAs, we refer to these symptoms as transient focal neurologic deficits and bear in mind that there are a variety of other conditions (i.e., seizures, neoplasms, arteriovenous malformations, subdural hematomas, metabolic derangements, demyelinating conditions, migraines, and vestibulopathies) that share these symptoms, mimicking TIAs. If the initiation or resolution of symptoms of a transient neurologic event is indistinct, the diagnosis of TIA should be questioned. A migration or "march" of symptoms from one body part to another is rare during a TIA and suggests a focal seizure or a migraine. Positive phenomena such as visual scintillations, fortification spectra, involuntary movements, or "seizurelike" activity are unusual during a TIA, as are loss of consciousness, confusion, sphincter incontinence, isolated episodic vertigo or wooziness, or dropattacks. Although TIAs are often referred as "painless" episodes, headache occurs in approximately one-fifth of patients and is occipital in location with vertebrobasilar events, and hemicranial with carotid circulation TIAs.

Identification of the involved arterial territory influences investigation and management. Because of the several mechanisms responsible for the development of TIAs, we strive to determine the primary pathophysiologic mechanism of each case. Most patients with TIAs have atherosclerotic lesions of the carotid or vertebrobasilar arteries, and the mechanisms of ischemia are the result of either artery-to-artery embolization of atherosclerotic debris or fibrin-platelet emboli, or are hemodynamic distur-

Table 1 Symptoms of TIAs

Transient Focal Neurologic Deficits	Symptoms	
	Carotid Artery Territory	*Vertebrobasilar Artery Territory**
Motor deficit	Contralateral weakness, clumsiness or paralysis (primarily hands and face)	Bilateral or shifting weakness, clumsiness or paralysis Ataxia, imbalance or dysequilibrium not associated with vertigo
Sensory deficit	Contralateral numbness, paresthesias (including loss of sensation—primarily of hands and face)	Bilateral or shifting numbness, paresthesias (including loss of sensation)
Speech/language deficit	Dysphasia, dysarthria	Dysarthria
Visual deficit	Ipsilateral monocular blindness (amaurosis fugax), contralateral homonymous hemianopia	Diplopia, partial or complete blindness in both homonymous visual fields
Other	Combination of the above	Combination of the above

* Transient vertigo, diplopia, dysarthria, or dysphagia by themselves are insufficient to establish a diagnosis of vertebrobasilar artery territory TIA.

bances causing focal hypoperfusion in areas of compromised circulation. Cardiac-to-artery embolism, small vessel (lacunar) disease, nonatherosclerotic vasculopathies, and a variety of hypercoagulable states account for the remainder of TIAs. Evaluation of a patient is aimed at excluding other conditions that may be causing the neurologic symptoms, establishing the mechanisms of the ischemic symptoms, and determining the presence of co-developing vascular diseases. The neurologic, neurovascular, and cardiovascular examinations are emphasized. Between TIAs, the neurologic examination will be normal. Ophthalmoscopic examination may detect embolic retinal particles. An audible cervical bruit may be the first indication of extracranial atherosclerotic vascular disease. A cervical bruit ipsilateral to a carotid TIA is suggestive of an underlying arterial disease. Auscultation of the orbit, temple, or mastoid may disclose a bruit in a patient with stenosis of an intracranial artery. However, there is poor correlation between a bruit and underlying carotid stenosis. A bruit and atypical symptoms are not sufficient for diagnosing a carotid TIA. The absence of a bruit does not mean that the carotid artery is normal. The cardiac examination concentrates on the detection of structural cardiac lesions or rhythm abnormalities that may potentially account for the patient's symptoms. The blood pressure is measured in both arms. Orthostatic blood pressure changes are sought.

Figure 1 summarizes our approach to the diagnosis and management of patients with TIAs. Computed tomographic (CT) evaluation should be done in all patients because it detects hemorrhagic or mass lesions that can present as a TIA. The majority of TIA patients have a normal CT, although hypodense lesions are often found, particularly among those with protracted (>1 hour) events. Patients with TIAs should have a complete blood cell count with differential and platelet count, which may iden-

tify an underlying polycythemia or thrombocytosis. Coagulation studies including prothrombin time and activated partial thromboplastin time should also be performed. An abnormally prolonged, activated partial thromboplastin time that does not correct with the addition of normal plasma (1:1 mixing) suggests a circulating anticoagulant. The association between a circulating anticoagulant and clinical thrombosis should lead to the determination of anti-phospholipid antibodies. Other investigations include serologic tests for syphilis, erythrocyte sedimendation rate, blood glucose, and lipid profile. Selected patients are evaluated for tests of platelet hyperfunction (platelet aggregation, circulating platelet aggregates, platelet factor IV activity, and platelet survival studies), antithrombin-III levels, protein-C levels, protein-S levels, fibrinogen, and hemoglobin electrophoresis.

Patients with TIAs should undergo chest roentgenography and baseline electrocardiography. Echocardiography and Holter monitoring are low-yield screening procedures that should be reserved for patients with clinical clues of cardiac disease. Noninvasive neurovascular testing in patients with TIAs is controversial. We use duplex scanning in combination with pressure oculoplethysmography as a complement to, although not as a replacement for, arteriography. These studies can be valuable during the follow-up evaluation.

Cerebral arteriography remains the most accurate means of determining the extent and site of atherosclerotic lesions. Selective cerebral arteriography is necessary to evaluate reliably the intracranial vasculature or to detect tandem large arterial lesions. Arteriography is not without complications. The risk of developing any complication (half of which are minor groin hematomas) is approximately 1 to 5 percent. The risk of developing permanent neurologic disability is 0.2 percent, whereas the risk of death is approximately 0.05 percent. Intra-arterial

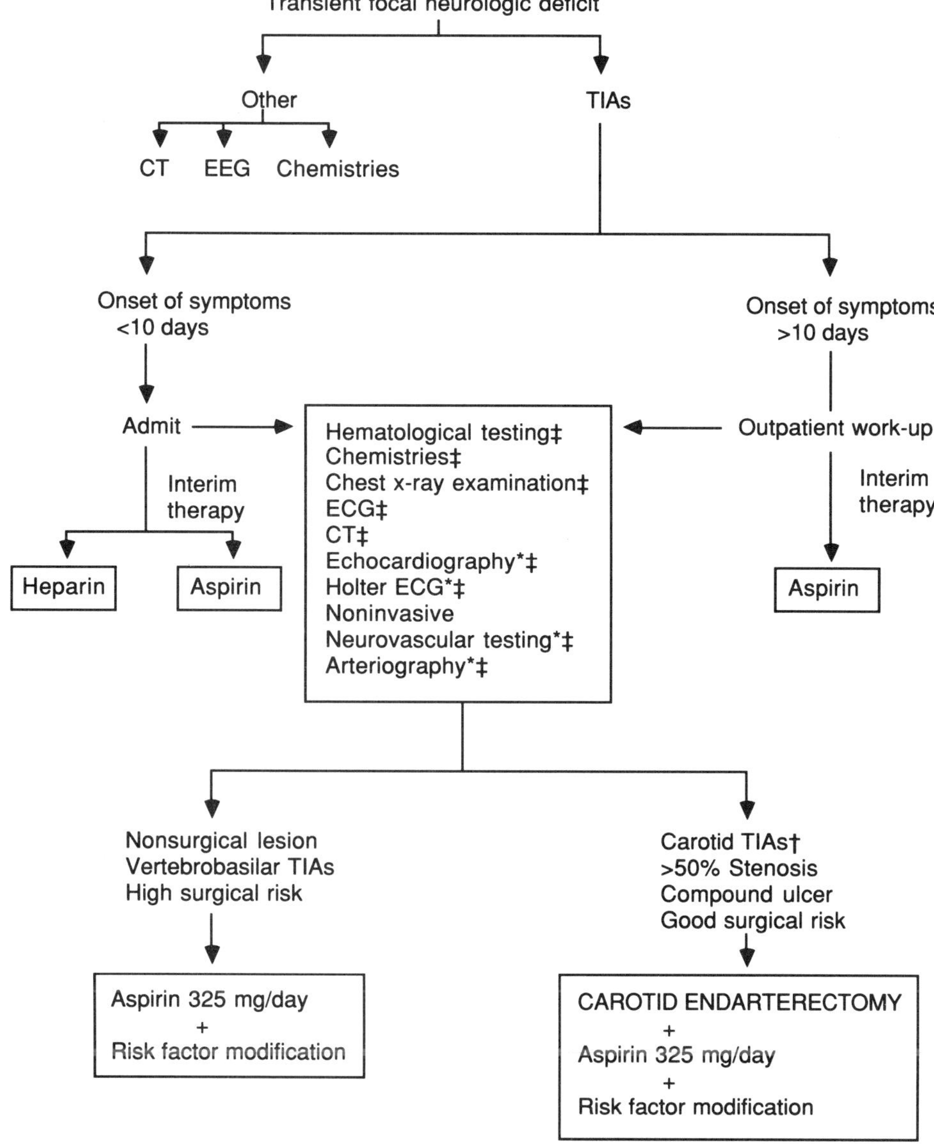

Figure 1   Diagnosis and management of patients with TIAs.
* Optional tests.
† For patients unwilling to participate in ongoing endarterectomy trial.
‡ See text for selected indications of anticoagulant therapy.

digital subtraction angiography (IA-DSA) provides adequate resolution for detection of extracranial disease and is generally useful for evaluating the intracranial circulation. IA-DSA is more economic than conventional film screen angiography and requires smaller volumes of contrast, although two injections are required for biplane views because most units are single plane. We favor conventional film screen angiography except for selected instances when we use IA-DSA. We undertake arteriography in good surgical–risk patients with bona fide carotid TIAs, selected cases in which we find it difficult to determine if the site of ischemia is the carotid or vertebrobasilar circulation, and in selected patients with vertebrobasilar TIAs in whom medical treatment with platelet antiaggregating agents has failed.

MANAGEMENT

Strategies for the treatment of TIAs include the use of platelet-antiaggregating agents, anticoagulants, and surgical revascularization and modification of atherosclerotic risk factors.

Modification of Atherosclerotic Risk Factors

Although the predisposing risk factors for ischemic stroke are not necessarily the same as the risk factors for coronary atherosclerosis, we avoid making a distinction because the main cause of death in patients with TIAs is cardiac disease. Advancing age, gender (male), and positive family history are fixed risk factors. A number of predisposing atherosclerotic risk factors such as arterial hypertension, diabetes mellitus, hypercholesterolemia, a low level of high-density lipoproteins, cigarette smoking, and obesity should be treated with a combination of drugs, dietary modification, and changes in lifestyle.

Platelet Antiaggregating Therapy

At present, aspirin is the best medical therapy in the management of TIAs. We currently use aspirin in a daily dose of 325 mg for both male and female patients. Aspirin inhibits platelet function by blocking cyclooxygenase, which converts arachidonic acid to prostaglandin endoperoxides and ultimately to thromboxane A_2. Several studies have evaluated the effectiveness of aspirin and other platelet antiaggregants in treating patients with threatened stroke. In most of these studies, doses of aspirin ranging from 900 to 1,300 mg daily were used.

The Canadian Cooperative Study Group evaluated 585 patients with TIAs or minor strokes and showed a 19 percent overall reduced incidence of TIAs, stroke, and death in all male patients. The use of aspirin yielded better results when overall stroke and death rates alone were analyzed, demonstrating a decrease in these rates of 31 percent, and even more favorable results in men without history of myocardial infarction (a 62 percent decrease in the incidence of stroke and death). This study did not show a benefit for women who received aspirin therapy.

A French study evaluated the effects of aspirin alone, aspirin in combination with dipyridamole, or placebo on 604 patients with either TIAs or stroke. At the end of the study, the cumulative rate of fatal and nonfatal stroke was 18 percent in the placebo group and 10.5 percent in each of the active-treatment groups. Dipyridamole did not provide additional benefit. Gender was not shown to influence the efficacy of aspirin in this study.

The American-Canadian Cooperative Study evaluated 890 patients with carotid TIAs to determine the potential benefit of a combination of aspirin plus dipyridamole versus aspirin alone. Dipyridamole did not supplement the effect of aspirin in reducing the risk of stroke, retinal infarction, or death.

The United Kingdom Trial evaluated the effects of two different dosages of aspirin (1,200 mg per day vs. 300 mg per day) and placebo among 2,435 patients with TIAs or minor strokes. The results of this study demonstrated that aspirin decreased the risk of myocardial infarction, major stroke, or death by 18 percent, and the risk of disabling stroke or vascular death by 7 percent. Aspirin benefited men only. No clear differences were noted between the two dosages of aspirin, except that fewer gastrointestinal side effects were associated with the lower dosage.

Ticlopidine hydrochloride, a new platelet antiaggregant, has been recently compared with aspirin in a study of more than 3,000 patients with TIAs or minor strokes. Ticlopidine hydrochloride appears to be approximately 15 percent better than aspirin in reducing strokes. The future role of this agent in the management of high-risk patients is yet to be defined.

Anticoagulant Therapy

The effectiveness of oral anticoagulant therapy is unknown. Anticoagulant therapy is risky and, in our opinion, should not be the first line of treatment, except in selected circumstances.

Although several nonrandomized and randomized trials have demonstrated a reduced incidence of cerebral infarction and TIA in treated patients, they have also shown a greater number of hemorrhages among them. Studies have failed to show a difference in the survival rates of the treated and control groups. The number of patients in these studies have been quite small, and all of the studies have had several flaws in their design.

We currently recommend warfarin therapy only for patients with a well-established cardiac source for TIA and for selected patients who continue to have TIAs despite treatment with platelet antiaggregants. If the TIAs are related to embolization from a left ventricular thrombus associated with a myocardial infarction, we use a 3- to 6-month course of warfarin to maintain the prothrombin time at 1.5 to 2 times control. In patients with rheumatic valvular heart disease, chronic atrial fibrillation, or dilated cardiomyopathy, we use a similar intensity of anticoagulation for the remainder of the patient's lifetime. In patients with mechanical prosthetic heart valves, we again use long-term anticoagulation of a similar intensity and add 300 to 400 mg of dipyridamole if the TIAs continue despite an adequate level of warfarin anticoagulation. When TIAs are attributed to mitral valve prolapse, we administer aspirin at a dosage of 325 mg daily.

Surgical Revascularization

There has been only one large controlled study evaluating the effectiveness of carotid endarterectomy, and it was inconclusive. At present, a large multicenter controlled trial underway in North America is comparing the efficacy of carotid endarterectomy supplementing best medical management with that of best medical management alone in the treatment of patients with TIAs or minor strokes in the carotid distribution and who have greater than 30 percent (but less than 100 percent) diameter stenosis with or without ulceration of the internal carotid artery. Until the results of this study and related trials are known, carotid endarterectomy is recommended only after careful consideration based on clinical judgment.

At present, we advise carotid endarterectomy on an "instinctual" basis for a suitable surgical–risk patient who has bona fide carotid distribution TIA and an ipsilateral carotid stenosis of greater than 50 percent diameter or a compound ulcerated lesion.

A recently completed trial of a superficial temporal-middle cerebral artery (extracranial-intracranial) bypass procedure demonstrated that the addition of surgery to medical therapy did not improve outcome for symptomatic patients with stenosis of the distal internal carotid artery, internal carotid artery occlusion, or middle cerebral artery stenosis or occlusion. We do not recommend this operation for patients with atherosclerotic cerebrovascular disease.

Interim Management for Patients Who Have Had Recent TIAs

We admit patients who have had recent TIAs (within the last 10 days) to the hospital for expeditious evaluation and treatment. We have been testing the usefulness of early medical therapy by randomly assigning these patients to receive either intravenous heparin or aspirin while evaluation is underway and until final recommendations can be made. For patients who are to receive heparin, we administer an intravenous bolus dose of 5,000 U followed by a constant maintenance infusion. The hourly dose of heparin is started at 1,000 U and is adjusted to maintain the activated partial thromboplastin time in the range of 1.5 to 2 times the preheparin controlled values. In patients undergoing cerebral arteriography, we discontinue the administration of heparin for 6 to 8 hours before the procedure.

SUGGESTED READING

The American-Canadian Co-operative Study Group. Persantine aspirin trial in cerebral ischemia. Part II: endpoint results. Stroke 1985; 16:406–415.

Bauer RB, Meyer JS, Fields WS, et al. Joint study of extracranial arterial occlusion. 3. Progress report of controlled study of long-term survival in patients with and without operation. JAMA 1969; 208:509–518.

Biller J, Bruno A, Adams HP Jr, et al. A randomized trial of aspirin or heparin in hospitalized patients with recent transient ischemic attacks: a pilot study. Stroke 1989; 20:441–447.

Bousser MG, Eschwege E, Haguenau M, et al. "AICLA" controlled trial of aspirin and dipyridamole in the secondary prevention of athero-thrombotic cerebral ischemia. Stroke 1983; 14:5–14.

Brust JC. Transient ischemic attacks: natural history and anticoagulation. Neurology 1977; 27:701–707.

The Bypass Study Group. Failure of extracranial-intracranial arterial bypass to reduce the risk of ischemic stroke: results of an international randomized trial. N Engl J Med 1985; 313:1191–1200.

The Canadian Cooperative Study Group. A randomized trial of aspirin and sulfinpyrazone in threatened stroke. N Engl J Med 1978; 299:53–59.

Hass WK, Easton JD, Adams HP Jr, et al. Randomized trial comparing ticlopidine hydrochloride with aspirin for the prevention of stroke in high-risk patients. N Engl J Med 1989; 521:501–507.

UK-TIA Study Group: United Kingdom Transient Ischemic Attack (UK-TIA) aspirin trial: interim results. Br Med J 1988; 296:316–320.

ATHEROTHROMBOTIC CEREBROVASCULAR DISEASE

ALASTAIR BUCHAN, M.D., FRCPC
VLADIMIR HACHINSKI, M.D., D.Sc., FRCPC

DEFINITIONS

Cerebral ischemia can be either focal (i.e., in an arterial territory) or global, implying hypoperfusion of the entire brain. Ischemia is a reduction of cerebral blood flow either locally or globally. The outcome of ischemia depends on the severity of the reduced blood flow and its duration. Histologically, selective neuronal necrosis may occur after even brief periods of global ischemia, and after focal ischemia there may be regions of pan-necrosis in the territory of the affected artery.

The symptoms of ischemia define its location, severity, and duration. Patients may present with transient ischemic attacks, a progressing stroke, or a completed stroke. Although a *transient ischemic attack (TIA)* has by tradition been defined as symptoms of ischemia that last for 24 hours or less, most true TIAs that do not cause cerebral infarction last a few minutes and probably less than 1 hour. Deficits lasting longer than 1 hour are increasingly likely to be associated with cerebral infarction, although the patient may make a complete symptomatic recovery. *Minor stroke* and TIA are similar in terms of etiology and outcome, and for the purposes of treatment and investigation can be considered to be the same. *Progressing stroke* is an observed deterioration after the initial insult that can occur for as long as 48 hours if the stroke affects the anterior circulation and sometimes for as long as 96 hours in those of the posterior circulation. Progression is seen in about half of those patients whose stroke is partial at the outset. In a *partial stroke,* only a portion of the arterial territory has been afflicted, while in a progressing stroke, further thrombosis is occurring. A *completed stroke* occurs if the entire cerebral tissue perfused by an artery (e.g., the middle cerebral artery) is damaged at the onset of the stroke or if a partial stroke progresses to completion. Deterioration, however, may have several causes (Table 1) and should not be assumed to be the result of progressive thrombosis.

CAUSES

The causes of TIAs and stroke are best thought of in an anatomic context. They are embolic, resulting from either cardiac lesions, major arterial lesions (most commonly atherosclerotic disease at the carotid bifurcation), and (rarely) intracranial lesions such as aneurysm or arteriovenous malformation (AVM), which can give rise to distal embolization. Focal ischemia may also arise from small vessel disease or from diseases that promote a hypercoagulable state (e.g., the paradoxical lupus anticoagulant).

Table 1 Causes of Deterioration in Stroke

Cerebral factors
  Infarction
    Cerebral edema
    Hemorrhagic infarction
    Recurrent embolism
    Progressive thrombosis
    (Postictal states)

  Hemorrhage
    Cerebral edema
    Rebleeding
    Acute hydrocephalus
    (Postictal states)

Systemic factors
  Cardiac
    Heart failure
    Cardiac arrhythmias
  Pulmonary
    Pneumonia
    Pulmonary embolism
  Metabolic
    Renal/hepatic failure
    Syndrome of inappropriate antidiuretic hormone
    Septicemia
    Psychological
    Drug use

Episodes of hemodynamic ischemia may occur in watershed territories in the cortex between anterior, middle, and posterior cerebral artery territories and are being recognized increasingly in the white matter.

MANAGEMENT DIAGNOSIS

When the patient is admitted, a clear-cut diagnosis is necessary as to location, both in terms of central nervous system structure and the location of the vascular lesion. The clinical syndrome is then classified as a transient ischemic attack, a minor stroke which may become a progressive stroke or even a completed stroke. Investigations are based on the clinical evaluation, and include both essential routine investigations and "special" investigations that are needed to answer specific questions (Table 2).

A computed tomographic (CT) scan should be performed as soon as possible to rule out hemorrhage or an unsuspected space-occupying lesion that may mimic the sudden deficit resulting from vascular disease. Subsequent serial CT scans and magnetic resonance images (MRIs) are obtained if the location, existence, or nature of a lesion is in doubt. Frequent sensory symptoms result from seizures, hence the occasional need for an electroencephalogram (EEG), or from thalamic dysfunction, which is best demonstrated by MRI. In most instances, CT ensures that there is no hemorrhage or hemorrhagic conversion of an infarct and can demonstrate the evolution of the new lesion, or in the case of a TIA, the absence of cerebral infarction.

Table 2 Investigations for Stroke

Affected Area	Routine	Special
Central nervous system	CT	MRI Lumbar puncture EEG
Vessels	Doppler	Angiography
Heart	ECG CXR Echocardiography	LV Wall Catheter Holter monitor
Systemic	CBC ESR VDRL Glucose Lipids Urea Liver function tests Urinanalysis	As needed

CBC = complete blood count; CXR = chest x-ray examination; ECG =electrocardiography; ESR = erythrocyte sedimentation rate; LV = left ventricle; VDRL = syphilis serology.

As can be seen in Table 2, most of the investigations revolve around the cause of the cerebral ischemia; although a careful clinical examination, normal chest x-ray examination, and electrocardiography might exclude the vast majority of potential cardiac emboli, we routinely perform echocardiography since it is cheap and noninvasive and since a large proportion of patients with cerebral ischemia have a source of cardiac emboli. Still more patients have coexistent coronary artery disease, even if their stroke is not related to abnormal structure and function of the heart. Only if there are paradoxical emboli through a patent atrial septal defect or the suggestion of dyskinesis on the echocardiogram do we go on to perform radionuclear angiography or angio-catheterization. In patients who have severe carotid artery disease as a cause of their cerebral symptoms (rather than heart disease), it may well be prudent to perform coronary stress tests, especially if the patient complains of angina.

Cerebral vessels are imaged in a variety of ways. Contrast-enhanced CT scans and MRI are indirect ways of looking for intracranial emboli and thrombosis. Although ultrasonography has proved to be a useful screening test for carotid artery disease, the use of transcranial doppler cannot yet be fully recommended. Cerebral angiography is the surest way of defining vascular lesions in both the extracranial and intracranial circulation. It allows us to see not only potential arterial sources of emboli, but if performed acutely, may show the distal occlusions. Patients with branch occlusions or hung-up vessels who have no arterial disease can then be investigated intensively from a cardiologic and hematologic standpoint. Hematologic tests are ordered on clinical suspicions, but a complete blood count, erythrocyte sedimentation rate, prothrombin time, partial thromboblastin time, VDRL, fasting glucose, and lipids are all deemed essential.

TREATMENT

Asymptomatic patients who are seen because of potential embolic sources such as atrial fibrillation or carotid stenosis are evaluated and treated for their risk factors. If appropriate, they are entered into prospective studies.

Transient Ischemic Attack

Patients who have been evaluated for a TIA or a minor stroke are treated with platelet anti-aggregants once cardiac and hematologic causes have been excluded. The arteries are then visualized with cerebral angiography, and if there is occlusive extracranial carotid disease appropriate to the symptom, and if there is no intracranial disease, these patients are then seen in consultation with either a vascular surgeon or a neurosurgeon. Carotid endarterectomy is an unproven prophylaxis against stroke in the ipsilateral territory, and we currently enter all of our appropriate patients into the North American Symptomatic Carotid Endarterectomy Trial (NASCET). We do not believe that there is any indication to operate on patients outside the study, (i.e., if they do not meet study criteria); we think it best that they be treated medically. There is no indication for prophylactic extracranial-intracranial bypass.

Aspirin, through its ability to acetylate platelet cyclooxygenase, thereby blocking thromboxane A_2 synthesis, inhibits platelet aggregation. Although the trials performed in patients with TIA and minor stroke have yielded mixed results, the overview as published by the antiplatelet trialists suggests through meta-analysis that there is a marked reduction in the risk of stroke or death for those patients treated with platelet anti-aggregants. New trials using Ticlopodine hydrochloride suggest that this agent is superior to aspirin, but the drug has not yet been approved by the Food and Drug Administration. Only in those patients whose carotid TIAs are uncontrolled by aspirin or whose angiography reveals intraluminal thrombus do we proceed to anti-coagulation, initially with heparin and subsequent maintenance with warfarin sodium crystalline (Coumadin).

Completed Stroke

The treatment of completed stroke is essentially the prevention of further episodes, the detection and treatment of any complications, and ensuring that a complete cardiologic assessment has been made. Neurologically the only treatment that can be offered is supportive and rehabilitative. The prevention of recurrent stroke is essentially that of prevention after minor stroke or a TIA with the proviso that if the stroke is devastating, angiography, surgery, or anticoagulation should probably not be performed.

Progressive Stroke

Progressive stroke afflicts perhaps 30 to 40 percent of all patients being admitted urgently. It is essential to define the location and nature of the process. Although there are no good prospective trials assessing treatment for the progressing stroke, in the absence of contraindications such as hemorrhagic conversion on the CT, uncontrolled hypertension, or a potential source of hemorrhage, one may consider careful anticoagulation. However, the data supporting this are weak, and although a recent double-blind trial purported to show that there was no significant difference between those treated with heparin and those treated with placebo, the therapy was delayed until the stroke had been stabilized for at least 24 hours, negating the suggestion that heparin was not indicated in progressing stroke. Patients who have a partial stroke, particularly if they are progressing, can be treated with anticoagulation with minimal risk. The treatment of progressing stroke is limited to considering anticoagulation. Interestingly there are no studies to show the effects of aspirin on progressing stroke.

If angiography demonstrates intraluminal thrombus, then although the decision is empirical, we usually anticoagulate for at least the short-term before restudying the patient.

Complete Stroke

If there is a complete stroke, anticoagulation is of no benefit unless the stroke is of cardiogenic origin, in which case anticoagulation is performed after a 72-hour interval to ensure that spontaneous hemorrhagic conversion does not occur.

Hyperacute Stroke

Perhaps of most interest is the management of the patient with a hyperacute stroke. CT scanning and MRI or rapidly obtained angiography allow visualization not only of the brain but also of the vessels and the disease process underlying the deficit. Two strategies are currently being investigated: on the one hand, the return of cerebral perfusion through the use of a new generation of thrombolytic drugs such as *tissue plasminogen activator,* and on the other, the return of cerebral function through the treatment of ischemic tissue itself with both *calcium channel blockers* and *glutamate antagonists.* There may also be some scope during reperfusion for *lipid peroxidation inhibitors,* and during the recovery phase, for gangliosides.

Although hyperacute treatment of atherothrombotic cerebrovascular disease is still in the experimental stages, an understanding of the natural history of the acute stroke during the first 24 hours is evolving. A determined attempt is being made to learn how to manage patients with stroke more swiftly. Only through the development of such programs will it be possible to evaluate patients promptly so that active intervention can be attempted before the stroke is completed.

From clinical studies we now know that most patients with TIAs recover in less than an hour—an important fact given that treating TIAs with thrombolytic agents would be wholly undesirable. Angiography during the first 3 hours demonstrates that as many as 80 percent of patients will have evidence of embolic phenomena in the cerebral circulation. Two

safety studies with tissue plasminogen activator are underway, one employing intravenous administration after CT but without angiography, and the other involving an arterial infusion of TPA after selective angiography. Both studies suggest that improvements can be achieved, but neither study has as yet involved a controlled group. The development of cytoprotective agents that block voltage-sensitive calcium channels (such as nimodipine) and glutamate-gated calcium channels (such as MK-801) mean that a combination of thrombolytic and cytoprotective agents may be used to resuscitate cerebral tissue. At present, however, these experimental strategies are not employed except under the auspices of experimental protocols.

It is not known whether aspirin on its own may be useful acutely, but we do have information suggesting that hemodilution, steroids, and barbituates are unnecessary. It makes sense to ensure that the blood pressure is judiciously stabilized and that the patient is normoglycemic. There is no evidence to suggest a deliberate reduction of blood sugar with insulin, unless hyperglycemia is producing hyperosmolar or ketotic states. At present, we have no reason to suggest that drugs such as mannitol should be given to prevent the formation of cytotoxic edema. If the stroke goes on to be large with consequent swelling of the hemisphere, the control of raised intracranial pressure with hyperventilation and mannitol may prove life-saving but we cannot recommend hemicraniectomies.

Cerebral venous stroke is now increasingly diagnosed with MRI showing sagittal and other sinus thromboses. Provided that significant cerebral hemorrhage is excluded, early anticoagulation is warranted and is effective in reducing the risk of both morbidity and mortality.

SUGGESTED READING

Anti-platelet Trialists Collaboration. Secondary prevention of vascular disease by prolonged anti-platelet treatment. Br Med J 1988; 296:320–331.

Buchan AM, Gates P, Pelz D, Barnett HJM. Intraluminal thrombus in the cerebral circulation. Stroke 1988; 19:681–687.

Cerebral Embolism Study Group. Brain hemorrhage and embolic stroke. Stroke 1984; 15:779–789.

Chambers BR, Norris JW, Shurvell B, Hachinski V. Prognosis of acute stroke. Neurology 1987; 37:221–225.

Delzopo G, Zeumer H, Harker L. Thrombolytic therapy in stroke: possibility and hazards. Stroke 1986; 17:595–607.

Duke RJ, Bloch RF, Turpie AGG, et al. Intravenous heparin for the prevention of stroke progression in acute partial stable stroke: a randomized controlled trial. Ann Int Med 1986; 105:825–828.

The EC/IC Bypass Study Group. Failure of extracranial-intracranial bypass to reduce the risk of ischemic stroke: results of an international randomized trial. New Engl J Med 1985; 313:1191–1200.

Levy DE. How transient are transient ischemic attacks. Neurology 1988; 38:674–677.

World Health Organization. Recommendations on stroke prevention: diagnosis and therapy. Stroke 1989; 20:1407–1431.

PATIENT RESOURCES

American Heart Association
7320 Greenville Avenue
Dallas, Texas 75231

Canadian Heart and Stroke Foundation
160 George Street, Suite 200
Ottawa, Ontario
Canada K1N 9M2

The Chest, Heart, and Stroke Association
Tavistock House North
Tavistock Square, London
United Kingdom WC1H 9JE

EMBOLIC STROKE OF CARDIAC ORIGIN

MERRILL C. KANTER, M.D.
DAVID G. SHERMAN, M.D.

Approximately 15 percent of all ischemic strokes are attributed to an embolus arising from the heart. The importance of cardiogenic embolus may in fact be much greater when one considers that several strokes are considered to be of "undetermined" etiology. The Stroke Data Bank found that one-third of their 1,805 patients had to be classified as "infarct, unknown cause." Approximately 30 percent of patients with an ischemic stroke have evidence of heart disease, and one-third of these have atherosclerotic cerebrovascular disease sufficient to have produced the stroke.

DIAGNOSIS

The diagnosis of a cardiogenic embolus to the brain is based on the best accumulated clinical and laboratory evidence. At times the nature of the heart disease and the patient's age and clinical presentation leave little doubt that the heart produced the stroke. Quite often, however, cardiac and noncardiac conditions coexist, making diagnosis difficult. The features of value in determining which strokes are caused by cardiogenic emboli and which strokes have other causes are outlined in Table 1. As demonstrated in the table, few features are both sensitive and specific for making this determination. Certain vascular-territory strokes are particularly suggestive of a cardiogenic embolism. In the middle cerebral artery territory, an isolated Wernicke's aphasia or global aphasia without hemiparesis appears to be a common sequela of embolic occlusion of the middle cerebral artery. The top of the basilar and posterior cerebral artery are sites of embolic occlusion in the vertebrobasilar territory.

Table 1 Clinical Features of Cardiogenic Embolism

Clinical or Investigative Feature	Frequency (%)		Likelihood of CE* (%)	
	CE	*Non-CE*	*Present*	*Absent*
Abrupt onset of maximal neurologic deficit	70	43	26	06
Loss of consciousness at onset	19	3	53	13
Concomitant systemic embolus	2.8	0	99	15
Prior transient ischemic attack	11	42	4	19
Past history of atrial fibrillation	37	6	52	10
History of myocardial infarction	33	15	28	12
History of congestive heart failure	36	7	48	10
CT scan showing hemorrhagic infarct	22	10	28	13
Cerebral angiography or noninvasive studies showing absent or insignificant disease	87	47	25	04

CE = Cardiogenic embolism.

* The likelihood of a cardiogenic embolism if the particular feature is "present" or "absent" is calculated using Bayes' theorem and assuming a pretest probability of cardiogenic embolism of 15% and of noncardiogenic embolism of 85%.

CARDIAC EVALUATION

One of the first management questions confronting the physician caring for a stroke patient is how extensive a cardiac evaluation does this patient need? The cardiac studies most readily available are echocardiography and Holter monitoring. Most patients with a stroke do not need an extensive cardiac investigation unless the history, physical examination, chest roentgenogram, or electrocardiogram suggest a cardiac disorder. Patients older than 60 years of age with no clinical heart disease and a stroke onset and pattern suggestive of an atherothrombotic stroke are rarely (only 1 to 6 percent of such patients) found by echocardiography to have a possible cardiac abnormality. On the other hand, 11 to 25 percent of stroke patients who are younger than 50 years of age or have clinical evidence of heart disease or cardioembolic features suggestive of a cardiogenic embolus are found by echocardiography to have a possible source of embolus. Other promising technologies, as yet not widely available, for identifying intracardiac abnormalities include ultrafast cardiac computed tomography (CT), transesophageal echocardiography, cardiac magnetic resonance imaging (MRI), and labeled platelet scintigraphy.

CAUSES OF CARDIOGENIC EMBOLI

There are several cardiac abnormalities that can lead to intracardiac thrombus and embolization (Fig. 1). Atrial fibrillation with or without associated valvular disease accounts for approximately 45 percent of all cardioembolic strokes. Ischemic heart disease is the next most common cause, with 15 percent of cardioembolic strokes associated with an acute myocardial infarct and 10 percent related to intraventricular thrombi remote from a myocardial infarct. Rheumatic heart disease and prosthetic valves each cause 10 percent of cardiogenic emboli. The remaining 10 percent arise from any of several less common cardiac abnormalities whose propensity to embolize varies widely.

EVALUATION AND TREATMENT

Management decisions concerning antithrombotic therapy for patients with a potential or already demonstrated cardiac source of brain embolus are based on estimates of how great the risk of embolism is and how long this risk is apt to persist, as well as on the estimated degree of the risk involved in anticoagulant or antiplatelet therapy. We have attempted to estimate the risk of embolism associated with each of the most common cardiac abnormalities, and basing our guidelines on this estimate, determine whether the patient needs high-range or low-range anticoagulation or antiplatelet therapy, and how long such therapy should be continued (Table 2). Low-intensity warfarin therapy is that dose that prolongs the prothrombin time to 1.3 to 1.5 times the control value (International Normalized Ratio [INR] of 2 to 3). High-intensity warfarin therapy is that dose that prolongs the prothrombin time to 1.5 to 2 times the control value (INR of 3 to 4.5).

Each feature listed in Table 2 adds to the risk of embolism. Certain factors, such as intracardiac thrombi and atrial fibrillation, carry a higher risk of embolism. Patients with atrial fibrillation often have significant atherosclerotic cerebrovascular disease. The evaluation of the stroke mechanism is of paramount importance in selecting prevention strategies, as it determines whether treatment should be aimed at a cardioembolic event with anticoagulation or a stroke secondary to coexistent atherosclerotic vascular disease. In the latter case, platelet anti-aggregating agents are often advocated. The severity of embolic strokes and the recurrence rate, particularly during the first 2 weeks, determine the need for immediate intervention.

Nonvalvular Atrial Fibrillation

In patients with nonvalvular atrial fibrillation (NVAF), the underlying heart disease is treated and conversion to normal sinus rhythm is performed, thus eliminating the atrial fibrillation. Conversion to normal sinus rhythm should be approached cautiously, as the procedure itself may induce a cardioembolic event. We recommend low-range anticoagulation for 2 to 3 weeks before the electrical cardioversion of patients who have had atrial fibrillation for more than 3 days. This should be continued until the patient has had normal sinus rhythm for 2 to 4 weeks. Anticoagulation is not indicated for cardioversion of atrial flutter or supraventricular

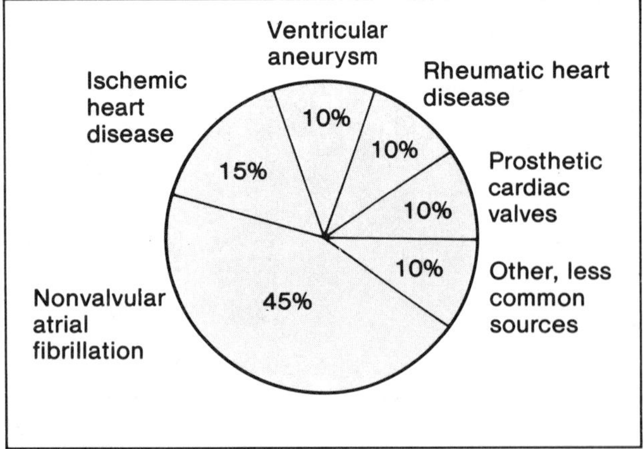

Figure 1 Sources of cardioembolism.

Table 2 Features and Treatment of Cardioembolic Stroke

Cardiac Disorder Features	Primary Prevention	Secondary Prevention	Risk of Stroke/TIA (Untreated)*
Nonvalvular atrial fibrillation			
High risk	APA or AC (L)	AC (L)	6% per yr
SSS	LR	HR	
CHF			
LA thrombus			
LA >5.5 cm			
LV segmental wall			
dysfunction			
Cardiomyopathy (dilated/hypertrophic)			
Recent onset of sustained AF			
Thyrotoxicosis†	AC (S)	AC (L)	
	LR	HR	
Low risk	None	AC (L)	0.5% per yr
<60 yrs old		HR	
"Lone AF"			
Acute myocardial infarction			
High risk	AC (S)	AC (L)	2–6% per yr
Anterior MI	LR	HR	
LV thrombus			
AF			
CHF			
Apical akinesis/dyskinesis			
Low risk	None	AC (S)	1–3% per yr
Inferior MI		LR	
>6 weeks post-MI			
Ventricular aneurysm			
High risk	AC (S)	AC (L)	5% per yr
LV thrombus (protruding/freely mobile)	LR	HR	
<6 weeks post-MI		(+/−	
		aneurysmectomy)	
Low risk	None	AC (S)	1–2% per yr
LV thrombus (flat/nonmobile)		LR	
No thrombus			
>6 weeks post-MI			
Rheumatic heart disease			
High risk	AC (L)	AC (L)	>5% per yr
Mitral stenosis	LR	HR	
AF		(+/− dipyridamole	
Left atrial diameter >5.5 cm		(225–400 mg/day)	
>45 yrs old			
Low risk	None	AC (L)	<2% per yr
Mitral regurgitation		HR	
NSR			
<45 yrs old			
Infective endocarditis			
High risk	Treat infection	Reassess antibiotic R_x	20%
Staphylococcus aureus	(+/− valve surgery)	Valve surgery	
<48 hrs (i.e., uncontrolled infection)	AC (L)	AC (L)	
Mechanical valve	HR	HR	
Low risk	Treat infection	Reassess antibiotic R_x	6%
Streptococcus	(+/− valve surgery)	Valve surgery	
>48 hrs after antibiotics			
Native valve			
Prosthetic Valves			
High risk	AC (L)	AC (L)	15% (?)
Mechanical	HR	HR	(−AC)
Mitral valve		dipyridamole	3–4%
Bioprosthetic valve and AF, CHF, or LA		(400 mg/day)	(+ AC)
>5.5 cm			

Table continues on the following page

Table 2 (continued)

Cardiac Disorder Features	Primary Prevention	Secondary Prevention	Risk of Stroke/TIA (Untreated)*
Low risk	AC (S) LR, then	AC (S)	2–4%
Bioprosthetic valve	APA (L)	LR	
Mitral			
Nonmitral	APA (L)	AC (S)	
		LR	
Mitral valve prolapse			
High risk	None‡	APA (L)	?
>45 yrs old			
Male			
Redundant/thick or myxomatous valve			
Low risk	None‡	APA (L)	<0.01%
<45 yrs old			
Female			
Valvular Calcification			
High risk	Treatment of	Treatment of	10%
Mitral annulus	underlying disease	underlying disease§	
Atherosclerosis			
HTN			
AF			
IE			
Low risk	APA (?)	APA (?)	?
Aortic stenosis			
Nonbacterial thromboembolic endocarditis			
High risk	APA or AC (?)	APA or AC (?)	0.5–1%
Coagulation abnormality			
Valve vegetation			
Atrial myxoma			
High risk	Surgical removal	Surgical removal	27–55%
All atrial myxoma (intracavitary location/ friability)			
Cardiomyopathy			
High risk	AC (L)	AC (L)	5–10%
CHF	HR	HR	
AF			
Thrombus			

High- and low-risk subgroups are based on the best available information (Cerebral Embolism Task Force).

* The percentages are based on a review of the literature. In several cases they may be modified by treatment and/or selection; however, we believe these are representative figures and have indicated where there is significant question.

† AC 2–4 weeks after conversion to NSR.

‡ General precautions against endocarditis.

§ Re-evaluate underlying disease as the cause of the infarct.

AC = Anticoagulation (Coumadin); AF = atrial fibrillation; APA = antiplatelet agent (ASA 1,300 mg/day divided dose); CHF = congestive heart failure; HR = High-range anticoagulation—PT ratio of 1.5–2 using a typical North American thromboplastin (INR of 3–4.5); HTN = hypertension; IE = infective endocarditis; (L) = long-term (indefinitely); LA = left atrium; LR = low-range anticoagulation—PT ratio of 1.3–1.5 using a typical North American thromboplastin (INR of 2–3); LV = left ventricle; MI = myocardial infarction; NSR = normal sinus rhythm; (S) = short-term (3 months); SSS = sick sinus syndrome.

tachycardia. When it coexists with any of the cardiac problems listed, atrial fibrillation increases the risk of embolism. It is postulated that this increased risk correlates with the presence of left atrial thrombi, although this relationship has not been proved. The sensitivity of current noninvasive methods of thrombus detection (i.e., traditional echocardiography) is limited. Transesophageal echocardiography may enable us to detect atrial thrombi with a greater sensitivity, especially in the atrial appendage. Left atrial enlargement usually exists when thrombi are present, although it is sometimes seen when there is no evidence of thrombus or embolism. Left atrial enlargement of greater than 5.5 cm is associated with atrial fibrillation and is considered a high-risk factor for embolism because of this correlation with the atrial arrhythmia.

Cardiomyopathy

All patients with cardiomyopathy are at high risk for thromboembolism as the dilated hypokinetic ventricle predisposes them to form thrombi. Those patients at highest risk are those with secondary atrial fibrillation and/or identifiable thrombi in addition to the global wall abnormalities.

Mitral Valve Prolapse

Mitral valve prolapse (MVP) is the most common cardiac valvular abnormality in adults. Despite its frequency, the overall risk of thromboembolism is low and ischemic events are often transient. In the future, primary prevention for the high-risk group may include platelet antiaggregating agents. These patients appear to be at higher risk for developing platelet-fibrin emboli. Other potential causes of stroke should be sought, particularly in patients who are at low risk for thromboembolism. Specifically active endocarditis, the use of oral contraceptives, protein C and protein S deficiencies, and coexistent paroxysmal atrial fibrillation should not be overlooked.

Endocarditis

In patients with infective endocarditis, control of the infection dramatically decreases the risk of embolism. There is no correlation between emboli and the site of the valve affected in native valve endocarditis. Recurrent emboli are not common after adequate treatment of the underlying infection. Anticoagulation in patients with infective endocarditis is limited to those patients with mechanical prosthetic valves.

Embolism secondary to nonbacterial thromboembolic endocarditis (NBTE) is probably related to an underlying hypercoaguable hematologic state. The use of anticoagulation, at least on a short-term basis, is reasonable in patients with a prothrombotic state.

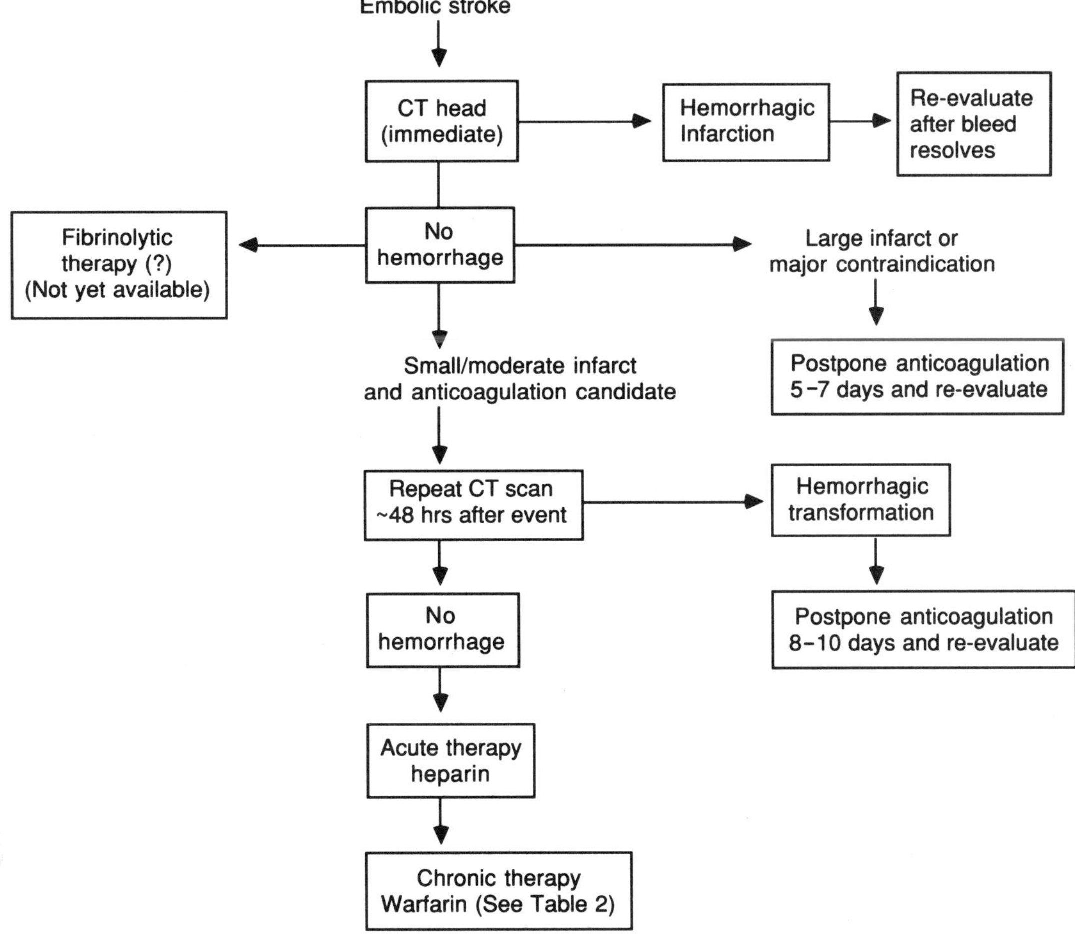

Figure 2   Anticoagulation of acute embolic stroke.

Atrial Myxomas

Atrial myxomas are friable intracardiac tumors and are the most common primary cardiac tumors to cause embolism. Approximately 1 percent of strokes that occur in young adults are caused by atrial myxomas. This tumor carries a high risk of embolism, although the overall incidence of atrial myxomas makes them an uncommon cause of cardiogenic brain embolism. Surgical therapy is usually curative. There is no clear indication for medical therapy in these patients.

Anticoagulation of Acute Cardioembolic Stroke

Approximately 20 percent of cardioembolic strokes undergo secondary hemorrhagic transformation. In the majority of cases, this occurs during the first 48 hours. In an untreated patient with a known source of embolus, the risk of re-embolization during a 2-week period immediately after an embolic stroke is about 1 percent per day. Reviewing the risks versus the benefits of anticoagulation of an acute embolic stroke, we have developed the management plan outlined in Figure 2.

If cerebral hemorrhage is identified on the initial CT scan, the patient is re-evaluated after the hemorrhage has resolved. This difficult situation necessitates an individualized decision. Therapies that carry less risk, such as dipyridamole for the treatment of valvular disease, are often considered.

If no hemorrhage is identified on the initial CT scan, there are currently two possible approaches to treatment. The first is used for patients with a large infarction or serious contraindication to anticoagulation. These patients are re-evaluated after 5 to 7 days. If they are candidates for anticoagulation therapy, their treatment is guided by their underlying cardiac disease (see Table 2). The second approach is used for patients with a small to moderate infarction and no serious contraindications to anticoagulation. We repeat the CT scan at approximately 48 hours after the event. If there is no hemorrhagic transformation, we begin acute anticoagulation followed by warfarin therapy. We begin with continuous infusion–heparin because of the higher risk of hemorrhagic complications and the lack of evidence for additional benefit with bolus therapy. Heparin should be administered via a continuous infusion pump to ensure accurate delivery. The partial thromboplastin time (PTT) should be maintained at 2 to 2.5 times the control value. Patients should continue to receive this level of anticoagulation while warfarin therapy is begun. Daily levels should be checked and used to adjust the infusion of heparin to maintain the therapeutic anticoagulated state. There are several options for changing from heparin to warfarin anticoagulation. We begin warfarin approximately 48 hours after heparin therapy. Warfarin started at a dosage of 10 to 15 mg per day usually brings the prothrombin time (PT) to near-therapeutic levels within 2 to 3 days. Heparin can then be tapered over 2 to 3 days. To ensure adequate anticoagulation, most physicians overlap the heparin and warfarin therapy for 2 to 6 days after the PT has reached therapeutic levels. We use low-intensity anticoagulation (PT = 1.3 to 1.5 times the control value) with warfarin after approximately 1 year of higher intensity therapy (PT = 1.5 to 2 times the control value) in patients who need anticoagulation indefinitely. This decreases the risk of serious side effects.

If hemorrhagic transformation has occurred, anticoagulation is postponed for 8 to 10 days. The source of embolization is sought and the patient is re-evaluated after the hemorrhage has resolved. The re-evaluation includes a repeat CT scan of the head and reassessment of the patient's medical, neurologic, and social risk factors for anticoagulation.

In the future we will have a third alternative that may include therapy with thrombolytic agents. It appears that this will carry the caveat of early detection and intervention. This approach is similar to the early use of fibrinolytic agents in acute coronary artery thrombosis. If therapy can be started within a therapeutic window (probably within 6 hours after the stroke), there is great promise for such intervention. Problems associated with early thrombolytic treatment include the potential for increased hemorrhagic transformation occurring most often during the first few days after embolic stroke. Controlled investigations are needed before there is widespread use of this therapy.

SUGGESTED READING

Dalen J, Hirsh J, eds. Second ACCP Conference on antithrombotic therapy. Chest 1989; 95(suppl).

PATIENT RESOURCES

Patient Information Guide for Neurology
American Academy of Neurology
(E. Wayne Massey, M.D.,
Coordinator AAN Practice Committee)
2221 University Avenue S.E., Suite 335
Minneapolis, Minnesota 55414

American Heart Association
7320 Greenville Avenue
Dallas, Texas 75231
Telephone: (214) 750-5300

National Stroke Association
1420 Ogden Street
Denver, Colorado 80218
Telephone: (303) 839-1992

INTRACEREBRAL HEMORRHAGE

MONROE COLE, M.D.

Decisions regarding the treatment of intracerebral hemorrhage must be based on acute appraisal of the clinical state; the site of the hemorrhage; the etiology of the hemorrhage; and the wishes of the patient (if able to act on his own behalf) or the patient's family.

ACUTE CARE

Cerebellar Hemorrhage

Typically the patient with cerebellar hemorrhage is first seen in the emergency room with coma and evidence of brain stem compression. The patient is hypertensive, and an adequate history of hypertension is obtained. No other causes of intracerebral hemorrhage (e.g., anticoagulation, antiplatelet agents, trauma) appear to play a role. If the hemorrhage is in the cerebellum, preparation should be made for immediate surgical evacuation of the cerebellar hematoma despite evidence of brain stem compromise (Fig. 1). While such preparation is being made, the following steps should be taken:

1. The patient should be intubated and supported by ventilator (i.e., hyperventilated) to reduce intracranial pressure.

2. A large-bore intravenous line should be inserted and kept open with 5 percent dextrose in water administered at a rate of 25 ml per minute, unless the patient is hypovolemic.

3. Blood pressure should be stabilized. I prefer a level of 140–160/80–100. If the pressure is much greater than these levels, a sodium nitroprusside drip is titrated under constant supervision (50 ml per 250 ml of 5 percent dextrose in water administered via an infusion pump at a rate of 3 μg per kilogram per minute ranging from 0.5 to 10 μg per kilogram per minute) (Table 1). The solution should be protected from light and freshly prepared. Hypotension is controlled by an infusion of dopamine (2 to 20 μg per kilogram per minute) or norepinephrine bitartrate (Levophed bitartrate) (4 ml per 1,000 ml in 5 percent dextrose in water at a rate of 0.5 to 1 ml per minute, average dose) (see Table 1).

4. Evidence of increasing intracranial pressure is treated with an infusion of a 20 percent mannitol solution (100 g of mannitol in 500 ml 5 percent dextrose in water) at a rate of 100 ml per hour or, more urgently, a bolus of 25 to 50 g of mannitol. I also immediately administer dexamethasone, 10 mg IV, although this treatment is controversial.

5. An indwelling urinary catheter should be placed and a baseline urinalysis and urine culture obtained.

6. Finally, the patient should be observed (by telemetry) for an arrhythmia while awaiting transfer to the operating room. Lidocaine (as a 50- to 100-mg bolus) should be administered for runs of premature ventricular contractions of three or more, or more than six per minute, followed by a drip of 2 mg per minute. Atropine, 0.5 to 1 mg IV, should be administered for a bradycardia of less than 50 beats per minute (see Table 1).

By the time these steps have been taken, preparations will have been made for the evacuation of the hematoma. If they have not, the patient should be transferred to an appropriate facility.

I have discussed the emergency treatment of a significant hypertensive intracerebellar hematoma first because it is a *treatable* lesion, often with a good prognosis for survival and acceptable function. The above scenario illustrates, with some exceptions (see below), the emergency neuromedical treatment necessary to support a patient in whom surgical treatment is indicated. However, the indications for surgical treatment may be uncertain or even contraindicated if the hypertensive hemorrhage is located at any of the other common sites.

Putaminal Hemorrhage

The comatose patient requires an intravenous line, stabilization, regulation of blood pressure, and an indwelling urinary catheter, and should be watched for cardiac arrhythmias, all as noted above. In addition I begin administering diphenylhydantoin (Dilantin) with a loading dose of 500 mg IV (if no seizures have occurred, otherwise 1,000 mg IV), specifying a rate of 50 mg per minute or less by direct push. A maintenance dose of 100 mg every 6 hours IV, by direct push, is continued with the same caveat, and serum Dilantin levels are obtained within 4 to 5 days. Finally, cimetidine, 300 mg every 6 hours IV, is administered to prevent a Cushing's ulcer.

Should the comatose patient with a putaminal hemorrhage be intubated and receive ventilatory support? In my experience, patients with a hypertensive putaminal hemorrhage severe enough to require artificial ventilation have such a poor prognosis that ventilatory support is not indicated. An airway (preferably) or intubation may be indicated for tracheal toilet only. This is, of course, an ethical as well as a medical (and medicolegal) decision and must be made after a frank discussion with the family, guardian, or attorney, if a "living will" is available indicating the wishes of the patient. I personally advise against the institution of ventilatory support. Frequently, however, this decision is moot, since

Table 1 Drugs Used in the Treatment of Intracerebral Hemorrhage

Drug	Usual Dose	Range	Purpose
Sodium Nitroprusside	3μ/kg/min (50 ml/250 ml 5% D/W)	0.5–10 μg/kg/min	Lower BP
Dopamine		2–20 μg/kg/min	Raise BP
Norepinephrine bitartrate (Levophed)	(4 ml/1,000 ml 5% D/W)	0.5–3 ml/min	Raise BP
Mannitol	20 g/hr (100 g/500 ml 5% D/W) or a 25–50-g bolus		Lower IICP
Dexamethasone	10 mg IV stat, then 4–6 mg IV or IM q6h		Lower IICP
Lidocaine	50–100-mg IV bolus, then 2 mg per min IV		Ventricle arrhythmia
Atropine	0.5–1 mg IV		Treat bradycardia
Dilantin	500–1,000 mg IV stat, then 100 mg IV q6h		Seizure Px
Carbamazepine (Tegretol)	200 mg via NG tube q6h		Treat seizure Px
Cimetidine	300 mg IV q6h		Treat ulcer Px
Alupent	0.3 ml in 2 ml saline q4h		Aerosol
Methyldopa	250–500 mg IV q6–8h		Lower BP
Ensure	Half-strength or full-strength at 75–100 ml/hr		Nutritional
Ensure Plus	75–100 ml/hr		Nutritional
Osmolite	Half-strength or full-strength at 75–100 ml/hr		Nutritional
Prochlorperazine	10 mg IM q4–6 h p.r.n.		Treat nausea
Vitamin K_1	25 mg IM		Reverse Coumadin
Nifedipine	10 mg SL q6h		Lower BP

BP = blood pressure; D/W = dextrose in water; IICP = increased intracranial pressure; NG = nasogastric; Px = prevention; SL = sublingual.

the patient has already been intubated and is receiving ventilatory assistance by the time evaluation is made by a neurologist.

Similar considerations exist for surgical evacuation of a putaminal hematoma, which often involves more than the putamen, especially the internal capsule. If the patient is comatose and the brain stem embarrassed, evacuation of the hematoma is *not* indicated. If the patient is comatose, or consciousness is declining but the brain stem is intact, evacuation of the hematoma *may save life but functional recovery is usually poor.* I advise against surgery, but discuss the option frankly with the patient's family. I advise against evacuation of the hematoma as a means of improving a hemiparesis, aphasia, or other focal neurologic deficit.

Thalamic Hemorrhage

I do not consider evacuation of the hematoma indicated for preservation of life or for improving neurologic function. Considerations for respiratory support are the same as for putaminal hemorrhage. Blood pressure should be controlled as described above. Mannitol should be infused in an attempt to reduce intracranial pressure. I also continue to administer dexamethasone (a 10-mg IV bolus followed by 4 to 6 mg every 6 hours, IV or IM for the first 24 to 72 hours) in an attempt to reduce cerebral edema.

Pontine Hemorrhage

Usually a hypertensive pontine hemorrhage is a devastating event. The patient enters the hospital comatose, quadriplegic, with severe gaze palsies and bilateral Horner's syndrome. Because the prognosis is so poor, I do not advise surgery or respiratory support. If, however, the patient is already receiving ventilatory support, this should be continued. Once rapport is established with the family and the grave prognosis is outlined, the question of continuing ventilatory support may be addressed. Control and stabilization of blood pressure should be continued. Increased intracranial pressure is not a problem. The question of control of life-threatening cardiac arrhythmias should be agreed upon with the family as soon as possible.

SUBACUTE CARE

Hypertensive Intracerebral Hemorrhage

Cerebellar Hemorrhage

Of the common sites of hypertensive intracerebral hemorrhage, in my opinion only a cerebellar hemorrhage should be considered a surgically treatable disease. However, if the patient with a cerebellar hematoma remains alert with flexor plantar responses, neuromedical treatment with close observation is indicated. A diminution in level of consciousness and/or a reversion to extensor plantar responses (indicating brain stem compression) should lead to hematoma evacuation.

Putaminal Hemorrhage

If the level of consciousness of a previously alert patient with a putaminal hemorrhage deteriorates,

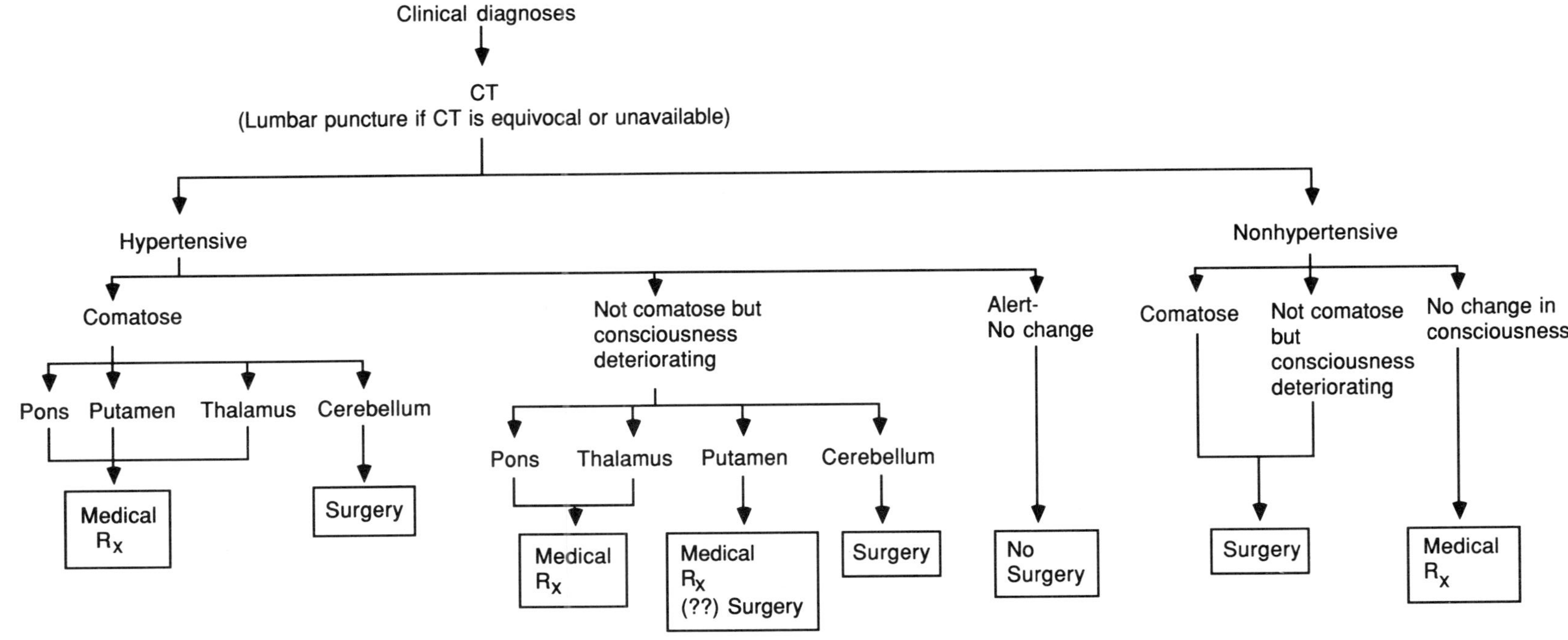

Figure 1 Treatment algorithm for intracerebral hemorrhage.

evacuation of the hematoma may be offered to the family. I stress, however, that in my experience, functional results of surgery have been poor.

Thalamic Hemorrhage

If alertness diminishes because of thalamic hemorrhage, obstruction of the third ventricle of the cerebrum should be searched for by computed tomographic (CT) scan, and if it is documented, lateral ventricular shunting should be considered. Patients with hematomas large enough to obstruct the third ventricle usually have a poor prognosis, even if life is sustained.

Nonhypertensive Hemorrhage

Except for the intracerebral hemorrhage (or hemorrhages) of amyloid angiopathy, the other causes of nonhypertensive intracerebral hematoma warrant a more aggressive approach to treatment. Considerations including the patient's neurologic condition, the site of the lesion, the age of the patient, and the etiology of the hemorrhage should enter into the decision-making process.

Patient's Neurologic Condition. Deterioration of the level of consciousness warrants hematoma evacuation. Coma or other levels of seriously impaired consciousness, with intact pupillary responses, intact extraocular movements (demonstrable, if necessary, by caloric stimulation), and spontaneous respirations, also warrant hematoma evacuation. If the patient is reasonably alert, however, and remains so, surgical treatment is not indicated.

Site of Lesion. Cortical-subcortical or cerebellar hematomas are eminently suitable for evacuation. The hematoma of pituitary apoplexy may need transsphenoidal evacuation to relieve upward compression on optic chiasm or nerves, hypothalamus, or mesencephalon. Thalamic or pontine hematomas should be evacuated, particularly in the younger patient, if there is neurologic deterioration.

Age of Patient. The child or young adult is especially likely to benefit from hematoma evacuation.

Etiology of Hemorrhage. Intracerebral hematoma caused by aneurysm, arteriovenous malformation, idiopathic thrombocytopenic purpura, leukemia, trauma, vasculitis, anticoagulation, antiplatelet agents, clot-dissolving enzymes, or unknown cause all indicate hematoma evacuation, depending on the neurologic status and course. Decisions regarding hemorrhage into a known primary or secondary cerebral malignancy depends, at least to some degree, on the prognosis of the underlying tumor.

NEUROMEDICAL CARE

Respiratory

Nasopharyngeal or oropharyngeal suctioning should be performed every 1 to 2 hours, or more often if necessary. An aerosol of metaproterenol sulfate (Alupent), 0.3 ml in 2 ml saline every 4 hours (except during sleep), is ordered to prevent atelectasis. If the patient is alert, the aerosol is administered via a mouthpiece; if the patient is stuperous, it should be administered via a mask.

Blood Pressure

After 24 hours, an attempt is made to discontinue sodium nitroprusside, and methyldopa (250 to 500 mg every 6 to 8 hours IV) is started, unless oral medication (e.g., diuretics, captopril, nifedipine) can be taken and proves effective. Sublingual nifedipine, 10 mg every 6 hours, may be sufficient to control hypertension.

Activity

The patient is prescribed bedrest until vital signs and neurologic conditions are stable, and the patient is alert for at least 24 hours. Bedside range of motion is also ordered when the patient is neuromedically stable. If the patient is alert, a trapeze is put over the bed to enable him to change his own position. Unless the duration of bedrest is minimal, sitting in a chair is not permitted until vascular reflexes have proven adequate on a tilt table.

Increased Intracranial Pressure

Mannitol is used only on an urgent basis. If clinical evidence of increased intracranial pressure persists for more than 12 to 24 hours, the continuation of mannitol therapy is of little use. Rebound may occur when it is discontinued. Dexamethasone is continued at 4 to 6 mg every 6 hours for 3 to 5 days, and is then gradually discontinued by halving the dose every 2 days.

Anticonvulsants

Dilantin is continued intravenously until the patient can take medication by mouth, nasogastric tube, or percutaneous esophagogastrostomy (PEG). If an allergic rash develops, carbamazepine (Tegretol), 200 mg every 8 hours is administered via a nasogastric tube. In all patients with lesions involving cerebral cortex or subcortex, I continue to administer anticonvulsants for at least 1 year.

Nutrition

Intravenous fluids provide the sole source of nutrition for the first 96 hours. Thereafter, one must consider more adequate nutrition via oral, nasogastric, or PEG feeding. If the patient is alert and able to swallow, oral feeding is started as a liquid diet, advancing to mechanical soft, bland, and regular diets (in that order). I try to provide nourishment of at least 1,500 to 2,000 cal per day. If the patient is unable to swallow safely, feeding is accomplished by nasogastric tube or PEG. If the patient appears able to survive but the prognosis for oral feeding in the near future seems poor, a PEG is advised. If the prognosis for recovery is hopeful, nasogastric feeding is started.

There are several liquid feeding systems available. I usually start with Ensure or Osmolite (1.06 cal per milliliter) in equal parts with water by constant drip at a rate of 75 to 100 ml per hour. This is advanced to full strength, then to Ensure Plus (1.5 cal per milliliter) at a rate of 75 to 100 ml per hour.

Headache and Nausea

Headache is usually controllable with codeine, 32 mg IM every 4 to 6 hours; nausea with prochlorperazine 10 mg IM every 4 to 6 hours, as necessary.

Skin Care

It is the physician's responsibility to prevent the occurrence of a decubitus ulcer (bedsore). This must *never* occur. I order the following: (1) sheep's wool under torso and heels (inflatable pads or mattresses, in my opinion, are worse than useless, as most only make the patient perspire and thus contribute to the problem); (2) that the patient be turned *every hour;* and (3) that the patient's back be dry and powdered, with the skin inspected daily for erythema or other color change.

Specific Therapy

If hemorrhage is caused by warfarin sodium (Coumadin) therapy, vitamin K_1, 25 mg IM (not IV), should be administered. If it is caused by thrombocytopenia, platelet transfusion is indicated. If the cause is unknown, angiography should be performed, especially in younger patients, to search for an arteriovenous malformation, which, if demonstrated, requires surgical treatment. An aneurysm, demonstrated by angiography, requires definitive surgical treatment.

Rehabilitation

In my opinion, rehabilitation is more than a means of psychological support for the patient and family. A frank discussion of what neurorehabilitation is likely to accomplish in the individual patient is warranted. The family should not, for example, expect a hemiplegic arm to be restored to complete usefulness by the rehabilitation process. However, increased general strength and endurance, adaptation, substitution, bracing, the use of aids and appliances, and the alteration of the home environment may be expected to improve function. Intensive speech therapy is indicated in motivated individuals. I send my patients for physical, occupational, and if they are dysphasic, for speech therapy, starting at the bedside as soon as the patient is stable. Regular rounds in the rehabilitation department prove instructive to the physician and helpful to the patient.

SUGGESTED READING

Fisher CM, Picard EH, Polak A, et al. Acute hypertensive cerebellar hemorrhage: diagnosis and surgical treatment. J Nerv Ment Dis 1965;140:38.

McKissock W, Richardson A, Taylor J. Primary intracerebral hemorrhage: a controlled trial of surgical and conservative treatment in 180 unselected cases. Lancet 1961;2:221.

Humphreys RP, Hockley AD, Freedman MH, Saunders EF. Management of intracerebral hemorrhage in idiopathic thrombocytopenic purpura. J Neurosurg 1976;45:700.

Zervas NT, Mendelson G. Treatment of acute haemorrhage of pituitary tumours. Lancet 1975;1:604.

PATIENT RESOURCES

Stroke support groups:

National Stroke Association
1420 Ogden Street
Denver, Colorado 80218
Telephone: (303) 839-1992

Stroke Club International
805 12th Street
Galveston, Texas 77550
(Will give location of state or local chapter.)

INTRACRANIAL ANEURYSM

DAVID O. WIEBERS, M.D.

The most common mode of presentation of intracranial aneurysms is rupture resulting in subarachnoid hemorrhage (SAH) with or without intracerebral hemorrhage. Intracranial aneurysms are not congenital but rather develop with increasing age. The average annual incidence of aneurysmal rupture is approximately ten per 100,000 people in the same general population in which the autopsy prevalence of aneurysm is approximately 5 percent. These figures suggest that the vast majority of intracranial aneurysms never rupture or cause any other symptoms. Nevertheless, physicians are discovering more and more unruptured aneurysms from computed tomographic (CT) scans, magnetic resonance imaging (MRI) scans, and cerebral angiograms obtained for reasons other than aneurysmal rupture.

The management of intracranial aneurysm is quite different, depending on whether the aneurysm is discovered before or after the rupture. These two courses of action will therefore be addressed separately.

RUPTURED ANEURYSM

It is very important to be aware of the clinical picture of aneurysmal rupture, because as many as half of patients with fatal aneurysmal ruptures may have had previous warning leaks consisting of a partial or milder version of a typical SAH. The typical clinical picture of SAH includes the sudden onset of severe headache with or without stiff neck. Key diagnostic points are the suddenness of onset, the unusual quality of the headache for that particular patient, and the stiff neck, which is not merely a tightness or tenderness to direct palpation but usually includes meningismus and an inability to move the neck anteroposteriorly. In addition, the level of consciousness may be diminished, and focal neurologic signs, particularly cranial nerve palsies, such as a palsy of the third cranial nerve, may be present. Other recognized clinical features of SAH are nausea and vomiting, diffuse intellectual impairment, photophobia, seizures, and hemispheric symptoms, often related to hemorrhage extending into the brain parenchyma. Occasionally, SAH from an intracranial source may produce neck or low back pain with radicular features, particularly if the patient is sitting or standing and blood has pooled in the spinal subarachnoid space. A similar presentation may occur with spinal SAH.

Physical examination may reveal neck meningismus (especially if the examination is performed within hours of onset of even a minor leak), preretinal and subhyaloid hemorrhages, papilledema, fever, and other neurologic deficits, such as those mentioned above, depending on the location and severity of the hemorrhage. Patients with symptoms that raise the possibility of SAH should be examined with caution; specifically, the neurologic examination should not include strenuous muscle testing or Valsalva maneuvers that could precipitate another rupture.

Patients with symptoms consistent with SAH should undergo a CT scan of the head in an attempt to detect subarachnoid blood, which can be seen without the use of contrast medium in approximately 80 percent of patients. If the CT scan is negative for subarachnoid or intraparenchymal blood, a lumbar puncture should be performed. If the CT scan shows evidence of subarachnoid or intraparenchymal hemorrhage, a lumbar puncture need not be done, since it will not contribute significant additional diagnostic information and can sometimes be dangerous, particularly when intraparenchymal blood is present.

Traumatic lumbar puncture must be differentiated from true SAH. Three or four successive tubes of cerebrospinal fluid are collected, and if the specimens show progressively less blood, a traumatic puncture is suggested. Clotting of the specimen virtually never occurs with true SAH. Xanthochromia is present in the supernatant within hours of SAH and remains in the spinal fluid for an average of 3 to 4 weeks. Red blood cells often disappear within several days after SAH. The cerebrospinal fluid may not show xanthochromia if small numbers of red blood cells are present from SAH (approximately 400 or fewer), and xanthochromia has been reported in rare instances with traumatic lumbar puncture if the red blood cell count is more than 200,000.

After the diagnosis of SAH is established, patients are prescribed bedrest in a quiet, darkened room, and if the patient is to undergo operation, bedrest is continued for at least 2 to 3 weeks. The patient should be kept under close observation for at least the first few days, either in an intensive care unit or at least in a hospital room close to a nursing station. Vital signs and neurologic checks are recorded at least every 4 hours, and careful attention is placed on fluid and electrolyte balance.

If the patient is agitated, I often administer a sedative in the form of phenobarbital, 30 to 60 mg twice daily, or chloral hydrate, 500 mg three times daily. It is important not to oversedate since the effect of the medication may be indistinguishable from depressed level of consciousness caused by rehemorrhage or other complications of SAH.

It is important to provide analgesia for pain relief because extra pain often leads to agitation and an increased likelihood of additional hemorrhage. I usually use codeine, 60 mg IM or orally every 3 to 4 hours, as needed. The use of morphine should be avoided because it may depress respiration and level of consciousness.

Overhydration may produce cerebral edema and increased intracranial pressure, while underhydration can lead to cerebral vasospasm. Consequently, I recommend fluid replacement with approximately 2 L of 5 percent dextrose in ¼ isotonic saline per day. Patients are given laxatives to avoid straining when passing stool. For patients clearly suffering from increased intracranial pressure, mannitol (1 to 1.5 g per kilogram IV in 20 percent solution over 30 minutes) and glycerol (1 g per kilogram via a nasogastric tube) are sometimes used as temporary antiedema agents. Smaller doses of mannitol may be used at 4- to 6-hour intervals, and the glycerol dose may be given at these intervals if longer-term control of intracranial pressure is desired.

One must be very cautious about the use of antihypertensive agents in this situation, because at least part of the hypertension observed is often the result of Cushing's reflex, in which intracranial hypertension leads to peripheral hypertension to maintain cerebral perfusion. Most of the time, increased systemic blood pressure gradually decreases as the patient rests in the hospital with or without mild sedation and analgesia. Patients with previously treated hypertension should maintain their previous therapy. For patients who continue to have considerable hypertension (greater than 180/110 mm Hg) despite the general measures already mentioned, blood pressure can be controlled rather precisely by a continuous intravenous infusion of sodium nitroprusside titrated to pressures slightly below this level.

The use of antifibrinolytic agents, such as epsilon-aminocaproic acid (Amicar), may decrease mortality from rebleeding of aneurysms, but it also increases thrombotic side effects, including cerebral infarction, deep vein thrombosis, and pulmonary embolism. A delayed myopathy occurring with the use of epsilon-aminocaproic acid has also been reported. I generally do not administer antifibrinolytic agents after a single SAH, but I do recommend such treatment if there is any evidence of continued or recurrent hemorrhage after initial hemorrhage. Epsilon-aminocaproic acid is usually administered in a dosage of 24 to 36 g in 1,000 ml of 5 percent dextrose solution every 24 hours.

Another important complication of SAH is cerebral vasospasm, which involves spasm of one or more cerebral arteries, particularly in the area of extravasated blood. This may lead to focal cerebral infarction and sometimes to a more generalized or multifocal decreased cerebral perfusion. The peak time for the occurrence of vasospasm is between 4 and 14 days after SAH. When vasospasm occurs, I

recommend blood volume expansion with plasma and whole blood transfusions. Human albumin (Albuminar) may also be used for this purpose. When central venous pressure is monitored, it is usually maintained between 8 and 12 cm H_2O. Dopamine infusion titration starting at doses of 5 to 10 μg per kilogram per minute to increase systolic blood pressure by 40 to 50 mm Hg may also be helpful in this circumstance, particularly if the patient is hypotensive. Recent studies have suggested that calcium-channel-blocking agents such as nimodipine and nicardipine hydrochloride may also be useful in this condition, but convincing confirmation of their efficacy awaits the completion of randomized clinical trials currently underway.

Surgical clipping of the ruptured aneurysm remains the definitive treatment for these lesions, and this is generally the ultimate goal in management. The overall mortality from aneurysmal SAH is approximately 59 percent at 30 days for each rupture, and the prognosis is clearly related to the patient's level of consciousness at the time of the first visit with the physician. Operative morbidity and mortality rates are much higher in patients who have depressed levels of consciousness or other severe neurologic deficits besides cranial nerve palsies. The peak time for rebleeding from intracranial aneurysm is 7 to 10 days after initial rupture, and as already mentioned, the peak time for vasospasm is 4 to 14 days after the initial rupture. Consequently, if at the time of the first examination patients with SAH have a normal or near-normal level of consciousness and no severe neurologic deficit other than cranial nerve palsy, I suggest that they undergo cerebral arteriography as soon as feasible so that the source for SAH may be clearly identified. When an intracranial aneurysm is identified, surgical clipping should be undertaken as soon as possible, preferably within the first 2 to 3 days after aneurysmal rupture to avoid the peak times for vasospasm and rebleeding. It is important to involve a neurosurgeon who is experienced and skilled in aneurysmal surgery, since these procedures are exceedingly difficult.

For patients with depressed levels of consciousness and severe neurologic deficits at the time of admission, medical management is generally undertaken until there is stabilization and improvement, at which time definitive surgical treatment has a lower probability of complications.

UNRUPTURED ANEURYSMS

Intracranial aneurysms may cause symptoms other than intracranial hemorrhage, particularly if they are 10 mm or greater in diameter. These symptoms may result from cranial nerve compression (most commonly compression of cranial nerves II, III, IV, V, and VI) or compression of other central nervous system structures, such as the pituitary on the brain stem. Seizure foci may result from impingement on supratentorial brain structures. In addition, aneurysms may rarely cause cerebral ischemia from embolization of a clot within the aneurysm to distal sites in the same arterial tree. When headache is caused by unruptured aneurysm, it may be produced by a sudden dilatation of the aneurysm or by chronic compression of pain-sensitive structures, such as the ophthalmic and maxillary divisions of the trigeminal nerve. Such headaches are often focal and unilateral, frontal, or orbital in location and may be associated with cranial nerve palsies.

Because the vast majority of intracranial aneurysms never rupture or cause any other symptoms, ideally the selection of patients for surgical treatment should depend on predicting which unruptured aneurysms will subsequently rupture. It is important to emphasize that this part of the discussion does not apply to patients with any suggestion of SAH (including warning leaks) before the discovery of the intracranial aneurysm.

Patients with unruptured aneurysms discovered by CT scan or MRI scan who are suitable surgical candidates should be considered for cerebral arteriography as soon as possible. Unruptured aneurysms 10 mm in angiographic diameter or larger have a fairly high probability of subsequent rupture, and many of these ruptures occur within a few months of identification of the aneurysm. Consequently, for patients with unruptured aneurysms of this size, an intracranial operation should be considered by a neurosurgeon experienced in aneurysmal surgery to isolate the aneurysm from the circulation as soon as possible.

For unruptured aneurysms less than 10 mm in diameter, there appears to be little likelihood of subsequent rupture. Only one such rupture has ever been reported (a 6-mm aneurysm), and it occurred after an ipsilateral carotid endarterectomy, which may have predisposed the aneurysm to rupture. Because there are no documented cases of clearly spontaneous subarachnoid hemorrhage in natural history studies for this patient group, it is difficult to recommend surgical intervention, particularly for patients with lesions 5 mm or less in diameter. Even in experienced hands, significant morbidity is associated with such aneurysmal surgery. Although data are limited, it also appears that carotid endarterectomy should be approached with increased caution in patients with unruptured intracranial aneurysms, particularly those that are >5 mm in diameter in the ipsilateral carotid system.

If compressive or embolic symptoms from an aneurysm develop after the original diagnosis, the aneurysm probably has enlarged and thus has a higher probability of rupture. In this circumstance, the patient should be restudied with cerebral arteriography and considered for neurologic surgery if enlargement has occurred. In recent years, high-resolution, dynamic, multiplane CT scanning techniques have made it possible to identify most intracranial aneurysms relatively noninvasively. Consequently, detection of aneurysmal enlargement has become easier and safer in many patients not treated surgically, even if they remain asymptomatic. In patients with normal renal function and no history of dye allergy who have not undergone operation, it seems reasonable to restudy at yearly intervals for 3 years, particularly if unruptured aneurysms are 6 to 9 mm in diameter. If no enlargement has occurred and no symptoms have developed after 3 years, it may be adequate to restudy at 5-year intervals.

SUGGESTED READING

Sengupta RP, McAllister VL. Subarachnoid haemorrhage. Berlin: Springer-Verlag, 1986.
Wiebers DO, Whisnant JP, Sundt TM Jr, O'Fallon WM. The significance of unruptured intracranial saccular aneurysms. J Neurosurg 1987; 66:23–29.

BRAIN ARTERIOVENOUS MALFORMATION

GERARD M. DEBRUN, M.D.

This chapter considers true arteriovenous malformations (AVMs), with a nidus of abnormal vessels interposed between the arterial feeders and the draining veins, and the fistulas with one direct communication between one artery and one vein, whether associated with a varix or not. It is interesting to note that there are also true fistulas inside the nidus of brain AVMs. The treatment of venous angiomas, cavernomas, and telangiectasias is not discussed in this chapter.

The therapeutic alternatives are conservative treatment, surgical excision alone, embolization alone, radiosurgery alone, embolization followed by surgical excision or radiosurgery, surgery followed by radiosurgery, and failure of radiosurgery followed by one of the previous therapeutic approaches. The decision of which approach to employ depends on many factors, most of which are objective, but some of which are subjective and have a psychological basis. We obviously need guidelines. In brief they are derived from: (1) the clinical presentation, (2) the location, size, anatomy and physiology of the AVM, and (3) the age and risk factors.

CLINICAL PRESENTATION

Patients who have already bled have a 2 percent chance of rebleeding per year. The cumulative risk increases if the patient's first occurrence of bleeding has taken place early in his life. It is therefore acceptable to be more aggressive in the treatment of young patients who have already bled.

If patients present with seizures that are well controlled with medical therapy without major side effects, conservative treatment should be considered whenever the risks of treatment seem to be greater than those associated with the natural history of the disease. Patients who have poorly controlled or uncontrollable seizures despite serious medical treatment are candidates for further treatment, if possible. Therapy is also indicated in patients with progressive neurologic deficit. Headaches and migraines are highly subjective factors; when they are isolated, the AVM should be treated only if the risks are low.

LOCATION, SIZE, ANATOMY, AND PHYSIOLOGY OF THE AVM

I have found it useful to use Spetzler's classification. This grading system is easy to apply and emphasizes the importance of whether or not the location of the AVM is in an eloquent area of the brain. The polar AVMs may be treated with less risk than a rolandic, internal capsule, basal ganglia, or brain stem AVM. The size of the AVM is also important, especially when radiosurgery is considered. The percentage of anatomic cure of an AVM at 2 years after radiotherapy is between 80 and 85 percent if the nidus is not larger than 2 cm. The dose to be delivered to the nidus and to its edge is controversial, but the number of cures percent at 2 years is probably dose dependent. The next decades will bring the answer when the results will be compared in function of the size of the nidus, the dose of radiation delivered, and the type of radiation used: cobalt ring, heavy particles, proton beam, or linear accelerator.

The geometry of the feeders and draining veins is an important factor when we consider embolization or surgical resection. The caliber and number of feeders are important to consider before attempting an embolization. When we consider embolization as a presurgical step, it is especially useful to embolize the feeders to which the neurosurgeon has difficulty obtaining access, while the feeders on the surface of the brain can be easily clipped and do not always need to be embolized, or sometimes cannot be embolized safely because they are too tortuous and distal.

The exact determination of the size of the nidus is probably the most difficult part of the radiologic evaluation. There is often a collateral circulation in the watershed areas with a highly tortuous abnormal network that should not be confused with the nidus and should be respected during embolization or surgery. Puck films with good subtractions, computed tomography (CT), and magnetic resonance imaging (MRI) need to be juxtaposed in order to determine the nidus with accuracy.

The rapidity of blood shunting through the AVM is an important physiologic factor but also difficult to quantify. The vein is almost invariably reached within 2 seconds of the beginning of the filling of the carotid artery, and often within 1 second. The merit of recent superselective angiography with microcatheters advanced into the feeder of an AVM immediately before entering the nidus is to show direct fistulae inside the nidus of a brain AVM. This important discovery explains why particulate embolization might be contraindicated in this situation or should be performed only after closure of this fistula. It is difficult to determine whether there is relative ischemia of the surrounding normal tissue, even in the presence of an intense steal. The concept of normal pressure breakthrough phenomenon is controversial, as is the concept of loss of autoregulation of the normal adjacent tissue. Acute clipping or occlusion of the feeder of an AVM immediately increases the blood pressure into this feeder and may be putting the normal tissue fed by this artery at risk.

AGE AND RISK FACTORS

It seems that the older the patient, the less is the risk of bleeding if he has never bled before. This is why the patient's age at the onset of the first bleed is important to consider. A patient who first bled in early life should be treated whenever there is a reasonable degree of risk.

Other risks should be considered as in any surgical candidate (e.g., high blood pressure, diabetes, myocardial infarction, atheromatous disease). When all of the possible risks have been determined, a team made up of a neurologist, vascular and stereotaxic neurosurgeon, neuroradiologist, and a radiotherapist should discuss the indications for treatment in each particular case.

Conservative treatment is sometimes the only alternative for patients with hemispheric, basal ganglia, internal capsule, or brain stem AVMs. One difficult therapeutic decision is in advising a young patient, who is neurologically intact and has never bled and in whom an AVM has been discovered incidentally, after the first seizure or for unexplained headaches. We usually follow the patient unless his AVM is suitable for radiosurgery (the nidus is no larger than 2 cm) or operable with very low risk (a small polar AVM). The natural risk of bleeding is difficult to determine in this category of patients. However, some patients refuse the idea of living with the threat of rupture of their AVM and say that they want to take the risk of treatment. This is certainly one of the subjective factors that I was mentioning which may lead to a more aggressive therapeutic plan than what was initially considered.

SURGICAL RESECTION ALONE

Small AVMs in a noneloquent area of the brain are surgically resected with 0 percent mortality rate and a morbidity rate of almost 0 percent. The mortality and morbidity rates increase with the grading of the AVM. Very large AVMs (larger than 6 cm in diameter) in eloquent areas of the brain cannot be resected at one sitting and are usually not operated on without obliteration of the nidus with embolization as complete as possible.

RADIOSURGERY ALONE

We have already mentioned the ideal indications of radiosurgery. The size of the nidus should not be larger than 2 cm. For AVMs larger than 2 cm, radiosurgery is probably not the procedure of first choice but may be offered if no better choice for treatment is available. The dose delivered to the AVM is the second most important factor and is in fact closely related to the size of the nidus: the smaller the nidus, the larger the dose.

When one is considering radiosurgery as the only treatment, it is very important to know whether the patient has experienced any previous bleeding. Since in 80 percent of the patients with good indications it takes 2 years for an AVM to be cured after radiosurgery, this treatment is least attractive for a patient who has recently bled or has bled several times. A more expeditious way to cure the AVM should be considered in this particular situation.

EMBOLIZATION ALONE

Embolization alone may cure a brain AVM. The smaller the nidus, the better the chance of complete obliteration. Also, an AVM with one or a few feeders is easier to cure with this method than a larger one with multiple feeders coming from the three major trunks (middle, anterior, and posterior cerebral arteries). The materials used for embolization are also an important factor. There are actually three different techniques; the first technique uses cyanoacrylic glue (N Butyl Cyanoacrylate or Bucrylate), the second technique uses particles of IVALON (Polyvinyl alcohol foam) mixed with or without 30 percent ethanol, and the third technique uses coils. Only embolization with Bucrylate can offer a chance of complete occlusion of the nidus. I am not aware of a single case of brain AVM treated with any of the other materials that did not recanalize the previously occluded vessels or did not recruit "new" feeders from enlargement of tiny vessels that were present before embolization.

The highest complete cure rate of embolization alone of brain AVMs using Bucrylate that has been reported is 18 percent with an overall morbidity rate of 10 percent and a mortality rate of 1 or 2 percent (all AVM types are included). The main reason for this relatively low cure rate is that small AVMs with one or two feeders are rarely addressed to the neuroradiologist for embolization, but rather are surgically resected or treated with radiosurgery. Whatever materials are to be used for embolization, there are several strict rules to follow. The embolic material must be delivered into the nidus of the AVM from a microcatheter positioned into the feeder 1 or 2 cm proximal to the nidus. The presence or absence of a balloon at the tip of the catheter makes a great difference in the embolization. The presence of a balloon with a distal hole makes it possible to stop the flow into the feeder, to perform selective angiography under flow control, and to inject the glue in the same condition. More glue stays and solidifies into the nidus. There is less risk of gluing the vein or having part of the glue embolize to the lungs. The injection of glue is also sometimes done under moderate hypotension with a mean arterial pressure of approximately 60 mm of Hg. It is difficult to lower the blood pressure more in the sedated patient without risking nausea and an impossibility of injecting the glue. The inconvenience of using a balloon is the risk of rupturing the feeder with catastrophic subarachnoid or intracerebral hemorrhage. There is a 3 percent risk of mortality associated with this technique. Without a balloon at the tip of the catheter, injection of glue can be done without control of the flow. Therefore the injection is done when there is a true nidus interposed between feeder and vein. When there is a true fistula with fast shunting, the fistula can be closed with a small injection of 0.1 ml of pure nonradiopaque glue. Then embolization can be pursued with radiopaque glue as usual.

EMBOLIZATION FOLLOWED BY SURGICAL RESECTION OR RADIOSURGERY

The goal of the treatment of a brain AVM is to achieve a complete obliteration of the nidus with complete disappearance of any arteriovenous shunting. When we fail to achieve this goal, the risk of devastating hemorrhage is unchanged, even if only 1 percent of the nidus is left. The embolization is performed in patients with large AVMs, with multiple feeders from two or three major arterial trunks used as presurgical step. Several sittings of embolization separated by 3 or 4 weeks are often necessary. After embolization with glue, the feeder is closed. After embolization with particles, the feeder remains open. It is wise to occlude the feeder at the end of the embolization with a detachable balloon or with coils. The embolic material is delivered through a microcatheter with its tip positioned immediately proximal to the nidus. The same principles apply whatever the material used. The goal is to fill the nidus as much as we can with solid particles, glue, or coils. Obviously it is more difficult to fill the nidus with coils than with particles or glue. The use of coils is more likely to occlude the feeders and at a distance of the nidus than the nidus itself.

After embolization, surgical resection becomes easier and safer. When radiopaque glue has been used, the feeders of the AVM close to the nidus are filled with black material that helps the surgeon find the nidus. It has been said that an AVM embolized with glue is like a piece of rock, making surgical dissection more difficult and risky. This has not been my experience. The N Butyl Cyanoacrylate that we use today is less solid than isobutyl cyanoacrylate was. I wonder if the negative attitude held by a few neurosurgeons concerning this treatment is because they have operated on AVMs that were completely obliterated with a large amount of glue. It is questionable whether these AVMs should be operated on. I believe that it is dangerous and unnecessary to resect an AVM that has been totally cured with glue.

There is no doubt in my mind that performing embolization before surgery is extremely beneficial, allowing complete surgical resection of large AVMs and decreasing the mortality and morbidity rates of surgery. I have not seen any normal pressure breakthrough syndrome in any of the large AVMs resected after reduction of the shunt and the nidus size by embolization. This syndrome is controversial and may be rare. However, it is seen by neurosurgeons who have the experience of resection of very large AVMs of high grade in Spetzler's classification. It is unlikely to occur in patients with AVMs of smaller size and lower grade.

This category of AVMs treated with embolization and surgical resection corresponds to large AVMs. Neuroradiologists and neurosurgeons have a common commitment: first, to reduce the size of the nidus and the speed of arteriovenous shunting as much as possible, and second, to accept the risks of complete surgical resection after completion of the embolization.

The risks of embolization and surgical resection are higher in patients with large AVMs, carrying a mortality rate of 5 percent and a morbidity rate of 15 to 20 percent. We must always consider the quality of life that the patient will have at the completion of the treatment. Most patients are able to resume their professional activity, with few being greatly disabled. Most large AVMs of the occipital lobe involving the calcarine cortex will be left with a permanent hemianopic defect. We explain to the patient that he will almost certainly be left with a cortical field defect. I consider that it is an excellent result when the patient is totally cured despite his hemianopsia.

EMBOLIZATION, SURGICAL RESECTION, AND RADIOSURGERY

After embolization and surgical resection, a small remnant of the AVM may be left because it is located in an eloquent and highly risky area of the brain, as the internal capsule, the thalamus, or the deep cerebellar nuclei. Radiosurgery of this remnant of AVM may cure an AVM which cannot be cured by any other approach.

FAILURE OF RADIOSURGERY

More and more patients with large AVMs (i.e., with a nidus larger than 3 cm in every dimension) are not cured at 2 years postradiosurgery. This is because small doses of radiation were given in order to avoid brain radiation necrosis. Radiosurgery is not the first choice in large AVMs. Embolization and surgical resection should be considered first and radiosurgery second or as an adjunct to embolization and resection.

SUGGESTED READING

Batjer HH, Devous MD, Seibert GB, et al. Intracranial arteriovenous malformation: relationships between clinical and radiographic factors and ipsilateral steal severity. Neurosurgery 1988; 23:322–328.

Batjer HH, Devous MD, Seibert GB, et al. Intracranial arteriovenous malformation: relationship between clinical factors and surgical complications. Neurosurgery 1989; 24:75–79.

Brown RD, Wiebers DO, Forbes G, et al. The natural history of unruptured intracranial arteriovenous malformations. J Neurosurg 1988; 68:352–357.

Fisher WS. Decision analysis: a tool of the future—an application to unruptured arteriovenous malformations. Neurosurgery 1989; 24:129–135.

Fults D, Kelly DL. Natural history of arteriovenous malformations of the brain: a clinical study. Neurosurgery 1984; 15:658–662.

Graf CJ, Perret GE, Torner JC. Bleeding from cerebral arteriovenous malformations as part of their natural history. J Neurosurg 1983; 58:331–337.

Luessenhop AJ, Rosa L. Cerebral arteriovenous malformations: indications for and results of surgery, and the role of intravascular techniques. J Neurosurg 1984; 60:14–22.

Picard L, Moret J, Lepoire J. Endovascular treatment of cerebral AVM's. J Neuroradiology 1984; 11:9–28.

Spetzler RF, Martin NA. A proposed grading system for arteriovenous malformations. J Neurosurg 1986; 65:476–483.

Spetzler RF, Martin NA, Carter LP, et al. Surgical management of large AVM's by staged embolization and operative excision. J Neurosurg 1987; 67:17–28.

Troupp H, Marttila I, Halonen V. AVM's of the brain: prognosis without operation. Acta Neurochir 1970; 22:125–128.

Vinuela FV, Debrun GM, Fox AJ, et al. Dominant-hemisphere arteriovenous malformations: therapeutic embolization with isobutyl 2-Cyanoacrylate. AJNR 1983; 4:959–966.

TEMPORAL ARTERITIS AND VASCULITIS OF THE CENTRAL NERVOUS SYSTEM

HAROLD P. ADAMS, Jr., M.D.
JOSÉ BILLER, M.D.

TEMPORAL ARTERITIS

Temporal arteritis (giant cell arteritis) is a leading cause of preventable blindness in persons older than 55 years of age. Monocular or binocular visual loss results from granulomatous inflammation and reduced blood flow to the posterior ciliary arteries (anterior ischemic optic neuropathy) or, infrequently, the central retinal artery (retinal infarction.) Because loss of vision usually occurs suddenly and without warning, the diagnosis and treatment of patients with temporal arteritis is an ophthalmic emergency.

Patients with temporal arteritis usually reach a neurologist with a complaint of new onset temporal, occipital, or generalized headache. The likelihood of temporal arteritis increases if the patient also reports a low-grade fever, malaise, diffuse muscle aches or weakness, or jaw claudication. Other, less frequent neurologic symptoms are stroke, hearing loss, vertigo, diplopia, or peripheral neuropathy. Non-neurologic manifestations include limb claudication, scalp or tongue gangrene, angina pectoris, or myocardial infarction.

The general medical examination of most persons with temporal arteritis yields normal results. The superficial temporal artery may be normal or swollen, firm, nonpulsatile, or tender to palpation. Limb-girdle muscles are often sore on palpation or painful on movement. Signs of anterior ischemic optic neuropathy are diminished visual acuity, visual field defects, afferent pupillary response, a pale or swollen optic disk, or splinter retinal hemorrhages. Patients with central retinal artery infarction will have reduced visual acuity, visual field deficits, amaurotic pupillary response, and a pale retina with a red fovea (cherry red spot.)

The proposed evaluation of a patient with suspected temporal arteritis is outlined in Figure 1. The most important study is the Westergren erythrocyte sedimentation rate (ESR). Rarely, temporal arteritis is accompanied by a normal ESR, but usually the study is markedly elevated. The C-reactive protein (CRP), another acute phase reactant, provides complementary information and should be tested serially in all suspected cases of temporal arteritis. In addition, some patients will have a normocytic, normochromic anemia or leukocytosis. Other blood abnormalities that may occasionally be found are decreased serum albumin and elevated alpha-2-globulin fractions, alpha-2-glycoprotein, fibrinogen or von Willebrand's factor.

Patients with suspected temporal arteritis should have a long (2.5- to 4-cm) temporal artery biopsy on the symptomatic side to allow for adequate pathologic analysis. Serial sections should be done throughout the length of the specimen. Because the arteritis is segmental and skip areas are frequent, a negative biopsy by itself does not exclude the diagnosis. Sampling the contralateral artery may be useful in "negative" cases because the arteritis can be unilateral. Properly performed bilateral temporal artery biopsies have a sensitivity approaching 100 percent, and a unilateral biopsy has a sensitivity of 75 percent. Although arteriography might demonstrate segmental narrowing, which would help in selecting a biopsy site, it is rarely performed. Doppler ultrasonography may be used to localize an involved arterial segment.

Long-term daily administration of high doses of oral corticosteroids (usually prednisone) is the basis of therapy (see Fig. 1). Treatment is aimed at relief of symptoms and prevention of visual loss. Most visual complications occur within 12 weeks of diagnosis. Alternate-day corticosteroid therapy has not been effective. Corticosteroids should be prescribed immediately for any patient who has a presentation

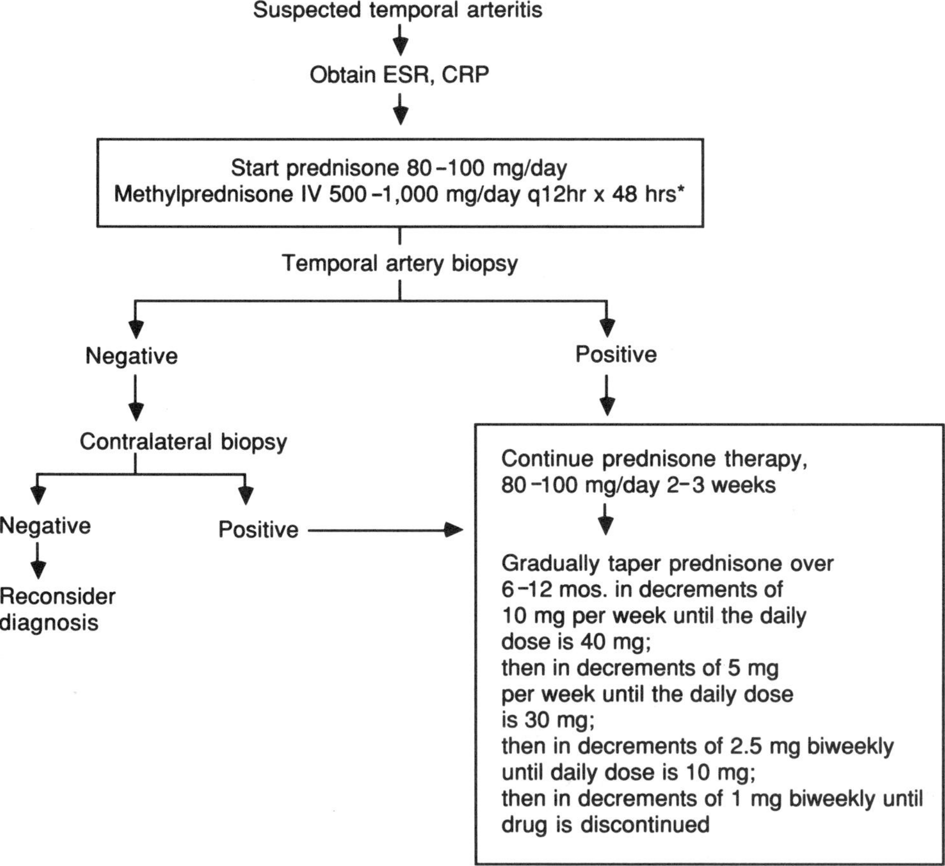

Figure 1 Evaluation of patients with suspected temporal arteritis.
* In the event of loss of vision.

compatible with temporal arteritis and should not be withheld pending the results of a temporal artery biopsy. The results of a biopsy will not be affected by a 1- to 2-day course of high-dose corticosteroid treatment, and the risk of blindness is greatest at the time of diagnosis. Because of the very high risk of complete blindness in patients with acute monocular visual loss or in those with impending visual loss of the contralateral eye, patients are admitted to the hospital and high-dose intravenous methylprednisone (1,000 mg every 12 to 24 hours) is administered for 2 days before the oral corticosteroids are instituted.

High-dose corticosteroids (80 to 100 mg prednisone per day) should be continued for at least 2 to 3 weeks and then gradually tapered pending the patient's response and the results of serial measurements on ESR and CRP (see Fig. 1). If a patient responds well to the treatment, the tapering of steroids will continue over several months. Most patients require 6 to 12 months of treatment, and in exceptional cases, may need medication for 2 to 3 years. The prednisone dose should be increased by an increment of 20 to 40 mg per day after any recurrence of symptoms or after there has been an increase in either the ESR or CRP. Although there is no absolute normal value of the ESR or CRP that can be used as a standard, a sudden jump from previously "normal" values for a particular patient should be considered a warning of reactivation of the arteritis. After the higher dose has been administered for 2 to 3 weeks, a taper can be reinstituted. Major adverse effects from corticosteroids may prompt consideration of therapy with dapsone, cyclophosphamide, or azathioprine. However, there is inadequate experience to determine the usefulness of these agents in the treatment of temporal arteritis.

CEREBRAL VASCULITIS COMPLICATING MULTISYSTEM AUTOIMMUNE DISEASES

Several noninfectious, multisystem inflammatory disorders can be complicated by cerebral vasculitis (Table 1). A variety of disorders, including infections, neoplasms, or idiosyncratic reactions to drugs can cause "vasculitis." However, these conditions, which may cause neurologic symptoms, are

Table 1 Disorders Complicated by Cerebral Vasculitis

Necrotizing Vasculitis
   Classic polyarteritis nodosa
   Churg-Strauss angiitis
   Necrotizing systemic vasculitis-overlap syndrome
   Wegener's granulomatosis

Vasculitis associated with collagen vascular disease
   SLE
   Rheumatoid arthritis
   Scleroderma

Giant cell vasculitis
   Takayasu's arteritis
   Temporal arteritis

Noninfectious granulomatous angiitis of the central nervous system

Table 2 Evaluation of a Patient with Suspected Cerebral Vasculitis

Serologic testing
  ESR
  CRP
  Antinuclear antibodies
    Antibody to single-stranded DNA
    Antibody to double-stranded DNA
  Rheumatoid factor
  Serum protein electrophoresis
  Serum immunoelectrophoresis
  Cardiolipin antibodies (IgG/IgA/IgM)
  Luetic serology
  C3, C4
  Granulocyte cytoplasmic antibody (Wegener's syndrome)
  Hepatitis B–surface antigen (polyarteritis nodosa)
  Coomb's test
Neurologic/biochemical evaluation
  Complete blood count
  Differential white blood cell count
  Platelet count
  Prothrombin time and partial thromboplastin time
  Bilirubin, AST, gamma GT
  BUN, creatinine
  Urinalysis
Tissue diagnosis/potential biopsy sites
  Skin
  Nasal mucosa
  Muscle
  Nerve
  Lung
  Kidney
  Brain/meningeal

AST = aspartate aminotransferase; BUN = blood urea nitrogen; GT = glutamyl transpeptidase.

beyond the scope of this chapter. The diagnosis of cerebral vasculitis is often inferential, based on clinical presentation, evidence of multisystem organ involvement, and abnormal serologic tests of blood. Caution should be exercised before attributing neurologic symptoms to cerebral vasculitis in a patient with multisystem vasculitis because they are often complicated by metabolic, hematologic, or cardiac disorders that result in brain dysfunction.

Most of the multisystem vasculitides have stereotyped, non-neurologic presentations. Neurologic symptoms are nonspecific and include headache, personality change, encephalopathy, seizures, intracranial hemorrhage, or ischemic stroke. Peripheral neuropathy or spinal cord dysfunction may also occur. Vasculitis is important in the differential diagnosis of stroke in children or young adults and is a cause of stroke that is accompanied by encephalopathy, fever, or unexplained skin lesions.

The evaluation of a patient with suspected cerebral vasculitis secondary to a multisystem disorder of altered immunologic activity is outlined in Table 2. Arteriography is an important component of the diagnostic evaluation, but because the vasculitis is often restricted to small-caliber or medium-caliber vessels, it may yield normal results. Arteriographic abnormalities include beading, segmental or tapered narrowing, microaneurysms, or occlusion. These changes are nonspecific and can be detected in a variety of arterial diseases including intracranial atherosclerosis. Cerebrospinal fluid examination may provide evidence of an inflammatory process. Brain and/or meningeal biopsy are needed for a definite diagnosis of cerebral vasculitis. Unfortunately, because the inflammatory process is often patchy, a random biopsy may yield false-negative results.

Because most physicians have treated only a few patients with cerebral vasculitis, no medical regimen has been established as useful for treating this condition secondary to a multisystem autoimmune disease. The variable natural history and myriad symptoms also hamper determination of any therapeutic response. In general, the condition of patients with cerebral vasculitis deteriorates if there is no treatment and the overall prognosis is poor.

Because the efficacy of some treatments for cerebral vasculitis is subject to dispute and because of major toxicities or side effects, major immunosuppressive drugs should not be prescribed unless there is (1) strong clinical evidence of a multisystem vasculitis and, usually, arteriographic evidence of cerebrovascular involvement, or (2) biopsy evidence of cerebral vasculitis.

The drug most commonly used for treatment of multisystem disorders caused by altered immunologic activity complicated by cerebral vasculitis is prednisone or cyclophosphamide. Prednisone is usually administered in an initial daily dose of 1 mg per kilogram. After 2 to 3 months, prednisone can then be converted to an alternate-day regimen. Thereafter, once the patient has improved, the dosage can gradually be tapered over 3 to 6 months. For critically ill patients, corticosteroid treatment may be instituted with intravenous methylprednisone.

Cyclophosphamide is initially given in a single daily dose of 2 mg per kilogram accompanied by large volumes of fluids in an effort to prevent urinary tract side effects. The dosage of cyclophosphamide is altered to maintain a white blood cell count of 3,000 to 3,500 per cubic millimeter and a neutrophil count of at least 1,000 to 1,500 per cubic millimeter. Maintenance therapy is continued for 6 to 12 months after complete remission. Thereafter, the dose can be tapered by decrements of 25 mg every 1 to 2 months.

Hemorrhagic stroke is the most common neurologic presentation of cerebral vasculitis with classic polyarteritis nodosa. Treatment usually consists of the use of prednisone combined with cyclophosphamide. Churg-Strauss angiitis is rarely complicated by neurologic involvement. High doses of prednisone are usually prescribed, while azathioprine or cyclophosphamide is used in resistant cases.

Neurologic complications of Wegener's granulomatosis are intraparenchymal or subarachnoid hemorrhage, arterial or venous thrombosis, cranial or peripheral neuropathy, and myopathy. In patients with these complications, cyclophosphamide is the drug of choice and treatment is usually initiated with an intravenous or oral dosage of 4 mg per kilogram for 2 to 3 days and then converted to a lower dosage of 2 mg per kilogram per day administered orally. Prednisone or azathioprine can be given to patients who cannot tolerate cyclophosphamide.

True immune complex–mediated cerebral vasculitis is an uncommon complication of systemic lupus erythematosus (SLE). Neurologic symptoms are more commonly the result of metabolic derangements. Cerebral infarction may result from thrombosis secondary to circulating anticoagulants or cardiolipin antibodies, or from embolism secondary to Libman-Sacks endocarditis. When diagnosed, cerebral vasculitis caused by SLE is treated with high doses of prednisone. The efficacy of either azathioprine or cyclophosphamide is difficult to ascertain. Rare cases of ischemic or hemorrhagic stroke may complicate cerebral vasculitis associated with rheumatoid arthritis. Cerebrovascular symptoms may also result from vertebral or basilar artery compression secondary to atlantoaxial subluxation or from thrombosis secondary to hyperviscosity. Cyclophosphamide appears to be the most useful drug for managing cerebral vasculitis complicating rheumatoid arthritis. While prednisone appears to be ineffective, penicillamine may be an alternative to cyclophosphamide.

Few patients with scleroderma develop cerebral vasculitis. These exceptional patients should be treated with prednisone. Takayasu's arteritis may lead to ischemia of the brain, eyes, face, or upper limbs. Prednisone may be helpful during the inflammatory phase of the disease.

NONINFECTIOUS GRANULOMATOUS ANGIITIS OF THE CENTRAL NERVOUS SYSTEM

Noninfectious granulomatous angiitis of the central nervous system is a rare granulomatous, necrotizing angiopathy with predominant or exclusive involvement of the central nervous system. Presentations include stroke, a mass lesion, or multifocal encephalopathy. Patients usually have normal blood serologic studies, an inflammatory response in the cerebrospinal fluid, and a segmental arterial narrowing on arteriography. Brain or leptomeningeal biopsy is the standard for diagnosis. Because of the focal nature of the angiitis, however, a negative biopsy does not preclude the diagnosis. In the absence of histologic confirmation, the diagnosis of granulomatous angiitis must be inferential. Early recognition and management are important because of the progressive and often fatal course of the disease. Therapy is based on long-term treatment with high doses of prednisone. Cyclophosphamide is added if the disease progresses or if the patient is steroid resistant.

SUGGESTED READING

Adel T, Andrews BS, Cunningham PH, et al. Rheumatoid vasculitis: effect of cyclophosphamide on the clinical course and levels of circulating immune complexes. Ann Int Med 1980; 43:407–413.

Elliot DL, Watts WJ, Reuler JB. Management of suspected temporal arteritis: a decision analysis. Med Decis Making 1983; 3:63–68.

Fauci AS, Katz P, Haynes BF, et al. Cyclophosphamide therapy for severe systemic necrotizing vasculitis. N Engl J Med 1979; 301:235–238.

Moore PM, Cupps TR. Neurological complications of vasculitis. Ann Neurol 1983; 14:155–167.

Rosenfeld SI, Kosmorsky GS, Klingle TG, et al. Treatment of temporal arteritis with ocular involvement. Am J Med 1986; 80:143–145.

TRAUMA

CLOSED HEAD INJURY

ANDRES M. SALAZAR, M.D., COL., M.C.

Traumatic brain injury (TBI) is currently the principal cause of death and disability in Americans younger than 35 years of age. It is estimated that a head injury occurs every 15 seconds in the United States; every 5 minutes one of these TBI victims will die and another will be permanently disabled. Because disabled TBI survivors are generally young and have a normal life span, the emotional and economic costs are staggering; the latter alone is estimated at $25 billion per year. Penetrating head injuries (PHIs) (gunshot wounds to the brain) are less common, with (30,000 occurring per year, but the incidence is rising and the overall fatality rate is much greater (40 to 50 percent) than for closed head injury. While the incidence of TBI is far greater than that of most common neurologic diseases, neurologists have traditionally shown little interest in it. Yet the background and training of neurologists are particularly well suited for dealing with TBI, not only in the postacute and chronic phases, but in the acute phase of injury as well.

The effects of so-called "minor" head injury have also received increasing attention from the neuroscientific and medical communities in recent years. Not only has permanent structural brain damage been documented pathologically after minor concussion in animals, but newer clinical techniques such as magnetic resonance imaging (MRI) and positron emission tomography (PET) have repeatedly shown structural and metabolic changes in humans that correlate with documented neurobehavioral changes after even very minor head injury without loss of consciousness. Partly as a result of such studies, the "postconcussion syndrome" is increasingly recognized by clinicians as resulting primarily from structural brain damage. The failure to recognize the causes of this syndrome and to institute proper, prompt management have almost invariably prolonged the resulting incapacitation and complicated the treatment severalfold. Given that minor head injury constitutes approximately three-quarters of all head injuries sustained in the United States, its economic and social impact are considerable.

PATHOGENESIS AND DIAGNOSIS

Although a detailed discussion of the pathogenesis and diagnosis of head injury is beyond the scope of this chapter, a brief review is warranted. An understanding of the various pathologic components of this condition is only now beginning to emerge, and is rapidly evolving; it is particularly important to the present-day management of the patient with head injury. First, it is important to realize that head injury is a dynamic process. Not only does the pathologic picture continue to evolve, often with devastating consequences, over the first few hours and days after an injury is sustained, but the physiologic and clinical aspects of the recovery process itself can continue for a period of years. Thus the notion of a "dynamic prognosis" is especially relevant to the patient with head injury. Over the past few decades, we have moved from conceptualizing closed head injury (CHI) in terms of hematomas and coup-contrecoup contusions to a three-level classification of the pathology that divides the injuries into three categories: (1) focal injury, (2) diffuse axonal injury (DAI), and (3) superimposed hypoxia/ischemia. More recently, diffuse microvascular injury with loss of autoregulation has been implicated as playing an important role in the acute stage of the injury. All of these pathologic features can be reproduced in animal models of acceleration-deceleration injury without impact.

Focal Injury

While focal contusions often occur under the site of impact and thus result in focal neurologic deficits referable to that area (e.g., aphasia, hemiparesis), by far the most common location is the orbitofrontal and anterior temporal lobes, where the brain abuts on bony edges. Thus a relatively typical pathologic and clinical picture is often seen in patients with CHI, and the most troubling clinical sequelae are usually behavioral and cognitive abnormalities referable to these areas of the brain. Usually caused by the rupture of bridging veins, hematomas are most common with rapid decelerations such as those which occur with falls and impact, especially in the elderly. Delayed hematomas, often within a contused area, are particularly important in the so-called "talk and die" patient, who may initially appear to be at low risk but then decompensates rapidly.

Diffuse Axonal Injury

DAI is probably the principal cause of persistent severe neurologic deficit in CHI today. It was initially conceptualized as a "shearing" injury of axons in the centrum semiovale, corpus callosum, and brain stem, and was characterized by axonal "retraction" balls microscopically in fatal cases. Recent work with animal models, however, shows that the typical pathology of DAI can be seen even after mild concussion and may not appear until 12 to 24 hours postinjury. The only early abnormality is a relatively subtle intra-axonal disruption on electron microscopy, with an intact axon sheath. This apparently leads to a disruption of axonal flow, accumulation of transport material proximal to the injury, and eventual severing of axons as a *secondary* phenomenon. One obvious clinical implication is that there may be a 12- to 24-hour window of therapeutic opportunity postinjury in which total axonal disruption may be prevented. Another important conclusion one can make from these studies is that DAI can be demonstrated even after minor head injury, thus providing one possible organic basis for the postconcussion syndrome and for the cumulative effects of repeated concussion, such as those seen in professional boxers. Interestingly, the pathology of dementia pugilistica includes neurofibrillary tangles (NFTs) but not Alzheimer plaques. NFTs associated with Alzheimer's disease have been postulated to result from abnormalities in axonal flow.

Diffuse Microvascular Damage

The pathology of hypoxia and/or ischemia includes border-zone necrosis and hippocampal changes; it has been well detailed elsewhere and will not be further discussed here. Diffuse microvascular damage, on the other hand, has been increasingly implicated as a major component of TBI. The vascular response appears to be biphasic. Depending on the severity of the trauma, early changes include an initial transient systemic hypertension (probably caused by massive release of catecholamines), an early loss of cerebrovascular autoregulation (decreased response to changes in CO_2, increased reactivity to circulating neurotransmitters), and a transient breakdown of the blood-brain barrier, (probably caused by endothelial changes). These changes result in a rapid swelling of perivascular astrocytes that peaks at approximately 1 hour postinjury but begins to recover by 6 hours. Somewhat later endothelial changes include the formation of intraluminal microvilli or blebs and craters, which peak at approximately 6 hours postinjury but can persist for as long as 6 days. The clinical significance of these intraluminal changes is still unclear, but may relate to the loss of autoregulation, to delayed edema, or to the delayed hyperemia with brain swelling that is often seen, especially in younger patients. Both cyclooxygenase inhibitors and oxygen-free radical scavengers prevent or reverse these arteriolar changes experimentally, suggesting that such drugs may come to play an important role in the management of TBI patients in the near future.

Secondary Injury

Delayed secondary injury at the cellular level has come to be recognized as a major contributor to the ultimate tissue loss that occurs after TBI. A cascade of physiologic, vascular, and biochemical events already alluded to is set in motion in injured tissue. This process involves a multitude of systems, including possible changes in neuropeptides, electrolytes such as calcium and magnesium, excitatory amino acids, arachidonic acid metabolites such as the prostaglandins and the leukotrienes, and the formation of oxygen-free radicals. Free iron, as found in contusions and hematomas, is particularly toxic, probably by catalyzing the formation of hydroxyl radicals. These products may result in progressive secondary injury to otherwise viable brain tissue through several mechanisms–e.g., by producing further ischemia or altering vascular reactivity, by producing brain swelling (edema or hyperemia), by injuring neurons and glia directly, or activating macrophages that result in such injury, or in the case of PHI, by establishing conditions favorable to secondary infection. In other words, much of the ultimate brain loss may be caused not by the injury itself, but by an uncontrolled vicious cycle of biochemical events set in motion by the trauma. The control of this complex cascade of cellular events remains one of the most important challenges in the acute management of head injury. As with DAI, it offers a potential therapeutic window of opportunity during which brain swelling and nerve cell death may be prevented during the first few hours after an injury has been sustained.

MANAGEMENT OF ACUTE TBI

Initial Evaluation and Resuscitation

An organized team approach to the acute management of the TBI patient is essential, from before the time the patient is admitted to the hospital through the time the patient enters the intensive care unit (ICU) and receives postacute care (Fig. 1). The cornerstone of early neurologic evaluation and care is the use of the Glasgow coma score (GCS), along with checks of lateralization and pupillary response. Such a simple, reproducible evaluation should be sufficient to determine whether the patient's condition is deteriorating and to identify the need for more specific interventions. A more detailed neurologic examination is probably not necessary until the patient is well stabilized in the ICU. Some system to record easily sequential changes in the GCS, pupils, and other vital parameters is an integral part of care. A history should be obtained from witnesses, particularly with regard to the onset of coma; an initial "lucid" or "semilucid" interval in a patient who later becomes comatose makes a diagnosis of severe diffuse axonal injury highly unlikely and that of hematomas or expanding contusions more likely.

The importance of cardiopulmonary resuscitation and management in trauma patients with acute head injury cannot be overstated; airway and shock management should be the top priority in the treatment of any trauma patient. Animal experiments have demonstrated that the traumatized brain is particularly sensitive to hypoxia/ischemia. Similarly, levels of hypercarbia tolerated by the normal brain may lead to critical marginal increases of intracranial pressure (ICP) in the patient with head injury. The majority of prehospital deaths after TBI are probably caused by vascular and/or respiratory failure, whether they are induced by initial anatomic or physiologic disruption of the brain stem or are a consequence of associated injuries not related to the central nervous system. Superimposed hypoxia/ischemia may be the single-most important predictor of ultimate outcome in patients with severe head injury. The importance of this aspect of care is highlighted by the marked improvements in survival achieved by emergency care systems into which early prehospital intubation and resuscitation have been incorporated.

Comatose TBI patients are often hypoxic or hypercarbic, even though they may appear to be ventilating normally. Comatose patients (GCS <8) should therefore be hyperventilated, via intubation if possible, to a Pco$_2$ of about 35. (This has the added advantage of decreasing lactic acidosis and can be maintained for several days, if necessary.) Hyperventilation at a lower level, however (i.e., to a Pco$_2$ of 25), should be avoided, although it can be used to control ICP for brief periods. Sedation with morphine, 4 to 12 mg IV every 2 to 4 hours, to prevent

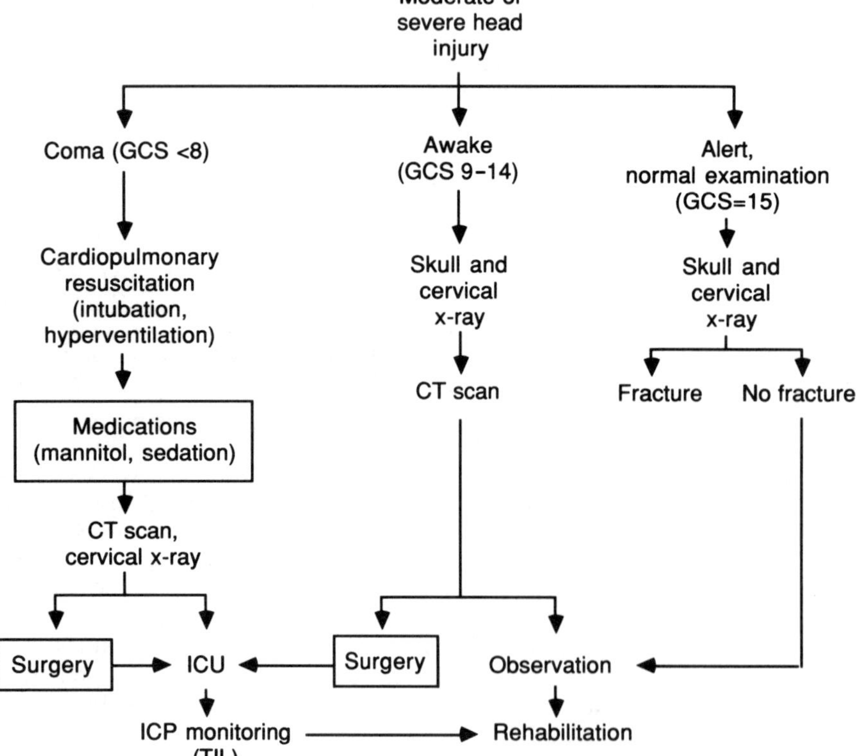

Figure 1 Management of closed head injury.

systemic hypertension, or paralysis with pancuronium bromide, 4 mg every 2 to 4 hours, should be used when necessary. The stomach should be emptied with a nasogastric tube to prevent emesis with aspiration. The head should be immobilized in the plane of the body, not only because of the possibility of associated cervical fracture (approximately 5 percent), but for airway maintenance and prevention of venous occlusion which might raise the ICP. Elevation of the head will further facilitate cranial venous return.

Shock is usually an indication of hemorrhage elsewhere, rather than a result of the head injury itself. Fluid resuscitation should rely on normal saline or Ringer's lactate solution, but TBI patients should not be overhydrated; central venous pressure should be monitored. Dextrose in water should be avoided, not only because it is hypotonic, but because of the potential for increased lactic acidosis and cerebral necrosis in the hypoxic and/or ischemic patient with hyperglycemia. For this reason, I also prefer to avoid early maintenance with dextrose solutions, although formal studies on this effect of dextrose solutions have not been done in patients with head injuries.

Laboratory tests should include a CBC, testing of electrolytes, glucose, arterial blood gases, blood alcohol, and liver, renal, and drug screens. In addition, because of the frequency of coagulopathies after TBI, we recommend evaluation with platelet count, prothrombin time (PT) and partial thromboplastin time (PTT), thrombin time, fibrinogen, and fibrinogen split products.

Radiologic Examination and Mass Lesions

Computed tomography (CT) has revolutionized the management of mass lesions in the patient with head injury, and when it is available, should be used in all patients with a GCS less than 13 ("does not obey commands") or when focal signs are present. CT is usually obtained as soon as possible after the patient has been resuscitated and stabilized. In the evacuation of hematomas, delays of more than 4 hours postinjury have been associated with a significant deterioration of the patient's condition. Comatose patients, however, must remain accompanied by a physician or critical care nurse; it is all too common to hear of a "stabilized" patient who suffers arrest or irreversible brain damage because of a simple airway problem that occurs while the patient is in the elevator on the way to the CT suite. Similarly, in the acute management of TBI, the usefulness of magnetic resonance imaging (MRI) is limited by the difficulty of managing the comatose patient in most present-day scanners.

In conscious patients experiencing mild confusion and who have no lateralizing signs, skull and cervical x-ray examinations and observation may be sufficient. However, a linear fracture as shown on the radiograph markedly increases the risk of a surgical lesion and is indication for CT, even in the alert TBI patient. In any case, it is imperative that one maintain a high index of suspicion for delayed hematomas or expanding intracerebral contusion. My bias at present is to be relatively aggressive in recommending surgical debridement of large, accessible expanding contusions. One recent study found that the large differences in the mortality rates of TBI patients of a variety of hospitals with different resources was accounted for not by the high-risk comatose ICU patients, but by patients who initially followed instructions and were considered to be at low risk, who later developed a mass effect.

Medical Therapy

Several drugs have been used to prevent secondary injury. Theoretically such drugs should be started as soon as possible after trauma. Mannitol is the most valuable of those presently available. In addition to its osmotic effect, it is also an oxygen-free radical scavenger. The usual initial dose for adults is 1 g per kilogram given in the emergency room. As long as the serum osmolarity is less than 310 mOsm per kilogram, patients are then administered 0.25-g boluses every 4 hours as necessary to control ICP. Some surgeons advocate the continued use of low-dose mannitol. Other diuretics such as furosemide are also used by some practitioners in specific situations.

The use of corticosteroids for acute TBI remains all too common. Approximately 42 percent of more than 1,000 neurosurgeons responding to a recent United States Army survey used steroids routinely in patients with head injuries. Nevertheless, repeated recent, well-conducted studies have failed to show that steroids at various doses have any benefit in acute TBI, and other studies have shown them to have a deleterious effect on the metabolism of the TBI patient. Consequently, I do not use steroids in the treatment of these patients.

Other promising medical approaches that are still in the experimental stage include the use of nonglucocorticoids such as the 21-amino steroids or "lazaroids" to inhibit lipid peroxidation; cyclooxygenase inhibitors such as indomethacin; superoxide dismutase with or without catalase and iron chelators to prevent or scavenge oxygen-free radicals; calcium antagonists; THAM to counter lactic acidosis; thyrotropin-releasing hormone (TRH) or naloxone analogs; or dextromethorphan hydrobromide or other NMDA receptor blockers.

Intensive Care Unit

Once a surgical mass lesion has been treated or excluded, the comatose patient should be managed in the ICU. The avoidance of secondary insults to the brain remains the principal goal of therapy. The principles of care and treatment used for the earlier stages of TBI are generally continued, but better monitoring is available. As before, organization, training, and adherence to relatively simple principles are the mainstay of care.

Although many physicians, in particular neurologists, may be reluctant to give up the neurologic examination as the principal measure of patient progress, recent studies suggest that the ICP, which is one determinant of cerebral perfusion pressure, is a more sensitive parameter. For example, the classic Cushing triad has been shown to occur less than 25 percent of the time in patients with an ICP greater than 30 mm Hg, a level that almost invariably proves fatal if not controlled. Yet it is much easier to prevent a rise to that level by treating the patient when the ICP is 15 mm Hg than it is to lower an ICP of 25 to 30 mm Hg. The ICP has repeatedly been shown to correlate significantly with outcome, and its monitoring is increasingly used in the care of the comatose TBI patient. In one recent study, the survival rate was 92 percent for patients whose ICP was controlled, as opposed to 17 percent for those whose ICP was not controlled. The particular monitoring technique used is determined by the neurosurgeon and by what facilities are available. Choices include an intraventricular catheter, a subarachnoid screw, or the more recent fiberoptic epidural transducers.

The relatively simple algorithm of the therapeutic intensity level (TIL) for treating increases in the ICP has the advantage of providing a standard measure of severity of ICP elevations in TBI patients (Table 1). It describes an orderly increase in therapeutic vigor from simple sedation through barbiturate coma. Although some measures such as sedation, hyperventilation, and administration of mannitol will have already been started in the emergency room, in general, each new level of therapy is instituted when the previous level has failed to keep the ICP at less than 20 mm Hg, and each is assigned a point value. The TIL score at any given point in time is the sum of the points for the interventions then in use. It should be emphasized, however, that using the TIL algorithm must not lull the physician into ignoring the possibility that progressive ICP elevations may also be caused by surgical lesions such as delayed hematoma, contusion with focal edema, or hydrocephalus. Similarly, seizures, hyponatremia, and airway problems raise the ICP.

Barbiturate coma has recently been shown to significantly improve outcome in patients younger than 45 years of age with otherwise uncontrolled ICP; it is the last step in the recommended nonsurgical control of ICP. In a recent large study, patients randomized to receive barbiturates were almost twice as likely to have a controlled ICP; in the ab-

Table 1 Management of Intracranial Pressure in Severe Head Injury: Therapeutic Intensity Level (TIL)*

Treatment	Dosage/Amount	TIL†
Sedation (morphine)		1
Paralysis (as needed) (pancuronium bromide)		1
Hyperventilation	P_{CO_2} >30	1
	P_{CO_2} <30 (for brief periods)	2
Ventricular drainage	<4 ml/hr	1
	>4 ml/hr	2
Mannitol	<1 g/kg/8 hrs	3
	>g/kg/8 hrs	6
Barbiturate coma (pentobarbital)	1	3

* Each new level is generally instituted when the previous level fails to control ICP below 15 to 20 mm Hg (see text).
† Minimum level = 0; maximum level = 15.

sence of cardiovascular complications, barbiturate therapy was more than five times as likely to control ICP than was nonbarbiturate therapy. Barbiturate coma is induced with pentobarbital at an initial loading dose of 10 mg per kilogram IV over 30 minutes. An additional 5 mg per kilogram is then given every hour for 3 hours, always with close monitoring of blood pressure. Serum levels should then be maintained at 3 to 4 mg percent at a dosage of approximately 1 mg per kilogram per hour. Barbiturate coma can be maintained for days, if necessary.

The overall risk of epilepsy in patients with CHI is relatively low: 2 to 5 percent overall, and approximately 11 percent for patients with severe CHI. Some studies, however, have shown a higher incidence in patients with hematoma (31 percent), depressed skull fracture (15 percent), or penetrating brain wounds (50 percent). In all cases, the risk decreases markedly as time passes. Although the risk of developing epilepsy after sustaining a PHI is still 25 times greater than it is for the normal age-matched population at 10 to 15 years postinjury, most patients with PHI can be 95 percent certain of remaining seizure-free if they have no seizures for the first 3 years postinjury.

There has been some confusion as to the role of anticonvulsants in the treatment of TBI. The most important reason for using these agents is to prevent seizures and secondary injury to the already fragile traumatized brain acutely. The second reason is hypothetical and is based on the experimental phenomenon of kindling; early anticonvulsants have been postulated to have an extended prophylactic effect on post-traumatic epilepsy. However, there is no good evidence at this time that the early use of phenytoin has any such prolonged prophylactic effect, although one recent, well controlled study suggests a protective effect during the 1st week postinjury only. Other anticonvulsants, including carbamazepine, need to be tested in this regard. Thus, in order to protect the traumatized brain, we recommend that anticonvulsants be used in high-risk CHI and PHI patients for several weeks only. Because of the sometimes subtle cognitive effects of phenytoin, however, we recommend switching patients to carbamazepine if they have had at least one seizure and require continued prophylaxis.

POSTACUTE AND LONG-TERM REHABILITATION AND CARE

The postacute care and rehabilitation of patients with head injury is an area that has traditionally been ignored by neurosurgeons and neurologists, specialists whose diagnostic skills and knowledge of the central nervous system could be particularly valuable in this important phase of management. Over the past few years, coincident with the growing involvement of third-party payors, the field of TBI rehabilitation has blossomed with a profusion of therapies such as coma stimulation, reality orientation, cognitive rehabilitation, speech therapy, occupational therapy, and recreation therapy. Yet their use has been largely empirical, and there has been a paucity of scientific validation for these sometimes expensive interventions (including comparison with minimal care, supportive models). The most important present-day challenge in the field is the development of reproducible, universally accepted measures of function and ultimate outcome with which to compare and refine various interventions.

Perhaps the most encouraging aspect of recovery is the amazing ability of the young adult brain to compensate naturally for many aspects of injury. Disabilities such as hemiparesis, seizures, and certain language disorders may appear more dramatic initially, but the most devastating long-term impairments are the cognitive and, in particular, the attentional and behavioral deficits that often persist after TBI. The goal of therapy should be the independence and community reintegration of the patient within his or her limits, rather than the specialized treatment of specific deficits simply because "they are there." All too often, scarce resources are used up during the early acute and postacute phases for the evaluation and therapy of deficits that will improve anyway or which are of marginal significance to the ultimate goal of independence. Some therapies may actually be counterproductive by fostering continued dependence on the therapy. Interventions that may be more cost-effective, such as training in decision making and specific community reintegration skills and certain forms of behavioral modification, may end up being omitted.

Third-party payors and rehabilitation facilities have increasingly turned to the use of "case managers" or "care managers" in this field. The care manager is a physician or health care professional who is responsible for the integration of various modalities of care and the allocation of resources for the patient with head injury. One of the principal roles of the neurologist or neurosurgeon should be to help place the entire rehabilitation process on a firm footing by providing care managers with an accurate pathologic diagnosis (i.e., DAI, focal contusions, and hypoxia and/or ischemia) and an *ongoing* assessment of status and prognosis in terms that are useful to the entire rehabilitation team. In addition to the history and examination, MRI may be especially useful at this stage by showing clinically significant focal contusions missed on CT. Somatosensory-evoked potentials correlate with outcome and may prove helpful in defining the extent of the DAI. Particular attention should be paid to input from family and attendants who spend much time with the patient. No less important is the identification of neurologic complications such as delayed hematoma or hydrocephalus, and the monitoring of other medical conditions and medications that may be impacting on recovery.

Psychometric testing is an important part of the evaluation but is of very limited value in the treatment of the confused patient and should be focused on the measurement of expected deficits for guiding therapy and evaluating progress (attentional deficits, post-traumatic amnesia), rather than on the standard batteries that are used to confirm anatomic deficits already identified on MRI and which include cognitive domains of little practical interest to the case.

Pharmacologic intervention at this stage of care remains an area of great interest, but the sensitivity of the traumatized brain or of the confused patient to medication must always be considered, and treatment must be tailored to each individual. Overmedication with anticonvulsants, sedatives, or stimulants is more often a problem than not; in confused patients, paradoxical responses to sedation are particularly common. Nevertheless, judicious use of adequate sedation can help re-establish sleep-wake cycles; and methylphenidate hydrochloride (Ritalin), dextroamphetamine, or bromocriptine may be useful as adjuncts in the management of the lethargic or apathetic patient. Recent unconfirmed studies have suggested that the combination of dextroamphetamine with physical therapy during the early phases of rehabilitation can improve ultimate motor scores. Finally, carbamazepine is beginning to emerge as a possible useful adjunct in the management of certain behavioral problems.

"Minor" Head Injury

One group of patients that has been mismanaged frequently in the past is that with so-called "minor" head injury. The most important element in the management of these patients is the recognition that there is usually an organic, pathologic basis for their complaints, at least during the early postinjury period, and that it usually resolves over a few months. If mismanaged, however, these patients often develop an overlying neurosis that makes evaluation and management infinitely more difficult. There is nothing more frustrating to the intelligent minor head injury victim than to be told by his physician, his family, and his employer that there is "nothing wrong." Proper counseling should therefore include not only the patient, but also the family, school, or employer. Early in the course of treatment, MRI, auditory-evoked potentials, and specific neuropsychologic tests such as choice reaction time can help delineate the deficits.

The basic elements of the postconcussion syndrome are cognitive, somatic, and affective. Clinically significant neuropsychologic impairments have been documented repeatedly, even after minor "dings" without loss of consciousness. In one large recent study, the most frequent somatic complaints were headache (71 percent), decreased energy or fatigue (60 percent), and dizziness (53 percent), all of which markedly improved at 3 months. The proper management of the "fatigue" element is a major factor in recovery which may relate to orbitofrontal injury and which requires the cooperation of the school or employer. We suggest a graded return to a full work load over a period of 4 to 8 weeks.

PATIENT RESOURCE

National Head Injury Foundation, Inc.
P.O. Box 567
Framingham, MA 01701
Telephone: (617) 879-7473

POSTCONCUSSIONAL SYNDROME

BARRY GORDON, M.D., Ph.D.

DEFINITION, PATHOPHYSIOLOGY, AND CLINICAL COURSE

Postconcussional syndrome (PCS) describes the clusters of symptoms that frequently occur after minor closed head injury or other causes of head acceleration-deceleration. PCS is somewhat misleadingly named. An individual need not have had a concussion to develop PCS. No loss of consciousness or temporary lapse of cerebral function is necessary. Any sufficient blow, fall, or acceleration-deceleration movement of the head (such as whiplash) can cause PCS. Nor is PCS a single syndrome. Instead, it represents the co-occurrence of a variable mixture of symptoms caused by distinct underlying problems (Table 1). Although different combinations of these symptoms appear in different individuals, overall, headache, fatigue, and dizziness are the most common symptoms.

PCS is not usually a nonorganic "compensation neurosis" or "accident neurosis," or frank malingering. Many of the symptoms of PCS can be plausibly related to organic pathology. This has been established by animal studies, occasional human clinicopathologic correlations, and human clinical research. Although exact correlations are uncertain, it does appear that different types of injury give rise to different types of lesions, which in turn may have characteristic symptomatology (Table 2).

Table 1 Symptoms of Postconcussional Syndrome*

Headaches
Blurred vision
Double vision
Dizziness
Unsteadiness
Vertigo
Poor coordination
Neck pain, aching, stiffness
Slowed thinking
Effortful thinking
Difficulty concentrating
Difficulty sustaining concentration
Inability to divide attention
Distractibility
Sensitivity to noise
Increased sensitivity to lack of sleep, fatigue, stress
Increased sensitivity to drugs, alcohol
Poor memory (new learning)
Poor memory (recall of old information, such as names)
Lack of energy
Decreased drive or initiative
Easy fatigability
Depression
Anxiety
Poor appetite
Emotional lability
Irritability
Impatience
Loss of libido

*Symptom checklist. These include both primary and secondary symptoms of PCS.

Table 2 Clinicopathologic Consequences of Mechanical Injury

Nature of Force	Type of Injury	Site(s)	Symptoms
Acceleration-deceleration (esp. rotational)	Diffuse axonal injury (axonal shearing, tears)	Midbrain Superior cerebellar peduncles Corpus callosum Central white matter	Loss of consciousness Impaired concentration, ataxia
	Cortical contusions	Site of injury (coup) Opposite side (contrecoup) Bilateral but asymmetric	
		Frontal lobes	Distractibility
		Polar, orbital	Personality change
		Temporal lobes	
		Anterior pole	
		Lateral	
		Inferior	
Acceleration-deceleration		Labyrinth Cervical mechanoreceptors Central vestibular connections	Dizziness, vertigo, unsteadiness in space
Acceleration-deceleration	Stretch, strain	Blood vessels Sympathetic vasoregulatory systems (also, 2° to structural effects)	Headache
		Cervical ligaments Cervical muscles Cervical spine	Neck aches, pain, dizziness
Impact trauma			

As expected, in minor head trauma, there is a rough proportionality between the severity of the mechanical injury and the severity of the resulting tissue injury. A sufficiently small mechanical force will be buffered enough so that the brain escapes injury. However, once a force is great enough to cause unconsciousness, the duration of unconsciousness, whether momentary or as long as 20 minutes, seems to have little relation to the incidence and severity of any subsequent PCS.

Psychic problems can result from the mechanical injury as well. Some of the psychic components of the PCS may well prove to have a primary, organic basis; irritability and decreased drive are perhaps among the most likely candidates. However, many problems are secondary, a reaction to the primary impairments and to the disruptions they have caused. Patients develop an understandable sense of anxiety, depression, frustration, hopelessness, irritability, and a tendency toward withdrawal. These may be aggravated by misinformation and inaccurate expectations. Patients may be misleadingly told their brains are irreversibly damaged or that every problem of daily living can be blamed on their injury.

After the injury, several days may pass before headaches, dizziness, and vertigo become apparent; it may take days to weeks for anxiety, depression, and irritability to appear. The frequency and time course of recovery are still debated in the literature. However, it appears that in most patients (>70 percent) and perhaps in the vast majority of those with uncomplicated head injury, problems resolve within 3 months, and often sooner. In those individuals with longer-lasting problems, improvement can still occur within months and even 1 to 2 years or more after the injury is sustained.

Some of these patients with persisting problems may represent those with more significant injury, while some may simply have greater biologic susceptibility. In others, recovery is delayed because of emotional reactions to the disruptions the injury has caused. This situation does not as a rule resolve when any legal or compensation issues are settled. Psychological stress caused by reaction to the other components of PCS is one of the major causes of the persisting disability that can occur.

Prior head injury also increases the likelihood of more severe, longer-lasting problems. Alcohol or drug abuse compounds the problems and may even aggravate them.

PREREQUISITES FOR TREATMENT

Time is generally the best healer for patients with PCS, and for some, the only effective one. The physician's task in treating PCS is threefold: (1) to make an accurate diagnosis; (2) to educate the patient about his condition so that he or she can better cope with it while it resolves (and also so that he or she can resist external influences that may magnify the problems); and (3) to treat symptoms when possible and to suggest ways in which the patient may mitigate the effects of those that cannot be treated.

History

The patient's own recollection of the injury is often suspect; corroboration is necessary from witnesses and from the early observations of the ambulance crew and emergency room team. Pertinent questions include the following: What was struck and how? Was the patient unconscious? If so, for how long? If the patient could not remember new events after the injury (post-traumatic amnesia), how long did it take for connected, day-to-day memory to return? (The latter is the usual measure of the duration of post-traumatic amnesia.) What are the patient's symptoms, and how did they evolve? What was done to diagnose the condition (e.g., skull x-ray examination, computed tomography [CT], magnetic resonance imaging [MRI], or electroencephalography [EEG])? Does the patient have any predisposing factors (prior head injury, a history of drug or alcohol abuse)?

It is also critical to understand the patient's mental state and social and emotional environment. What is the patient's understanding of his or her condition? What has the patient been told (by concerned friends as well as by health professionals)? What does he or she think is "going wrong?" Does the patient believe he or she is crazy? (Not infrequently, patients will start recounting their problems with, "I know you won't believe me, but. . . .") What are the patient's expectations regarding recovery? Has he or she set a timetable to go back to work? What does the patient's employer and/or family expect from him or her? (A professional can often delegate or defer the demands of his job; a blue-collar worker usually cannot.)

I have patients complete an extensive written history before their visit or in the waiting room. This includes a history of present illness, a symptom checklist (see Table 1), a past medical history, an education and employment history, and a mood assessment. This questionnaire gives the patients a chance to organize their thoughts and to tap other sources (such as their family) for information they may not remember. It also gives them a chance to checklist a detailed review of symptoms and expand on positive areas. During the direct interview, this information is rechecked and augmented as necessary.

An accurate history may support the diagnosis of PCS by establishing the occurrence of a significant head injury and early symptoms and signs. Conversely, some patients presenting with what at first seems like PCS may never have had a head injury or only truly trivial mechanical taps. Other etiologies should be suspected in these patients.

Physical and Laboratory Examinations

The basic rule of the physical and laboratory examinations is that the earlier they are performed, the more likely they are to confirm evidence of organic impairments. Although it may not be crucial to document physical abnormalities, it is often useful to do so. Patients will thus have reassuring confirmation that they are not imagining their symptoms. This may be equally reassuring for their physicians, since the symptoms of PCS are so subjective and subtle. Also, it is useful to perform an evaluation early to rule out other conditions, such as intracranial hematomas (for which there is a risk of approximately 3 percent). Finally, since a large percentage of cases raise legal questions regarding the nature and extent of the injury, the objective evaluation is often more persuasive evidence than the patient's subjective complaints.

The neurologic examination of these patients should include mental status testing, testing of extraocular movements and vestibulo-ocular suppression, and the Bárány maneuver. I obtain an MRI in essentially all patients. CT is less sensitive for demonstrating the direct results of injury, although it is still a good screen for other conditions. For those patients with complaints of blurring of vision, dizziness, vertigo, and unsteadiness or ataxia, I recommend vestibular function testing (including testing for visual fixation suppression of the vestibulo-ocular reflex) and brain stem auditory–evoked responses (BAERs).

For patients who complain of impaired attention and/or concentration, slowness of thinking, poor memory, or other mental complaints, I recommend a formal neuropsychologic examination. The main purpose of the neuropsychologic testing is to distinguish the deficits directly related to the injury from those caused by depression and anxiety. Less commonly, the testing helps establish malingering or a nonorganic cause for the patient's distress. Such would be the case, for example, if the patient claims near-total memory loss, yet is found to be deliberately choosing the wrong answers on memory tests. The testing is also useful in providing a baseline, should the patient's symptomatology worsen. It is worth noting that because the primary deficits expected from PCS are relatively subtle changes in attention and/or concentration, new learning ability, word retrieval, and judgment, valid problems may not register on the testing. Also, many of the complaints of PCS, such as difficulty with divided attention, are not well tested by current clinical examinations. In this case, a negative examination cannot count as evidence against there being an organic cause of the patient's symptoms.

Although regional cerebral metabolism and/or blood flow measurements may prove to have clinical utility in the study of PCS patients, at present they are still experimental tools. Because of uncertain standards for normalcy, brain electrical activity mapping (BEAM) and long latency cognitive–evoked potentials (P300's and similar measures) are not yet clinically useful in any individual patient. Thermography may be useful in making the subjective complaint of headache more plausible.

TREATMENT OPTIONS

I use the approach to evaluation and treatment of PCS outlined in Figure 1.

Patient Education

Patients are typically bewildered by their condition. Their overt injury was mild and their bruises are disappearing, but they are plagued by headaches, a lack of energy, dizziness, and an inability to concentrate or to handle their usual schedule. It is not surprising that patients are frequently frustrated and angry with themselves and their medical care.

After I am convinced that I am dealing with

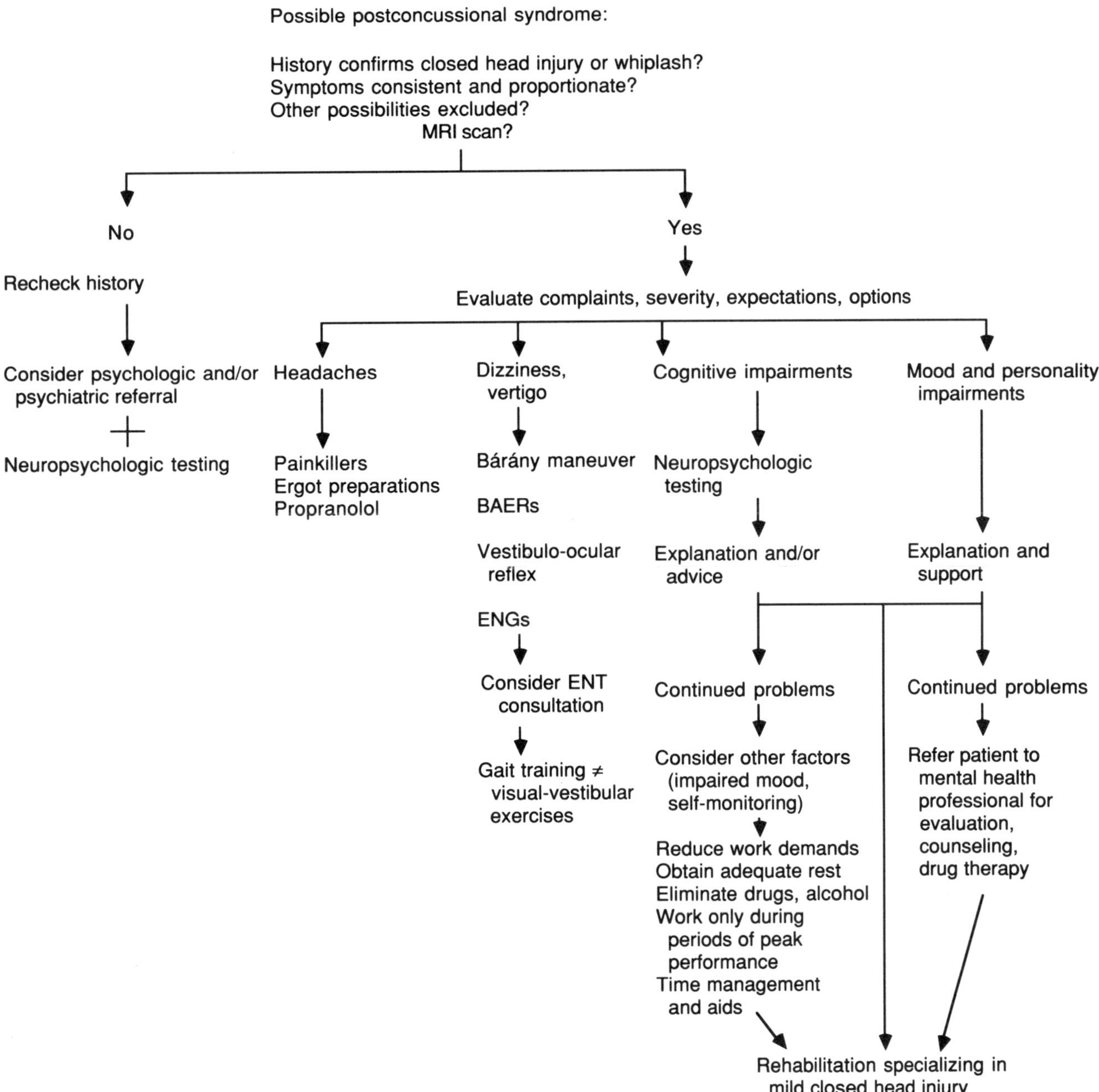

Figure 1 Evaluation and treatment of PCS.

PCS, I have found that it helps to explain to patients what has happened to them, how their apparently disparate complaints may have a single pathophysiologic explanation, and that although almost everybody recovers, the recovery usually takes longer (weeks to months) than the patient would expect.

Headache, Dizziness, and Vertigo

The headache of PCS may not have many characteristics of vascular headache, but most of these headaches are probably the result of vascular causes. Many respond to treatment with simple painkillers. Those with clearly defined onsets may be aborted by ergot preparations (ergotamine tartrate) (Ergostat, Ergomar). More frequent or more continuous headaches may respond to propranolol (Inderal) and other beta-blockers, or to antidepressants. (A more detailed strategy for treating headache is discussed elsewhere in this book.)

Dizziness and vertigo arise from several different sources in PCS. Unfortunately, the dizziness and vertigo of PCS are often highly resistant to therapy. Drugs such as meclizine 12.5 to 25 mg twice per day or three times per day can be tried, although these are usually not helpful. Gait training and visual-vestibular exercises may help promote adaptation. (A detailed treatment plan is discussed elsewhere in this book.)

Impaired Mentation

Therapy begins by cataloging what the patient must accomplish and what problem(s) he seems to be having. Typically, the patient himself is aware that he is not functioning as efficiently, that it takes him longer to do his work, and that he cannot juggle as many projects as he once could. Frequently there is also increased sensitivity to stress or fatigue. Often, these failings are subjective only; no one else has noticed them. But because they are no less real, the patient needs to be reassured that his perceptions are plausible if the physician believes they are.

Although the cognitive impairments cannot yet be directly treated, often patients have several of the following contributory problems.

Mood Impairments

Thinking is never as smooth when one is frustrated, angry, depressed, and irritable. I question patients about any similar prior mood problems. Based on their past experience, they may appreciate how much of their mental impairment is due to their mood per se. It often relieves them to understand that their current mood with its share of problems will pass, just as previous episodes did. More serious problems require professional referral (see below).

Excessive Self-Monitoring

Normally, thinking and speaking are done without much self-consciousness. If too much attention is given to monitoring what is being done, performance suffers because resources are diverted, and the normal pacing of mental operations is disrupted. (Public speaking is a good example.) Self-consciousness in thinking and speaking is common in patients with PCS, and a frequent cause of further disruption. Sometimes, patients become so wary of making errors, they set too high a standard. For example, they may remember someone's name, but since they are not *completely* sure, they will not say it.

For many patients, it is enough for the clinician to point out that their self-monitoring does not help their condition, but rather is itself a cause of the problem. Even those patients who cannot stop monitoring and doubting themselves can be reassured that the problems related to speech and thinking are not the result of direct brain malfunction; this component of their problem can be transient.

After these approaches have been considered, there are several work-around strategies for the cognitive deficits: optimizing the patient's mental capacity, increasing his or her efficiency with time management and mechanical aids, and reducing the demands on him or her during this period.

Optimizing Mental Capacity

Everyone has good and bad days, and many people know their periods of peak performance (morning, afternoon, or evening). It is no surprise that mentation is less efficient when an individual is tired or stressed, and this is frequently magnified in patients with PCS. Ideally, then, patients with PCS should try to get enough rest (both physical and mental). They should also try to engage in important or difficult work during their periods of maximal competency only. Again, professionals are generally better able to rearrange their work schedules than are blue-collar workers.

Increasing Work Efficiency

Time management techniques can be as useful for the patient with PCS as they are for others. Small pocket notebooks and appointment books can also be tried. An electronic watch with a reminder alarm is another inexpensive (approximately $15 to $50) adjunct. More complicated electronic notebooks (such as Casio's SF-4000 Digital Diary [$89] and its larger version, the Business Organizer Scheduling System [about $270]) are available. It must be realized, however, that using any of these strategies and tools demands self-discipline, which is often harder to enforce in PCS patients than it would be otherwise.

Reducing Demands

Since the patient's mental abilities are temporarily reduced, it makes sense to try to reduce his need for these abilities. Professionals in particular can often reduce their work load (if they absolutely have to), spread it out over longer periods of time (for example, work at a more leisurely pace into evenings or weekends), or delegate it.

Depression and Other Psychic Complaints

In most of my patients, depression and other psychic complaints are annoying but relatively mild. They often respond well to an explanation, and many of these patients eschew drug therapy. If drug therapy or psychotherapy is warranted, I prefer to refer this aspect of care to a psychiatrist, psychologist, or other mental health professional. In making the referral, it is important to convey an accurate impression of your assessment of what is structural and what is secondary in your patient. Since many consultants will not be able to evaluate the primary data, there is a danger that they may overemphasize the brain injury or, conversely, magnify the role of the psychic factors. Psychiatric referral is particularly warranted when complaints appear late, since those individuals in whom this occurs are the most likely to be suffering from marked depression and the real or imagined consequences of their injury.

Other Options

Drugs such as Inderal or carbamazepine (Tegretol) have been claimed to ameliorate the irritability or anxiety of patients with closed head injury. Since there is little or no statistical evidence for this, I do not prescribe these agents for this purpose.

Many centers now have specialized cognitive rehabilitation programs for patients with mild head injury. Referral to such centers is indicated for the patient with persisting problems, in large part because they provide emotional and psychiatric support. Patients should not expect these centers to alleviate primary symptoms directly (although these will often get better over time), since there is not yet any scientific proof that such programs benefit these. If such a program is available, early referral is usually warranted. If the program is *not* geared for mild cases, there is a risk that patients with mild head injury will experience demoralization and embarrassment from being around those with far more serious handicaps. Cost is also a concern.

SUGGESTED READING

Auerbach SH. Neuroanatomical correlates of attention and memory disorders in traumatic brain injury: an application of neurobehavioral subtypes. J Head Trauma Rehab 1986; 1:1–12.

Levin HS, Eisenberg HM, Benton AL. Mild head injury. New York: Oxford University Press, 1989.

Levin HS, Grafman J, Eisenberg HM. Neurobehavioral recovery from head injury. New York: Oxford University Press, 1987.

PATIENT RESOURCES

The National Head Injury Foundation, Inc.
333 Turnpike Road
Southborough, Massachusetts 01772
Telephone: (617) 485-9950

The National Head Injury Foundation is a full-service organization dedicated to serving as an informational clearing house, support group, and advocate for those with head injury. There are many active state chapters, which may have support groups for individuals with PCS. The NHIF offers several articles of special interest for PCS patients from their catalog of more than 250 items, such as:

"Disability Caused by Minor Head Injury" (C #81-001, $1.50)
"Minor Head Injury in Children—Out of Sight But . . ." (#83-003, $1.00)
"Postconcussional Symptoms and Syndrome" (#81-003, $1.00)
"Persisting Symptoms after Mild Head Injury" (#85-007, $8.00)
"Post-Concussion Syndrome" (#82-001, $1.00)

SPINAL INJURY

DAN S. HEFFEZ, M.D., FRCS

Injuries to the spinal cord and column are tragically common causes of morbidity and mortality among young and active people. The majority of these injuries are caused by motor vehicle accidents, often as a consequence of drug or alcohol intoxication. Especially among teenagers, spinal injuries may be related to sports such as wrestling, diving, and football. As spinal injuries disable more often than kill, the cost in terms of medical expenditure and lost potential is enormous. In this chapter, I deal exclusively with the general principles of the treatment of patients with spinal injuries.

The three principle goals of therapy in all cases are:

1. Prevention of additional neurologic injury by immobilization of the spine.
2. Reduction of fracture dislocations to allow for possible recovery of existing neurologic

deficits caused by spinal cord or nerve root compression.

3. Maintenance of skeletal realignment by internal or external fixation to promote bony healing.

Until the initial evaluation of the spine is complete, the patient is kept immobilized on a spinal board. The neck is further immobilized with a rigid collar or sandbags. In the case of the multiple trauma victim, attention is paid first to the life-threatening injuries and appropriate trauma resuscitation measures are instituted. If tracheal intubation is required for securing the airway, nasotracheal intubation is performed so that the cervical spine is not moved. Intravenous access is secured and infusion of crystalloid, usually Ringer's lactate or 0.5 N saline, is begun.

The evaluation of the spine begins with the neurologic examination. In the alert cooperative patient, the history is of great value; complaints of spinal pain and subjective neurologic deficits should be noted. In addition, external evidence of trauma to the face or forehead, chest or abdomen will implicate the likely level of injury. This is of particular importance in the patient who is intoxicated and uncooperative. Motor and sensory examination of the upper and lower limbs is performed. The pattern of neurologic injury is carefully noted, as this often guides the radiologic investigation. The neurologic examination may suggest a central cord syndrome, a Brown-Séquard hemisection, an anterior spinal artery syndrome, involvement of the cauda equina or conus medullaris or may indicate a deficit limited to a single nerve root. Alternatively, the patient may be paraplegic or quadriplegic, in which case the level of preserved function will suggest the approximate level of injury. Anal tone, the anal wink reflex, and the abdominal cutaneous reflexes are tested. Horner's syndrome is noted.

Once the neurologic condition has been determined, the radiologic investigation is initiated. In all cases of trauma, anteroposterior and lateral cervical roentgenography is performed. If the entire cervical spine from the cranio-cervical junction to the first thoracic vertebra is visualized, no additional films are required unless a cervical injury is suspected based on the clinical examination. In heavy or muscular individuals, the arms must often be pulled down in order to prevent the shoulders from obscuring the view of the cervicothoracic junction. If this fails, a swimmer's view, taken through the axilla with the patient's aim over his or her head, will usually visualize the C-7 to T-1 level.

CERVICAL INJURY

If cervical spine injury is suspected, a more detailed roentgenologic evaluation includes oblique views and an open-mouth view of the odontoid process. If no abnormality is diagnosed, dynamic flexion and extension x-ray examinations are performed to exclude instability caused by ligamentous injury. If no motion can be detected, the cervical spine is considered stable. If the patient is neurologically intact, spinal injury has been safely excluded. The presence of a neurologic deficit in the absence of a radiologic abnormality occurs in as many as 67 percent of children younger than 10 years of age who suffer spinal injury. In the pediatric population, injury is attributed to transient subluxation of the hypermobile bony spine. These children are treated by protecting the neck with a rigid external orthosis for 6 to 8 weeks. A similar situation is encountered in the adult patient with cervical spondylosis who suffers a hyperextension injury. Hyperextension reduces the anteroposterior diameter of the spinal canal that is already encroached upon by spondylotic bars; this results in spinal cord contusion. The neurologic findings in these patients usually indicate a central cord syndrome. In such cases, I prefer to exclude spinal cord compression by performing computed tomography (CT) before confirming spinal stability with dynamic x-ray examination. The neck is then protected by the use of an external orthosis such as a two-poster brace. The neurologic deficits, which often principally involve the upper limbs, usually improve. Semi-elective CT myelography or magnetic resonance imaging (MRI) is indicated to evaluate spinal cord and canal anatomy, as these patients usually require an elective anterior or posterior cervical decompression to reduce the risk of future injury.

If an unstable fracture such as a severe vertebral body burst or a facet subluxation or dislocation is diagnosed, no dynamic x-ray examination is performed. The patient is transferred on the spinal board to a rotating wedge frame, and Gardner-Wells tongs are applied. Weights are applied for traction in order to immobilize the spine and bring it into alignment. Weight is added in an incremental fashion and lateral cervical radiographs obtained after the addition of each increment to confirm alignment. Closed reduction can be facilitated by the use of muscle relaxants such as diazepam. If alignment can be achieved through this means of closed reduction, attention is paid to the need for additional investigation using CT, CT myelography, or MRI. In general, these tests are advised in order to exclude ongoing spinal cord or nerve root compression by retropulsed bone, disc, or (in the younger patient) cartilaginous end plate. These investigations are particularly important in the patient with a partial neurologic injury, as the presence of ongoing spinal cord compression necessitates a decompressive procedure. Standard laminectomy is seldom indicated; anterior cervical decompression by discectomy or vertebrectomy with arthrodesis using autologous or bank bone is more appropriate since spinal cord compression is usually ventral. Because the spine is further destabilized by this procedure, a posterior cervical fusion is recommended in order to allow for prompt mobilization of the patient. Alternatively, external immobilization can be achieved with a halo orthosis worn for 3 to 6 months. If closed reduction fails, open surgical reduction followed by arthrodesis with bone and wire is required. After recovery from the surgery the patient can be mobilized and aggressive rehabilitation initiated.

THORACIC, THORACOLUMBAR, AND LUMBAR INJURIES

Unlike the cervical or lumbar spine and thoracolumbar junction, the upper thoracic and midthoracic spine are stabilized by the chest wall. Fractures may be stable or unstable. The diagnosis of the exact nature of the fracture can be made by standard lateral and anteroposterior roentgenograms. Unenhanced CT scans of the spine supplemented by three-dimensional and sagittal reconstruction are necessary to assess the degree of canal compromise and the need for surgical decompression. Anterior wedge compression fractures and stable burst fractures should be treated with bedrest and analgesics followed by immobilization in a rigid orthosis such as a thoracolumbar-sacral orthosis (TLSO) for 3 to 6 months. If multiple vertebral levels are involved, especially at the cervicothoracic junction, a progressive kyphosis may develop, ultimately leading to spinal cord compression. Under such circumstances, a posterior stabilization with Harrington instrumentation is indicated. An unstable burst fracture is one in which severe vertebral body compression ($>$40 percent) is associated with disruption of the posterior spinal elements. This injury as well as the flexion distraction and flexion rotation injury are highly unstable. Stabilization by internal fixation to allow for prompt patient mobilization is the treatment of choice. If the posterior longitudinal ligament is believed to be intact, posterior spinal instrumentation can be used to correct any kyphosis and reduce retropulsed bone fragments. If repeat CT myelography performed immediately postoperatively demonstrates persistent spinal cord compression, a transthoracic anterior decompression by vertebrectomy, discectomy, and fusion is indicated.

Spinal injuries of the thoracolumbar junction and lumbar spine are frequently unstable and are associated with neurologic injury to the cauda equina and/or conus medullaris. With the exception of simple wedge compression fractures, these injuries should be treated by operative stabilization. An anterolateral retroperitoneal or posterior approach is chosen, depending on the need for decompression of the neural structures. As with upper thoracic injuries, posterior instrumentation can often realign the spine and promote the reduction of retropulsed bone fragments. Follow-up CT is necessary to confirm neural decompression. If this has not been achieved, retroperitoneal exploration is indicated. If, based on the radiographic studies, anterior decompression and fusion alone are prescribed, external immobilization is necessary until solid bony union is demonstrated on standard roentgenograms.

MEDICAL TREATMENT

Medical management of the *acute* spinal injury patient takes place in an intensive care setting.

During the early treatment of the spinal injury patient, especially those who are quadriplegic or high-level paraplegic, special attention must be paid to cardiopulmonary instability. Hypoventilation is likely if respiration is entirely diaphragmatic. Aggressive chest physical therapy is instituted to minimize atelectasis and prevent pneumonia. Nasotracheal intubation and mechanical ventilation may be indicated. Cardiovascular instability, which results from the interruption of sympathetic outflow after a high cervical injury, may persist for 2 to 3 weeks. If bradycardia results in hypotension, treatment with atropine is indicated. If hypotension is the result of depressed myocardial contractility or reduced preload, aggressive treatment with volume expansion and sympathomimetic drugs is indicated. I prefer to use the combination of dopamine and phenylephrine hydrochloride (Neo-Synephrine) because of the positive effect on both cardiac contractility and peripheral vascular resistance. I monitor the effect of this therapy using a Swan-Ganz catheter and aim for a mean arterial pressure of 80 to 100 torr. Prolonged hypotension can aggravate the traumatic spinal cord injury by superimposing an ischemic insult. Surgical intervention should be postponed until the patient's vital functions are stabilized. The use of corticosteroids in acute spinal injury is controversial. Because no definite therapeutic value has been demonstrated, I do not prescribe them.

The spinal shock that follows acute spinal injury resolves within approximately 3 weeks. Thereafter, automatic spinal reflexes are re-established. Mass spinal reflexes consisting of flexor spasms, hypertension, bradycardia, diaphoresis, and cutaneous vasodilatation may be precipitated by such stimuli as bladder distention, palpation, or catheterization and rectal examination. *Extreme care must be taken to avoid precipitating such reflexes,* as the associated cardiovascular disturbances can be fatal.

Good bladder care to prevent urosepsis is an integral component of the global care that these patients require. Initially, an indwelling catheter is placed. Thereafter, intermittent catheterization to promote bladder emptying should be performed every 4 to 6 hours. When the spinal shock resolves, the patient should be instructed in the technique of self-catheterization and of bladder emptying by the Credé maneuver.

A regimen of stool softeners and bulk-forming laxatives is instituted to maintain bowel function. Intestinal obstruction caused by ileus or fecal impaction are dealt with accordingly.

In the paraplegic or quadriplegic patient, meticulous skin care is imperative.

The patient with a spinal cord injury is always at risk for developing a pulmonary embolus. Regular examination is necessary to exclude thrombophlebitis and to evaluate any sudden change in respiration. If indicated, definitive diagnostic studies such as a venography or an isotope lung scan are performed before therapeutic anticoagulation is instituted. Prophylactic therapy with subcutaneous heparin or with antithrombotic pumps or antithrombotic stockings can reduce the risk of this complication.

Open injuries are uncommon in civilian practice. Attention is paid to spinal realignment and stability to preserve neurologic function, and to wound debridement to repair the dura in order to prevent meningitis. Removal of retained foreign bodies and bone fragments from within the spinal canal is indicated but often does not lead to significant neurologic improvement. As in the case of closed injuries, complete paraplegia or quadriplegia seldom improves.

The outlook for patients with spinal injury correlates with the extent of the neurologic deficit. Those with a partial spinal cord syndrome should be expected to undergo some improvement. In these patients, spinal realignment and immobilization ensure against recurring neural trauma. The neurologic prognosis for the paraplegic or quadriplegic patient who makes no improvement within the first 24 hours is very poor. In these patients, aggressive physical and psychological rehabilitation is the key to achieving functional independence.

SUGGESTED READING

Allen BL, Ferguson RL. Cervical spine trauma in children. In: Bradford D, Hensinger R, eds. The pediatric spine. New York: Thieme Inc., 1985: 89.

Bohlman HH. Acute fractures and dislocations of the cervical spine: an analysis of 300 hospitalized patients and review of the literature. J Bone Joint Surg 1979; 61-A:1119–1142.

The Cervical Spine Research Society. The cervical spine. Philadelphia: JB Lippincott Co., 1988.

Dunsker SB, Schmidek HH, Frymoyer J, Kahn A, eds. The unstable spine (thoracic, lumbar, and sacral regions). Orlando: Grune and Stratton, 1986.

Pang D, Wilberger JE. Spinal cord injury without radiographic abnormalities in children. J Neurosurg 1982; 57:114–129.

PERIPHERAL NERVE INJURY

EARL R. HACKETT, M.D.

Injuries to the peripheral nerves manifest themselves in a variety of ways, depending on the manner of injury and the pathophysiologic factors occurring within the damaged nerve. It is important to understand these changes in order to select the most appropriate therapy (Fig. 1). In treating the patient with peripheral nerve injury, the neurologist has several courses he can follow; he may choose to observe the deficit over a certain period of time while treating the associated disability, or he may send the patient for surgical repair. Factors that influence this choice include (1) the cause of the injury, (2) the location of the injury (accurately identified by clinical examination and electrophysiologic tests), (3) time factors, and (4) the availability of a surgeon trained in peripheral nerve surgery and the availability of rehabilitation facilities and specialists.

CAUSES

When injured, a nerve may be divided or may remain "in continuity." Nerve injuries may be caused by sharp lacerations, crush injuries, and penetrating wounds, or by blunt trauma. Each type of injury presents its own problems which guide management.

Lacerations generally divide the nerve, although sometimes they may sever only part of the nerve. Separated nerves require surgical repair. If the cause of the laceration is a sharp object (a knife, razor, or glass), the wound should be explored and the nerve should be primarily repaired. This approach provides the best chance for a quicker and more satisfactory recovery.

Crush injuries and penetrating wounds are more complex, as there may be separation and/or contusion of nerve elements or stretch of the nerve. These changes may occur in relatively short segments or may be widespread. In the latter setting, surrounding tissue is also damaged; often, bones, arteries, and soft tissues must be reconstructed before the nerve can be assessed. During this reconstruction, it is important that the surgeon identify nerve struc-

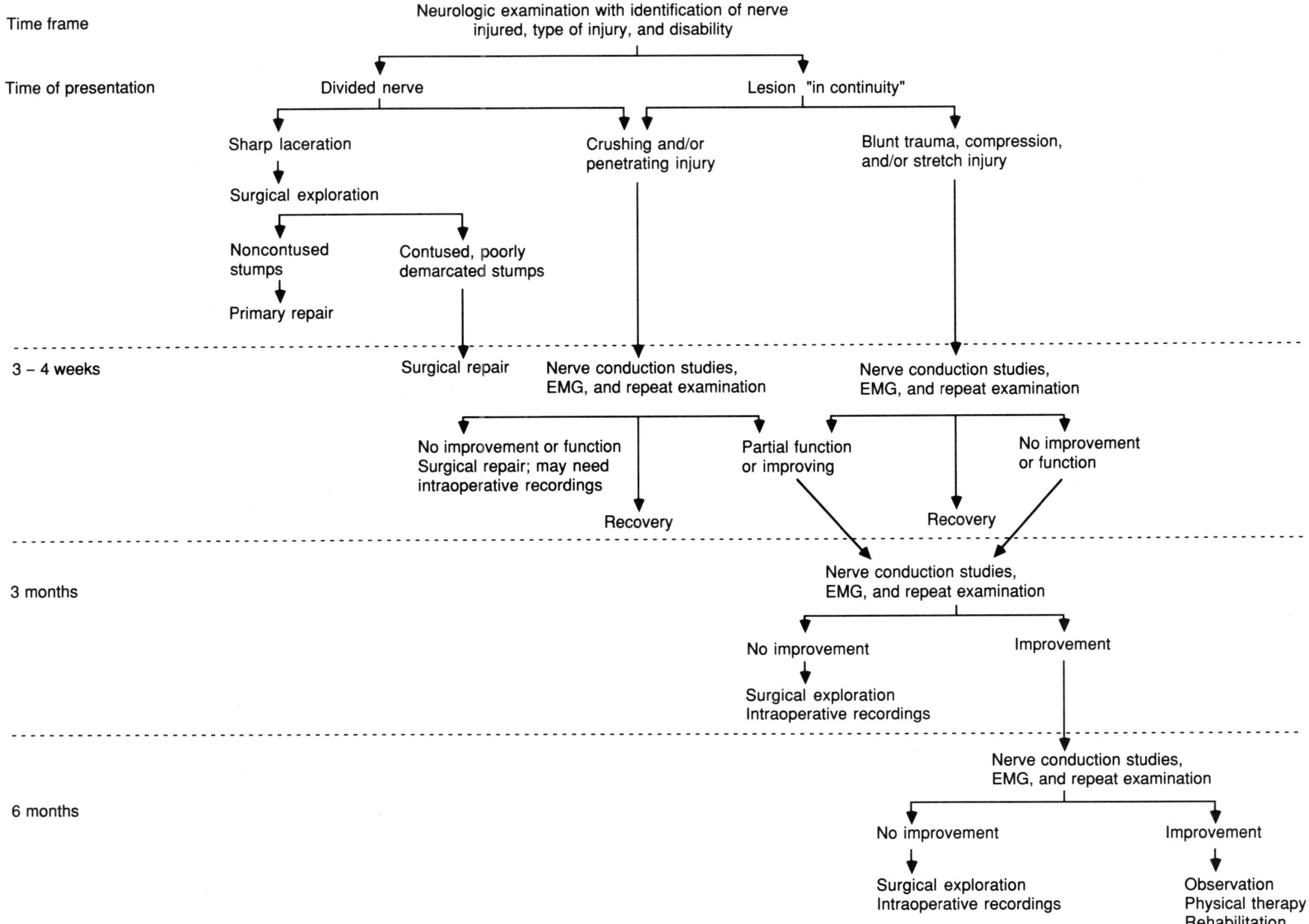

Figure 1 Management of peripheral nerve injuries.

tures, especially those not in continuity, and tag the loose ends. The nerve ends will retract, and if nerve repair is attempted later, they can be identified easily amidst the scarring that is so frequently found.

Blunt injuries, including compression and stretch injuries, rarely divide the nerve structures but cause contusions and/or stretching over variable lengths of the nerve. Severe injuries may cause avulsion of the nerve roots, particularly in the brachial plexus. It is usually best to delay surgical intervention in patients with blunt injuries, as there is frequently recovery of nerve function.

LOCATION OF INJURY

It is most important to identify accurately the location of the lesions(s) on the nerve. Knowledge of the anatomy of the nerve, its sensory distribution to skin, and its motor distribution to muscles is essential. There are many excellent manuals and books devoted to the examination of the peripheral nervous system and these should be consulted if there is some doubt regarding the findings of the examination. Careful evaluation at the time of injury and on subsequent follow-ups can give important information as to recovery. It should be noted that some traumatic nerve injuries progress during the initial 12 hours, but beyond 24 hours one should not expect to see further loss of function. Loss of function after 24 hours requires immediate attention to prevent permanent changes in the nerve. Entities such as hematoma, entrapment, pseudoaneurysm, or a compartment syndrome need to be ruled out.

Electrophysiologic tests are helpful. Nerve stimulation tests (conduction velocities, H-reflexes, F waves, sensory evoked potentials [SEPs]) are often helpful in identifying the level of the lesion. The presence of a sensory nerve action potential in a flail extremity points to a nerve root lesion (avulsion). The presence of motor action potentials when the nerve is stimulated below the suspected lesion suggests a neurapraxia with its better prognosis. The presence of a motor response when the nerve is stimulated above the injury points to a partial lesion and indicates that surgical intervention should be delayed. Needle electromyography (EMG) delineates which muscles have lost innervation and provides the clinician with some idea of the degree of loss. Needle EMG is also helpful in localizing the lesion in the nerve. On repeat examinations, the presence of new motor units in an area previously denervated suggests regeneration of the nerve. EMG is not useful during the first few weeks after injury.

The nerve involved and the level of involvement guides therapy to some extent. In general, proximal lesions have less functional recovery than distal lesions. When brachial plexus injuries resolve, they usually only reinnervate the shoulder and proximal arm. In the arm, radial nerve recovery is more likely than recovery of the ulnar or median nerves. In the leg, injury of the posterior tibial nerves has a better prognosis than that of the peroneal nerves. This does not mean that ulnar, peroneal, or plexus injuries should not be aggressively pursued, but only that expectations of success should be less. Superficial sensory nerves are usually not approached surgically unless a painful neuroma is present.

TIME FACTORS

A nerve injury should be assessed immediately. The clinical examination provides information on the cause of injury, the extent of involvement of the surrounding tissues, the level of nerve involvement, and the degree of disability. Electrophysiologic testing is rarely indicated at this time. As mentioned before, a sharp laceration should be explored if there is a significant functional loss and if it is believed that a nerve has been divided.

Many nerve injuries are seen several days after the injury is sustained. In this case, a more leisurely ''wait and see'' approach may be taken. The clinical examination should be thorough, including examination of both the motor and sensory functions in order to establish a baseline for comparison with follow-up examinations. Nerve conduction studies should be postponed for 3 to 4 weeks so that denervation changes (i.e., fibrillations, positive sharp waves) can develop and neurapraxia can reverse. Patients with penetrating and crush injuries should be reassessed at 3 to 4 weeks. If there is evidence of a severed nerve, exploration and reanastomosis or nerve grafting should be carried out.

In patients with blunt injuries, I perform a follow-up evaluation involving both clinical and electrophysiologic examinations at 3 months. If no recovery is seen, surgical exploration is advised. If there is some evidence of nerve regeneration, I re-evaluate the patient at 5 to 6 months. If there is no evidence of recovery at that time, surgery is advised. If some degree of recovery is noted at 3 months but has not improved further by the time of the re-evaluation at 5 to 6 months, surgery should be done. Delaying surgery beyond this point leads to a diminishing degree of recovery because of changes that occur in the target muscles.

PERIPHERAL NERVE SURGERY AND MEDICAL THERAPY

Increasing numbers of surgeons are being trained to deal with peripheral nerve injuries. The advent of the operating microscope, better nerve grafting procedures, and the use of intraoperative records of the exposed nerves has improved the ability of surgeons to manage the nerve lesion appropriately, and special training in these techniques is a necessity. Often, finding a surgeon with this background is difficult and may require that the patient be sent to a locale where these procedures are done. Intraoperative stimulation and recordings provide the surgeon with the best information as to how to proceed, and I believe that this should be used in all patients with lesions "in continuity."

Rehabilitation measures are needed for most patients with a nerve lesion. To obtain optimal results, splinting for protection, passive and active exercises, exquisite skin care, and procedures to improve total body functioning are necessary, whether surgical management or conservative management is used. The use of staff with training in the rehabilitation of patients with nerve injuries provides a greater degree of recovery.

Pain is a common symptom after nerve injury and may occur at any time. Often it may be quite debilitating and requires medical management. Amitriptyline, usually administered in doses of 50 to 100 mg, helps the patient sleep and tolerate his pain better. Carbamazepine (Tegretol) and phenytoin (Dilantin) may be helpful in reducing nerve irritability. Analgesics and even narcotics often do little for the pain and should be used judiciously. Intractable pain may require surgical exploration of the injured area. This is one of the few indications for surgery in patients with partial nerve injury or who are recovering from an injury.

SUGGESTED READING

Gentili F, Hudson AR. Peripheral nerve injuries: types, causes, grading. In: Wilkins RH, Rengachary SS, eds. Neurosurgery. New York: McGraw-Hill, 1985: 1864.

Kline DG, Hackett ER. Management of the neuroma in continuity. In: Wilkins RH, Rengachary SS, eds. Neurosurgery. New York: McGraw-Hill, 1985: 1864.

Kline DG, Hackett ER, Happel LH. Surgery for lesions of the brachial plexus. Arch Neurol 1986; 43:170–181.

Lundborg G. Nerve regeneration and repair. Acta Orthop Scand 1987; 58:145–169.

Millesi H. Reappraisal of nerve repair. Surg Clin North Am 1981; 61:321–340.

Seddon HJ. Medical research council report, No. 282. H.M. London: Stationary Office, 1954.

NEOPLASTIC DISEASE

BRAIN TUMORS IN CHILDREN

PETER C. PHILLIPS, M.D.

Brain tumors are the most common solid tumors among children, occurring with an estimated incidence of 1,500 cases per year. One in five children with cancer have a brain tumor, and one in four deaths due to cancer in children result from brain tumors. As such, they represent a major cause of morbidity and mortality during childhood.

The diagnostic and treatment issues posed by pediatric brain tumors are often different from those for adults. First, the frequency of metastasis to distant sites within the neuraxis or to extraneural systemic sites is often greater with brain tumors seen in childhood. Second, problems of late complications of treatment, including neurotoxicity, endocrinopathies, and secondary malignancies, are greater for children than for adults. Finally, pediatric brain tumors are histologically diverse. Whereas malignant gliomas represent more than 50 percent of all brain tumors in adults, no tumor constitutes more than 25 percent of all pediatric brain tumors. The most common pediatric brain tumors include medulloblastoma, cerebellar astrocytoma, brain stem and malignant supratentorial gliomas, ependymoma, and craniopharyngioma. The diversity of pediatric brain tumor types (each with a distinctly different biologic behavior), the rapidly evolving diagnostic and therapeutic approaches, and the need for multidisciplinary care from specialists in neurology, neurosurgery, oncology, radiation therapy, and endocrinology provide strong arguments for the management of these patients in regional childhood cancer centers.

MEDULLOBLASTOMA

Medulloblastoma, also termed cerebellar primitive neuroectodermal tumors, represents approximately 20 percent of pediatric brain tumors. Recent advances in medulloblastoma therapy emphasize the importance of determining metastatic spread and other high-risk factors in establishing the most appropriate treatment. The clinical signs and symptoms of medulloblastoma include vomiting, headache, lethargy, and papilledema, all consequent to obstructive hydrocephalus. Ataxia, nystagmus, and dysmetria suggest primary cerebellar dysfunction. Computed tomography (CT) or magnetic resonance imaging (MRI) studies typically show hydrocephalus and a midline cerebellar mass with homogenous contrast enhancement.

The initial management of medulloblastoma is surgical. For patients with severe hydrocephalus and increased intracranial pressure, emergency placement of an external ventricular drain may be necessary before tumor resection. A direct surgical approach by suboccipital craniotomy is essential for determining the histologic diagnosis. The primary surgical objective should be gross total resection; biopsy and limited resection adversely affect prognosis and should be avoided. Complete or generous tumor resection often re-establishes normal cerebrospinal fluid (CSF) flow without the need for ventricular shunts. Ventricular shunts should be avoided whenever possible, as they increase the risk for systemic metastasis.

Postoperative tumor staging for all medulloblastoma patients should include (1) a contrast medium–enhanced CT or MRI (within 72 hours after surgery) to determine residual tumor, (2) a complete myelogram (or CT myelogram) and CSF cytology examination to determine metastatic tumor within the subarachnoid space, (3) a radionuclide bone scan and bone marrow examination to identify systemic metastasis. At the time of the initial diagnosis, the risk for metastasis within the neuraxis ranges from 10 to 35 percent; the risk for systemic metastasis ranges from 3 to 5 percent. The major risk factors associated with poor prognosis in medulloblastoma are the patient's age at the time of the diagnosis (i.e., <3 years), any metastasis, the presence of large tumor before surgery, and the presence of large postoperative residual tumor. Based on these risk factors, treatment should be individualized such that patients with no high-risk factors are treated with radiotherapy only and those with one or more high-risk factors are treated with radiotherapy and chemotherapy.

Radiation therapy for children with medulloblastoma is complex and should not be undertaken at a local hospital or by a radiation oncologist inexperienced with childhood brain tumors. Extreme precision is essential to avoid overlapping ports or undertreated regions. Cumulative doses of 5,500 rad to the tumor and 3,600 rad to the craniospinal axis are standard. Doses of less than 4,500 to the tumor are inadequate. Conventional radiation treatments are administered as daily 180 rad fractions for 6 weeks.

The role of adjuvant chemotherapy is under active investigation. It is widely recognized that patients with systemic metastasis should be treated with adjuvant chemotherapy. However, two large cooperative studies failed to demonstrate that chemotherapy (CCNU and vincristine with or without prednisone) after radiotherapy versus radiotherapy alone significantly benefits the treatment of childhood medulloblastoma. Further analysis of these studies suggests that adjuvant chemotherapy may be beneficial for certain high-risk subgroups. Current cooperative group studies are treating only poor-risk patients with chemotherapy and radiotherapy. The Children's Cancer Study Group (CCG) is using a multidrug regimen ("eight-in-one") before and after radiation; the Pediatric Oncology Group (POG) is using preradiation cisplatin, vincristine, and cyclophosphamide. For low-risk patients, CCG and POG will randomize patients to receive lower craniospinal radiotherapy doses of 2,340 rad versus conventional craniospinal radiotherapy of 3,600 rad.

Despite improvements in treatment, approximately 40 percent of all medulloblastoma patients will relapse within 5 years of diagnosis. After relapse, there is no reasonable hope for cure. In most patients who relapse, the tumor recurs at the original tumor site, although 15 to 20 percent of these patients have isolated relapses at distant sites, including intracranial metastases, spinal intradural or intramedullary metastases, or extraneural metastases. Prolonged remissions with good quality of life can be achieved with various chemotherapeutic agents, and strong consideration should be given to further treatment when the relapse is identified. Effective agents include cisplatin, carboplatin, and cyclophosphamide. Combination chemotherapy with cisplatin, VP-16 (etoposide), and cytosine arabinoside, Mustargen, Oncovin, procarbazine, and prednisone (MOPP), continuous infusion vincristine sulfate and doxorubicin hydrochloride (Adriamycin) or "eight-in-one" have shown effectiveness. Investigations are ongoing to identify other single agents and drug combinations effective in the treatment of medulloblastoma.

CEREBRAL ASTROCYTOMA AND MALIGNANT GLIOMA

Cerebral astrocytoma (low-grade) and malignant glioma (including glioblastoma multiforme) represent opposite ends of the clinical and treatment spectrum. However, their clinical presentation may be identical, since signs and symptoms are more dependent on the tumor's location within the brain than on its histology. The clinical signs and symptoms of these supratentorial tumors include headache, papilledema, focal motor or sensory deficits, seizures, and tremor. CT and MRI scans are of critical diagnostic importance; nevertheless, some common radiographic misconceptions must be clarified: (1) in pediatric astrocytomas, there is no direct relationship between the degree of contrast medium enhancement used and malignancy, and (2) in malignant gliomas, the peritumoral low-density regions on CT (increased signal on T2 weighted MRI), often attributed to edema, frequently contain microscopic regions of malignant glioma.

The surgical approach to cerebral astrocytoma and malignant glioma depends on the location of the tumor. Tumors at or near the cortical surface may be resected in their entirety or biopsied under direct visualization. In some circumstances, intracranial subdural grid monitoring with stimulation for functional assessment may assist in the determination of brain regions that may be removed without significant neurologic deficit. Tumors located in the basal ganglia or thalamus are often best diagnosed by stereotaxic needle biopsy, although debulking of these tumors may be achieved through a transcallosal approach when they extend into the lateral ventricle.

The treatment of cerebral low-grade astrocytomas is changing. In many institutions, local radiotherapy after surgery has been advocated, regardless of the degree of tumor resection. This policy is being re-evaluated by CCG and POG national cooperative studies. For children with cerebral juvenile pilocytic astrocytoma, particularly the cystic-nodular type, the benefit of radiotherapy is uncertain, and every effort should be made to remove these tumors surgically. The role of radiotherapy in childhood diffuse fibrillary astrocytomas is not well defined. Because of the slow growth rate and benign clinical course for most cerebral low-grade astrocytomas in children, it is reasonable to withhold radiotherapy for all completely resected or nearly completely resected astrocytomas and follow closely with CT or MRI for evidence of tumor regrowth. If there is evidence of tumor regrowth, a second surgical resection should be performed. If a complete resection is obtained, radiotherapy may be withheld. If significant tumor remains, radiotherapy should be considered. Additional factors which may favor radiotherapy include rapid tumor regrowth, increased cellular atypia, or small stereotaxic biopsy specimens that may not be representative of the entire tumor. Chemotherapy is generally not appropriate for low-grade astrocytomas, except in patients with unresectable symptomatic tumors that continue to grow after radiotherapy and in patients for whom no additional radiotherapy is feasible.

In contrast to the conservative management of low-grade astrocytoma, the treatment for malignant glioma and glioblastoma should be aggressive and should include both radiotherapy and chemotherapy. Metastatic spread to CSF or spinal cord is not as common for malignant glioma at initial diagnosis as it is for medulloblastoma. However, a postoperative myelogram is recommended. Positive CSF cytology is uncommon; evidence of metastatic spread is almost always identified by myelography.

Local radiation therapy is usually administered to the tumor in a cumulative dose of 5,500 rad. Unless there is evidence of metastasis within the neuraxis, whole brain or spinal cord radiotherapy is not recommended. A recent cooperative study by CSG indicates a significant survival advantage for patients treated with chemotherapy (CCNU, vincristine, and prednisone) after radiotherapy versus those treated with radiotherapy alone. Cooperative group studies are currently evaluating the role of preradiation chemotherapy for these tumors.

Although early recurrence in patients with malignant glioma is most commonly caused by failure to control local tumor, there is growing appreciation that late CSF spread is a significant problem. Treatment at the time of recurrence may include single-drug or combination chemotherapy. Radiation treatment with implantation of radioactive seeds or stereotactic implantation may be appropriate for patients without disseminated disease.

BRAIN STEM GLIOMA

Brain stem gliomas generally carry an extremely poor prognosis, with the expected survival significantly less than that for patients with cerebral malignant gliomas. The characteristic triad of clinical findings in brain stem glioma includes (1) cranial nerve palsies, most commonly involving the abducent, facial, or lower cranial nerves, (2) long-tract signs, including spasticity, hyper-reflexia, and extensor plantar responses, and (3) ataxia. The finding of hydrocephalus at diagnosis is atypical. Signs and symptoms usually precede diagnosis by 1 to 3 months; however, longer intervals are often noted. Other causes for acute brain stem disease in childhood must be carefully considered in order to exclude brain stem encephalitis, abscess, arteriovenous malformations, or metabolic diseases (e.g., Leigh's disease).

MRI is the radiographic procedure of choice for brain stem glioma, providing excellent anatomic detail without the bony artifacts that complicate CT images of the posterior fossa. The majority of brain stem gliomas appear as a diffuse enlargement of the pons with prominently increased signal on T2 weighted images. Although distinctly less common than the radiographically diffuse brain stem gliomas, three variant types have been described: (1) cystic—nodular tumors similar in appearance to those found in the cerebellum; (2) dorsally exophytic tumors that extend and may obstruct the fourth ventricle, causing early hydrocephalus; (3) focal, sharply demarcated tumors in the cervico-medullary junction.

The role of surgery in the treatment of brain stem gliomas, traditionally limited to biopsy, has been expanded to include tumor resection for a select few tumors. Biopsy should be limited to cases in which the history, clinical course, or radiographic appearance is atypical. Although when the biopsy is performed by an experienced surgeon, the morbidity is acceptably low, other factors provide arguments against the use of routine biopsy. Usually only small superficial biopsies are obtained, and these may underestimate the degree of histologic malignancy. Aggressive therapy is given to all patients with typical diffuse brain stem gliomas regardless of the histology, and therefore histologic confirmation adds nothing to the therapeutic plan. By contrast, patients with the brain stem glioma variants described above are more likely to have a greater prediagnostic symptomatic interval and an extended post-treatment survival. These tumors are frequently low-grade, and histologic diagnoses including those of ganglioneuroma, ganglioglioma, or juvenile pilocytic astrocytoma have been made. For patients with brain stem glioma variants, major or complete surgical resection may provide a significant therapeutic contribution.

Radiation therapy is the standard and conventional treatment for patients with brain stem glioma. Usual cumulative doses administered to a posterior fossa port range from 5,000 to 5,500 rad. No therapeutic advantage has been identified for standard fractionation radiotherapy at 6,000 rad as compared with those at lower doses. In the absence of documented leptomeningeal metastases, an extremely uncommon occurrence at the time of the diagnosis, there is no role for routine craniospinal radiation. Most children show symptomatic improvement during or soon after radiation therapy; the absence of clinical response is a poor prognostic sign. After radiotherapy, the median survival ranges from 9 to 15 months, and the 5-year survival rate ranges from 10 to 30 percent in most series; however, a median survival of 2 years and a 5-year survival rate as great as 50 percent have been reported.

Hyperfractionation radiation therapy, which uses lower single treatment doses two or more times per day (i.e., 110 rad twice each day), has permitted the delivery of cumulative doses as high as 7,800 rad without serious radiation injury to normal brain stem structures. This approach is currently being investigated in single-institution and cooperative group studies for brain stem glioma. Preliminary results suggest that, compared with hyperfractionation radiation therapy using 6,600 rad or conventional radiotherapy, hyperfractionation radiation therapy using 7,200 rad may prolong survival.

Chemotherapy is of uncertain benefit in the treatment of brain stem gliomas. To date, several large studies have not shown adjuvant chemotherapy to have a significant survival advantage compared with radiation therapy alone. For patients with recurrent or progressive disease after radiotherapy, single-agent or combination chemotherapy trials may produce objective or clinical responses of limited duration. In one series, high-dose cyclophosphamide resulted in a tumor reduction of greater than 50 percent in four of five brain stem glioma patients.

Two important problems are often apparent late in the course of brain stem glioma management. First, hydrocephalus from pontine enlargement and compression of the fourth ventricle may exacerbate pre-existing symptoms and give the clinical impression of acute tumor progression. Hydrocephalus should be treated promptly by ventriculoperitoneal shunting. Second, the complications of chronic corticosteroid use, including severe obesity, painful osteoporosis, diabetes mellitus, hypertension, and gastrointestinal hemorrhage, are often incapacitating. Every effort should be made to taper corticosteroids *during* radiation therapy. Patients who do not require corticosteroids before radiotherapy should not receive them on a "prophylactic" basis. Later in the course of management, when corticosteroid treatment is necessary for symptomatic control, efforts should be made to find the lowest effective dose.

PINEAL REGION TUMORS

Pineal region tumors were once considered surgically inaccessible, and clinical diagnoses based on radiographic features or response to radiotherapy were common. The obsolete term "pinealoma" indicated the tendency to treat all pineal tumors as one, with histologic types identified only at autopsy. Pineal region tumors are now recognized as an extremely diverse group. The extreme differences in tumor biology and response to treatment among these tumors requires a histologic diagnosis. Pineal tumors may be broadly classified into four groups: (1) pure germinomas, (2) nongerminoma germ cell tumors (choriocarcinoma, embryonal carcinoma, teratoma, endodermal sinus tumor), (3) pineal parenchymal tumors (pineoblastoma and pineocytoma), and (4) miscellaneous tumors including glioma, dermoid, primary lymphoma, and others.

The signs and symptoms of pineal tumors are referable to the location and include those of increased intracranial pressure: headaches, nausea, vomiting, papilledema, and Parinaud's syndrome. Despite claims to the contrary, accurate histologic diagnosis cannot be made by CT or MRI. MRI is the imaging modality of choice for these tumors. CSF tumor markers, including alpha-fetoprotein (elevated in teratoid tumors), beta-HCG (elevated in choriocarcinoma), and placental alkaline phosphatase (elevated in germinoma), may provide additional diagnostic information but should not be considered sufficient for diagnosis in themselves.

Surgery plays an important role in the treatment of pineal region tumors. Histologic confirmation may be accomplished by stereotaxic biopsy or open biopsy. Tumor resection may not be as important for pure germinomas (extremely radiation-sensitive and chemotherapy-sensitive) as it is for the highly malignant germ cell tumors; however, benign teratomas, meningiomas, dermoid cysts, and astrocytomas are best treated by complete resection when possible. It is important to recognize that germinomas may contain small areas of malignant teratoma or other germ cell tumors that may be missed by limited biopsy. This may result in undertreatment of these highly aggressive tumors.

Whereas an extent-of-disease work up is unnecessary for patients with benign or low-grade tumors, all patients with germinoma or other malignant germ cell tumors, pineal parenchymal tumors, and malignant gliomas should undergo complete myelography and CSF cytology examination after surgery. In addition, in patients with highly malignant germ cell tumors and pineoblastoma, bone marrow aspirates, bone scans, and chest radiographs should be obtained.

Radiation therapy is highly effective for children with germinoma. Rapid and complete tumor regression is the rule, and 5-year survival rates of greater than 75 percent have been reported. Routine craniospinal irradiation for germinoma is controversial and is often reserved for patients with documented metastasis within the neuraxis. Germinomas are also highly sensitive to chemotherapy regimens used for testicular seminoma (cisplatin, bleomycin, vinblastine sulfate). By contrast, nongerminoma germ cell tumors are highly malignant and metastasis to CSF or spinal cord is common. Systemic metastases are especially common with choriocarcinoma. Because of the uniformly poor prognosis for these patients, multimodality therapy including craniospinal radiation and chemotherapy is warranted.

Although pineocytomas in adults tend to be slow-growing tumors with little tendency to neuraxis metastasis, a recent report suggests that pineocytomas in children may have a greater metastatic potential. Standard treatment includes local radiation. The need for routine craniospinal radiotherapy is controversial. The role of chemotherapy in the treatment of this tumor has not been defined. By contrast, pineoblastomas are highly malignant tumors that frequently metastasize to the neuraxis. After diagnosis, treatment should include craniospinal radiation and chemotherapy. Pineoblastomas are uncommon tumors; however, limited experience with chemotherapy indicates that tumor regression can be seen when cisplatin, cyclophosphamide, and high-dose methotrexate are used.

SUGGESTED READING

Allen JC, Bloom J, Ertel E, et al. Brain tumors in children: current cooperative and institutional chemotherapy trials in newly diagnosed and recurrent disease. Semin Oncol 1986; 13:110–122.
Cohen ME, Duffner, PK. Brain tumors in children: principles of diagnosis and treatment. New York: Raven Press, 1984.
Packer RJ, Seigel KR, Sutton LN, et al. Efficacy of adjuvant chemotherapy with poor-risk medulloblastoma: a preliminary report. Ann Neurol 1988; 24:503–508.

PATIENT RESOURCE

The Association for Brain Tumor Research provides patient-oriented clinical brochures, computerized literature searches, and a referral list of physicians who specialize in neuro-oncology:

Association for Brain Tumor Research
3725 North Talman Avenue
Chicago, Illinois 60618
Telephone: (312) 286-5571

GLIOMA

EDWARD J. DROPCHO, M.D.

Glioma represents one of the most common and difficult problems in clinical neurology. As a group, gliomas are the most common primary intracranial tumors of adults and are diagnosed in approximately 8,000 persons in the United States every year. The majority of these lesions are histologically malignant and clinically aggressive; unfortunately, a "benign" glioma can often be equally devastating. It is difficult to make confident dogmatic statements about the proper treatment of either benign or malignant gliomas since there is controversy regarding nearly every aspect of management of these patients.

BENIGN GLIOMA

Histologically, benign glioma carries a much better prognosis than malignant tumors, but the management of this tumor is complicated by the absence of well-designed clinical trials on which to base treatment decisions. No prospective or controlled studies have addressed key treatment questions such as: What is the desired extent of surgical resection? Which (if any) patients should be given radiation therapy after surgical diagnosis? What are the optimal doses and ports of radiation? What quality of life can be expected in these patients after treatment? Magnetic resonance imaging (MRI) has significantly improved the ability to diagnose these tumors early, but it has also presented the dilemma of how best to manage patients with a single seizure or well-controlled seizure disorder, a normal neurologic examination, and an abnormal MRI scan.

Astrocytomas

A distinction should be made between pilocytic ("juvenile") astrocytomas and the more common "fibrillary" tumors. Although pilocytic astrocytomas occur most commonly in the cerebellum or diencephalon of children and young adults, they can arise at any age and in any location. The tumors often consist of a gross cyst with a mural tumor nodule and are characterized histologically by elongated (pilocytic) tumor cells, microcystic change, and Rosenthal fibers. Gross total surgical resection is possible in many patients and results in long survival or even in cure; the outlook is also quite favorable even for patients with less than total tumor resection. Radiation therapy is therefore generally not recommended unless a postoperative tumor burden remains or tumor progression occurs after surgery.

Despite the obvious hazards of basing treatment recommendations on nonrandomized retrospective data, several tentative conclusions regarding low-grade ("benign" or "grades I and II") fibrillary astrocytomas can be derived from the existing literature:

1. There is probably a survival advantage for younger patients and for patients who undergo ex-

tensive surgical resection as compared with patients who have only biopsy or partial tumor excision.

2. There is a consensus that patients who receive postoperative radiation therapy (RT) have modestly better 5-year and 10-year survival rates than patients who undergo surgery only, although some studies indicate that RT delays tumor recurrence without actually affecting the eventual long-term (greater than 10-year) survival. The optimal radiation volume and ports are not known, although "standard" treatment generally consists of 5,000 to 5,500 cGy given focally to the tumor plus a 2- to 4-cm "margin" as defined by CT or MRI. In the age of safe stereotaxic biopsy there is no justification for irradiating a supratentorial lesion without histologic confirmation of the diagnosis. For patients fortunate enough to have a gross total resection, RT can probably be withheld and the patient followed closely by serial imaging studies. Almost no published studies have addressed the issue of neurologic impairment and quality of life of long-term survivors who received RT. The major controversy revolves around the growing recognition that a significant proportion of patients develop cerebral atrophy and cognitive impairment—sometimes severe—after receiving doses of cranial irradiation previously believed to be safe.

3. At the time of recurrence, 50 to 75 percent of initially benign astrocytomas show histologic and clinical evidence of malignant transformation. There are no data to suggest that radiation therapy either prevents or accelerates the degeneration of these tumors into a more malignant histology, nor is it known whether RT given "up front" or at the time of tumor recurrence yields better-quality survival of greater duration.

Oligodendrogliomas

As with tumors of astrocytic derivation, oligodendrogliomas exhibit a spectrum of histologic malignancy. A postoperative survival of more than 10 years is not unusual for patients with histologically benign oligodendrogliomas. Complete resection, when feasible, should be the goal of surgery. All of the published studies addressing the usefulness of postsurgical RT in the treatment of oligodendrogliomas are retrospective and nonrandomized, and they arrive at conflicting conclusions regarding the effect of RT on the time to tumor progression and on the duration of survival. A compromise approach to benign oligodendrogliomas is to administer focal irradiation (5,000 to 5,500 cGy) to patients with a large postsurgical residual tumor burden and to defer RT in patients who undergo complete or nearly complete tumor excision.

There is still no widely accepted grading system for oligodendrogliomas, but recent evidence suggests that dense cellularity, marked pleomorphism, a high mitotic rate, endothelial proliferation, and necrosis have a negative impact on survival. The distinction between a "benign oligodendroglioma with some anaplastic features" and an "anaplastic oligodendroglioma" is a subjective one made by the pathologist; the former tumor probably warrants treatment with focal RT, while the latter tumor should be managed in the same manner as the other malignant gliomas discussed below.

MALIGNANT GLIOMAS

Recent studies from the Brain Tumor Study Group (BTSG) and Radiation Therapy Oncology Group (RTOG) support the usefulness of classifying malignant astrocytic neoplasms into two main groups: anaplastic astrocytoma (AA) and glioblastoma multiforme (GBM). The term "malignant gliomas" also includes anaplastic oligodendroglioma and gliosarcoma. The BTSG and RTOG trials have clearly demonstrated three major independent prognostic factors for malignant gliomas that are useful as general predictors of individual patient outcome and are critically important in designing and interpreting clinical trials:

1. *Patient age.* This is probably the single-most powerful predictor of outcome; median survival is inversely proportional to age throughout all decades of adult life.
2. *Tumor histology.* The median survival of patients with intratumoral necrosis (which distinguishes AA from GBM) is less than half that of patients without necrosis. Only about 10 percent of patients with GBM are alive at 24 months, while the 24-month survival rate for AA patients approaches 50 percent.
3. *Performance status.* Not surprisingly, patients with a better performance status at the time of diagnosis have a better survival outlook than those who present with severe neurologic impairment.

Surgery

Skillful and aggressive surgery remains the foundation for the treatment of malignant gliomas. The rationale for extensive surgical resection of these tumors includes the alleviation of increased intracranial pressure, removal of necrotic tissue, "buying time" for subsequent therapy, and cytoreduction, which theoretically leaves behind fewer tumor cells to become resistant to radiation and/or chemotherapy. Recent studies have clearly shown that subtotal or gross total resection is more likely to improve than to worsen neurologic deficits, and that the amount of residual tumor remaining after surgery is an important independent predictor of survival. The general goal of surgery should therefore be the maximal tumor resection consistent with preservation of neurologic function; a "biopsy only" approach should be restricted to tumors located in deep or critical locations.

Surgery also has an important role at the time of tumor recurrence or progression. In selected, relatively young patients with good performance status and accessible lesions, a second debulking or resection can "set up" further chemotherapy and has a good chance of improving neurologic function and of increasing the duration of survival. In addition, serious consideration should be given to biopsying recurrent tumors in patients in whom the recurrence occurs after a relatively long interval (a year or more) since the time of the initial treatment, because (in the absence of positron-emission tomography scanning) there are no clinical or neuroimaging features that reliably distinguish tumor recurrence from radiation necrosis.

Radiation Therapy

The BTSG has shown that the addition of external RT to surgery doubles the median survival of patients with malignant gliomas from 14 months to 36 months. Standard RT regimens deliver 4,000 cGy to the whole brain and an additional focal boost so that the "tumor volume" receives 6,000 cGy. Tumor doses less than 6,000 cGy probably yield inferior survival rates, while doses exceeding 6,000 cGy are more neurotoxic and do not improve the outlook for survival.

Malignant gliomas occasionally spread through the leptomeninges or recur far from the initial tumor site, but for the vast majority of adult patients, the ultimate cause of death is tumor recurrence at the primary site. In addition, as many as 30 to 40 percent of malignant glioma patients who survive for more than 18 or 24 months after whole brain RT develop cognitive impairment, sometimes progressive, associated with diffuse cerebral atrophy and abnormal hemispheric white matter on central nervous system (CNS) imaging studies. These observations have led some neuro-oncologists to question the need for whole brain irradiation in all patients and to recommend limited field RT with generous margins based on CT or MRI scans. On the other hand, in a significant proportion of patients, glioma cells have been found infiltrating the "brain around the tumor" well beyond the area of enhancement on CT scans and even beyond the area of increased T2 signal on MRI scans; this makes it difficult to outline the true "tumor margin" with any certainty. Until the controversy is resolved by a randomized comparison of focal RT and whole brain RT it seems prudent to continue to give the whole brain/tumor boost regimen to patients with large or clearly diffuse tumors, and to use limited field RT (5,500 to 6,000 cGy with wide margins) for patients with unusually small or "well circumscribed" lesions.

Brachytherapy using interstitial radionuclide implants is one of the more promising recent developments in the treatment of malignant gliomas. This technique consists of stereotaxtic placement of one or more removable catheters into the tumor, which are then afterloaded with high-activity iodine-125 sources; the implants deliver a very high radiation dose to the tumor with a rapid decrease in the dose absorbed by surrounding normal brain. Nonrandomized studies of brachytherapy in highly selected patients with recurrent gliomas have shown encouraging results. Patients with tumors that are large, highly irregular, bilateral, or located in critical areas of the brain (e.g., those areas involving speech and motor function) are generally not candidates for brachytherapy. Another practical problem concerning brachytherapy is the high incidence of focal radiation necrosis that confounds the assessment of response and causes clinical deterioration requiring surgical debulking in as many as 50 percent of patients. The major theoretical objection to brachytherapy is that many malignant gliomas are diffuse lesions and that local treatments cannot kill the tumor cells that infiltrate far from the central tumor mass. Until the proper role of brachytherapy (including proper patient selection and possible combination with external RT for newly diagnosed patients) is better understood, this treatment should remain experimental.

Chemotherapy

As with many other solid tumors, the progress in finding effective chemotherapy for malignant gliomas has been painstakingly and disappointingly slow. The large number and wide diversity of published chemotherapy trials for malignant gliomas attest to the absence of a regimen with dramatic effectiveness and acceptable toxicity. The therapeutic resistance of gliomas to chemotherapy is probably the result of a combination of factors, including limited drug delivery into tumors, the relatively low tolerance of normal brain tissue, and the poorly understood intrinsic resistance of the tumor cells to currently available agents.

Postoperative treatment with a nitrosourea remains the conventional chemotherapy for malignant gliomas against which newer therapies should be compared. A large randomized study by the BTSG has demonstrated statistically significant increases in the median survival (from 36 weeks to 51 weeks) and in the proportion of long-term survivors (24 percent at 18 months) for patients receiving intravenous carmustine (BCNU) in addition to surgery and RT. The modest effect of this treatment on total median survival is due to the fact that only a minority of patients clearly respond to BCNU, while in a larger number of patients the chemotherapy probably has little or no effect on tumor progression or survival. There is unfortunately no way of predicting with confidence which patient will benefit from BCNU (or any other agent), even taking into account the known prognostic factors outlined above.

Intravenous BCNU (200 mg per square meters of body surface area [m^2] infused over 1 to 2 hours) for newly diagnosed patients is generally begun during the 1 week of RT and administered every 8 weeks, depending on the recovery of blood counts. The drug is also effective in some patients with recurrent tumors. The only common acute toxicity of BCNU is mild to moderate nausea and vomiting, and most patients tolerate outpatient treatment quite well. The most frequent (and often dose-limiting) side effect is a delayed, cumulative myelosuppression characteristic of all nitrosoureas. Progressive interstitial pulmonary fibrosis is a serious concern but is rare unless patients have preexisting lung disease or receive a cumulative BCNU dose exceeding 1,400 mg per m^2; the drug should be discontinued if serial pulmonary diffusion capacities fall below 60 to 70 percent of the predicted value. Procarbazine hydrochloride given in monthly oral courses is probably as effective as BCNU and is a reasonable alternative for patients who cannot receive nitrosoureas.

The search for better chemotherapy regimens for malignant gliomas has included trials of single agents, multiple agents, and improved delivery techniques. Several agents, most notably cisplatin and the lipid-soluble drug diaziquone (AZQ), have shown some effectiveness in patients with recurrent tumors, but no single agent has been proven to be superior to BCNU for newly diagnosed patients. There have been numerous trials of multi-agent regimens, generally combining cell cycle–nonspecific drugs (such as the nitrosoureas or cisplatin) with cycle-specific drugs (such as hydroxyurea, vincristine, or 5-fluorouracil), but to date none have been convincingly shown to be superior to BCNU or to other single agents, either for newly diagnosed patients or for those with recurrent tumors.

Intra-arterial (IA) chemotherapy is capable of delivering several times more drug into the infused tumor (and normal brain) than is the same dose of drug given systemically. BCNU has pharmacokinetic properties that are particularly well suited to IA therapy, but unfortunately there have been no well-designed studies showing IA BCNU to be more effective than conventional intravenous BCNU. In addition, interest in IA BCNU has greatly diminished after several study groups encountered an unacceptably high incidence of severe, often fatal leukoencephalopathy in the infused normal brain. Intracarotid cisplatin has shown promising efficacy in some patients with recurrent tumors; side effects include visual and/or hearing loss, seizures, and acute neurologic deterioration after infusion, but to date the devastating delayed neurotoxicity seen with BCNU has not been reported with cisplatin. The role of IA cisplatin or other IA drugs in the treatment of newly diagnosed patients is still unknown. IA chemotherapy has been combined with hyperosmotic disruption of the blood-brain barrier; pilot trials of IA methotrexate administered after barrier disruption are encouraging, but experimental studies show that barrier disruption proportionally increases the delivery of the drug into surrounding normal brain much more than it increases delivery into the tumor. The ultimate usefulness and toxicity of barrier disruption remain to be determined. Until more extensive data are available, it is strongly recommended that IA chemotherapy be restricted to a research setting.

Immunotherapy

The theoretical promise of specific antitumor cytotoxicity with little or no damage to normal brain has spurred recent interest in immunotherapy of malignant gliomas. Current studies fall into one of four main groups:

1. Active immunization with irradiated autologous tumor cells or cultured human glioma cells. This is based on the (unproven) assumptions that tumor-specific (or relatively specific) antigens exist and that patients can mount an effective cytotoxic response.
2. Adoptive immunotherapy using intravenous or intratumoral injections of immune cells, such as specifically sensitized cytotoxic T lymphocytes or lymphokine-activated killer (LAK) cells. Preliminary studies have shown that large numbers of LAK cells can be injected into malignant gliomas without undue toxicity; the efficacy of this approach remains to be demonstrated.
3. Humoral immunomodulators or biologic response modifiers, particularly the interferons. Interferons have multiple effects on the immune system, but their main activity against gliomas is probably a direct antiproliferative effect on tumor cells. Alpha-interferon has produced promising responses in patients with recurrent tumors (at least in some studies); current research is centered around possible synergistic effects between interferons and chemotherapeutic agents.
4. Monoclonal antibody therapy with antibodies conjugated to biologic toxins or radioisotopes. Several serious practical problems have thus far prevented monoclonal antibodies from becoming the ''magic bullets'' of brain tumor treatment; these include the difficulty in producing even relatively tumor-specific antibodies, the consid-

erable antigenic heterogeneity between the tumors of different patients and among cells within an individual tumor, and the problem of delivering macromolecules into brain tumors.

Supportive Therapy

The mainstay of supportive treatment of gliomas is the use of corticosteroids to control cerebral edema. Most patients receive a starting dose of 8 to 16 mg dexamethasone per day (admittedly an arbitrary dose) before surgery, and the dose is increased as necessary. The effects of beginning or changing the dose are generally seen within 48 to 72 hours. Continual efforts should be made to gradually taper the dose, although most patients require at least a low dose to minimize the acute side effects of radiation therapy (headache, nausea, worsening of focal symptoms). In patients with recurrent tumors that are unresponsive to treatment, the dexamethasone may be increased to 32 mg per day or even higher in order to improve (transiently) the patient's quality of life. For the obtunded patient with terminal disease, one should seriously consider (in consultation with the patient's family) abruptly discontinuing the steroids.

Seizures occur in 20 to 50 percent of malignant glioma patients at some time during their illness. The same basic principles regarding single-drug therapy and anticonvulsant pharmacokinetics used for the management of seizures apply to brain tumor patients just as they apply to other epileptic patients. "Prophylactic" anticonvulsants (usually phenytoin) are often administered to patients before craniotomy, but there is no hard evidence to support the efficacy of this practice. In addition, there are recent reports of life-threatening erythema multiforme and Stevens-Johnson syndrome occurring in patients who take phenytoin and in whom doses of dexamethasone are tapered during cranial irradiation, suggesting that anticonvulsants and especially phenytoin should not be given routinely to patients with brain tumors.

Despite intensive laboratory and clinical research efforts, malignant gliomas continue to exert a terrible impact on patients and their families. The painfully slow progress in developing better treatment for these patients should not, however, lure physicians into a nihilistic attitude. Conventional treatment and careful attention to supportive care can certainly help patients maintain their quality of life for significant periods. Whenever possible, patients should be encouraged and assisted to enter well-designed and carefully conducted investigational treatment programs. Future advances will be made only through the perseverance of researchers and the courage of patients.

SUGGESTED READING

Burger PC. Malignant astrocytic neoplasms: classification, pathologic anatomy, and response to treatment. Semin Oncol 1986; 13:16–26.
Dropcho EJ, Mahaley MS. Chemotherapy for malignant gliomas in adults. In: Thomas DGT, ed. Management of malignancies of the brain. London: Edward Arnold Ltd (in press).
Kornblith PL, Walker M. Chemotherapy for malignant gliomas. J Neurosurg 1988; 68:1–17.
Leibel SA, Sheline GE. Radiation therapy for neoplasms of the brain. J Neurosurg 1987; 66:1–22.
Morantz RA. Radiation therapy in the treatment of cerebral astrocytoma. Neurosurgery 1987; 20:975–982.
Vick NA, Bigner DD, eds. Symposium on neuro-oncology. Neurol Clin 1985; 3:703–917.

PATIENT RESOURCE

The Association for Brain Tumor Research is an excellent source of information for patients and families and maintains a listing of major treatment centers and support groups.

Association for Brain Tumor Research
3725 North Talman Avenue
Chicago, Illinois 60618
Telephone: (312) 286-5571

The National Cancer Institute also provides a cancer information service for patients and families. The telephone number is: 1-800-4-CANCER

BRAIN METASTASIS

ROY A. PATCHELL, M.D.

Metastases to the brain constitute approximately half of all intracranial tumors and occur in 20 to 40 percent of patients with systemic cancer. With the possible exception of metabolic encephalopathies, brain metastases are the most common neurologic complication of systemic cancer. There is evidence that as patients with systemic cancer live longer (because of improved treatment of the primary tumor), both the frequency and clinical importance of brain metastasis will increase.

In most instances, the metastasis reaches the brain by hematogenous spread through the arterial circulation. Brain metastases may appear anywhere in the brain, but in general, the distribution is proportional to the blood supply to specific brain areas.

Therefore more than 80 percent of metastases occur in the cerebral hemispheres, with approximately 10 to 15 percent occurring in the cerebellum and 2 to 3 percent in the brain stem. Brain metastases are "single" in approximately 50 percent of patients. The term "single brain metastasis" refers to patients with one metastasis in the brain and implies nothing about the extent of cancer that may be present elsewhere in the body. The term "solitary brain metastasis" refers to a relatively rare subgroup of patients with single brain metastases in whom the brain metastasis is the only known cancer in the body. Metastases from colon, breast, and renal cell carcinoma are more often single, while malignant melanoma and (to a lesser degree) lung cancer have a greater tendency to produce multiple metastases. Primary tumors located in the pelvis are more likely to produce posterior fossa metastases.

In most patients with brain metastases, the neurologic history is one of headache followed over a period of days to weeks by progressive focal neurologic symptoms and signs (especially hemiparesis). Headaches may be mild, are often bilateral or diffuse, and rarely have localizing value. Early morning headache (usually believed to be associated with raised intracranial pressure) occurs in only about 40 percent of patients who present with headache. Headaches are more common in patients with multiple metastases or with single metastases in the posterior fossa. Although headaches usually imply raised intracranial pressure, since the advent of computerized tomography (CT), papilledema is present in only about 25 percent of patients with brain metastases at diagnosis. Approximately 10 percent of patients have seizures as the first sign of the metastasis. An additional 5 to 10 percent of patients may present with acute neurologic symptoms caused by hemorrhage into or sudden expansion of the metastasis, and 1 to 2 percent of patients have a nonfocal encephalopathy as the only sign of the brain metastasis.

The best diagnostic tests for brain metastases are CT and magnetic resonance imaging (MRI). If the history is typical and the lesions are multiple, there is little doubt as to the diagnosis. However, there are other diagnostic possibilities that should be considered, such as primary brain tumor, brain abscess, and cerebral infarct or hemorrhage. Usually the scans will be able to differentiate these entities, although recent studies have shown the false-positive rate for the diagnosis of suspected brain metastases to be as high as 10 to 15 percent. Other diagnostic tests, including arteriography or biopsy, may be needed to establish the diagnosis.

A question often arises as to how far to pursue a metastatic work-up in patients with a brain mass on CT or MRI and no previous history of systemic cancer. Since most metastases reach the brain by hematogenous spread through the arterial circulation, the lung is an important source of brain metastasis. If the primary tumor is not pulmonary, it has probably metastasized to the lung before seeding into the arterial circulation and reaching the brain. More than 60 percent of patients with brain metastases will have a mass demonstrated on chest radiograph that is caused by either a primary lung cancer or a lung metastasis from a primary located elsewhere. A careful chest x-ray examination is therefore one of the most important diagnostic tests for patients with suspected brain metastases. When the chest x-ray examination fails to demonstrate a lesion, CT or MRI of the lung may reveal metastases and suggest the cause of the neurologic disorder. Further search for a primary is seldom fruitful, especially if there are no positive findings on physical examination (e.g., a breast mass) and no features of the history that suggest a specific primary tumor.

MEDICAL AND RADIATION TREATMENT

Even after more than 60 years of clinical experimentation, the optimal treatment of brain metastases (whether single or multiple) is still controversial. Several methods of treatment are available for patients with intracranial metastases. Corticosteroids, radiation therapy, and surgery all have a place in the management of metastases. Chemotherapy is also useful for a few individual patients. In determining the optimal treatment for each patient, several factors must be considered, including the patient's neurologic status, the extent of systemic disease, and the number and site of metastases. All patients should begin receiving corticosteroids at the time of diagnosis. The usual dexamethasone dose is 4 mg taken orally four times daily. Corticosteroids should be continued until patients complete radiation therapy.

Brain metastases are associated with a poor prognosis regardless of therapy. Patients with brain metastases who do not receive treatment have a median survival of only about 1 month. Virtually all patients who do not receive treatment die as a direct result of the brain tumor. With corticosteroid treatment alone, the median survival is increased to approximately 2 months, but without more aggressive treatment, again, most patients die as a direct result of the brain metastases. Whole brain radiation therapy (WBRT) increases the median survival to 3 to 6 months, and data from large retrospective studies have shown that more than half of the patients treated with WBRT ultimately die of progressive systemic cancer and not as a direct result of the brain metastases.

Typical radiation doses used for brain metastases are usually short courses (5 to 10 days) with relatively high doses per fraction (150 to 400 cGy per day). Total doses are usually in the range of 3,000 to

5,000 cGy, and several large multicenter trials conducted by the Radiation Therapy Oncology Group have shown that there is no significant difference in results when the lower range of doses are used. However, recent reports have suggested that many long-term survivors have some degree of dementia and leukoencephalopathy related to high dose/ fractionation schedules. Therefore, in patients with expected survivals of greater duration, a longer course of radiation with smaller doses per fraction should probably be used. A reasonable schedule would be a total dose of 4,500 to 5,000 cGy given in doses of no more than 200 cGy per fraction.

In the subgroup of patients whose only metastases are to the brain, it has been shown that death is more likely to be the result of the brain metastasis than of progressive systemic disease. Therefore, in patients with controlled systemic cancer who develop brain metastases, the treatment of the brain disease is the factor that is the most likely to determine the duration of survival. In these patients, the question of whether more aggressive therapy (e.g., surgery) should be instituted is usually raised. There are theoretical reasons for believing that the combination of surgery followed by postoperative radiation therapy may be more effective at eradicating brain metastases than WBRT alone. Radiation therapy is most successful when used against small tumor volumes. In patients with larger tumors, radiation is usually effective at the periphery of the tumor where there are relatively fewer cells and where the cells are well oxygenated; however, in the center of the tumor, where tumor cells are more numerous and more hypoxic conditions usually exist, radiation may fail to destroy the tumor completely. Although there are documented reports of sterilization of brain metastases by radiation therapy alone, in most cases, residual tumor probably remains. Surgery is most successful at removing large volumes of tumor; however, small numbers of malignant cells may be left behind. Rational treatment plans combining surgical debulking and radiation therapy have been developed to overcome the deficiencies of both types of treatment, and combined therapy has shown promise in a variety of tumor types.

SURGICAL TREATMENT

Despite the theoretical advantages of surgical treatment, until recently the actual role of surgery has been unclear because of an absence of any controlled trials showing the efficacy of surgical treatment. Two independent, prospective randomized trials have now been performed to evaluate the efficacy of surgery in the treatment of single brain metastases. One recently completed study was done at the University of Kentucky Medical Center in Lexington, Kentucky. A second study, being performed under the auspices of the Comprehensive Cancer Center West in the Netherlands, is nearing completion. Both studies were similar in design. Patients with known systemic cancer and single brain metastases were administered steroids and then randomized into one of two treatment groups. The treatment groups consisted of patients receiving either (1) complete surgical resection of the brain metastasis plus postoperative WBRT, or (2) WBRT alone. In the Kentucky Study, patients randomized to receive WBRT alone had stereotaxic needle biopsies of the brain lesion to confirm the diagnosis of metastasis before radiation therapy. In the Dutch Study, patients randomized to receive WBRT alone did not undergo biopsies. In both studies, there was prerandomization stratification for tumor type and extent of systemic disease. (Stratification ensured roughly equal distribution of important prognostic variables between the two treatment groups.) The radiation doses in both groups were similar, with the Kentucky Study using 3,600 cGy and the Dutch Study using 4,000 cGy.

The results from the Kentucky Study are now available. Fifty-four patients were entered in the study. Of those, six (11 percent) were found to have no metastatic brain tumors after resection or biopsy. (The nonmetastatic lesions consisted of two glioblastomas, one low-grade glioma, two abscesses, and one sterile inflammatory reaction.) Of the remaining 48 patients, 25 were in the surgery + WBRT group, and 23 were in the group that received radiation alone. Local recurrence of the brain metastasis was more common in the group that received radiation alone, 52 percent versus 20 percent (p < 0.02). Overall survival was significantly longer (p < 0.01) in the surgery + WBRT group (median of 10 months versus 4 months). Quality of life (as measured by the length of time after treatment that Karnofsky performance scores remained ≥ 70 percent) was also significantly (p < 0.005) better in the surgery plus WBRT group (median of 8 months versus 2 months). The 30-day mortality rates were 4 percent in both treatment groups; therefore, no excess mortality was associated with surgical resection. Surgery reduced the number of local recurrences and this resulted in a subsequent reduction in morbidity and mortality resulting from neurologic causes. Patients with single brain metastases treated with surgical resection plus WBRT lived longer and had a better quality of life than patients treated with WBRT alone. The Dutch Study is still accruing patients, but preliminary results also show a benefit from surgery.

Although surgery + WBRT is superior to WBRT alone in the treatment of single brain metastases, WBRT alone is still the treatment of choice for most patients with brain metastases. This is because only about half of brain metastases are single and, therefore, potentially resectable. Also, nearly half of patients with single metastases are unfortunately not

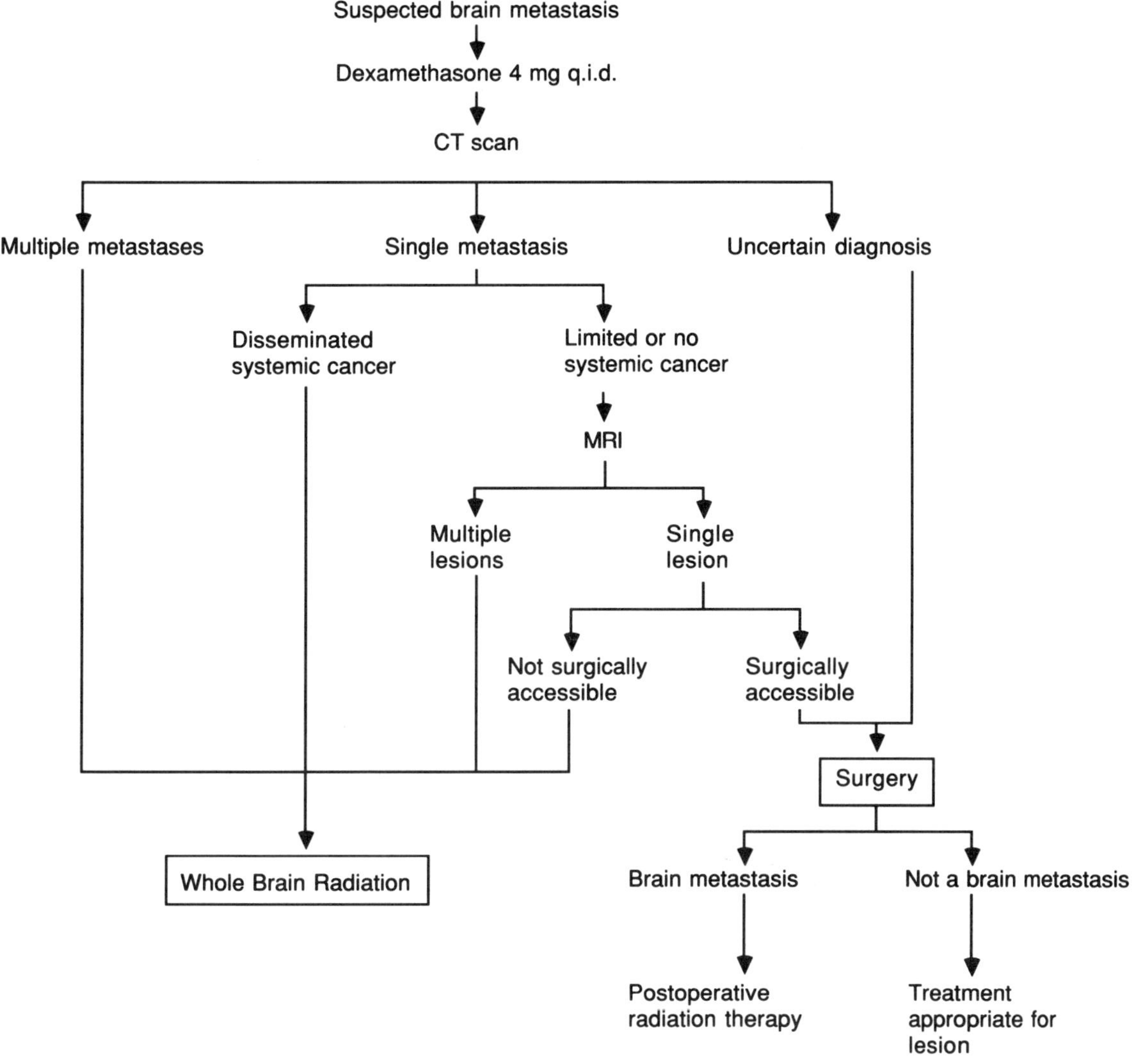

Figure 1   An approach to the patient with a suspected brain metastasis.

surgical candidates because of extensive systemic disease, inaccessibility of the tumor, and other factors. Only about 25 percent of all patients with brain metastases benefit from surgical resection; the rest should be treated with WBRT alone.

The patients with brain metastases who are most likely to benefit from surgical resection are patients with a single surgically accessible lesion and either no remaining systemic disease (true solitary metastasis) or with controlled systemic cancer limited to the primary site only. Candidates for this treatment should also have life expectancies of at least 2 months. In the Kentucky study, it was found that the median time that Karnofsky scores were maintained at pretreatment levels was about 2 months in patients treated with WBRT alone. Patients with life expectancies less than 2 months therefore receive adequate palliation from radiation alone and are unlikely to gain any benefit from surgery. Surgery should also be performed in patients in whom the diagnosis of systemic cancer has not been made (to obtain a tissue diagnosis) and in those with impending herniation to relieve pressure. An approach to the treatment of brain metastases is given in the accompanying algorithm (Fig 1).

SUGGESTED READING

Cairncross JG, Posner JB. The management of brain metastases. In: Walker MD, ed. Oncology of the nervous system. Boston: Martinus Nijhoff, 1983:341.

Patchell RA, Cirrincione C, Thaler HT, et al. Single brain metastases: surgery plus radiation or radiation alone. Neurology 1986; 36:447–453.

EPIDURAL SPINAL CORD COMPRESSION AND CARCINOMATOUS MENINGITIS

MARK R. GILBERT, M.D.

EPIDURAL SPINAL CORD COMPRESSION

Epidural spinal cord compression (ESCC) occurs in approximately 5 percent of patients with systemic malignancy, making it the second most common neurologic complication. The term ESCC implies that there is spread of cancer into the epidural space, causing deformation of the spinal cord or the cauda equina. Compression of the spinal cord and the resultant neurologic dysfunction, however, often occur weeks to months after the onset of the initial symptoms of metastatic spread to the epidural space. The initial symptom in 95 percent of patients is pain, either localized or occurring in a radicular pattern. Moreover, patients generally have *no* neurologic dysfunction with the onset of pain. Despite the early presence of pain in most patients with epidural metastases, three-quarters of these patients have significant neurologic dysfunction *at the time of diagnosis*. The most common neurologic findings in patients with ESCC are weakness in the extremities, sensory loss (often with a dermatomal sensory level), and ataxia. Urinary and fecal incontinence are also frequent complaints at the time of diagnosis.

The most common types of primary malignancy that cause epidural metastases are breast cancer, lung cancer, prostate cancer, sarcomas, melanoma, and gastrointestinal cancers, primarily that of the colon. Virtually all types of metastatic cancer have been reported to cause ESCC. The relative frequency of a specific tumor type resulting in ESCC may be related to three factors: (1) the overall incidence of the tumor, (2) the propensity of the tumor to spread to bone (i.e., vertebrae), and (3) the overall duration of survival for patients with the malignancy. ESCC is often a late complication not commonly seen in patients with malignancies associated with a short expected survival, such as those who have pancreatic cancer.

There are two routes by which the tumor infiltrates into the epidural space. The more common route is taken by direct extension of a metastatic lesion from the vertebral bones through the cortical margin of bone that surrounds the spinal canal and into the epidural space. In taking the second route, the tumor spreads into the epidural space through the intervertebral foramina. This occurs most commonly with tumors in the retroperitoneal region or tumors that have metastasized to the periaortic lymph nodes. Once the tumor has reached the epidural space, the fatty tissue and blood vessels in this region provide little barrier to rostral and caudal extension of the tumor. The tumor can extend several vertebral levels from the initial region of tumor infiltration.

Diagnosis

Patients with cancer, back pain, and neurologic dysfunction warrant an emergency evaluation (Fig 1). Plain spine radiographs are useful for directing computed tomographic (CT) myelography. I recommend an x-ray survey of the entire spine so that symptomatic but abnormal regions can be evaluated during CT myelography.

Patients with cancer and back pain who have a *normal* neurologic examination require an x-ray study of the symptomatic area. The finding of a lytic or blastic lesion in the vertebral bones indicates that there is a high likelihood (60 to 80 percent) of tumor being present in the epidural space. X-ray films of the remainder of the spine should then be obtained and the patient should undergo CT myelography to examine the regions with bone changes. Patients with normal spinal radiographs are more difficult to evaluate. If the patient's pain is radicular or if the tumor is retroperitoneal or is a lymphoma (both such tumors being likely to have spread into the epidural space through the intervertebral foramina), I proceed with CT scanning of the symptomatic region of the spine. The CT scan is obtained to look for a paraspinous mass or evidence of vertebral bone metastases eroding through the cortical margin of bone surrounding the spinal canal. If the CT scan is positive, the patient should undergo myelography. If it is negative, the patient is observed.

Combined with CT scanning, myelography using water-soluble agents (metrizamide, iohexol) provides excellent detail of the epidural space with a very low incidence of side effects. The finding of ESCC mandates the delineation of the full extent of the tumor because rostral or caudal extension of tumor greater than five vertebral levels commonly occurs. Complete block often necessitates a second installation of the contrast agent from the other side of the block to determine the extent of the lesion. Cerebrospinal fluid (CSF) should be cytologically evaluated at the time of myelography because carcinomatous meningitis can occur concurrently with ESCC or present with similar symptoms.

The role of magnetic resonance image (MRI) scanning, with or without magnetic "contrast" agents (i.e., gadolinium), in the diagnostic evaluation of ESCC is controversial. A direct comparison of MRI and CT myelography has not been made. Nevertheless, I have had several cases in which

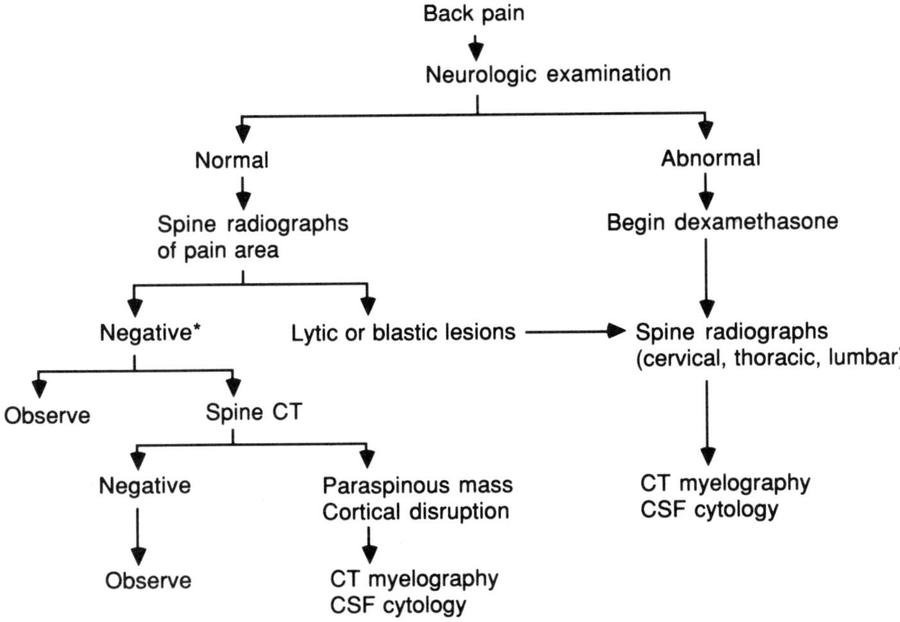

Figure 1 Evaluation of epidural spinal cord compression. *See text.

large epidural deposits of tumor that were found by CT myelography were not demonstrated by MRI scans. In addition, it is unclear whether MRI is able to detect small deposits of tumor in the epidural space at the extending edge of the tumor; if it is not, this limits its usefulness in determining the full extent of disease.

Other diagnoses to consider are carcinomatous meningitis, intramedullary metastases, epidural abscess or hematoma, fungal or tuberculous meningitis, and radiation myelopathy. Rarely, a patient with a parasagittal brain metastasis may present with bilateral (usually asymmetric) lower extremity weakness. Similar findings occur in cases of sagittal sinus thrombosis. Paraneoplastic myelopathy remains a diagnosis of exclusion, as there is no diagnostic test for this condition at present.

Treatment

Corticosteroids

Corticosteroids are highly useful in decreasing edema in the peritumoral region. Prompt institution of steroid therapy for patients with ESCC may prevent vascular compromise of the cord and irreversible dysfunction, thereby allowing time for more definitive treatment of the tumor. In patients presenting with neurologic dysfunction, I recommend high-dose dexamethasone, beginning with a 100-mg bolus, and thereafter 96 mg per day for 3 days. The steroid dose is then tapered off over the next 2 to 3 weeks. In patients with back pain, a normal neurologic examination, and abnormal x-ray studies, I recommend dexamethasone at a dose of 4 mg every 6 hours. This often provides prompt pain relief while diagnostic evaluation is underway.

Surgery

Several studies have shown that a posterior surgical decompression (laminectomy) combined with radiation therapy offers no advantage in outcome or duration of response when compared with radiation treatment alone. There are, however, several indications for surgical intervention:

1. ESCC without a known malignancy. These patients may require a tissue diagnosis before treatment can be initiated. In this case, a needle biopsy may be sufficient.
2. Vertebral instability, particularly of the cervical spine. This may necessitate a debulking and stabilizing procedure.
3. Progression of symptoms during radiation treatment. This may necessitate a surgical decompression to permit completion of the radiation therapy.
4. Recurrence of epidural tumor in a previously irradiated region. This may necessitate surgical decompression to alleviate pain and allow sufficient time for chemotherapy to reduce tumor volume.
5. The possibility of an epidural abscess. This warrants a biopsy procedure.

The most promising surgical technique for treating ESCC is an anterior or anterolateral resection. Most tumors arise from the vertebral body; therefore the most effective debulking procedure would involve resection of the vertebral body and replacement of the bone with a methacrylate prosthesis. Several studies using this technique have yielded promising results, showing that it provides good symptomatic relief and, in some cases, reversal of dense neurologic dysfunction. The procedure is complex, however, and in patients with widely metastatic disease it is associated with high morbidity and mortality rates. I therefore reserve this technique for patients with limited vertebral involvement who also have a long life expectancy.

Radiation Therapy

Radiation therapy is the primary treatment for patients with ESCC. Radiation ports are carefully defined to prevent recurrence of tumor at the edge of a previous treatment field. Local recurrence would preclude treatment of the new lesion because of overlap of the radiation exposure to the previously treated area of the spinal cord. To prevent this problem, I insist on full delineation of the extent of tumor in the epidural space by myelography and often request a second injection of contrast agent if there is a complete block. Evaluation of other regions of the spine that show abnormalities on x-ray films but are asymptomatic may uncover small epidural deposits of tumor that may benefit from early treatment and assist in planning the radiation treatment port(s).

Chemotherapy

The role of chemotherapy in the treatment of epidural spinal cord compression is limited for most solid tumors, but I have used chemotherapy effectively in patients who have undergone previous irradiation and cannot receive more radiation therapy to that area of the spinal cord. I have had some dramatic success with chemotherapy-sensitive tumors, such as lymphomas, where improvement in neurologic function was noted within days of beginning treatment. For other tumors that are less sensitive to chemotherapy, I recommend a surgical decompression, if cord compression exists, in order to allow time for chemotherapy-induced tumor reduction to occur.

Outcome

The outcome of treatment is directly related to the patient's functional status at the time of diagnosis. Generally, patients who are ambulatory at the time of diagnosis will remain so after treatment. Paraplegic patients rarely regain neurologic function after surgical resection and postsurgical radiation treatment. The key to successful management of epidural tumors, therefore, is early diagnosis. Patients with malignancy who develop back pain warrant an evaluation as outlined in Figure 1. It is through the prompt recognition and treatment of epidural metastases that we can alleviate the associated pain and prevent neurologic dysfunction.

CARCINOMATOUS MENINGITIS

Carcinomatous meningitis is defined as the presence of free-floating tumor cells in the CSF. These cells can cause neurologic dysfunction by local infiltration of nerve roots and brain parenchyma, by obstructing the normal flow of the CSF, and by irritating the surface of the cortex, causing seizures. The evaluation and management of carcinomatous meningitis are appropriate for lymphomatous and leukemic meningitis. Management of the spread of primary brain tumors into the spinal fluid, such as in medulloblastoma and glioblastoma multiforme, requires special consideration and is beyond the scope of this discussion.

The most common manifestation of carcinomatous meningitis is an alteration in cognitive function. This symptom may be related to diffuse infiltration of the brain surface by tumor or to increased intracranial pressure. Patients with carcinomatous meningitis frequently complain of headache, which is also often related to increased intracranial pressure. An increase in intracranial pressure is caused by either communicating or noncommunicating hydrocephalus or a combination of both. Communicating hydrocephalus results from tumor cells infiltrating the arachnoid granulations and preventing CSF resorption. Noncommunicating hydrocephalus results from a collection of tumor cells, usually in the cerebral aqueduct, preventing the outflow of CSF.

Patients with carcinomatous meningitis may also present with isolated cranial nerve or spinal radicular findings. Often, nerve dysfunction may be evident at several levels, indicating the diffuse nature of this process. Symptoms of cranial nerve involvement may include blindness (infiltration of the optic nerve or chiasm), diplopia (usually involvement of cranial nerve III or VI), peripheral facial palsy, and less commonly, facial numbness and hearing loss. Spinal cord involvement tends to show predominantly lumbosacral signs and symptoms because tumor cells have a propensity to collect in the thecal sac. This collection may be caused by gravity-related settling of the tumor cells. Patients may also present with low back pain that often has a radicular component similar to sciatica. Lower extremity weakness, dermatomal pattern sensory loss, incontinence, and selected loss of deep tendon reflexes are common.

Seizures, relatively rare occurrences, may be either focal or generalized. Seizures are believed to be caused by meningeal irritation or infiltration of cortical parenchyma by tumor.

Carcinomatous meningitis is primarily caused

by adenocarcinomas, most commonly those of the breast, lung, and melanoma. Leukemic meningitis is common in patients with acute leukemia, particularly those with acute lymphocytic leukemia. Lymphomatous meningitis occurs with nonHodgkin's lymphomas, with a few reported cases occurring with Hodgkin's lymphoma. Lymphoma cells in the CSF are a common finding in primary CNS lymphoma.

Diagnosis

The definitive diagnostic test for carcinomatous meningitis is the demonstration of malignant cells in the CSF. This may require repeated lumbar puncture. The diagnostic yield of a single cytologic analysis of CSF has been reported to be 50 percent. Three CSF analyses increase the sensitivity cytologic examination to approximately 85 percent. Five CSF samples increase the yield of cytology to 95 percent. The spinal fluid, however, is abnormal in almost all patients. Most commonly, the CSF total protein is elevated (80 percent). Other abnormal findings include a pleocytosis (predominantly mononuclear), elevated opening pressure, and a low glucose concentration.

Radiologic studies are often helpful in supporting a diagnosis of carcinomatous meningitis. MRI scanning, particularly with gadolinium administration, may show enhancing deposits along the walls of the ventricles or the cortical sulci. Similar cortical enhancement is sometimes noted on contrast CT scans. Additionally, communicating and noncommunicating hydrocephalus may often be seen with either MRI or CT scanning. CT myelography of the cauda equina region often detects nodular tumor deposits on the nerve roots.

Infectious meningitis, usually a subacute infection such as tuberculosis or a fungal process, may present with findings similar to those of carcinomatous meningitis. Brain metastases, bland or hemorrhagic infarct, or cerebral abscess may present with signs and symptoms of increased intracranial pressure, altered mental status, and headache, which are similar to the common clinical features of carcinomatous meningitis. Other processes that can cause isolated spinal symptoms include ESCC, brachial or lumbar plexopathy, intramedullary metastases, and radiation myelopathy.

Treatment

Radiation Therapy

Radiation therapy was the original means of treating carcinomatous meningitis. Cranial-spinal irradiation, encompassing the entire neuraxis, is necessary if radiation therapy is the only treatment used. However, irradiation of the vertebrae, which provide much of the bone marrow in adults, is asso-

ciated with significant myelosuppression. Myelosuppression severely limits any future chemotherapeutic treatment and is often severe enough to make the patient dependent on transfusions of blood products. Radiation treatment to the brain is also associated with a chronic neurotoxic syndrome known as leukoencephalopathy. This syndrome usually occurs months to years after treatment and is characterized by a slowly progressive change in personality, leading to changes in cognitive function and often ultimately leading to coma or death. Patients who receive intrathecal chemotherapy after brain irradiation are at a particularly high risk for developing leukoencephalopathy.

As indicated in the following sections of this chapter, I use radiation therapy only for control of local symptoms or to alleviate ventricular outflow obstruction if noncommunicating hydrocephalus exists. This approach usually provides some reversal of local neurologic dysfunction, particularly if cranial nerve palsies are prominent findings. Relief of ventricular outflow obstruction is critical for safe installation of chemotherapy into the lateral ventricles through a reservoir.

Chemotherapy

Intrathecal administration of chemotherapeutic agents is the predominant treatment modality for carcinomatous meningitis. Chemotherapeutic agents administered systemically do not cross the blood-brain barrier in sufficient amounts to achieve tumoricidal levels in the CSF. Chemotherapy can be instilled into either the lumbar thecal space or into the lateral ventricles through a subcutaneous reservoir (i.e., Ommaya reservoir). Lumbar injections can be done with standard lumbar punctures, although studies using radiotracer have shown that 10 to 15 percent of these injections end up in the epidural space or in the subcutaneous fat. Moreover, repeated injections can lead to local scar formation, making subsequent punctures difficult and uncomfortable. Placement of the ventricular reservoir system requires a neurosurgical procedure, but once the ventricular reservoir system is in place, it provides a well-tolerated method of instilling drug into the CSF. I use the reservoir also to obtain an [111]Indium DTPA ventriculogram before injecting the drug to ensure that ventricular outflow is not obstructed. Outflow obstruction causes pooling of drug in the lateral ventricles, which can result in a rapidly progressive, often fatal degeneration of brain parenchyma. Patients with outflow obstruction undergo local radiation treatment; clearance of the obstruction is then confirmed with a repeat ventriculogram.

It is unclear whether an advantage exists for either lumbar or ventricular injections. Some recent data from studies of drug delivery in animal models indicate that combined lumbar and ventricular administration of drug is best for achieving adequate concentrations of drug throughout the neuraxis. Ventricular injections provide high concentration of drug in the CSF surrounding the brain, but the levels are significantly lower in the spinal cord region. The reverse, however, is true with lumbar injections. For this reason, I favor a combination of both lumbar and ventricular injections.

Methotrexate is the most commonly used drug for intrathecal injections. It has tumoricidal activity against most solid tumors, leukemias, and lymphomas. Cytosine arabinoside (ara-C) is useful only for leukemias and lymphomas. Thiophosphoramide (Thiotepa) can also be administered intrathecally. This alkylating agent is useful for solid tumors, particularly for breast and lung cancers. I usually administer intrathecal drugs two times per week for 8 to 12 weeks or until the tumor is cleared from the CSF. I continue a maintenance regimen of biweekly injections for 1 year or until there is evidence of progressive disease. The standard dose of methotrexate for adults is 12 mg per injection; ara-C is administered in a dose of 50 mg per injection; and Thiotepa is given in doses of 10 mg.

As described above, intrathecal chemotherapy is associated with a high incidence of leukoencephalopathy. Prior cranial radiation therapy significantly increases the incidence of developing leukoencephalopathy. In my experience, almost all patients who receive both radiation and intrathecal chemotherapy develop leukoencephalopathy within 1 year of completing treatment.

Outcome

Carcinomatous meningitis carries a grave prognosis. The duration of survival is related to the type of primary malignancy and to the extent of neurologic dysfunction at the time of diagnosis. For all tumor types, if the patient is not treated, survival is generally a few weeks. Patients with melanoma have the worst prognosis; despite radiation and chemotherapy, low treatment response rates (20 percent) and short median survival times (3.6 months) have been reported. Patients with carcinomatous meningitis from lung cancer fare only slightly better than patients with melanoma; the treatment response rate is 20 percent and the median survival is 4 months. Patients with breast cancer have the best prognosis, but even in those who are treated, the median survival is only 7.2 months. There are, however, several reports of patients with breast cancer surviving more than 2 years after the diagnosis of carcinomatous meningitis. Unfortunately, most of these patients develop severe neurologic dysfunction from leukoencephalopathy caused by chemotherapy and radiotherapy.

SUGGESTED READING

Findlay GFG. Adverse effects of the management of malignant spinal cord compression. J Neurol Neurosurg Psych 1984; 47:761–768.

Grossman SA, Chen CDP, Thompson G, et al. Cerebrospinal fluid abnormalities in patients with neoplastic meningitis: an evaluation using [111]Indium-DTPA ventriculography. Am J Med 1982; 73:641–645.

Harrington KD. Anterior cord decompression and spinal stabilization for patients with metastatic lesions of the spine. J Neurosurg 1984; 61:107–117.

Rodichok LD, Harper GR, Ruckdeschel JC, et al. Early diagnosis of spinal epidural metastases. Am J Med 1987; 70:1181–1187.

Wasserstrom WR, Glass JP, Posner JP. Diagnosis and treatment of leptomeningeal metastases from solid tumors: experience with 90 patients. Cancer 1982; 49:759–772.

Weissman DA, Gilbert MR, Wong H, Grossman SA. The use of computed tomography of the spine to identify patients at high risk for epidural metastases. J Clin Oncol 1985; 3:1541–1544.

PARANEOPLASTIC SYNDROME

MICHAEL SWASH, M.D., FRCP, MRC Path
MARTIN S. SCHWARTZ, M.D.

The paraneoplastic syndromes that affect the nervous system (Table 1) are disorders that result from the presence of malignant disease, either overt or occult, that is remote from the involved neural tissue; these syndromes are not caused by primary or secondary tumor in the nervous system. The association of these syndromes with malignant disease has been recognized from epidemiologic evidence, but other criteria are also important. In most, there is evidence of a specific humoral or cell-mediated immune mechanism, and clinical improvement may result when this immune disturbance is modified by appropriate treatment. In others (e.g., dermatomyositis), the immune basis of the syndrome has not yet been identified. Some paraneoplastic syndromes are characteristically associated with particular neoplasms—for example opsoclonus, ataxia, and myoclonus associated with neuroblastoma in childhood. Other paraneoplastic syndromes are not specific (e.g., peripheral neuropathy associated with paraproteinemia), and the association with particular neoplasms is recognized by appropriate immuno-

Table 1 Paraneoplastic Syndromes of the Nervous System

Paraneoplastic Syndromes	*Associated Neoplasms*
Peripheral nervous system disorders	
Neuropathies	
Subacute sensory neuropathy	SCLC
Symmetrical sensorimotor neuropathy	Carcinoma, lymphoma, myeloma
Motor neuropathy	Osteosclerotic myeloma
Guillain-Barré syndrome	Hodgkin's disease
Acquired amyloid neuropathy	Myeloma and other paraproteinemia
Mononeuritis multiplex	SCLC lymphoma
Neuromuscular junction disorders	
Myasthenia gravis	Thymoma
LEMS	SCLC
Muscle	
Polymyositis-dermatomyositis	SCLC, carcinoma, especially of the breast and ovary; lymphoma
Subacute necrotizing myopathy	Carcinoma and lymphoma
Chronic graft versus host disease	Bone marrow transplantation
Central nervous system	
Encephalomyelitis	SCLC, carcinoma of breast or ovary; lymphoma
Limbic	
Brain stem	
Subacute cortical cerebellar degeneration	
Opsoclonus/myoclonus	Neuroblastoma, carcinoma of the ovary or lung
Necrotizing myelopathy	SCLC, breast carcinoma
Retinopathy and uveomeningitis	SCLC, carcinoma of the breast
Vascular	Hypercoagulable states, carcinoma of the pancreas, other carcinomas and lymphomas
Marantic endocarditis	Various carcinomas
Hyperviscosity syndrome	Myeloma
Others	
Central pontine myelinolysis caused by inappropriate ADH secretion	SCLC
Inappropriate ACTH secretion	SCLC
Hypercalcemia	Metastatic carcinoma
Inappropriate parathormone secretion	
Progressive multifocal leukoencephalopathy	Immunosuppression associated with carcinoma
AIDS	Complex relation to carcinoma
POEMS	Myeloma
Hypoglycemia	Insuloma, retroperitoneal sarcoma
Carcinoid syndrome	Paraganglioma
Pheochromocytoma	Adrenal tumor

logic and radiologic investigation. These clinical syndromes may also occur without association with carcinoma, as idiopathic autoimmune disorders; for example, myasthenia gravis may occur with or without thymoma and Lambert-Eaton myasthenic syndrome (LEMS) with or without oat cell carcinoma of the lung (SCLC).

INCIDENCE

Although these disorders are uncommon, they have been recognized, often as subclinical phenomena, in as many as 6 percent of patients with cancer in a large series. About 50 percent of all paraneoplastic syndromes are associated with SCLC. These complications occur less commonly with carcinoma of the ovary, stomach, and breast; there are also frequent associations with lymphoma and with myeloma (Table 1 and Fig. 1), but reliable estimates of

their incidence are not available. In some patients, two or more paraneoplastic syndromes may coexist —for example, peripheral neuropathy with encephalomyelitis, and LEMS with subacute cortical cerebellar degeneration. Although paraneoplastic peripheral neuropathy is probably the most common of the paraneoplastic syndromes, peripheral neuropathy is frequently secondary to chemotherapy rather than directly caused by the tumor. Paraneoplastic central nervous system (CNS) syndromes are rare, but are more specifically associated with neoplasia than with the other paraneoplastic syndromes.

PATHOGENESIS

Lymphocytic infiltration in the affected tissue is a well established feature of most paraneoplastic syndromes. In addition, the CNS syndromes are frequently associated with cerebrospinal fluid (CSF)

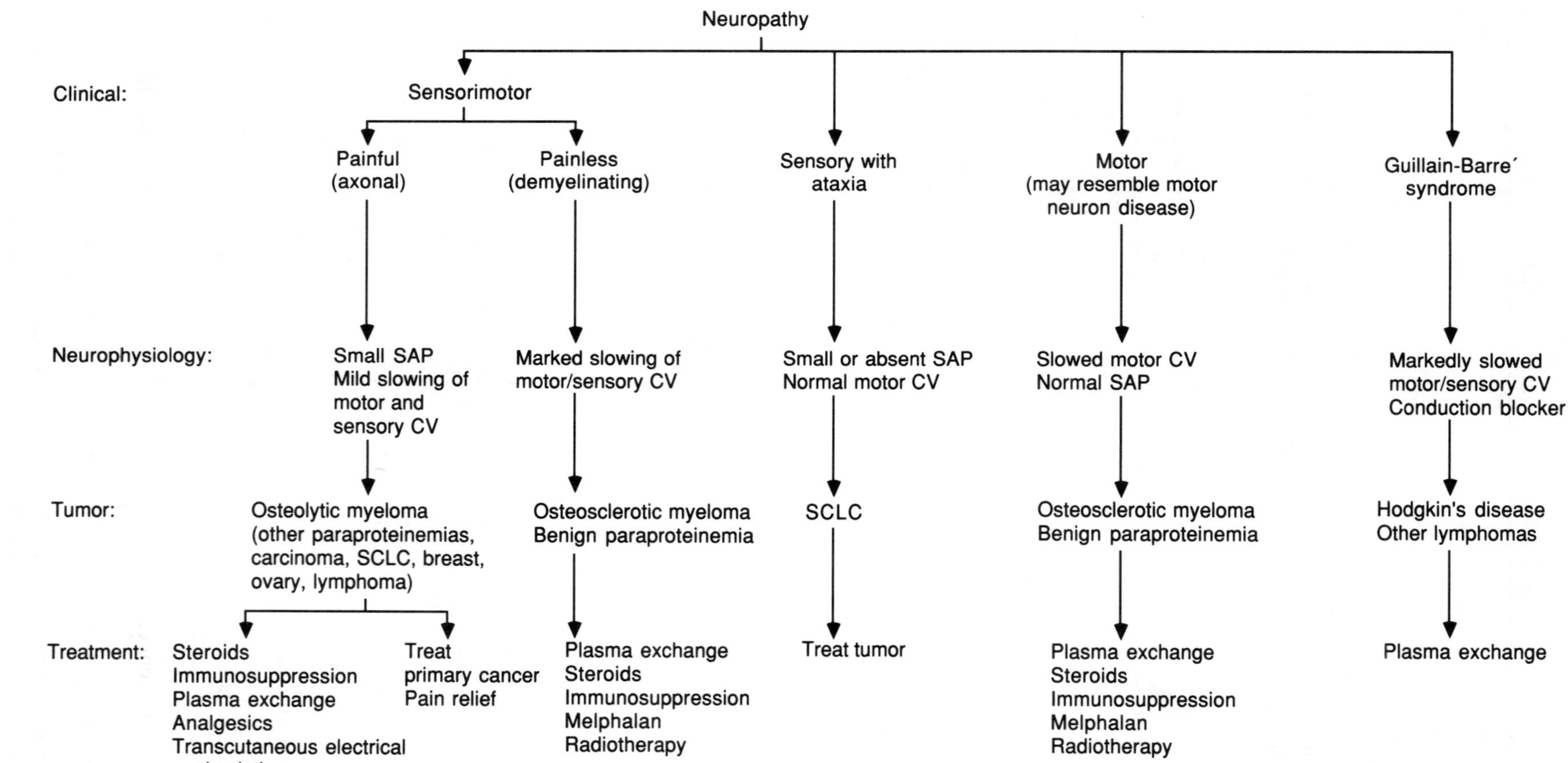

Figure 1 Management of paraneoplastic neuropathy. CV = conduction velocity; SAP = sensory action potential.

lymphocytosis and a raised CSF protein level, and the peripheral neuropathy that occurs with myeloma is associated with a circulating paraprotein, usually immunoglobulin M (IgM). Specific circulating immunoglobulin G (IgG) antibodies that react with antigens in the target tissue have been identified in most of these syndromes. In some, the antibody cross-reacts with tumor homogenates, (e.g., of SCLC cells). However, passive transfer experiments using these antibodies have replicated the features of paraneoplastic syndromes only in thymoma-associated myasthenia gravis, in LEMS, and in certain paraproteinemias associated with myeloma. Paraneoplastic syndromes may occur in syndromes with established malignant disease or may antedate discovery of the tumor, sometimes by a year or more. Successful treatment of the tumor is not usually accompanied by improvement in symptoms related to the paraneoplastic syndrome, except in myeloma and in myasthenia gravis associated with thymoma.

PERIPHERAL NERVOUS SYSTEM DISORDERS

Peripheral Neuropathies

Subacute Sensory Neuropathy

This disorder presents with a subacute or rapid onset of sensory ataxia, with profound posterior column sensory disturbance and with pseudoathetoid involuntary movements of the extremities. There is distal sensory impairment with dysesthesias that may be painful. Subacute sensory neuropathy may be associated with features of brain stem encephalomyelitis, especially nystagmus and dementia. The patient is unable to stand or walk. This neuropathy is strongly associated with SCLC. There is degeneration of cells in the posterior root ganglia with infiltration by lymphocytes, plasma cells, and macrophages, and axonal degeneration in the posterior columns. In most patients, symptoms of the neuropathy precede discovery of the carcinoma by about 6 months and death occurs approximately 1 year later. No treatment is available; steroids and immunosuppressant drugs are not effective. The neuropathy also fails to improve if the cancer is treated surgically, with radiation therapy, or with chemotherapy. Dysesthesias may be managed by treatment with clonazepam (200 mg twice daily) or carbamazepine (in a starting dose of 200 mg twice daily, which is increased incrementally to a maximum of 800 to 1,000 mg daily). However, often this is not effective, and treatment with nonsteroidal antiinflammatory drugs, particularly Diflunisal (250 to 500 mg twice daily), is worth trying. Tricyclic antidepressants and chlorpromazine may also be useful, as well as transcutaneous electrical stimulation and localized heat. Reducing afferent input by wearing rubber gloves or elastic stockings generally reduces the severity of dysesthesias. The neuropathy does not improve after surgical excision of the tumor or after radiotherapy or chemotherapy.

Symmetrical Sensorimotor Neuropathy

Distal sensorimotor neuropathy associated with carcinoma may be axonal or demyelinating in type.

Axonal Type. This is a symmetrical polyneuropathy that is predominantly sensory, presenting with distal sensory loss involving all modalities, and is the most common of the paraneoplastic syndromes. Dysesthesias may be severe and painful. Mild distal weakness and atrophy are also present. The neuropathy may be of rapid or insidious onset. Trigeminal involvement and bulbar signs with proximal weakness are features of some cases. This syndrome has been reported with many different types of carcinoma and lymphoma and with osteolytic myeloma. A relapsing and remitting form is particularly associated with SCLC.

This painful axonal neuropathy may improve with steroid therapy and the successful treatment of the underlying malignancy, especially when it is associated with seminoma of the testis or with renal carcinoma. If the clinical syndrome is severe or disabling, oral prednisolone (60 to 80 mg per day) is worth trying in a single daily morning dose for 4 weeks; if this agent is of benefit, the dose should be gradually changed to an alternate-day regimen (60 mg on alternate days) during the subsequent month, and then reduced to a maintenance schedule of 10 to 30 mg on alternate days, depending on the clinical response. Immunosuppressant drugs have also been used in the treatment of this syndrome, but based on our experience, we believe that these are probably not as effective as prednisolone. Dysesthesias may continue and should be managed as described earlier in this chapter.

Demyelinating Type. The sensorimotor neuropathy found in association with osteolytic myeloma and other malignant paraproteinemias (e.g., B-cell leukemia) responds to removal of the paraprotein by plasma exchange and to successful treatment of the malignancy by chemotherapy and/ or radiotherapy. Plasma exchange is probably not worthwhile when there is a low concentration of paraprotein, but this is a difficult clinical judgment. Steroid therapy, often used in conjunction with chemotherapy in order to prolong the survival of red and white blood cells in patients with extensive bone marrow infiltration, has a beneficial effect on the symptoms caused by the neuropathy. The effectiveness of therapy can be monitored by sensory and motor nerve conduction studies as well as by careful neurologic assessment and by measurement of paraprotein levels in the blood, but usually the patient's assessment of symptoms is the less sensitive measure. Approximately 20 percent of these patients have amyloidosis, and approximately 30 percent develop carpal tunnel syndrome, which may sometimes require decompression.

Motor Neuropathy

Painless motor neuropathy is associated with osteosclerotic myeloma and solitary plasmacytoma, including IgM, IgG, and immunoglobulin A (IgA) types. Some patients show features of the POEMS syndrome (polyneuropathy, organomegaly, endocrinopathy, IgM paraproteinemia, and skin manifestations), including hepatosplenomegaly, lymphadenopathy, diabetes mellitus, gonadal failure with gynecomastia in males, hirsutism, and hyperpigmentation. In most patients, there is a low concentration of paraprotein and the bone marrow is often nondiagnostic. Immunoelectrophoresis of plasma is often necessary to make the diagnosis, and a skeletal survey is required to locate the myeloma. "Benign" paraproteinemia evolves into myeloma in 30 to 50 percent of cases, and repeated investigation is therefore important.

Treatment of the causative neoplasm by radiotherapy produces remission, or at least arrest, of the neuropathy. Plasma exchange may be useful if the neuropathy is severe, but is unlikely to be helpful if there is only a low concentration of paraprotein in the blood. If the tumor recurs, the neuropathy often worsens. Electrophysiologic monitoring is helpful in assessing the disorder during both treatment and clinical relapses. If the neuropathy is severe, treatment with prednisolone (40 to 80 mg daily) for 1 month, followed by a gradually decreasing dose, depending on the clinical response, may initiate a remission. The role of immunosuppressant drugs in the treatment of this condition has not been adequately assessed, but it may be reasonable to try azathioprine (50 mg three times daily) in patients refractory to other forms of treatment.

Guillain-Barré Syndrome

This is a rare complication of malignancy. It occurs in Hodgkin's disease, angioimmunoblastic lymphadenopathy with dysproteinemia, and chronic lymphatic leukemia. Paraneoplastic Guillain-Barré syndrome does not differ from idiopathic Guillain-Barré syndrome in its clinical features, and management is identical. The onset is unrelated to remission or exacerbation of the malignancy.

Mononeuritis Multiplex

Immune-mediated paraneoplastic mononeuritis multiplex must be differentiated from local invasion of nerves, plexuses, or roots. Local invasion of roots may be accompanied by CSF pleocytosis, with malignant cells. Mononeuritis multiplex is particularly associated with SCLC. There is often a mild underlying sensorimotor neuropathy, the mononeuritis syndrome perhaps being related to nerve entrapment or pressure palsies, but vasculitis of the vasa nervorum has been found in some cases. Treatment with prednisolone (60 mg daily) may be effective. The dose should be reduced, and an alternate-day protocol should be used according to standard regimens (see above). Azathioprine (50 mg three times daily, adjusted according to body weight) should be given on the assumption that the disorder is caused by vasculitis.

Neuromuscular Junction Disorders

Myasthenia Gravis

Myasthenia gravis (MG) occurs in 30 percent of patients with thymomas, but only 10 percent of patients with myasthenia gravis have thymoma. Myasthenia gravis develops in 10 percent of patients after removal of a thymoma. Remission of myasthenia gravis after thymectomy is less likely if there is a malignant thymoma than if there is hyperplasia; its severity cannot be linearly correlated with levels of circulating acetylcholine receptor IgG antibody. Benign thymomas carry a good prognosis resembling that of thymic hyperplasia. The treatment of myasthenia gravis associated with thymoma does not differ from that of the disease associated with thymic hyperplasia.

Lambert-Eaton Myasthenic Syndrome

LEMS occurs in 3 percent of patients with SCLC, but 50 percent of patients with LEMS have or develop SCLC. Other paraneoplastic syndromes (e.g., cerebellar degeneration) may coexist. In patients with LEMS that is SCLC associated, the tumor will become apparent within 2 years of presentation of the neuromuscular syndrome; other cases are autoimmune in origin.

Muscle Disorders

Polymyositis-Dermatomyositis

The association of polymyositis and dermatomyositis with malignancy is well established, but its frequency remains controversial. Juvenile dermatomyositis is an autoimmune disease that is not associated with malignancy. Polymyositis of adult onset is less strongly associated with cancer than dermatomyositis, although estimates vary. Approximately 20 percent of patients older than 40 years of age with polymyositis-dermatomyositis syndrome show this association. Cancer may be found concurrently with, subsequent to, or before the onset of muscle disease. It is generally accepted that the strength of the association increases with increasing age, but since the prevalence of cancer in older patients also increases, there is doubt as to the significance of this finding. The association of inflammatory muscle disease with cancer is closer for SCLC and breast cancer, but it has been described for many different forms of neoplasm, including lymphomas.

The clinical response of patients with inflammatory muscle disease to steroids and immunosuppression is similar to that of patients with inflammatory myopathy not associated with cancer. Treatment of an underlying neoplasm or lymphoma has no effect on the course of the muscle disease. Investigation of patients with polymyositis or dermatomyositis for occult neoplasia is likely to be informative only in patients older than 50 years of age. We restrict this investigation to routine hematologic and liver function tests, chest x-ray examinations, mammography, and pelvic and rectal examinations unless there are any specific features suggestive of neoplasm in other organs.

Subacute Necrotizing Myopathy

This disorder is an acute fulminant myopathy that has been associated with cancer of the colon, stomach, bladder, and breast. Patients with subacute necrotizing myopathy do not respond to treatment with steroids, immunosuppressive drugs, or plasma exchange, and the disorder is rapidly fatal. It may mimic acute Guillain-Barré syndrome at presentation, but the creatine kinase is raised to 100 times the normal range.

Chronic Graft Versus Host Myositis

This rare disorder occurs months or years after bone marrow transplantation, usually in the treatment of leukemia. It is accompanied by muscle pain, tenderness, and weakness. Prednisolone (60 to 80 mg daily) following the protocol used for idiopathic polymyositis is effective in the treatment of these syndromes. Immunosuppressive drugs must be used with caution in order to avoid compromising the bone marrow graft. Graft versus host myasthenia gravis and polyneuropathy have also been described.

CENTRAL NERVOUS SYSTEM DISORDERS

Encephalomyelitis

There are three paraneoplastic encephalomyelitis syndromes: limbic encephalitis, brain stem encephalitis, and subacute cerebellar degeneration. These symptoms often overlap and many of the patients with these disorders also develop sensorimotor neuropathy.

Limbic Encephalitis

This syndrome is accompanied by progressive impairment of recent memory with mild dementia, often presenting with depression, hallucinations, and anxiety. Seizures may occur. The onset may be abrupt or subacute during several weeks. Dysarthria may also be a feature. After a period of progression, the disorder arrests. At autopsy, there is evidence of a loss of neurons and inflammation in the medial temporal structures with glial proliferation. The disorder is associated with SCLC, but this is usually occult and may be discovered only after death. IgG antinuclear antineuronal antibodies have been found, and plasma exchange may cause improvement with reductions in antibody titre. Steroid therapy and immunosuppressant therapy are ineffective. Anticonvulsant drugs should be used as necessary. The syndrome does not respond to treatment of the underlying neoplasm.

Brain Stem Encephalitis

Vertigo, nystagmus, ataxia, nausea, vomiting, and cranial nerve signs, especially ophthalmoplegia, develop with this syndrome and are associated with neuronal loss, lymphocytic and plasma cell infiltration, and gliosis in the brain stem, particularly in the pons. There may be involvement of the cervical cord, with loss of anterior horn cells, and mononuclear cells are often found in the CSF. This syndrome in particular is associated with occult SCLC, but also occurs with Hodgkin's disease. There is often an associated peripheral neuropathy which may precede the encephalitis. All forms of treatment are ineffective, but it is difficult to avoid trying a course of high-dose steroids. Although plasma exchange may also be tried, we have not observed any improvements with this treatment. Removal of a SCLC, if it can be detected, does not result in improvement.

Subacute Cortical Cerebellar Degeneration

In this disorder, there is loss of Purkinje cells from the cerebellar cortex without inflammation, but sometimes with degeneration also in the dentate nuclei. In a second, clinically identical form of the disorder, there is an associated inflammatory reaction. This syndrome presents with ataxia, cerebellar dysarthria, nystagmus, dysphagia, and dementia. Vertigo may be a prominent feature, and therefore it is often difficult to distinguish this syndrome from paraneoplastic brain stem encephalitis. The CSF may show a pleocytosis. This cerebellar degeneration is most frequently associated with SCLC, but many other tumors have been reported in an apparently causal relationship. In our experience, all treatments are ineffective, although improvement after resection of SCLC has been reported.

Opsoclonus/Myoclonus

This characteristic clinical syndrome consists of chaotic irregular movements of eyes and limbs (dancing eyes/dancing feet) and usually occurs in children. Cerebellar ataxia may coexist. In 50 percent of patients, there is an associated, often calcified adrenal neuroblastoma. The syndrome may be transient or remittent, and there may be improvement after resection or radiation treatment of the tumor. Steroid therapy often induces remission.

In older patients, the differential diagnosis includes viral encephalitis and multiple sclerosis, and the syndrome also occurs in association with SCLC. In patients in whom remission has occurred, the disorder may be exacerbated after incidental viral infection or immunization, but a remission can often be induced again by steroid therapy.

Necrotizing Myelopathy

This is the rarest and least well documented paraneoplastic syndrome. It has been reported to occur with SCLC and Hodgkin's disease and consists of a subacute progressive myelopathy leading to paraplegia and incontinence, often within a few days after onset. There may be brain stem involvement. Steroids and immunosuppressant treatment are ineffective.

Vascular Syndromes

Paraneoplastic Cerebrovascular Disease

Malignancy may be associated with hypercoagulable states (e.g., in association with carcinoma of the pancreas, stomach, or ovary) and may present with neurologic complications, especially cerebral infarction and sagittal sinus thrombosis. There may be features of thrombosis in other tissues, especially the great vessels of the abdomen and thorax, and in the subcutaneous veins. Often the diagnosis can be made only after exclusion of other hematologic causes of intravascular coagulation. Although treatment with steroids is ineffective, anticoagulation with intravenous heparin is an effective temporary measure. Its use is limited, however, by the complications or long-term intravenous heparin, especially bone necrosis. Oral anticoagulant therapy with warfarin (Coumadin) is less effective, and antiplatelet medication—for example aspirin (300 mg daily), dipyridamole (50 mg three times daily), and fibrinolytic drugs (e.g., Stenozalol, 5 mg daily) may have some beneficial effect. Sulfinpyrazone is not effective.

Malignant disease is also associated with *marantic endocarditis,* leading to arterial embolism and stroke. This can be managed with anticoagulants; treatment should be begun with intravenous heparin, and then Coumadin should be used. Septic embolism must be excluded. *Cerebral hemorrhage* or *infarction* also occurs with *hyperviscosity syndromes*—for example, in association with myelomatosis and paraproteinemia, and with carcinoma of the stomach or low platelet states, especially metastatic carcinoma in the bone marrow. Fresh platelet transfusion may be needed.

OTHER SYNDROMES

Other paraneoplastic syndromes may indirectly affect the nervous system (see Table 1). These include infections in immunocompromised patients, such as progressive multifocal leukoencephalopathy and herpes zoster encephalitis. In acquired immunodeficiency syndrome (AIDS), there are complex interactions between the primary retroviral infection and cancer. In other syndromes, the CNS is affected as a result of hormonal disturbance caused by the tumor.

Inappropriate Antidiuretic Hormone Secretion

This syndrome is accompanied by persistent hyponatremia. This is associated with central pontine myelinolysis, occurring spontaneously or during rapid correction of the hyponatremia. The hyponatremia itself causes confusion, muscle cramps, and seizures.

Inappropriate Adrenocorticotropic Hormone Secretion

This syndrome results in Cushing's syndrome and is sometimes associated with myopathy and encephalopathy. Removal of the adrenocorticotropic hormone (ACTH)-secreting tumor, usually found in the pulmonary cavity, results in improvement. ACTH-secreting adrenal tumors may cause the same syndrome.

Hypoglycemia

Profound hypoglycemia caused by insulinoma can cause an irreversible encephalopathy presenting with confusion, sweatiness, pallor, seizures, and coma. Severe disability may result if this disorder is not corrected. Hypoglycemia may also develop with retroperitoneal lymphomas, hepatocellular carcinoma, fibrosarcomas, and other mesenchymal tumors. Treatment of these lesions prevents further hypoglycemic episodes.

Hypercalcemia

Severe hypercalcemia, caused by bony metastases or ectopic parathormone secretion, may cause dementia, stupor, and coma, preceded by nausea, vomiting, muscular weakness, irritability, and renal failure. These features are reversible with correction of the hypercalcemia.

Pheochromocytoma

Paroxysmal hypertension, caused by secretion of vasoactive adrenergic compounds from the tumor, usually situated in the adrenal gland, may cause cerebral edema and headache, vomiting, anxiety, or even cerebral hemorrhage. Recognition of the syndrome may be difficult, but control of hypertension by beta- and alpha-blockade followed by excision of the tumor is effective in preventing the irreversible effects of paroxysmal hypertension. The tumor may be located by computed tomography or magnetic resonance imaging and by selective angiography.

SUGGESTED READING

Henson RA, Urich H. Cancer and the nervous system. Oxford: Blackwell Scientific Publications, 1982: 657.
Arnason BGW. Paraneoplastic syndrome of muscle, nerve, and brain: immunological consideration. In: Rose FC, ed. Clinical neuroimmunology. Oxford: Blackwell Scientific Publications, 1979: 421.
Antel JP, Moundjian R. Paraneoplastic syndrome: a role for the immune system. J Neurol 1989; 236: 1–3.
Layzer RB. Neuromuscular manifestations of systemic disease. Philadelphia: FA Davis, 1985: 253.
Kelly JJ, Adelman LD, Berkman E, Bhan I. Polyneuropathies associated with IgM monoclonal gammopathies. Arch Neurol 1988; 1355–1359.

PSEUDOTUMOR CEREBRI

LISSETTE JIMENEZ, M.D.
LEON D. PROCKOP, M.D.

Pseudotumor cerebri (PTC) is a clinical syndrome of uncertain etiology characterized by elevated intracranial pressure in the absence of any demonstrable structural central nervous system (CNS) lesion, localizing neurologic signs, or hydrocephalus. A variety of etiologic factors and related disorders are sometimes associated with the syndrome (Table 1).

Although the syndrome can occur at any age, the typical patient is a young obese female. Hypertension and obesity are the most consistent associated risk factors. Usual presenting symptoms are headache and visual disturbances. Headaches may be mild or severe, pressurelike or pounding, unilateral or bilateral, and they may be worse during or just after the patient is in the recumbent position.

Visual disturbances, occurring in 50 percent of patients, include transient visual obscurations, blurred vision, permanent visual loss, and horizontal diplopia caused by a false localizing sign as a result of increased intracranial pressure. Permanent visual loss, the most serious complication, reportedly occurs in 5 to 23 percent of cases. It may occur early or late in the course of the disease. Less common manifestations are aching of the neck, arms, and back; facial pain; retro-ocular pain; pulsatile tinnitus; low-frequency hearing loss; and facial paralysis.

The neurologic examination of these patients usually yields normal results except for papilledema and visual field abnormalities. Although an enlarged blind spot is common, a constricted visual field, nasal inferior visual field loss, and central and paracentral scotomata may also be seen. Visual acuity is normal in uncomplicated cases.

Pseudopapilledema, usually resulting from optic disc drusen, should be distinguished from papilledema. The former does not exhibit exudates and hemorrhage. Stereoscopic color fundus photography and fluorescein angiography may be needed for differentiation.

DIAGNOSIS

Because PTC is diagnosed through exclusion, in the diagnostic evaluation one should consider the many other etiologies for increased intracranial pressure presenting without localizing signs. Although some of these may represent coincidental associations, their identification may lead to therapeutic intervention (see Table 1).

Because of its greater sensitivity compared with brain computed tomographic (CT) scanning, magnetic resonance imaging (MRI) is the diagnostic imaging procedure of choice. Both CT and MRI are usually normal, or may show slitlike ventricles. MRI may show increased white matter signal. MRI can also demonstrate dural venous or sagittal sinus thrombosis as specific etiologies. Cerebral angiography may also be necessary when such thromboses are considered. In some patients, PTC causes sella turcica enlargement and empty sella syndrome.

If neuroimaging studies are normal or demonstrate slitlike ventricles, lumbar puncture to measure cerebrospinal fluid (CSF) pressure and com-

Table 1 Conditions Associated with Pseudotumor Cerebri

Intracranial venous drainage obstruction
  Mastoiditis and lateral sinus obstruction
  Congenital atresia or stenosis of venous sinuses
  Cervical or thoracic venous drainage obstruction
  Internal jugular vein ligation

Drugs
  Tetracycline
  Amiodarone
  Nalidixic acid
  Nitrofurantoin
  Lithium
  Sulfonamides
  Chlordecone (Kepone)
  Levothyroxine sodium

Endocrine and metabolic
  Obesity
  Menarche
  Menstrual irregularities, use of oral contraceptives
  Pregnancy and postpartum
  Sex hormones (male and female)
  Corticosteroid therapy and withdrawal
  Hypoparathyroidism
  Addison's disease
  Cushing's disease
  Hyperadrenalism
  Hyper- and hypovitaminosis A

Hematologic disorders
  Iron deficiency anemia
  Wiskott-Aldrich syndrome
  Infectious mononucleosis
  Cryoglobulinemia
  Polythemia vera

Other
  Rapid growth in infancy
  Systemic lupus erythematosus

position should then be performed. The opening pressure is elevated, usually from 250 to 600 mmH$_2$O. The protein content is normal or low, sometimes less than 20 mg per deciliter. No other abnormalities occur that might indicate infection, hemorrhage, or other disease.

Routine hematology and electrolyte profile plus ANA and Venereal Disease Research Laboratory (VDRL) should be sufficient unless there is clinical suspicion of endocrine abnormalities, in which case appropriate tests should be performed.

There are no predicting signs or symptoms of impending visual loss. A careful ophthalmologic evaluation, including testing of visual acuity, photography, and sequential quantitative perimetry should be done at intervals set by the clinical circumstances. Intraocular pressure (IOP) should be measured serially, especially in patients receiving steroids. A causal relationship between increased IOP and visual loss has been suggested.

TREATMENT

The natural history of untreated pseudotumor has not been defined. Except for the risk of loss of vision, the course is benign with a high spontaneous remission rate, although the recurrence rate is approximately 10 percent.

Because there are no prospective, randomized studies comparing different treatment modalities, it is impossible to make categorical statements about therapy for patients with PTC. Treatment goals are the preservation of normal vision and relief of symptoms (Fig. 1). Therapeutic intervention should include a weight loss regimen, treatment of hypertension, and modification of secondary factors causally implicated in PTC.

Treatment Modalities

Lumbar Puncture

Relief of symptoms is often achieved after a single lumbar puncture. Symptomatic remission after a first lumbar puncture has been noted in 25 to 30 percent of cases. Sufficient CSF (as much as 30 ml) is removed to achieve normal CSF pressure.

Repeated lumbar punctures, varying from once per week to once per day, should be performed for those patients with persistent symptoms. Postlumbar puncture headache, usually self-remitting or responsive to a blood patch, may occur.

Diuretics

Carbonic anhydrase inhibitors (e.g., acetazolamide in doses of 250 to 1,000 mg per day) may reduce intracranial pressure by decreasing CSF production. Side effects include tingling, nausea, anorexia, metabolic acidosis, and a distaste for carbonated beverages.

Thiazide diuretics in doses of 40 to 160 mg per day have also been used. Diuresis and potassium wasting may pose a disadvantage as compared with acetazolamide.

Steroids

Prednisone in doses of 20 to 80 mg per day has been associated with significant early symptomatic relief in patients not responsive to repeated lumbar punctures. Because they may induce systemic hypertension and intraocular hypertension with resulting visual compromise, corticosteroids should be tapered after 2 weeks, regardless of the response. Data regarding recurrence of symptoms after steroid withdrawal are equivocal.

Surgical Therapy

The outcome of therapy should be assessed by the relief of headache, elimination of transient visual

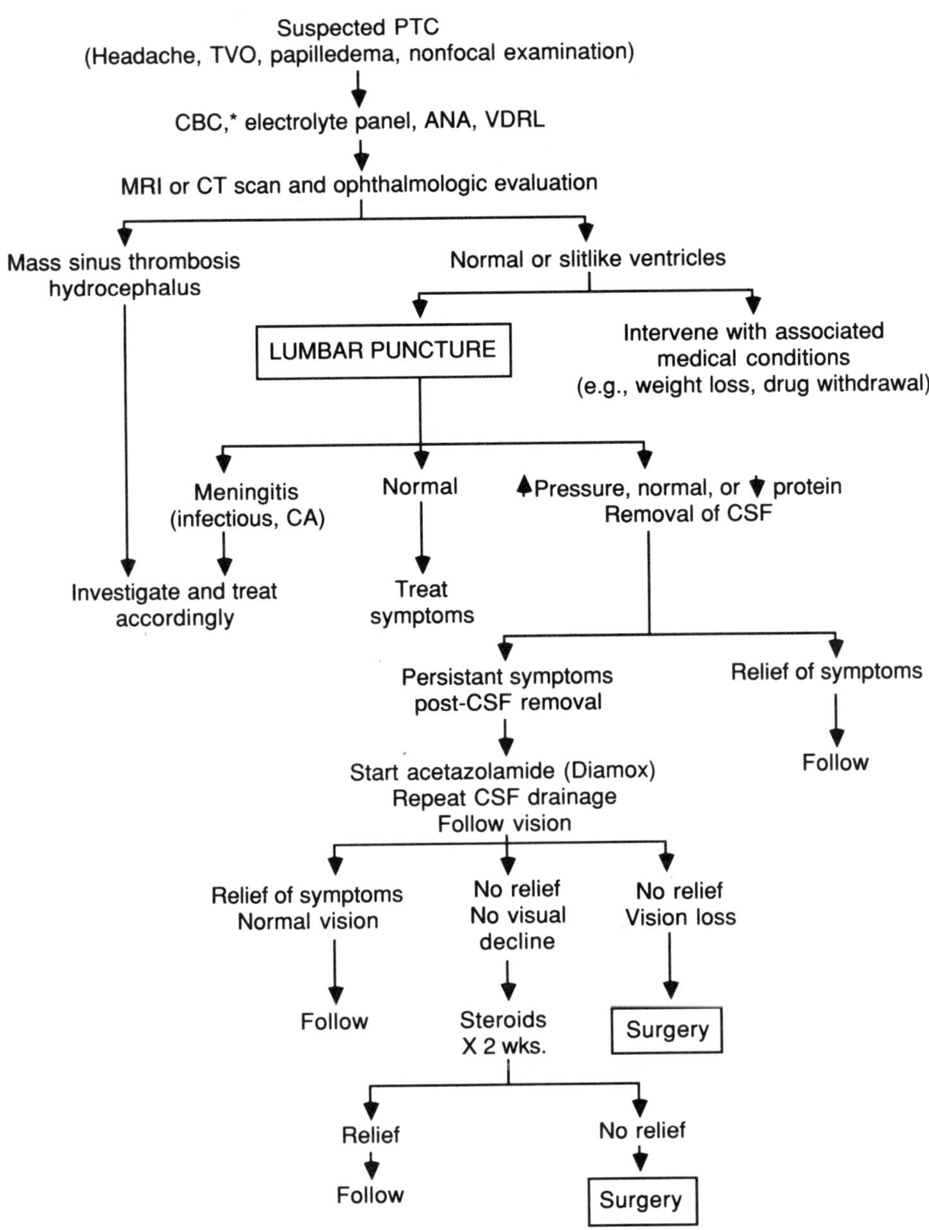

Figure 1 Evaluation and treatment of PTC. ANA = antinuclear antibodies; CBC = complete blood count; TVO = transient visual obscuration.

obscurations and diplopia, and resolution of papilledema, and not by the CSF pressure itself, which may remain elevated long after the resolution of other clinical signs and symptoms.

In cases of rapid loss of visual fields or acuity or disabling symptoms unresponsive to medical therapy, surgery should be considered. In those patients with severe headache without loss of vision, medical management including analgesics and migraine prophylactic medication is usually sufficient, whereas in those with progressive visual deficits, early surgical intervention is mandatory because severe loss

of vision or optic atrophy may be irreversible. Optic pallor is not a surgical contraindication for surgery, but rather an indication for rapid intervention.

Lumboperitoneal, ventriculoperitoneal (VP), cisternal-jugular CSF shunting, and subtemporal decompression have all been used. Lumboperitoneal shunting is preferred because a VP shunt may be technically difficult in a patient with small ventricles. Shunt malfunction is the most common complication, although infection is also known to occur.

Recently, optic nerve sheath decompression has been advocated. Sustained improvement of visual symptoms in the operated eye, and frequently in the nonoperated eye, is reported. Intraoperative and postoperative complications include disturbance of ocular motility, horizontal tropias, and irregular and transient atonic pupils. Visual improvement is reported in cases of shunt failure. Headache is also frequently alleviated. Optic nerve sheath decompression is now the procedure of choice for patients with rapid loss of vision, but should not be performed exclusively for headache relief.

Unilateral operation has been recommended except in those cases of severe bilateral vision loss or in patients who are poor surgical candidates for repeated general anesthesia.

SUGGESTED READING

Corbett JJ, Nerad MD, Tse DT, et al. Results of optic sheath fenestration for pseudotumor cerebri. Arch Ophthalmol 1988; 106:1391–1397.

Sørensen PS, Krogsaa B, Gjerris F. Clinical course and prognosis of pseudotumor cerebri: a prospective study of 24 patients. Acta Neurol Scand 1988; 77:164–172.

Weisberg LA. Benign intracranial hypertension. Medicine 1975; 54:197–207.

MOVEMENT DISORDERS

PARKINSON'S DISEASE

STEPHEN G. REICH, M.D.
MAHLON R. DeLONG, M.D.

Parkinson's disease (PD) is one of the most common movement disorders seen by primary care physicians and neurologists. The usual ease of diagnosis and the relatively few treatment options currently available suggest that management should be easy. However, the controversy about the optimal time to begin administering levodopa (Sinemet), the eventual emergence of motor fluctuations and drug-induced side effects in most patients, and the emotional and cognitive problems as well as the problems for the caregiver frequently encountered during long-term care of patients with PD present the physician with an intricate array of management options and dilemmas.

DIAGNOSIS

The classic signs of PD include tremor at rest, bradykinesia, stooped posture, masked face with diminished blink rate, cogwheel rigidity, shuffling gait, and postural instability. When all or most of these signs are present, the diagnosis is straightforward and is often made while the patient is observed in the waiting room; in his original essay *The Shaking Palsy* (1817) James Parkinson himself tells us that he encountered professionally only three of the six patients he reported, whereas the others were casually observed on the streets of London. We have observed three presentations of PD that occasionally lead to a delay in the diagnosis:

1. When the patient presents with a severe, dominant tremor without any other parkinsonian features or with other parkinsonian features that are subtle. In such patients, the essential tremor may be mistakenly diagnosed.
2. When tremor is absent in a patient presenting

with unilateral rigidity and bradykinesia (''pseudo-hemiplegic'' PD). In such cases, diagnoses of upper or lower motor neuron syndromes are entertained.
3. When patients with PD are younger than 50 years of age. PD may not be considered in the differential diagnosis, despite the fact that, while uncommon, PD may present as early as the fourth or fifth decade of life.

Although Parkinson's *disease* is the most common diagnosis among patients presenting with parkinsonian signs, there are a number of other diseases which must be considered in the differential diagnosis (Table 1). The appearance of cerebellar, corticospinal, lower motor neuron, autonomic, or ocular motor signs, particularly in patients with little or no response to antiparkinsonian medications, is a clue that another parkinsonian syndrome may be at hand.

GENERAL TREATMENT PRINCIPLES

The first step in effective treatment is education. Many patients are under the mistaken impression that the diagnosis of PD promises a future of complete dependency. We point out that although progressive, the rate is generally very slow, that effective treatment is available, and that most patients with PD live a normal life span and remain productive. Patient-oriented books and support groups should be prescribed with caution just after a patient is diagnosed, as they often serve only to emphasize the ''worst case scenario.'' But as the disease progresses, both are useful, sometimes as much to the caregiver as to the patient.

From the beginning, emphasis is placed on the *activities of daily living* (ADLs) as the ''barometer'' for deciding when to initiate treatment and when medication adjustments are needed in patients already receiving treatment. During routine follow-up visits, unless worsening symptoms translate into a *functional* decline, we do not make any changes in medication. The one exception to this rule is that when patients find the signs of PD embarrassing but not necessarily functionally limiting, we adjust antiparkinsonian medications accordingly. Before

Table 1 Differential Diagnosis of Parkinsonism

Toxins
  Manganese
  Carbon monoxide
  Carbon disulfide
  Cyanide
  Methanol
  MPTP

Drugs
  Neuroleptic
  Metoclopramide

Multisystem degenerations
  Progressive supranuclear palsy
  Shy-Drager syndrome
  Olivopontocerebellar atrophy
  Striatonigral degeneration
  Amyotrophic lateral sclerosis-PD-Dementia
    complex of Guam

Primary dementing illnesses
  Alzheimer's disease
  Creutzfeldt-Jakob disease

Heredofamilial diseases
  Wilson's disease
  Juvenile Huntington's disease
  Hallervorden-Spatz syndrome

Multi-infarct state

Calcification of the basal ganglia
  Idiopathic
  Hypoparathyroidism

starting treatment we emphasize to patients that the goal is not to eliminate all of the symptoms and signs of PD, but rather to maintain an effective degree of functioning.

ANTIPARKINSONIAN THERAPY

Drugs used for the treatment of PD fall into one of two classes: anticholinergics and dopaminergics (Table 2). The latter group includes levodopa, which is usually combined with a decarboxylase inhibitor, carbidopa, and the direct dopamine receptor agonists bromocriptine and pergolide mesylate. Amantadine has both anticholinergic and dopaminergic activity.

Our treatment strategy is to begin administering an anticholinergic or amantadine when there is minimal impairment of the ADLs. As the disease progresses, we add Sinemet and increase toward a total daily levodopa dose of 400 mg, at which point bromocriptine or pergolide is added as adjunctive therapy. The goal is to use the least amount of medication necessary to maintain a reasonable degree of functioning.

Anticholinergics

Anticholinergics are helpful in the treatment of early PD, particularly when tremor is a predominant sign. No single preparation has been shown convincingly to be superior to the others, and as a group, anticholinergics are the least expensive of the antiparkinsonian medications. Although in modest doses they are generally well tolerated by younger patients, side effects include dry mouth, blurred vision, constipation, urinary retention, memory loss, and confusion. We try to avoid the use of anticholinergics in elderly or demented patients.

Amantadine Hydrochloride

Originally marketed as an anti-influenzal drug, amantadine (Symmetrel) was discovered by chance to improve PD. Although useful in the treatment of early PD, its beneficial effect is generally short-lived, and most patients will require additional treatment within 6 to 12 months. Once the patient begins taking Sinemet, amantadine can often be discontinued with no deterioration of the patient's condition. Common side effects include pedal edema, confusion, hallucinations, and livedo reticularis. Like the anticholinergics, amantadine is best avoided in elderly or demented patients. In later stages of PD, the addition of amantadine is occasionally useful, but again, the beneficial effect wanes after several months.

Dopaminergics

Levodopa (Sinemet)

Dopamine depletion is the biochemical hallmark of PD and its replacement is the mainstay of treatment. The inability of dopamine to cross the blood-brain barrier led to the use of its precursor, levodopa. In order to avoid the peripheral conversion of levodopa to dopamine, Sinemet combines levodopa with the decarboxylase inhibitor carbidopa. The optimal time to begin administering Sinemet remains controversial—proponents for early treatment with this agent have shown that this approach leads to a longer life span, slower progression of disease, and better preservation of function; others insist that the usefulness of Sinemet is limited and therefore that its use is best delayed as long as possible rather than "wasted" when symptoms and signs are minimal. Our approach is to delay the use of Sinemet until there is significant impairment of the ADLs, but at that point we do not hesitate to initiate treatment, particularly if the symptoms and signs cannot be controlled adequately with anticholinergics and amantadine.

We start with the 25/100 tablet twice per day and, depending on the patient's response, gradually increase the dose by half or full tablets to a mainte-

Table 2 Drugs Used for Parkinson's Disease

Drug	Available Preparation	Dose (mg)	Schedule	Starting Dose (mg)	Maintenance Dose (mg)
Anticholinergic agents (representative examples)					
Trihexyphenidyl hydrochloride Artane)	Scored tablets Elixir	2 mg, 5 mg 2 mg/5 ml	3 to 4 times daily	2 mg	2–10 mg
	Timed-release capsule	5 mg	Once daily	(Timed-release capsule may be substituted for regular Artane after maintenance dose is determined)	
Benztropine mesylate (Cogentin)	Tablets	0.5 mg, 1 mg, 2 mg	Once or twice daily	1 mg	0.5–6 mg
Dopaminergic agents					
Carbidopa/levodopa (Sinemet)	Scored tablets 10/100, 25/100, 25/250		2 to 4 times daily	50/200 in two divided doses	400–500 mg levodopa
Bromocriptine (Parlodel)	Scored tablets Capsules	2.5 mg 5.0 mg	2 to 3 times daily	1.25 mg daily	7.5–30 mg
Pergolide mesylate (Permax)	Scored tablets	0.05 mg, 0.25 mg, 1.0 mg	3 times daily	0.05 mg daily	1–3 mg
Deprenyl (Eldepryl, selegiline hydrochloride)	Tablets	5.0 mg	2 times daily	5 mg daily	10 mg
Amantadine (Symmetrel)	Capsules	100 mg	2 times daily	100 mg daily	200 mg

nance dose of one tablet, administered 3 or 4 times per day. Most patients tolerate Sinemet well, with nausea being the most common early side effect. Although the nausea is generally self-limited, it can be prevented by having the patient take Sinemet with food and by making sure that at least 75 mg of carbidopa per day is used. Other side effects include orthostatic hypotension, confusion, hallucinations, and hypersexuality, but most resolve when the dose is reduced.

Dopamine Agonists

Bromocriptine and pergolide mesylate are ergot derivatives that have been shown to be useful adjuncts to Sinemet. To date, neither formulation has been shown to have a clear therapeutic advantage over the other. Although some advocate their use as initial monotherapy—and there is growing evidence that this may prevent or at least forestall motor fluctuations—our current approach is to add bromocriptine or pergolide mesylate when symptoms and signs cannot be controlled adequately by the use of 400 mg of levodopa per day. The starting dose of bromocriptine is 1.25 mg at bedtime; the dose is then increased by increments of 1.25 mg, with the goal being an initial maintenance dose of 7.5 mg per day. Depending on the response and tolerance, the dose can be increased gradually every 2 to 4 weeks to as much as 30 mg per day. Pergolide mesylate is started at 0.05 mg at bedtime and gradually increased until a maintenance dose of 1 to 3 mg per day in 3 divided doses is achieved.

Patients should be warned that the optimal effect of bromocriptine or pergolide mesylate may not be seen until several weeks after a stable dose is reached and that the benefit is typically subtle, unlike the dramatic effect many patients experience when they initially receive Sinemet.

The side effects of bromocriptine and pergolide are similar to those of Sinemet; however, these agents are less well tolerated in elderly and demented patients because of their greater propensity to cause confusion, hallucinations, and psychosis. Dopamine agonists are the most expensive of the antiparkinsonian agents.

MOTOR FLUCTUATIONS

Most patients maintain an obvious beneficial response to Sinemet for the first 3 to 5 years of treatment. After that time, not only does the beneficial effect wane, but motor fluctuations also appear, and from this point onward, the management of PD becomes more difficult as the therapeutic window of Sinemet narrows. Variables contributing to dose fluctuations include erratic gastric emptying and in-

testinal absorption, competition between levodopa and dietary amino acids for transport across the blood-brain barrier, loss of the ability of the remaining nigral neurons to metabolize and store dopamine, and changes in the number and sensitivity of postsynaptic dopamine receptors.

The most common early fluctuation is end-of-dose deterioration ("wearing-off"). This is treated by decreasing the dosing interval while attempting to maintain the same total daily dose of levodopa, often accomplished by using half-tablets and adding an agonist.

The second category of dose-related fluctuations are dyskinesias, which take the form of choreoathetosis or dystonia and can effect the limbs as well as the face and trunk. Although many patients are unaware of their dyskinesia or find them preferable to akinetic periods, their appearance generally heralds the beginning of more problematic fluctuations. Peak dose dyskinesias occur 1.5 to 2 hours after each dose and is treated by decreasing the dose of Sinemet and using an agonist to maintain adequate antiparkinsonian control.

More problematic than the dose-related fluctuations are random fluctuations known as *"on–off"*, characterized by sudden, unpredictable, and occasionally dramatic motor oscillations, often accompanied by freezing episodes and falling. These fluctuations are difficult to treat but may diminish with the addition of an agonist, frequent Sinemet dosing, the use of long-acting Sinemet (controlled release), or a brief drug "holiday" during which the dose of Sinemet is temporarily decreased and then reintroduced at a slightly lower maintenance dose. Despite their one-time popularity, we do not advocate complete drug holidays, as they are potentially dangerous and the beneficial effect is short-lived. Several investigators have shown that continuous duodenal infusion of Sinemet or subcutaneous apomorphine is helpful in controlling motor fluctuations and these techniques may eventually become more widely available.

DEPRENYL

Deprenyl (Eldepryl, selegiline hydrochloride) is a monoamine oxidase B inhibitor that prevents the catabolism and re-uptake of dopamine and has been shown to be an effective adjunct to Sinemet for patients with response fluctuations. Because only the "B" form of the enzyme is inhibited, which exists exclusively in the central nervous system, it is not necessary to restrict dietary tyramine since systemic hypertension is not encountered. Although dyskinesias may be exacerbated, necessitating a reduction in the Sinemet dose, deprenyl is otherwise relatively free of side effects. Nevertheless, side effects have been reported, including nausea, insomnia, dry mouth, dizziness, psychosis, and confusion. The maintenance dose is 5 mg twice per day.

In addition to its effectiveness in diminishing motor fluctuations, Deprenyl has also recently been shown to slow the progression of early Parkinson's disease, specifically, delaying the length of time before treatment with Levodopa is required. The mechanism involved is believed to be due to the ability of Deprenyl to block the toxic transformation of unknown potential environmental substances such as 1-Methyl-4-Phenyl-1,2,3,6-Tetrahyropyridine (MPTP), thereby limiting the death of nigral neurons.

SURGERY

Renewed interest in the surgical treatment of PD was aroused by the initial report of dramatic clinical improvement occurring after implantation of autologous adrenal medullary tissue into the caudate nucleus. Subsequent series, including those using fetal nigral tissue, have been met with less enthusiasm. The current procedure is associated with an unacceptably high morbidity rate, a lack of extended follow-up, and failure to demonstrate viability of the graft. We consider implantation to be a strictly experimental procedure that should be performed only in carefully selected patients as part of a research protocol. By contrast, stereotaxic thalamotomy, when performed at a center specializing in the procedure, is a safe, effective treatment for patients with disabling tremor unresponsive to medical therapy.

DEMENTIA

Based on the population studied, definition of dementia, and tools used to assess cognitive performance, the estimated frequency of dementia developing in patients with PD varies widely. A conservative estimate is that at least 15 to 20 percent of patients with PD develop dementia. Although the incidence of dementia in patients with PD is higher than in nonparkinsonian age-matched controls, it is crucial to appreciate that dementia is not an inevitable feature of PD and therefore must be approached with the same rigorous search for remediable causes as that used in patients without PD. All of the medications used to treat PD have cognitive and behavioral side effects, particularly the anticholinergics, and when dementia surfaces, an attempt should be made to reduce the dosages, and if possible, to discontinue the use of these drugs.

Dementia in patients with PD is occasionally complicated by bothersome hallucinations, agitation, and psychosis often coupled with insomnia or a reversal in the sleep-wake cycle. If these problems do not respond to a reduction in the dosage of antiparkinsonian medications or to the use of mild sedatives, a very low dose of a neuroleptic may be required. Although a worsening of parkinsonian signs may result, the suppression of intolerable behavior usually leads to an overall improvement in the patient's condition and eases the burden on the patient's caregiver.

DEPRESSION

Depression is common in PD, occurring in as many as 50 percent of patients. It is not clear to what extent depression is the result of an intrinsic neurochemical defect such as the mesolimbic loss of dopamine versus a reactive depression to the physical disability imposed by the disease. Patients (and physicians) commonly fail to recognize depression and often mistakenly ascribe a decline in function, particularly psychomotor retardation, to PD. Symptoms of depression, and specifically vegetative symptoms, should be rigorously sought during each outpatient visit. Psychiatric evaluation is helpful for most patients and essential for patients with severe depression.

Depression associated with PD can be effectively treated with tricyclic antidepressants. In severe cases, particularly when the depression is compounded by delusions or psychosis or when tricyclics are either ineffective or not tolerated, electroconvulsive therapy is the treatment of choice. As the depression resolves, there is often concurrent improvement of many parkinsonian symptoms and signs.

SUGGESTED READING

Brown RG, Marsden CD. How common is dementia in Parkinson's Disease? Lancet 1984; 1:1262–1265.

Jankovic J, Tolosa E, eds. Parkinson's disease and movement disorders. Baltimore: Urban & Schwarzenberg, Inc. 1988.

Koller WC, ed. Handbook of Parkinson's disease. New York: Marcel Dekker, 1987.

Lieberman AN. Update on Parkinson's disease. NY State J Med 1987; 87:147–153.

Marsden CD, Parkes JD. Success and problems of long-term levodopa therapy in Parkinson's disease. Lancet 1977; 1:345–349.

The Parkinson Study Group. Effect of Deprenyl on the progression of disability in early Parkinson's Disease. N Engl J Med 1989; 321:1364–1371.

PATIENT RESOURCES

Associations

United Parkinson Foundation (International)
360 West Superior Street
Chicago, Illinois 60610

The American Parkinson Disease Association, Inc.
116 John Street
New York, New York 10034

The Parkinson Disease Foundation
William Black Medical Research Building
640 West 168th Street
New York, New York 10032

National Parkinson Foundation, Inc.
1501 Ninth Avenue NW
Miami, Florida 33136

Literature

Duvoisin RC. Parkinson's disease: a guide for patient and family. New York: Raven Press, 1984.

ESSENTIAL TREMOR

WILLIAM C. KOLLER, M.D., Ph.D.

Essential tremor is a common disorder of the nervous system characterized by tremor of the hands, head, voice, and less often, the legs and trunk. Half of the cases occur sporadically and half are familial, transmitted as an autosomal dominant. Hand tremor is characteristically present during maintenance of a position (postural tremor) and during active movements (kinetic tremor). Patients complain of difficulty with handwriting, drinking liquids, and manipulative tasks. Hand tremor, and especially head tremor, result in embarrassment and potential social isolation. Essential voice tremor has a characteristic quavering intonation which results in a fluctuating and rhythmic dysphonia. Essential tremor is sometimes described as being benign. While the tremor may be a nuisance to some patients, the livelihood of others is threatened by it, and many experience functional disabilities. Effective treatment is available for many patients with essential tremor (Table 1).

ALCOHOL

Many patients relate that the ingestion of a small amount of alcohol will temporarily cause a substantial reduction of their tremor. Often patients find that a single glass of wine or even one beer will check their tremor for 45 minutes to 1 hour. In 1949, McDonald Critchley stated that patients with essential tremor note that "a heavy dose of spirits will temporarily check the tremor." The effect of alcohol on essential tremor appears to be unique to this disorder. Patients with parkinsonian or cerebellar tremor do not find a dramatic reduction in their symptoms with alcohol intake. In several controlled studies, alcohol administered both orally and intravenously has been found to cause a dramatic reduction in essential tremor. All patients tested responded, and almost 75 percent of the patients experienced a reduction in their tremor. Alcohol would appear to be one of the most effective drugs in the treatment of essential tremor. Alcohol probably works through a central mechanism, as the local intra-arterial infusion of alcohol does not decrease tremor. However, exactly how alcohol works is unclear. Alcohol has a variety of actions on the central nervous system and affects many neurotransmitter systems. Yet an understanding of alcohol's action in the reduction of essential tremor could lead to the development of better pharmacologic agents for the treatment of this disorder.

A major concern with the use of alcohol to treat essential tremor is the fear that some patients might become chronic alcoholics. Critchley warned that alcohol was used to treat essential tremor "apparently all too often to serve as an excuse for habits of intemperance." Some considered the risk of addiction as a contraindication for the use of alcohol. The rate of chronic alcoholism in patients with essential tremor has been recently defined. A retrospective chart survey of former patients yielded a relatively high alcoholic rate. According to three subsequent prospective studies done in the United States, Sweden, and Finland, however, the prevalence of pathological drinking among patients with essential tremor did not differ from that among patients with other tremor disorders or chronic neurologic disease without tremor. As essential tremor often gets worse when the effect of alcohol wears off or the morning after heavy alcohol ingestion, it seems reasonable to assume that heavy alcohol consumption would not

Table 1 Treatment of Essential Tremor

Drugs with proven efficacy
  Alcohol
  Beta-adrenergic blockers
  Primidone
Drugs with possible efficacy
  Phenobarbital
  Alprazolam
Drugs with limited efficacy
  Diazepam
  Clonazepam
  Clonidine
  Amantadine
  Alpha-adrenergic blockers

be a major problem for patients with essential tremor. Since chronic alcoholism and essential tremor are very common disorders, one would think that by chance alone these disorders may frequently coexist. Also, chronic alcoholism itself may result in a persistent tremor disorder lasting for as long as 1 year after complete abstinence. It can be concluded that the occasional use of alcohol in the treatment of essential tremor is not contraindicated and that the risk of alcoholism is low. The judicious use of small amounts of alcoholic beverages before meals or other events to reduce tremor appears reasonable. Many patients find that taking a glass of wine or some other alcoholic drink before meals helps them perform that task much more easily. Perhaps the recommendation of a glass of wine before dinner is a reasonable one for patients with tremor and those individuals without tremor alike.

BETA-ADRENERGIC BLOCKERS

Propranolol

In 1971, two groups independently reported that propranolol decreased essential tremor. Initially 24 patients were investigated in a double-blind crossover study using objective measurements. The average effective dose was 120 mg per day, with a range of 60 to 240 mg per day in divided doses. No side effects were encountered. Subsequent studies have also shown the efficacy of propranolol in the treatment of essential tremor. Some studies, however, have reported a lack of effect, but these results were probably due to inadequate dosage, small sample size, or lack of objective measures. Investigations that confirmed the efficacy of propranolol in reducing hand tremor used both subjective and objective (accelerometer recording) evaluations. According to these studies, tremor amplitude was decreased but tremor frequency was left unchanged.

Propranolol has become the drug of choice for the treatment of essential tremor. It is useful both for reducing essential tremor and for blocking stress-induced enhancement of the tremor. A sustained release preparation (long-acting propranolol) designed to be used in a once-daily dose is available and is preferred by many patients for ease of administration. Similar therapeutic results were obtained when this preparation was compared with multiple doses of propranolol. The drug is, however, somewhat more costly than generic propranolol. The clinical response of patients to propranolol is variable and often incomplete. A wide range of individual responses is to be expected. It is generally estimated that 50 to 70 percent of patients will have some symptomatic control. Dramatic improvement occurs in a much smaller percentage, and only in a rare individual is tremor totally suppressed. Unfor-

tunately, some patients will have no response to this agent. In those patients who do respond, average tremor reduction is usually 50 to 60 percent, often allowing a patient to perform writing, eating, drinking, and other activities of daily living. The effective dose varies widely among individuals. In a dose response study, 120 to 320 mg per day in divided doses was found to be optimal. Doses greater than 320 mg per day provided no additional benefits and were associated with a higher incidence of side effects. There is no correlation between plasma drug levels and therapeutic response. No clinical characteristics have been identified that allow one to predict who will respond to the drug. A reasonable starting dose is 80 to 120 mg per day. This can be given in divided doses or, if the long-acting preparation is used, as a single dose. One question that is not totally resolved is the long-term efficacy of propranolol treatment. Some have suggested that tolerance to the drug occurs over time. In one recent study, however, loss of drug effect occurred in less than 15 percent of patients who were followed for 1 year. Propranolol therefore appears to have both short-term and long-term benefit.

Propranolol therapy is usually fairly well tolerated. Relative contraindications for propranolol use are (1) heart failure, especially if poorly controlled, (2) second-degree and third-degree atrioventricular block, (3) asthma or other bronchospastic disease, and (4) insulin-dependent diabetes, where propranolol may block the adrenergic manifestations of hypoglycemia. Many side effects of propranolol are related to beta-blockade. The pulse will be lowered in most patients. A pulse of 60 beats per minute is usually well tolerated. However, if the pulse is less than 50 beats per minute, it is probably wise to reduce the dose or discontinue the drug, even if the patient is asymptomatic. Other less common adverse reactions include fatigue, lassitude, nausea, diarrhea, skin rash, and impotence. A variety of mental status changes (e.g., depression) may also occur. It is important for the clinician to ascertain if these side effects are present, since often the patient may not volunteer this information when simply asked whether they are suffering any adverse reaction. If a patient does have adverse reactions with one beta-blocking drug, it may be possible to switch to another beta-blocking drug and retain the therapeutic efficacy without incurring the same type of side effect. The mechanism of action of propranolol in the treatment of essential tremor is unknown. Initially it was proposed that a central site of action was necessary because of a delay in the effect of chronic oral therapy. However, recent studies have shown that the effect of an oral dose of propranolol is almost immediate in reducing tremor. Beta-adrenergic–blocking drugs that have poor penetration of the central nervous system also decrease essential tremor, as do drugs that have pure beta-2–

blocking properties. Therefore, it appears that propranolol acts at a peripheral site of action, probably through blockade of beta-2 adrenergic receptors, which are located on muscle spindles.

Other Beta-Adrenergic Blockers

Other beta-adrenergic blockers are currently available (Table 2). These drugs are also useful in the treatment of essential tremor. If essential tremor does not respond to propranolol, however, it will not respond to other beta-adrenergic–blocking drugs.

Metoprolol has been shown to reduce essential tremor. This drug differs from propranolol in preferentially antagonizing beta-1 adrenergic receptors. This selectivity for beta-1 receptors is, however, only relative. With higher doses, beta-2 adrenergic receptors are also blocked. Some degree of beta-2 blockade appears in patients receiving daily doses of more than 100 mg. Metoprolol is effective in the treatment of essential tremor in divided doses of 100 to 200 mg per day. It has been suggested that metoprolol is the preferred drug for patients with bronchospastic disease. Because of its relative lack of beta-2–blocking properties, metoprolol is theoretically better tolerated than propranolol or other nonspecific blockers. Several asthmatic patients with essential tremor have been reported to tolerate metoprolol but not propranolol. Metoprolol is also capable of causing respiratory distress, however, and should be used with caution in bronchospastic disease.

Because of its renal excretion, nadolol can be given in a single daily dosage and has been shown to significantly decrease essential tremor. Atenolol and timolol have been reported in several studies to have only a limited effect on essential tremor. Pindolol possesses partial agonist activity and may cause tremors.

PRIMIDONE

O'Brien and colleagues noted that when primidone was given to a patient with epilepsy and essential tremor, he reported marked reduction in tremor. They therefore gave the drug to 20 other patients, starting with a dose of 125 mg and increasing to 750 mg per day. In 1981, they reported that 12 patients had a good clinical response to the drug. Six patients, including four receiving the 125-mg dose, could not tolerate the drug because of side effects (vertigo, unsteadiness, and nausea). The addition of propranolol resulted in further clinical improvement in these patients. They concluded that primidone was more effective than propranolol, but that patients with essential tremor could not tolerate primidone as well as seizure patients. Several other studies have confirmed the efficacy of primidone in the treatment of essential tremor. It was found in one study that doses as low as 50 mg would reduce tremor and that doses of more than 250 mg were not associated with any greater reduction in tremor. The drug was given in a single night-time dosage. No correlation has been found between therapeutic response and serum drug levels. Several studies have found that primidone decreases essential tremor more than propranolol, and it is not uncommon to see very dramatic responses to primidone. However, some patients will not respond to the drug. There are no predictive factors that indicate which patients will respond to the drug. It has been suggested that the starting dose be 50 mg given at night-time, and that it then be increased, if necessary, to 125 mg and then to 250 mg taken as a single dose at night-time. The 50-mg dose is available as a pediatric dose form. The 250-mg tablet is scored and can be broken to provide the 125-mg dose. If the drug is taken before going to bed, there is less difficulty with daytime sedation and the therapeutic benefit tends to occur throughout the day.

A major problem with the use of primidone in the treatment of essential tremor is initial acute reactions. It has been estimated that 25 to 30 percent of the patients have a reaction the following day. This consists of an "ill" feeling involving nausea, malaise, and sometimes ataxia. This is a transient reaction that will last 1 to 3 days regardless of whether the drug is discontinued. This idiosyncratic reaction occurs even if a dose smaller than 50 mg is given. Many patients will attempt to discontinue the drug after the acute initial reaction. The patient should

Table 2 Pharmacologic Properties of Beta-Adrenergic Blockers

Drug	Beta-Blockage Potency	Cardioselectivity Relative Beta₁ Blockage	Partial Agonist Activity	Membrane Stabilization	Plasma Half-Life	Penetration Into Central Nervous System	Metabolism
Propranolol	1	−	0	+	5–12 hrs	Good	Hepatic
Metoprolol	1	+	0	−	3–4 hrs	Good	Hepatic
Nadolol	0.5	−	0	−	20–24 hrs	Good	Renal
Atenolol	1	+	0	−	6–8 hrs	Poor	Hepatic
Timolol	6	−	+	−	4–5 hrs	Good	Hepatic
Pindolol	6	−	+	+	3–4 hrs	Good	Hepatic

therefore be warned that such a reaction may occur; I often advise our patients to take the drug for the first time on a Friday when they have nothing planned for the weekend. If patients know that this reaction might occur and that it is transient and will not interfere with long-term drug treatment, they will probably not discontinue the drug. I ask that my patients call me if a reaction does occur, and encourage them to continue the drug and remind them that the reaction will soon go way. In a rare patient, adverse reactions may last for 1 week or longer, but the side effects often diminish quickly with time. Long-term side effects of primidone tend to be minimal when 250 mg at night-time is employed. There is also some controversy as to whether patients develop tolerance to primidone's effects. Some patients relate that their best tremor reduction occurs during the morning after the first night-time dose and that the tremor may still remain reduced below baseline levels thereafter. Some patients have been reported in whom the drug loses efficacy after several months of therapy. In one study, however, 85 percent of the patients still retained therapeutic benefit after 1 year of treatment. Tolerance does not appear to be a common problem with primidone therapy.

The mechanism of action of primidone's antitremor effect is unknown. Primidone is converted to two active metabolites: phenyethylmelomide (PEMA) with a half-life of 24 to 40 hours, and phenobarbital with a half-life of 50 to 120 hours. Primidone has a half-life of approximately 10 hours. PEMA has been administered to patients with essential tremor and has been found to have no effect. As discussed below, there is some controversy as to whether phenobarbital has an antitremor action. If primidone is given acutely, reduction of tremor is seen during the first several hours after administration. At this time, no phenobarbital is detected in the bloodstream, indicating that primidone's acute effect, at least, is not mediated through phenobarbital.

DRUG OF CHOICE

Both propranolol and primidone are effective drugs in the treatment of essential tremor. There is no concensus on the first drug that should be employed. For most patients, I prefer to start with primidone because it is effective in more patients and a greater degree of tremor reduction is often observed. The initial adverse reactions are problematic but, as I have discussed, if the patient is warned about this and encouraged to continue using the drug, the patient tends not to be deterred. The long-term side effects with primidone are generally minimal. Propranolol, on the other hand, is contraindicated in some patients, and the drug is not well tolerated by the many elderly patients. Mental changes that occur in some patients with proprano-

lol and side effects with chronic therapy are additional negative aspects of this drug. I therefore prefer to give patients primidone in an initial dose of 50 mg at night, which I then increase to 125 or 250 mg after several weeks. If the patient has no response to 250 mg of primidone, I discontinue the drug. However, if the patient has some tremor reduction but still has functional disability, I will add propranolol to the dosage regimen. I prefer long-acting propranolol because of its ease of administration and good patient compliance. I usually give patients the long-acting preparation in an initial dose of 80 or 120 mg taken immediately on arising in the morning. This dose can be increased to a total dose of 320 mg per day. Two drugs in combination will often cause tremor reduction and an increase in functional capabilities, with improvement in handwriting, drinking, and eating. Unfortunately, embarrassment and fine manual dexterity remain a problem for many patients even when tremor reduction can be demonstrated by objective measures.

PHENOBARBITAL

Phenobarbital has been used in the treatment of essential tremor for a long time and antedates the use of many other drugs. It is generally considered to have low efficacy. Although several studies have demonstrated that the drug does cause some tremor reduction, other studies have shown no effect. Sedation is often a major problem with the use of the drug. I therefore almost never employ this drug in the treatment of essential tremor.

ALPRAZOLAM

Recently a double-blind placebo-controlled parallel study of 24 patients was done showing that alprazolam (Xanax) causes reduction of essential tremor. However, mild fatigue and sedation occurred in 50 percent of these patients, and it is possible that tremor reduction could have been caused in part by the sedation. It was suggested that alprazolam may be effective in those needing only intermittent therapy. Further investigation is needed before this drug can be considered to have efficacy in the treatment of essential tremor. However, if propranolol and primidone have been found not to be effective, a trial of alprazolam may be indicated. The drug can be started at 0.25 mg twice per day and then slowly increased. Sedation often limits the ability to increase the dose to more than 1 to 2 mg per day.

OTHER DRUGS

Other benzodiazepines such as diazepam have often been employed in the treatment of essential tremor. Benzodiazepines may be more effective when used in combination with propranolol therapy and may block the enhancement of tremor by stress. However, these drugs have never been scientifically evaluated. It is my general impression that diazepam has very limited usefulness in the treatment of essential tremor and I never prescribe the drug. There are several anecdotal reports that clonidine and amantadine may be effective in reducing essential tremor. Similarly, there are reports of alpha-adrenergic blockers decreasing essential tremor. However, when studied in controlled trials, these drugs have been found to have no efficacy.

SURGERY

Surgical therapy (stereotaxic thalomotomy) is an option for those patients with severe tremor that causes marked functional disability that is unresponsive to all medications. Ablation of the ventral intermediate nucleus of the thalamus appears to alleviate parkinsonian, essential, and cerebellar type tremors equally well. Paresis, speech disturbances, hypertonus, and cerebellar dysfunction represent possible adverse reactions. Bilateral operations are rarely indicated because of the high incidence of speech abnormalities associated with this treatment. Tremor may recur in a certain percentage of patients. There has been no published long-term follow-up of stereotaxic thalomotomy in the treatment of essential tremor. My personal experience indicates that stereotaxic thalomotomy is efficacious in the treatment of essential tremor; however, not all patients will have good results. It is unclear how long the benefit will last. I have followed some patients for several years who have had continual benefit from the surgery. Therefore this option should be considered in patients with severe disabling tremor that has not responded to pharmacologic agents. With current technology, the procedure does appear to be associated with minimal risk only. Nevertheless, many patients are not inclined to undergo the procedure and refuse it when offered.

BEHAVIORAL THERAPY

A variety of behavior techniques including psychotherapy, biofeedback, and hypnosis have been employed in the treatment of movement disorders. Any benefit from these procedures has been minimal and short-lived. There is one anecdotal report of psychotherapy being helpful in the treatment of essential tremor. The reported improvement was believed to be caused by mental stabilization and relaxation of muscle tension. It is my opinion that behavioral therapy currently plays no role in the treatment of essential tremor.

ESSENTIAL TREMOR VARIANTS

A variety of atypical tremor disorders exist that appear to be related to essential tremor (Table 3). The association of these conditions with essential tremor is suggested by the high occurrence of a family history of essential tremor, the frequent presence of a mild postural tremor, and reduction in tremor noted to occur with alcohol ingestion. These tremor disorders have a different pharmacologic responsiveness than the more typical essential tremor. Most patients with essential tremor have varying degrees of postural and kinetic tremors. Marked dissociation occurs in what has been referred to as kinetic predominant tremor, where the postural component is minimal or absent. Cerebellar signs are also absent. Functional disability may be severe in patients with a marked kinetic tremor. These patients have been reported to have significant tremor reduction when taking clonazepam in doses of 1 to 2 mg per day. Drowsiness limits further dosage increase in many patients. Although propranolol is helpful in some of these patients, clonazepam appears to be the first drug of choice in the treatment of kinetic predominant essential tremor.

Primary writing tremor refers to a test-specific or selective action tremor in which pronation of the forearm elicits a pronation/supination tremor. Often it is not seen during other movements of the arm. The patient's chief complaint is "my hand shakes while writing." This disorder needs to be distinguished from writer's cramp or focal dystonia of the hand. Primidone or propranolol may be effective in some patients with this disorder. Anticholinergics have also been reported to reduce this tremor, and these drugs should be tried if the patient does not respond to primidone or propranolol.

Truncal tremors are sometimes observed in essential tremor as a late manifestation. An uncommon variant of essential tremor is orthostatic truncal tremor. In this condition, the sole symptom is a tremor of the trunk and proximal legs that occurs while standing. The tremor worsens the longer the patient stands, and may lead to falling. The tremor is absent when the patient is sitting, walking, or leaning against a firm support. Propranolol has been reported to be ineffective in the treatment of this disorder. However, clonazepam has been found to cause a marked reduction in a truncal tremor, and this has been confirmed by several reports. Clonazepam should be the first drug of choice in orthostatic truncal tremor.

Table 3 Variants of Essential Tremor

Kinetic predominant hand tremor
Primary writing tremor
Orthostatic truncal tremor

GENERAL APPROACH

Treatment of essential tremor of the hand or head should start with primidone in a dose of 50 mg at bedtime, with the dose increased gradually to 250 mg per day. Propranolol at 80 to 120 mg should be added and increased to a maximum of 320 mg per day if the response remains inadequate. Long-acting propranolol can be used if once-daily administration is desired. Hand tremor tends to respond the best, and although head tremor may be reduced, it may still cause embarrassment for the patient. Tremor of the voice appears to respond poorly to both propranolol and primidone therapy. Rare variants of essential tremor may respond to clonazepam therapy. The use of these drugs frequently results in tremor reduction and increased functional abilities. However, some patients do not respond to any therapy and remain disabled.

SUGGESTED READING

Critchley M. Observations on an essential tremor. Brain 1949; 72:113–139.
Larsen TA, Calne DB. Essential tremor. Clin Neuropharmacol 1983; 6:285–306.
Koller WC. Diagnosis and treatment of tremors. In: Neurology Clinics. Jankovic J, ed. Philadelphia: WB Saunders Co. 1984:499.
Koller WC. Dose response relationship of propranolol in essential tremor. Arch Neurol 1986; 35:42–43.
Koller WC, Royse VL. Efficacy of primidone in the treatment of essential tremor. Neurology 1986; 26:121–124.

PATIENT RESOURCE

The International Tremor Foundation provides information on essential tremor and other tremor disorders and publishes a quarterly newsletter for patients with tremor disorders.

The International Tremor Foundation
360 West Superior
Chicago, Illinois 60610

HUNTINGTON'S DISEASE

JOHN B. PENNEY, Jr., M.D.

Huntington's disease (HD) is a progressive, degenerative disease of the basal ganglia. The disease is inherited as an autosomal dominant disorder with complete penetrance. Persons who carry the gene will show symptoms of the disease if they live long enough. Five to seven individuals per 100,000 people have the disease, and the prevalence of the gene is believed to be three times greater than that of the disease. There are currently about 25,000 affected individuals in the United States. While the peak age of disease onset is approximately 40 years of age, the age of onset distribution is broad, ranging from 5 years of age to 80 years of age.

CLINICAL FEATURES

The disease is characterized by a movement disorder and progressive intellectual deterioration. The movement disorder is usually choreiform. Before the onset of symptoms, the patient or the patient's family may note that the patient has become fidgety, clumsy, has a tendency to drop things, and is experiencing difficulties balancing and driving as well as changes in the speech rhythm. These minor difficulties progress to obvious chorea as the disease becomes fully manifest. Early in the course of the disease, most patients do not have any associated rigidity, bradykinesia, or dystonia. However, these features become more prominent as the disease progresses. Patients whose onset is during their teenage years or their early 20's often have prominent parkinsonian features of rigidity, bradykinesia, and occasionally, tremor. In the youngest patients, seizures and cerebellar signs may be a problem, particularly late in the course of the disease.

The movement disorder is accompanied by slowness and irregularity of rapid repetitive movements, such as finger tapping and tongue movements. The patient also has difficulty generating ocular saccades. Early in the course of the disease, patients may have to blink or move their heads in order to generate a saccade. Later, there is limitation in the range of voluntary eye movements. Dysarthria is prominent, and dysphagia becomes a major late problem. Hyperreflexia is common, and clonus may be an early sign of the disease. Extensor plantar responses are not usually seen until very late in the course of the disease.

These patients have several psychological and intellectual difficulties. They have difficulty organizing and carrying through with a plan. As a result, they tend to neglect long-term and, later, short-term achievement of goals. This is frequently perceived as lack of motivation by their family and physicians. In addition, about half of the patients have severe depression. Suicide is seen early in the course of the disease. Many patients have difficulty with impulse control and are given to outbursts of anger. Schizophreniform and obsessive-compulsive disorders are less commonly seen.

All patients with HD undergo progressive intellectual decline. Even late in the course of the disease, however, questioning will reveal that patients can still recognize family and friends and have awareness of their surroundings, unlike those with Alzheimer's disease. Furthermore, intelligence as measured by formal psychological tests may remain normal well into the course of the disease.

The disease is inexorably progressive. The rate of progression is highly variable and may change. HD usually progresses more rapidly in younger patients. Patients become invalids between 5 and 15 years after the onset of the disease. Duration of survival ranges from 10 to 30 years. Patients in a vegetative state may have an extremely long survival.

Symptoms and signs of HD may develop before the onset of the movement disorder. Depression, conduct disorder, and (rarely) overt psychosis may be present. The presence of these psychological difficulties in a person who is at risk for Huntington's disease suggests that the gene may be present but is not diagnostic. In addition, most patients have the onset of rapid movement and saccadic eye movement difficulties before the development of overt chorea. The astute clinician may be suspicious of making the diagnosis of HD in individuals who have these signs and may wish to see them on an annual basis while waiting for the movement disorder to appear. A computed tomographic (CT) scan is usually not useful in such patients. It is not clear whether positron-emission tomography (PET) is useful in the diagnosis of HD. Some groups claim to have found abnormalities in patients before the onset of symptoms, while others are unable to confirm these findings. At best, PET scans yield abnormal results a few years before the onset of overt symptoms.

DIAGNOSIS

Positive Family History

The diagnosis is based on the presence of a movement disorder in the patient with a positive history of the disease, unless the movement disorder is due to some other cause. The most important step by far in establishing the diagnosis is defining the family history. It is best if the family history is known and there is autopsy confirmation of HD in at least one family member. When the family history is less clear, an extensive evaluation needs to be made. Hospital records should be checked for family members who were diagnosed as having HD. Autopsy records should also be checked. The presence of a movement disorder in a patient with a positive fam-

ily history almost certainly means Huntington's disease. In younger patients, Wilson's disease should be excluded since it is treatable. A history of neuroleptic treatment can confuse the diagnosis because tardive dyskinesia may mimic HD. However, tardive dyskinesia is not accompanied by the eye movement disorder seen in patients with HD. A CT scan or magnetic resonance imaging (MRI) may provide useful information in these circumstances. Atrophy of the caudate is usually present in patients who have been symptomatic for more than several years. The ratio between the intercaudate distance across the lateral ventricles and the distance between the outer tables of the skull at the level of the caudate should be less than 0.15 in normal patients. Because many patients with early HD do not have abnormalities on their CT scan, a normal CT scan does not exclude HD.

Until the last few years, it was impossible to make the diagnosis of HD in a patient with a positive family history but no movement disorder. However, persons who now wish to know their genetic status may be able to obtain this information.

The gene for Huntington's disease has been localized to the tip of the short arm of chromosome 4. A number of genetic markers have been found that are linked to the HD gene. These markers can provide greater than 99 percent accuracy of diagnosis in patients with a positive family history if it is possible to trace how the marker (which is not the gene) and the gene travel together through the family. At a minimum, blood from the individual at risk and two symptomatic patients is needed. Once the gene itself is found, however, it will be possible for the patient without a positive family history to receive genetic information. Currently, only one-third to one-half of those persons who are at risk have a family through which the markers and the gene can be traced.

Only a few people have actually taken this test. These have been mostly middle-aged women who wished to gain information for their families. Other reasons for taking the genetic test include the desire to make informed decisions on planning a career, a family, marriage, and financial arrangements. Although genetic testing originally was available on a research basis only, it is now available on a commercial basis in several centers. Those individuals who are tested are given extensive pretest and post-test counseling to be sure that emotionally they are able to handle the information they receive. The counseling and the need for analyzing many blood samples make this test extremely expensive. It is also feared that health and/or life insurance companies will cancel the policies of patients who carry the gene. Because many persons therefore do not wish their insurance company to know that they are being tested, problems with billing and keeping medical records result for those doing the testing.

All those who have tested positive for the gene

have become depressed after obtaining this information. It is believed that there is a high risk of suicide in this population. Any genetic testing program should therefore be part of an on-going counseling and psychiatric therapy program for those people who take the test.

It is also possible to provide prenatal information to ensure that patients at risk for HD who are planning a family will have normal children. The technique involves chorionic villus sampling, and must be planned before the pregnancy in order for an abortion to be performed.

Negative Family History

Not infrequently, patients present who appear to have HD but who have a negative family history. In these cases, it is extremely important to gather the best family history possible. Many families hide the diagnosis. Therefore, it is important for the clinician and the patient to talk to as many family members as possible. Because onset of symptoms may be delayed until late in life, it is important to examine the parents of anyone who appears to have HD, as one may be affected and not know it. Paternity testing is also appropriate, but it is frequently difficult to obtain.

Patients without a family history should be examined for other diseases that may present with a choreiform movement disorder. These include Wilson's disease, parkinsonism, multiple sclerosis, cerebellar disease (particularly olivopontocerebellar atrophy), Gilles de la Tourette's syndrome, cerebral vasculitis, Sydenham's chorea, choreoathetoid cerebral palsy, familial choreoathetosis, chorea-acanthocytosis, and essential tremor. One must search extensively for a past history of neuroleptic use, as tardive dyskinesia is an important consideration. Other diseases associated with chorea are hyperthyroidism, hypocalcemia and hypercalcemia, hypernatremia, hypomagnesemia, hypoglycemia and hyperglycemia, carbon monoxide poisoning, hepatic and renal encephalopathies, chorea gravidarum, and Addison's disease. Rarely, other infectious, immunologic, and cerebral vascular disorders including acquired immunodeficiency syndrome (AIDS) have been associated with chorea. The presence of minor hepatic, renal, thyroid, or electrolyte abnormalities does not rule out HD.

Benign familial chorea is extremely rare, with chorea present from childhood without causing disability. This condition is distinct from juvenile HD, which presents with parkinsonism. "Senile chorea" is probably either HD with an extremely late onset or the result of multiple cerebral vascular accidents.

Once one has searched extensively for a family history and a metabolic evaluation has been done, some patients still appear to have HD without a family history. Such patients have to face a progressive, degenerative disease in addition to the uncertainty regarding the diagnosis. While documentation of a spontaneous new mutation has never occurred, this remains possible.

When diagnosis is established, it is extremely important to begin counseling of both the patient and the patient's family. The clinician should meet with all the members of the immediate family to make certain that they understand the situation. The patient's spouse, children, parents, and siblings are now the patient's caregivers. Children now find themselves at risk for the disease. In counseling, it is important to determine what the person knows about HD. The following should then be explained to the patients: the signs and symptoms of the disease, the course of the disease (without an undue emphasis on the inevitable progression to death), the hereditary nature of the disease, the risk status of the individual patient, what is known about the pathogenesis of the disease, the late onset of the disease, and that although there is no cure for HD, treatment for specific symptoms is available and research to find the cure is on-going. Next one should assess what the person has learned and finally provide him or her with written information about the disease and a resource for further information, the Huntington's Disease Society of America (HDSA). Patients should be referred to the local HDSA chapter for further counseling and support groups.

ON-GOING CARE

Patients vary greatly in their response to the diagnosis. A few patients commit suicide, some patients deny the diagnosis, some accept it without emotion, while others are actually relieved to have had their uncertainty resolved. Regardless of the response, it is important to maintain on-going social work, psychological, and genetic counseling and support for the patients. As the disease progresses, one will need to provide disability papers for the patient, to stop the patient from driving, to handle their insurance and estate needs, and ultimately, to provide custodial care. Speech, occupational, and physical therapy are useful in keeping patients functional at their jobs and, later, in maintaining their activities of daily living. Eventually, patients require total care. Most patients die with aspiration pneumonia. Progressive swallowing problems develop, and at some point, an indwelling gastric tube for feeding becomes important for maintaining nutrition.

No known therapy alters disease progression. Patients inevitably lose weight and neurologic function. In patients who maintain their weight, the disease may progress less rapidly.

There are, however, medicines for specific symptoms, particularly for psychiatric symptoms.

Depression is extremely common. The patients respond to tricyclic antidepressants. Mood altering tricyclics such as nortryptiline hydrochloride or desipramine hydrochloride are useful in patients who are apathetic. Sedating tricyclics such as amitriptyline and doxepin are useful in agitated patients. All tricyclics have a tendency to increase chorea and to interfere with memory function. These are more prominent problems with highly anticholinergic drugs such as amitriptyline. The alleviation of the patient's depression is usually much more important than any temporary problem with the movement disorder or intellect, however. Lithium salts may be useful in patients with prominent mood swings. It may be necessary to treat patients with impulse control problems and angry or violent outbursts with neuroleptics. Many of these patients, however, may be maintained with benzodiazepines without any problem.

It has been common to use neuroleptics to treat chorea. However, it is not clear that this is anything more than a cosmetic treatment, and neuroleptics have many long-term side effects. The response of chorea to neuroleptics may only be temporary. Neuroleptics such as the phenothiazines and butyrophenones act by blocking the dopamine receptor in the basal ganglia. Reserpine can be used for similar effects by depleting the brain's stores of dopamine. While diminishing chorea, these drugs have several side effects that increase parkinsonian symptoms, cause akathisia, worsen dysphagia, and increase sedation. Some patients do have disabling chorea for which neuroleptics may be useful. The drugs should be used for a short time, as the chorea generally lessens with progression of the disease. Furthermore, the longer the drugs are used, the greater the chance of developing a superimposed tardive dyskinesia. Overall patient function correlates better with intellectual and emotional abilities than with lessening of chorea.

SUGGESTED READING

Folstein SE, Folstein MF, McHugh PR. Psychiatric syndromes in Huntington's disease. Adv Neurol 1979; 23:281–289.
Folstein SE, Franz ML, Jensen BA, et al. Conduct disorder and affective disorder among the offspring of patients with Huntington's disease. Psychol Med 1983; 13:45–52.
Hayden MR, Hewitt J, Kastelein JJP, et al. First-trimester prenatal diagnosis for Huntington's disease with DNA probes. Lancet 1987; 1:1284–1285.
Mazziotta JC, Phelps ME, Pahl JJ, et al. Reduced cerebral glucose metabolism in asymptomatic subjects at risk for Huntington's disease. N Engl J Med 1987; 316:357–362.
Meissen GJ, Myers RH, Mastromauro CA, et al. Predictive testing for Huntington's disease with use of a linked DNA marker. N Engl J Med 1988; 318:535–542.
Young AB, Penney JB, Starosta-Rubinstein S, et al. Normal caudate glucose metabolism in persons at risk for Huntington's disease. Arch Neurol 1987; 44:254–257.
Young AB, Shoulson I, Penney JB, et al. Huntington's disease in Venezuela: neurologic features and functional decline. Neurology 1986; 36:244–249.

PATIENT RESOURCE

The Huntington's Disease Society of America
220 West 22nd Street
New York, New York 10021
(Will provide information and location of local chapters.)

INHERITED ATAXIA

S.H. SUBRAMONY, M.D.
ROBERT D. CURRIER, M.D.

The inherited ataxias are a broad group of disorders with varying modes of inheritance and different biochemical mechanisms that share ataxia as the major clinical feature because of degeneration of the cerebellum, the cerebellar connections, or the proprioceptive pathways. In addition, in most of the ataxias, neurologic features other than ataxia and sometimes general systemic features occur. In some of the disorders discussed in this chapter, ataxia may be a relatively minor feature or it may occur as a major problem in only some of the patients. This is particularly true of some of the neurologic disorders with a known biochemical pathogenesis.

The therapy and research of inherited ataxias would be facilitated if one could classify these diseases into groups based on their genetics and the underlying biochemical mechanisms. However, the underlying genetic defect and the resulting biochemical abnormality are unknown for the majority of inherited ataxic syndromes. Therefore, the classification of inherited ataxias is still an evolving process. The wide variability of modes of inheritance and clinical features among different families with ataxia, the lack of uniformity of clinical and pathologic features among members of a single genetic entity, the occurrence of similar clinical and pathologic features in obviously different entities, and the lack of precise biochemical information have all created difficulties with regard to classification. Many of the disorders in which ataxia may be a prominent feature are shifted into other classification schemes once their precise biochemistry and genetics are known. This still leaves a core of ataxic syndromes that defy classification schemes. Nevertheless, classification is important for prognostication and genetic counseling. Some recent attempts at the classification of inherited ataxic disorders are shown in Tables 1 and 2.

Overall, perhaps approximately 5 percent of inherited ataxic syndromes have a known metabolic error and a potential for an appropriate medical treatment. Nevertheless, it is important to look for treatable causes in individuals presenting with a progressive ataxia. Such metabolic errors are probably more common in patients whose onset of disease occurs at a younger age than in those whose onset occurs during adulthood. Some of the laboratory studies that may be helpful in the work-up of patients include imaging procedures such as computed tomography (CT) and magnetic resonance imaging (MRI), peripheral nerve conduction studies and evoked responses, and a measurement of various biochemical parameters such as vitamin E levels, immunoglobulins, cortisol values, lactate levels, copper levels, and ceruloplasmin levels. Also, in selected cases with appropriate diagnostic clues, one may want to screen for deficiencies of lysosomal enzymes such as hexosaminidase and arylsulfatase A, perform muscle biopsy to document a mitochondrial disease or ceroid lipofuscinosis, and perform

Table 1 Classification of the Hereditary Ataxias

Type	Inheritance	Age of Onset (decade)
(I) Disorders with known metabolic or other cause		
Metabolic disorders		
Progressive, unremitting ataxia		
Abetalipoproteinemia (Bassen-Kornzweig disease)	AR	1st–2nd
Hypobetalipoproteinemia	AR	2nd–4th
Hexosaminidase deficiency	AR	1st
Glutamate dehydrogenase deficiency	AR	2nd–6th
Cholestanolosis	AR	Ataxia 3rd–6th
Intermittent ataxia		
Pyruvate dehydrogenase deficiency	AR	1st
Hartnup disease	AR	1st
Intermittent branched-chain ketoaciduria	AR	1st
Deficiencies of urea cycle enzymes (ornithine transcarbamyolase deficiency*, citrullinaemia, argininemia, argininosuccinicaciduria)	AR/XLD*	1st
Disorders characterized by defective DNA repair		
Ataxia telangiectasia (Louis Bar syndrome)	AR	1st
Xeroderma pigmentosum (de Sanctis-Cacchione syndrome)	AR	1st–2nd
Cockayne syndrome	AR	1st
(II) Disorders of unknown etiology		
Early onset cerebellar ataxia (onset usually before 20 years of age)		
Friedreich's ataxia	AR	1st–2nd
Early onset cerebellar ataxia with retained tendon reflexes	AR	1st–2nd
With hypogonadism ± deafness and/or dementia	AR	1st–3rd
With congenital deafness	AR	Ataxia 2nd–3rd
With childhood deafness and mental retardation	AR	1st
With pigmentary retinal degeneration ± mental retardation/dementia/deafness	AR	1st
With optic atrophy and mental retardation ± deafness/spasticity (Behr's syndrome)	AR	1st
Marinesco-Sjögren syndrome (with cataract and mental retardation)	AR	1st
With myoclonus (Ramsay Hunt syndrome)	AR/AD	1st–2nd
X-linked recessive spinocerebellar ataxia	XLR	1st–2nd
Cerebellar ataxia with essential tremor	AD	1st–3rd
Late onset cerebellar ataxia (onset usually after 20 years of age)		
Cerebellar ataxia with optic atrophy/ophthalmoplegia/dementia/amyotrophy/extrapyramidal features (? includes Azorean ataxia)	AD	3rd–5th
Cerebellar ataxia with pigmentary retinal degeneration ± ophthalmoplegia and/or extrapyramidal features	AD	Mid 2nd–4th
Pure cerebellar ataxia with later onset	AD	6th–7th
Cerebellar ataxia with myoclonus and deafness	AD	Ataxia 2nd–5th

* AD = autosomal dominant; AR = autosomal recessive; XLD = X-linked dominant; XLR = X-linked recessive. (Republished with permission from Harding AF. Classification of the hereditary ataxias and paraplegias. Lancet 1983; 1:1151–1155.)

Table 2   A Tentative Classification of Ataxia

I. Stationary or nonprogressive ataxias
   Congenital-cerebral palsy
   Injury—anoxia, stroke, heat, nutrition, toxic
II. Intermittent subtypes (very rare)
III. Progressive ataxias
   A. Secondary—cancer, multiple sclerosis, thyroid,
      seizures, others
   B. Sporadic—idiopathic (exist?)
   C. Hereditary—primary
     1. Common types
       a. Dominant Heredity
         (1) Usual age of onset: (20–50 yrs) (OPCA)
           (a) Usual symptoms (Marie, Nonne, Menzel,
              Schut) increased reflexes with
              cerebellar signs, dysarthria, and
              dysphagia
           (b) Common variants
             1. Decreased reflexes
             2. Extrapyramidal signs (Joseph)
             3. Spastic ataxia
             4. Others
         (2) Old Age (more than 50 years of age) at onset
         (3) Childhood onset: (exist?)
       b. Recessive heredity
         (1) Adult onset
           (a) Increased reflexes
           (b) Decreased reflexes
         (2) Old age onset
           GDH deficiency
         (3) Childhood
           (a) Increased deep tendon reflexes—
             Charlevoix
           (b) Decreased deep tendon reflexes—
             Friedreich's disease
     2. Rare types
       a. Neurologic—pathologic variations
         (1) Spinopontine
         (2) Posterior column
         (3) Cerebello-olivary
         (4) Anterior horn cell—peripheral nerve
         (5) With cerebral cortex changes—dementia
         (6) Infantile types—with broad CNS pathology
         (7) Others
       b. With sense organ abnormality
         (1) Ocular—retina, optic nerve, EOM weakness
         (2) Ear—deafness
         (3) Others
       c. Body abnormality in addition to ataxia
         (1) Gonadal
         (2) Skeletal
         (3) Others

Republished with permission from Currier RD. Classification of
ataxia. Ital J Neurol Sci 1984; (suppl 4): 55–64.

other esoteric biochemical measurements such as
measurements of cholestanol, ammonia, amino
acid, and very long chain fatty acid levels. Also,
when there is no clear family history, tests such as
CT or MRI, cerebrospinal fluid (CSF) studies, anti-
Purkinje cell antibodies and serum drug levels may
uncover acquired causes of cerebellar ataxia. Some
help in selecting appropriate laboratory tests can be
obtained from Tables 3 and 4.

MEDICAL TREATMENT

Ataxia of Known Pathogenesis

In many of these disorders, ataxia is often a
minor or variable feature, and other diagnostic clues
are often available. Appropriate replacement therapy or dietary manipulations not only can prevent
further neurologic progression, but often reverse established neurologic deficits in such diseases. Table
3 lists some ataxic disorders in which the metabolic
error is known and for which fairly effective treatment is available.

For several disorders, however, despite a
knowledge of an underlying metabolic or enzymatic
defect, an effective treatment is not yet available.
Some of the experimental approaches to treating
these disorders are listed in Table 4.

Ataxia of Unknown Pathogenesis

Treatment designed to arrest progression or reverse neurologic deficits in this group of disorders
remains disappointing. The commonly encountered
inherited ataxias in this group include Friedreich's
ataxia in children and dominantly inherited disorders often loosely included under the rubric of "olivopontocerebellar atrophies" in adults. Friedreich's
ataxia is characterized by onset during the early
teenage years, progressive gait ataxia, significant
proprioceptive loss, areflexia, and often an associated cardiomyopathy. It is recessively inherited.
The ataxias with onset occurring during adulthood
and which are dominantly inherited are characterized by progressive cerebellar signs as well as by
additional features such as hyperreflexia and up-
going toe responses during the early stages of
the disease, dysarthria, gaze palsies, and increased
tone in later stages. In selected families, additional
features such as retinal degeneration, myoclonus,
and deafness may occur as well. Although biochemical and neurotransmitter abnormalities have been
described in many of these disorders, strategies employed to alter transmitter function in the cerebellum have not been successful in treating them.
We believe that experimental treatments of this kind
should be offered only in the setting of a controlled
clinical trial and not in a random fashion. Table 5
lists some selected medications that have been tried
in some of these disorders with variable and generally disappointing results. We are as yet unable to
predict if there are selected subgroups of patients
that will respond to some of these drugs.

The only inherited ataxia of unknown etiopathogenesis that responds well to medical treatment is
familial paroxysmal ataxia. This autosomal dominant disorder is characterized by bouts of ataxia,
dysarthria, and nystagmus lasting 1 to 6 hours which
occur with variable frequency. Treatment with
acetazolamide (Diamox) in a dose of 250 mg 1 to 3

Table 3 Effective Treatment of Inherited Ataxias with Known Biochemical Pathogenesis

Disease	Diagnostic Clues	Laboratory Diagnosis	Treatment
Abetalipoproteinemia	Childhood onset, progressive ataxia, areflexia, proprioceptive loss, retinitis pigmentosa, malabsorption	Acanthocytes, low cholesterol/ triglyceride levels, low vitamin E levels, apolipoprotein B absent	Restrict long-chain fatty acid (C16-C24) intake, supplement vitamin A and K, vitamin E 100 mg/kg/day
Selective vitamin E malabsorption	Ataxia, areflexia, proprioceptive loss	Low vitamin E levels	Vitamin E 800–2,000 mg/day
Cerebrotendinous xanthomatosis	Progressive spastic ataxia during the 2nd and 3rd decades of life, tendon xanthomas, cataracts	Low/normal serum cholesterol levels, elevated plasma and bile cholestanol	Chenodeoxycholic acid 750 mg/day
Wilson's disease	Childhood onset/young adult, involuntary movements, behavioral and intellectual decline, ataxia, liver disease, hemolysis, renal tubular acidosis, Kayser-Fleischer ring	Low serum copper levels, elevated urinary copper levels, low/absent serum ceruloplasmin	D-penicillamine 1–3 g/day, oral zinc sulphate 600 mg/day, low copper diet (1.6 mg/day) Triethylene tetramine 1,200–2,400 mg/day
Partial hypoxanthine guanine phosphosribosyl transferase deficiency	Progressive ataxia, retardation and seizures (in some), gout	High serum uric acid; macrocytic RBCs	Allopurinol (does not affect CNS dysfunction)
Urea cycle defects	Episodic encephalopathy, ataxia, seizures, retardation in children	Hyperammonemia, abnormal serum amino acids, enzyme deficiency in liver biopsy/ cultured fibroblasts	Protein restriction with or without supplementation of essential amino acids
Aminoacidurias	Episodic encephalopathy, ataxia, unusual odor in children	Abnormal serum and urinary amino acids	Diet low in branched-chain amino acids and protein Niacin supplement in Hartnup disease
Pyruvate/lactate defects; biotinase deficiency	Episodic encephalopathy ataxia, Leigh's syndrome has progressive course	Metabolic acidosis, lactic acidosis, enzyme levels in WBCs, fibroblasts	Ketogenic diet, thiamine 100–1,000 mg/day, acetazolamine, lipoic acid, biotin

Table 4 Experimental Treatments in Inherited Syndromes of Known Biochemical Pathogenesis Often Associated with Ataxia

Disease	Diagnostic Clues	Laboratory Diagnosis	Experimental Treatment
Leukodystrophies (metachromatic, globoid cell)	Dementia, visual impairment, ataxia, spasticity	Abnormal peripheral nerve conduction, enzyme levels in WBCs, fibroblast Nerve biopsy	Enzyme delivery to brain, activators of enzymes
Hexosaminidase deficiency variants	Ataxia, dementia, seizures, spasticity	Abnormal enzyme levels in WBCs, fibroblasts	Enzyme replacement, bone marrow transplant
Mitochondrial encephalomyopathies	Ataxia, fatigable weakness, myoclonus, short stature, basal ganglia calcification	Muscle biopsy with ragged red fibers, respiratory transport defect in mitochondria	Riboflavin coenzyme Q_{-10}, pyridoxine, alpha-ketogluglutarate
Ceroid lipofuscinosis (adult, late infantile variants)	Visual failure, myoclonus, ataxia, dementia	Increased dolichols in urine sediment Lymphocytes, inclusions on electron microscopy Skin biopsy for inclusions	Antioxidant therapy (vitamins E and C)
Niemann-Pick disease	Ataxia and spasticity (in some), hepatosplenomegaly, childhood onset	Lipid-laden cells in bone marrow, sphingomyelinase assay in WBCs, fibroblasts	Implants of human amniotic tissue, bone marrow transplant
Ataxia telangiectasia	Ataxia of childhood onset, telangiectasias of skin, conjunctiva, recurrent respiratory infections	Low levels of IgA and IgE, increased alpha-fetoprotein	Plasma transfusion, thymosin, fetal thymic transplants

Table 5 Experimental Treatments for Inherited Ataxias of Uncertain Etiopathogenesis

Drug	Disorder	Selected References	Side Effects
Cholinergic system			
Physostigmine 6–8 mg/day p.o.	Different types	Kark RAP, et al. Neurology 1981; 31:288.	GI upset, bradycardia
Choline chloride 150 mg/kg/day p.o.	Different types	Lawrence CM, et al. J Neurol Neurosurg Psychiat 1980; 43:452.	GI upset, fishy odor
Lecithin 50–100 g/day p.o.	Friedreich's	Chamberlain S, et al. J Neurol Neurosurg Psychiat 1980; 43:843. Pentland B, et al. Br Med J 1981; 282:1197.	GI upset, depression, weight gain
Adrenergic system			
Propranolol 40–80 mg/day p.o.	Different types	Duhigg WJ. Arch Neurol 1985; 42:15.	Bradycardia, depression, lassitude
Amantadine hydrochloride (Symmetrel) 200 mg/day p.o.	Friedreich's	Peterson PL, et al. Neurology 1988; 38:1478.	Nausea, insomnia, livido reticularis
Serotonergic system			
L-5 hydroxytryptophan 200–300 mg/day p.o. (with carbidopa)	Different types	Trovillas P, et al. Rev Neurol 1982; 138:415.	Nausea, diarrhea, sleepiness, hypomania*
Amino acid system			
Gamma vinyl gamma-aminobutyric acid 250 mg b.i.d. p.o.	Different types	DeSmet Y, et al. Can J Neurol Sci 1982; 9:171. Bonnet AM, et al. Can J Neurol Sci 1986; 13:331.	Dizziness, drowsiness, nausea, facial clonus
Aspartate, asparigine	Dominant ataxia	Personal experience	GI upset
Peptides/Growth Factors			
Thyrotropin releasing hormone 0.5–6 mg IV	Different types	Sobve I, et al. J Neurol Sci 1983; 61:235. LeWitt PA, et al. Lancet 1982; 2:981.	Flushing, nausea, urinary urgency
Purified brain gangliosides (Cronassial) 40–100 mg/day IM	Friedreich's	Bradley WG, et al. Neurology 1988; 38:1731.	Pain, rash

* The FDA has advised consumers to discontinue L-tryptophan due to an outbreak of the "eosinophilia-myalgia" syndrome.

times per day abolishes these attacks. Long-term side effects of such treatment may include anorexia, weight loss, parasthesias, and occasionally nephrolithiasis and bone marrow suppression. Diamox is sometimes effective in the treatment of intermittent ataxia caused by a known error of pyruvate metabolism as well.

In some families with inherited ataxias, extrapyramidal features in the form of parkinsonism and dystonic posturings are common and may occur as major disabling problems. Extrapyramidal features appear to be more common in patients belonging to families with Joseph disease. Parkinsonian symptomatology in such patients may show significant improvement when treated with levodopa in a manner similar to that used in the treatment of idiopathic parkinsonism. Such a response occurs only in those members of the family exhibiting parkinsonian features. As the disease progresses and additional features become evident such as severe ataxia or amyotrophy, levodopa loses its effectiveness. Levo-dopa is not particularly effective in the treatment of typical dominantly inherited familial ataxia with olivopontocerebellar atrophy as its pathologic substrate.

Spasticity, usually seen during late stages of adult onset dominant ataxia, may respond to medications such as baclofen (Lioresal). Dosages of baclofen range from 5 to 10 mg 3 times per day and may be increased in gradual increments until a dosage of 60 to 100 mg per day is reached. As in multiple sclerosis, ambulatory patients with spasticity may experience greater gait problems when receiving baclofen. Thus, individual judgment needs to be exercised in the administration of this medication.

Cardiomyopathy and diabetes mellitus are systemic features that occur in Friedreich's ataxia. Cardiomyopathy initially is hypertrophic in type, and ambulatory patients can have angina. With decreased physical activity, angina disappears, and in late stages of the disease, arrhythmias and cardiac failure occur. Angina, cardiac failure, and arrhythmias respond to treatment with standard drugs such as propranolol, digitalis, and lidocaine derivatives. Electrocardiogram (ECG) and echocardiography are useful in documenting heart disease. Symptomatic heart disease should prompt referral to a cardiologist. Since nonambulatory patients do not complain of exertional dyspnea, clinical examination for rhythm disturbances and cardiac failure should be performed routinely. Diabetes occurs in approximately 40 percent of these patients, and about 20 percent of these are insulin dependent.

PHYSICAL AND
REHABILITATION MEASURES

The role of physical therapy in retarding progression of functional disability or reversing established neurologic deficits is not well established. However, physical therapy has a major role in preventing secondary problems that can increase functional disability such as joint contractures and postural abnormalities. Physical therapy also has a role in maintaining the mobility of the patient at each stage of the disease. Active and passive stretching exercises and gait training are important during the early stages. As ambulation deteriorates, periodic physical therapy evaluation is indicated to anticipate the use of appropriate walking aids such as a cane or walker. In selected patients, lower extremity orthotics may help maintain ambulation. Still later, the therapist should evaluate the patient for an appropriate wheelchair, keeping in mind such factors as the patient's lifestyle and the type of help he or she has at home.

Similarly, the occupational therapists have a role in maintaining the patients' activities of daily living. Suggestions regarding devices to maintain postural stability and aids for bathing, dressing, and feeding can all be given by an occupational therapist. Occupational therapists may also make recommendations regarding the design of the home environment, such as showers and wheelchair ramps. A significant number of assistive devices are available, and physical and occupational therapy departments have several catalogues of these.

Progressive scoliosis is more of a problem in childhood ataxias such as Friedreich's ataxia. The spine should be examined periodically in these patients. Thoracic lumbar sacral orthoses (TLSO) are useful if the curves are less than 30 degrees (or after spinal fusion). A thoracic orthosis, fitted to hold the lumbar spine in lordosis and limit lateral mobility, is often used. Spinal alignment is obtained by fitting the orthosis with the patient in cervical traction and elevating the ribs and forcing the shoulders back. Similarly, specialized wheelchair seating may be used to support a flexible deformity in preferred position or to accommodate a fixed deformity, although it should not be thought of as definitive spinal support throughout the day. Overall, the goal is to hold the lumbar spine in lordosis and limit lateral mobility. Surgery is often indicated if the curves are more than 40 degrees and unstable. However, pulmonary function should be good enough to permit surgery (more than 40 percent of predicted normal).

GENETIC COUNSELING IN
INHERITED ATAXIAS

As one can see from the classification schemes, commonly occurring inherited ataxias have autosomal dominant or recessive forms of inheritance. With autosomal recessive inheritance, the parents are clinically normal because both are heterozygotes for the defective gene. The disease often affects several siblings, however, and the risk for the siblings of an index case is 25 percent. There is often consanguinity between the parents; this is especially likely if the disorder in question is relatively rare. The risk to other relatives is negligible, including offspring of affected individuals, all of whom will be heterozygotes. This situation is typical of Friedreich's ataxia. Thus a couple who has already had one or more children with Friedreich's ataxia has a risk of 25 percent for each of their subsequent children. Preclinical detection is probably not of great relevance in the setting of this disorder, although parents of children at risk are often anxious. There is some suggestion that loss of tendon reflexes as well as abnormalities in sensory nerve conduction studies may be preonset clues to the occurrence of Friedreich's ataxia. The risk of transmission of the disease from a patient to his or her offspring is quite low in view of the general low prevalence of the Friedreich's gene in the population and thus the unlikelihood of the marital partner carrying the gene. Similarly, the risk that the siblings of affected patients will have children affected by Friedreich's ataxia is quite low. Recently the defective gene for Friedreich's ataxia has been located on chromosome 9 with the use of restriction fragment length polymorphism (RFLP) markers. Thus in selected families with informative markers, one can predict the risk of heterozygosity much more easily.

Autosomal dominant inheritance is commonly seen in the adult onset ataxias. The disease occurs in successive generations, and overall, 40 to 50 percent of the offspring of an affected person have the disease. The disorder is transmitted by both males and females and affects both males and females. One of the problems with dominant disease in general is the variability in clinical severity of disease, sometimes resulting in apparent "skipping" of a generation. Careful examination of family members is often needed to detect such disease in an apparently unaffected parent. Thus in straightforward autosomal dominant inheritance, an affected patient will have a 50 percent chance of transmitting the disease to each of his children. The search for genetic markers for this form of ataxia as well as for Joseph disease is intensifying. In several families with dominantly inherited adult onset ataxia, linkage to the HL-A locus on chromosome 6 has been established and RFLP markers will become available. As regards Joseph disease, evidence is accumulating that the disorder may be located on chromosome 1. In families in which linkage can be established, this data can be used to predict the risk of the children of affected parents developing the disease. The certainty of this prediction obviously depends on the closeness of the linkage between the selected marker and the disease gene. In addition, the age at the time of the onset of the disease must be considered in calculating the probability of developing the disease and counseling individuals at risk. Although in late onset dominant ataxia, the age at the time of onset is variable, ranging from the second to the sixth decade of life, the likelihood of developing the disease becomes smaller and smaller the longer the person at risk lives without developing any symptoms, since most individuals become symptomatic before the age of 40 years. Thus an individual at risk who is 35 years old and is as yet asymptomatic has only a 30 percent chance of developing the disease later on. This risk calculation can be further modified by adding linkage data, if available. As tightly linked markers become available in many of these families with dominantly inherited ataxias, better predictions can be made as to the risk at younger ages and preonset determination will become possible. This is particularly important in the adult onset ataxias since many of these disorders do not become symptomatic until after the patient has reached reproductive age and counseling may no longer be useful by the time the person becomes symptomatic.

We follow certain "rules" regarding genetic counseling for individuals at risk for hereditary ataxias. First, predictive risk counseling is done only at the request of the individual concerned and the information is given only to that individual. The counseling is done by the geneticist personally and alone with the person at risk or with his or her spouse. The information is not given to parents of children at risk. Usually such counseling is sought when a marriage or pregnancy is being planned. The information is discussed with the person more than once. No prior psychological preparation is performed before counseling. We have not had any formal follow-up of persons counseled; however, we are aware of only one major adverse reaction in the form of suicide among the many individuals counseled.

Currently there are no other accurate methods of preclinical detection available. We have found that clinical abnormalities of a subtle nature are prevalent before symptom onset in many of these patients. Similarly, a good neuro-ophthalmologic examination may be used to detect preclinical abnormalities in many of these individuals. However, at present none of these are accurate enough for prediction of risk.

SUGGESTED READING

Jackson JF, Currier RD, Martin NE. Dominant spinocerebellar ataxia: genetic counseling. J Neurogenetics 1983; 1:87–90.

Mangum BV. Recent advances in the treatment of cerebellar ataxias. Clin Neuropharmacol 1986; 9:508–516.

Stanbury JB, Wyngaarden JB, Frederickson DS, et al. The metabolic basis of inherited disease, 5th ed. New York: McGraw-Hill, 1983.

PATIENT RESOURCES

National Ataxia Foundation
600 Twelve Oaks Center
15500 Wayzata Boulevard
Wayzata, Minnesota 55391

Friedreich's Ataxia Group in America, Inc.
P.O. Box 11116
Oakland, California 94611

Muscular Dystrophy Association
810 Seventh Avenue
New York, New York 10019

DYSTONIA

PAUL GREENE, M.D.
STANLEY FAHN, M.D.

Dystonic syndromes are characterized by involuntary twisting movements and postures of a sustained nature. They can be classified into two groups: primary (idiopathic) and secondary (symptomatic) dystonia. Both types of dystonia can be subdivided into sporadic and hereditary forms and further subdivided in a variety of ways. Although treatment of dystonic symptoms may always be attempted, a rational approach to treatment is expedited by a specific diagnosis. Table 1 shows a brief classification system for dystonic conditions that is oriented towards specific treatment strategies and serves as an outline for this review.

Wilson's disease often presents as a dystonic syndrome in young people, and so all patients with dystonia who are younger than 50 years of age and who do not have a clear family history of dystonia should have a serum ceruloplasmin and slit lamp examination for Kayser-Fleischer rings. Because dystonic symptoms may result from structural lesions in the basal ganglia, thalamus, or brain stem, computed tomography (CT) or magnetic resonance imaging (MRI) of the head should be routinely done in patients with dystonia, especially when the symptoms are unilateral. Beyond this, a discussion of a systematic approach to the evaluation of dystonia is beyond the scope of this review.

PRIMARY DYSTONIA

Diurnal Dystonia

Levodopa-responsive dystonia (diurnal dystonia) often starts in childhood with gait disturbance, and is typically familial. Patients may have signs of parkinsonism (bradykinesia and loss of postural reflexes), corticospinal tract signs (including Babinski signs), and diurnal variation (dramatically better in the morning). These patients can be rendered symptom-free through treatment with 200 mg to 300 mg of levodopa daily in the form of carbidopa/levodopa (Fig. 1). Some patients may lack one or more of the typical features of this condition. We therefore initially treat all patients with idiopathic dystonia that has its onset during childhood and young adulthood with 400 mg daily of carbidopa/levodopa for at least 2 weeks. It is best to start with 100 mg daily and gradually increase the dose since some patients experience dramatic improvement when taking small doses but develop levodopa dyskinesias when taking higher doses.

Focal Dystonias

Most focal dystonias improve with injections of botulinum toxin type A (Botox). Botox interferes with the release of acetylcholine from cholinergic nerve terminals and creates muscle weakness lasting from 3 to 6 months. When Botox is injected intramuscularly or subcutaneously over a muscle, dystonic contractions may be dramatically reduced without severely compromising normal functioning. For best results, and to minimize side effects, techniques of injection require special training. No serious or long-lasting side effects of chronic Botox injections have been seen in almost a decade of use. Most focal dystonias occur during adulthood, and we prefer Botox to medicine for the treatment of focal dystonia in adults. Most childhood onset dystonias progress beyond focal dystonia to segmental, multifocal, or generalized dystonia. The safety of chronic Botox injections in children has yet to be established, and we still prefer pharmacotherapy as the initial treatment for the occasional child with focal symptoms.

Spastic dysphonia (laryngeal dystonia) improves dramatically in almost 100 percent of patients who receive low doses (2.5 to 3.75 U of toxin activity) injected into both vocalis muscles through a hollow core electromyogram (EMG) needle with EMG verification of needle tip placement. Blepharospasm improves in approximately 90 percent of patients after the subcutaneous injection of approximately 25 U per eye in a divided dose administered to five or six sites around each eye. EMG guidance is not required. Oromandibular and lower facial dystonia often improve after EMG-guided injections into the contracting muscles. Benefit from the injections lasts for 3 to 6 months, after which time patients can be reinjected. Local side effects only have been seen

---

Table 1 Classification of Dystonic Syndromes

Primary dystonia
   Levodopa responsive dystonia (diurnal dystonia, Segawa variant)
   Focal dystonia (torticollis, blepharospasm, oromandibular dystonia, occupational cramps, spastic dysphonia)
   Segmental, multifocal, and generalized dystonia
   Hemidystonia
   Paroxysmal kinesigenic and nonkinesigenic dystonia
Secondary dystonia
   Wilson's disease
   Intracerebral mass lesion (e.g., tumor, arteriovenous malformation)
   Tardive dystonia (after exposure to dopamine receptor–blocking agents)
   Acute dystonic reactions (after exposure to dopamine receptor–blocking agents)
   Other drug exposure (e.g., anticonvulsants, calcium channel blockers, levodopa, dopamine agonists)
   Psychogenic dystonia
   Other conditions

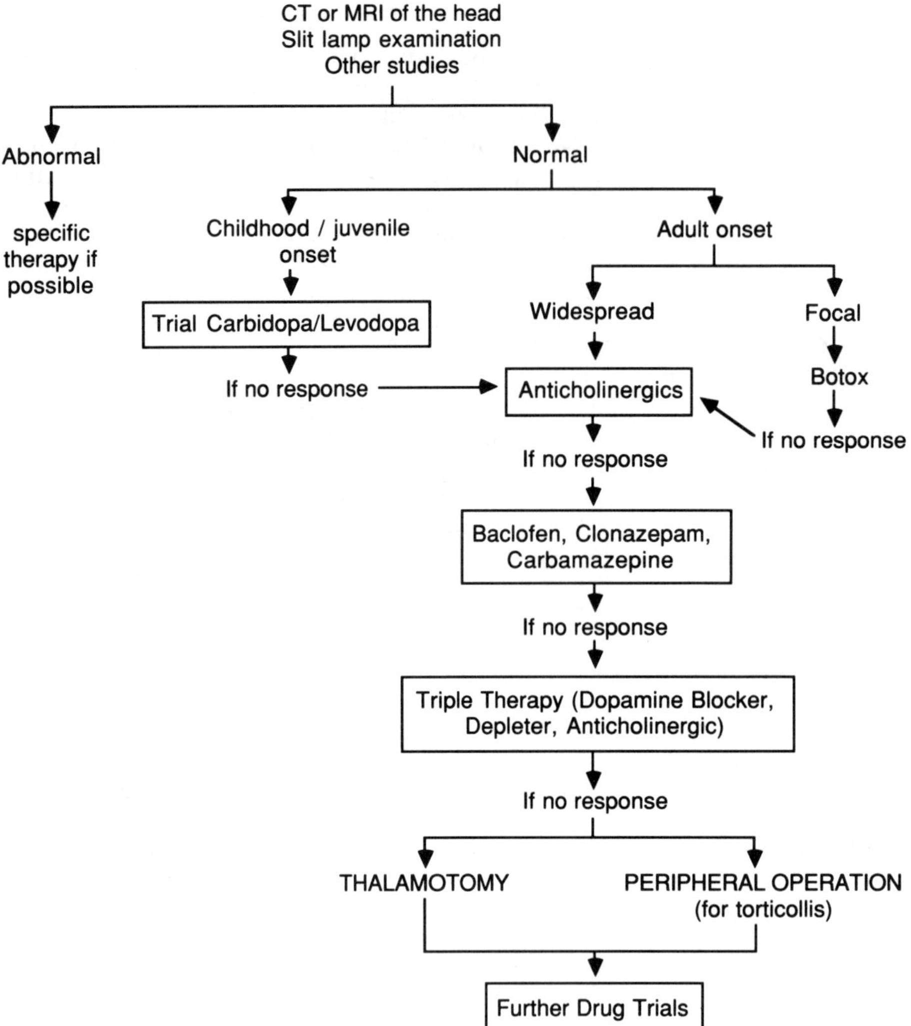

Figure 1 Treatment of primary dystonia.

with these injections; transient breathiness or swallowing difficulty after vocal cord injections, transient ptosis after eyelid injections, and excess local weakness after lower facial injections.

Torticollis requires much higher doses of toxin (as much as 450 U) injected into the sternocleidomastoid, splenius capitus, trapezius, and other contracting muscles to achieve reasonable benefit. Approximately 60 to 75 percent of patients experience substantial benefit lasting for approximately 3 months. Some patients experience systemic symptoms of malaise, generalized aching, nausea, and headache, although actual weakness of uninjected muscles has not been seen. Some patients may develop sufficient titers of antibotulinum toxin antibodies to block the effects of Botox, so we try to use the smallest doses possible and inject as infrequently as possible.

Patients with brachial dystonia (occupational cramps) may improve with EMG-guided Botox injections into contracting muscles when only a few muscles produce most of the disability. Carefully selected patients with writer's cramp have improved dramatically after receiving Botox injections. Doses must be determined empirically after repeated injections, starting with small amounts of Botox.

Patients with focal dystonia who fail to improve with Botox injections may be treated with pharmacotherapy.

Many operations that lesion the peripheral nervous system have been used to relieve the symptoms of a variety of focal dystonias. Most have been superseded by medical therapies. The only operation that we currently recommend is selective posterior ramisectomy for torticollis. We do not recommend surgery for any patient who is not extremely disabled, and even then, only if Botox injections and multiple medical trials have failed.

Segmental and Generalized Dystonia

Segmental, multifocal, and generalized dystonia can be treated with pharmacotherapy. If low doses of levodopa as described above are ineffective, we start treatment with anticholinergic agents. Children initially receive trihexyphenidyl hydrochloride in a dose of 2.5 mg once daily, which is increased by 2.5 mg per week and administered four times daily until adverse effects appear. In adults, ethopropazine hydrochloride often produces fewer side effects and can be increased on a similar schedule, with 25 mg of ethopropazine substituted for 2.5 mg of trihexyphenidyl hydrochloride. Because the benefit from anticholinergic agents may be delayed in onset, after each month or so of increasing doses, we observe the patients for several weeks while they are receiving a constant dose. Benefit may be seen when total daily doses of 20 mg or more of trihexyphenidyl (200 mg of ethopropazine) are used. Children tolerate high doses of anticholinergic medicine (> 80 mg/day of trihexyphenidyl), and approximately two-thirds of children experience improvement in their symptoms. Adults tolerate these agents poorly, and approximately two-fifths improve to some degree.

Peripheral anticholinergic side effects such as dry mouth, blurred vision, constipation, and urinary retention may be treated with oral pyridostigmine and pilocarpine eye drops. A few patients complain of the short duration of benefit after each dose of anticholinergic medicine or of having side effects shortly after taking the medicine. A timed-release preparation of trihexyphenidyl hydrochloride is available that has been helpful in such cases. Memory loss or confusion require a trial of the timed-release preparation or dose reduction.

If anticholinergic agents are of no benefit, other agents may be substituted. If anticholinergics are of partial benefit, they are continued and other drugs added. Many patients will get additive benefit from the use of multiple agents. Baclofen and clonazepam increased gradually until adverse effects appear produce some benefit in 10 to 20 percent of patients of all ages and with all types of dystonia. Baclofen seems to be of particular efficacy in patients with cranial dystonia. When receiving high doses of clonazepam, some patients have developed irritability as well as drowsiness. Patients may have fewer side effects with other benzodiazepines, which may be tried if clonazepam produces benefit but is not tolerated. Carbamazepine benefits a small percentage of patients with dystonia, but may occasionally produce dramatic improvement.

When these measures fail to produce significant relief of symptoms, dopamine depleters and dopamine receptor–blocking agents can be tried. Reserpine and metyrosine are antidopaminergics without dopamine receptor–blocking activity. They can cause drowsiness, orthostatic hypotension, depression, and parkinsonism, but they may benefit some patients with idiopathic dystonia. We use them as a last resort in combination with a dopamine receptor blocker and an anticholinergic agent. We try to avoid the use of dopamine receptor–blocking agents because of the risk of developing tardive complications with chronic use. We consider using these agents only after all other medicines have failed, and then only for the treatment of severe, disabling dystonia. We hope that addition of a dopamine depleter such as reserpine may reduce the risk of developing tardive complications.

Tetrabenazine is an investigational dopamine depleting agent with a small amount of dopamine receptor–blocking activity. It has never been associated with the development of tardive complications. Alone or in combination with lithium, it benefits some patients with dystonia. In addition to the complications associated with dopamine depleters, some patients develop acute akathisia (restlessness) when receiving tetrabenazine. The akathisia always resolves if tetrabenazine is discontinued.

Levodopa and dopamine agonists such as bromocriptine may worsen dystonia in some patients. Paradoxically, they may also reduce symptoms in a few patients who have dystonia. Because these patients do not have the levodopa-responsive dystonia mentioned earlier, they require high doses to achieve benefit.

Many other agents have been reported to be of benefit to an isolated patient with dystonia. Some patients are eager to continue therapeutic trials if the agents mentioned prove ineffective. As long as the patient desires further attempts at pharmacologic therapy, our policy is to continue medication trials with medicines that do not have significant risk and are known to affect brain transmitter systems.

Hemidystonia

Hemidystonia is most commonly found in patients with secondary dystonia, but occasional idiopathic patients have persistent hemidystonia or predominantly unilateral symptoms. If all measures described above fail, these patients may benefit from thalamotomy. Patients with bilateral dystonia or severe axial dystonia who fail medical therapy may also benefit from thalamotomy, but these patients require bilateral thalamotomies. In addition to a small risk of infarct or hemorrhage, bilateral thalamotomies involve a substantial risk of speech impairment. Thalamotomy should only be considered in the most disabled patients, after extensive conservative measures have failed.

Paroxysmal Dystonia

Paroxysmal dystonias can be divided into two groups: kinesigenic (brief, multiple attacks triggered by sudden movements) and nonkinesigenic (more prolonged attacks unrelated to movement). The kinesigenic variety usually improves dramatically with anticonvulsants such as carbamazepine or phenytoin. The nonkinesigenic is difficult to treat. In addition to clonazepam and anticonvulsants, acetazolamide should be tried. If these fail, any of the agents used for nonparoxysmal dystonia may be tried.

SECONDARY DYSTONIA

Some patients with secondary dystonia of any etiology respond to the measures outlined for idiopathic dystonia, but the response of secondary dystonia is, in general, inferior to the response of idiopathic dystonias. Nevertheless, there are some exceptions.

Some patients exposed to dopamine receptor–blocking agents develop dystonic spasms that persist after the agent has been discontinued. The movements appear while the patient is taking the drug or as late as approximately 3 months after the drug has been discontinued. These tardive dystonic movements may look identical to movements seen in patients with idiopathic dystonia. Approximately 50 percent of patients with tardive dystonia improve when treated with high-dose anticholinergic agents, dopamine depleters (reserpine or tetrabenazine), or a combination of the two. Patients requiring treatment with dopamine receptor–blocking agents for psychiatric reasons may benefit from the addition of these agents. Underlying depression is not an absolute contraindication to the use of dopamine depleters, since many patients become less depressed when their dystonic symptoms improve. Careful monitoring for depression is of course necessary. Some patients develop drug-induced parkinsonism as the dystonic symptoms improve. If these symptoms are mild, they may be better tolerated than the tardive dystonia. Patients who do not improve with this regimen should be treated as described for idiopathic patients.

After dopamine receptor–blocking agents are discontinued, acute dystonic reactions produced by these agents do not persist for long. When severe, they can be treated with anticholinergics, antihistamines, or benzodiazepines. These may be administered intramuscularly or intravenously for rapid control of severe symptoms.

Dystonic symptoms can be produced by the use of anticonvulsants, calcium channel blockers, levodopa, and dopamine agonists. The dystonic symptoms may resolve if the agent is discontinued. The possibility of drug-induced dystonia should be considered even when one is administering agents not known to be dopamine receptor blockers.

The approach to differentiating psychogenic dystonia from organic dystonia is beyond the scope of this chapter. Since dystonia is an unfamiliar condition in which emotional stress may precipitate unusual posturing, overdiagnosis of psychogenic dystonia is a danger. Because some patients with psychogenic dystonia benefit from psychiatric intervention, however, this diagnosis should not be missed.

SUGGESTED READING

Bertrand CM. Peripheral versus central surgical approach for the treatment of spasmodic torticollis. In: Marsden CD, Fahn S, eds. Movement disorders. London: Butterworth, 1981: 315.

Brin M, Fahn S, Moskowitz C, et al. Localized injections of botulinum toxin for the treatment of focal dystonia and hemifacial spasm. Movement Disorders 1987; 2:237–254.

Burke RE, Fahn S, Marsden CD. Torsion dystonia: a double-blind prospective trial of high-dose trihexyphenidyl. Neurology 1986; 36:160–164.

Fahn S, Williams DT. Psychogenic dystonia. Adv Neurol 1988; 50:431–455.

Greene P, Shale S, Fahn S. Analysis of open-label trials in torsion dystonia using high dosages of anticholinergics and other drugs. Movement Disorders 1988; 3:46–60.

Jankovic J, Orman J. Tetrabenazine therapy of dystonia, chorea, tics and other dyskinesias. Neurology 1988; 38:391–394.

Kang UJ, Burke RE, Fahn S. Natural history and treatment of tardive dystonia. Movement Disorders 1986; 1:193–208.

Marsden CD, Marion MH, Quinn N. The treatment of severe dystonia in children and adults. J Neurol Neurosurg Psychiat 1984; 47:1166–1173.

PATIENT RESOURCES

Dystonia Medical Research Foundation
8383 Wilshire Boulevard
Suite 800
Beverly Hills, California 90211
Telephone: (213) 852–1630

Benign Essential Blepharospasm Research Foundation
P.O. Box 12468
Beaumont, Texas 77726-2468
Telephone: (409) 832–0788

National Spasmodic Torticollis Association, Inc.
P.O. Box 873
Royal Oak, Michigan 48068-0873
Telephone: (313) 647–2280

Spastic Dysphonia Support Group
C/O Midge Kovacs
799 Broadway
Suite 640
New York, New York 10003

ESSENTIAL BLEPHAROSPASM AND MEIGE'S SYNDROME

GERALD G. STRIPH, M.D.
NEIL R. MILLER, M.D.

Essential blepharospasm is a chronic bilateral focal dystonia of the orbicularis muscles resulting in frequent involuntary eyelid closure. Blepharospasm is sometimes associated with spasms of other facial, lingual, or cervical muscles; in this case, the condition is called Meige's syndrome or orofacial dystonia. Although some cases of blepharospasm are caused by ocular irritation or mesencephalic lesions, the cause of essential blepharospasm and Meige's syndrome is unknown.

Essential blepharospasm usually begins as an increased frequency of blinking that seems to be exacerbated by certain stimuli such as wind or sunlight. It progresses to prolonged, spasmodic eyelid closure that occurs without obvious external provocation. One eye may be affected weeks to months before the other. The spasms are mild at first, but eventually they may become so severe that they prevent reading and driving. Many patients become occupationally and socially disabled. Such patients may shun social contacts and become depressed. Essential blepharospasm can become sufficiently severe that patients are functionally blind.

BOTULINUM TOXIN TREATMENT

As the underlying pathologic lesion is unknown, a variety of treatments active at different sites have been tried. We achieve the best response with the least morbidity through the use of botulinum A toxin (Oculinum), currently an investigational drug. During the past 6 years, we have treated more than 150 patients using a protocol approved by the National Institute of Health. It is anticipated that the Federal Drug Administration will approve botulinum for use by all physicians in the near future.

Botulinum toxin is produced by the bacterium *Clostridium botulinum.* Large amounts of the toxin that enter the bloodstream from ingestion of contaminated food or from a puncture wound produce the systemic disease botulism, a disorder characterized by muscle weakness. Six antigenically distinct toxins (A–F) with similar pharmacologic activity have been isolated. We use type A in the treatment of essential blepharospasm and other disorders characterized by involuntary facial movement (e.g., hemifacial spasm).

Botulinum toxin interferes with the release of acetylcholine from the presynaptic nerve terminals, thus producing temporary paralysis of the affected muscle. The paralysis resolves over several weeks to months as the terminals regenerate. The small doses used in the treatment of involuntary movement disorders such as blepharospasm have no known systemic side effects and do not seem to result in the formation of systemic antibodies.

Our approach to treating patients with blepharospasm begins with a thorough discussion of the natural history of the condition and the reassurance that it is not the harbinger of more serious underlying disease. The various treatment alternatives are discussed. The discussion emphasizes that injections of botulinum toxin provide *temporary,* symptomatic relief from the condition. Should the patient request botulinum injection, he or she is given additional reading material and is scheduled for treatment.

After giving informed consent, the patient receives the injection. The injections are given with a tuberculin syringe and 30-gauge needle while the patient sits in the examination chair. Neither anesthesia nor sedation is needed, although two patients have experienced vasovagal attacks at the time of the first injection. If a patient is particularly afraid of the injections, we have him lie supine while he receives the injections. Each injection consists of 2.5 to 3.75 U (2.5 U per 0.1 ml) of the toxin and is placed subcutaneously. The locations of the injections are shown in Figure 1. Two to three injections are placed medially, laterally, and (occasionally) centrally, just above the eyebrow. Two injections administered in the upper lid are placed at the level of the upper border of the tarsus. The toxin thus affects the pretarsal orbicularis but has little effect on the levator muscle (which at this location is represented by the aponeurosis). An injection is administered just above and below the lateral canthus. We inject in the lower lid unless the patient has previously developed local problems (entropion, ectropion). Although some investigators believe that lower lid injections, particularly those administered medially, are unnecessary, we have found them to be helpful. In patients with Meige's syndrome, one or more injections are also placed in areas of the midface and lower face affected by involuntary movements. Typically, these areas include the nasolabial folds and near the corner of the mouth. We are careful not to inject so much toxin that the patient develops a severe lower facial paresis. The total dose given ranges from approximately 50 U in patients with blepharospasm to 60 to 75 U in patients with Meige's syndrome. There is no apparent benefit from higher doses of botulinum, nor are there any systemic side effects from doses as high as 250 U.

Before and after injection, patients are reminded that there is a possibility of transient local side effects including ptosis, diplopia, entropion, ectropion, dry eyes, and facial drooping. These side effects usually last several days to several weeks.

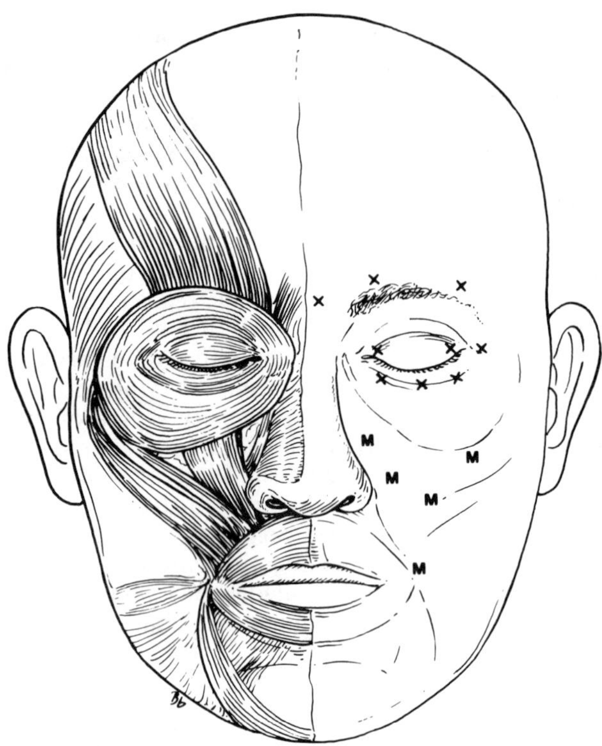

Figure 1 The injection sites used for a typical blepharospasm patient are indicated with an "X." Additional sites for patients with Meige's syndrome are shown with an "M." All injection sites are individually selected based on the location of the current spasms and the effects, both desirable and undesirable, of any previous injections.

Patients are told to use artificial tear solution, ointment, or both, for irritation. We tell patients who have received an injection for the first time to contact the office within 1 week to let us know how they are doing. We tell all patients to contact us immediately if they have any difficulties. Otherwise, they are to contact us when the blepharospasm begins bothering them again, at which time they may wish to schedule another injection. An important part of the therapy is that it is directed by the patient. Most patients elect to return for reinjection within 2 to 4 months. We currently have a success rate of more than 90% as measured both objectively by lid closure force grading and, more importantly, by patient satisfaction.

Complications of botulinum injections for blepharospasm are infrequent, mild, and usually related to the injections achieving more muscle paralysis than is desired. Entropion or ectropion may occur, sometimes resulting in an exposure keratopathy that may usually be managed with lubricants. Ptosis and weakness of other facial muscles may also occur, and diplopia from involvement of the inferior oblique muscle after deep lower lid injections has been reported. We have performed more than 1,000 injections in more than 150 patients and have never seen diplopia, entropion, or ectropion result.

MEDICAL TREATMENT

Before the introduction of botulinum injections, a variety of medical, surgical, and psychological therapies were commonly employed. They may still be helpful for those patients who hesitate to receive injections, who do not desire to return for reinjection periodically, or in whom the injections are unsuccessful. Blepharospasm and Meige syndrome may be associated with a central monoamine overactivity or a relative cholinergic deficiency. Drugs that target the transmitters in these systems may thus help some patients. For patients who prefer oral medical therapy, we initially prescribe clonazepam (Klonopin), 0.5 mg 2 or 3 times per day, and increase the dose slowly to 10 mg per day until the blepharospasm resolves or until the side effects (usually sedation) become problematic. Lorazepam (Ativan) may be used in the same way. Baclofen (Lioresal), an antispastic agent chiefly used in patients with multiple sclerosis, may also be tried. It is given in an initial dose of 5 mg 3 times per day and is then increased over several weeks to 120 mg per day. Ataxia and sedation are prominent side effects. At the conclusion of therapy, all of these medications should be tapered, rather than abruptly discontinued. In our experience, the medical treatment of blepharospasm is largely unsatisfactory. The medications all have significant side effects, particularly with chronic use, and they have a success rate of only approximately 30 percent.

SURGICAL TREATMENT

Numerous surgical techniques have been used in the treatment of blepharospasm. These procedures relieve spasm by reducing the innervation of the facial nerve or by removing the orbicularis oculi and adjacent muscles. Although they all have the advantage of providing a potentially permanent cure, they are long, complicated procedures that usually require general anesthesia and have significant, potentially *permanent* side effects, including facial paralysis and exposure keratopathy.

Partial avulsion of the peripheral seventh nerve may reduce the severity of blepharospasm. The results of the operation are simulated for the patient with local anesthetic and a regional block (e.g., Atkinson or O'Brien peripheral nerve blocks). The avulsion is generally performed with the patient under general anesthesia without the use of other local anesthetic agents or muscle relaxants that could affect the results of intraoperative nerve stimulation. A preauricular incision is made about 2 cm anterior to the tragus. Blunt and sharp dissection is carried out to the level of the parotid fascia. Meticulous hemostasis is required. Lobes of the parotid gland are retracted. A nerve stimulator may be used to locate branches of the facial nerve by watching for orbicularis contraction; once located, the branches can be traced back to their corresponding plexi. Branches are sectioned with small scissors. The distal nerve ending is grasped with a hemostat and the nerve is avulsed by retracting the peripheral branch in a hand-over-hand fashion for several centimeters, through the use of two hemostats. The proximal ends of the nerve may be clipped to retard regrowth. The nerve stimulator is used to verify that all branches innervating the orbicularis and buccal muscles are removed. Symmetric surgery is performed bilaterally for a better cosmetic effect. The wound is closed in layers and dressed. A drain is used if there is any residual oozing of blood. The procedure is difficult to titrate. It may result in profound periocular facial muscle paralysis and consequent exposure keratopathy, or there may be residual blepharospasm. In addition, recurrence of blepharospasm within 6 months after the procedure is common.

The most successful surgical procedure for the relief of blepharospasm is myectomy of the orbicularis, corrugator supercilii, and procerus muscles. This procedure must be extensive to be successful, and the duration (several hours) of surgery makes general anesthesia desirable although not mandatory. Supplemental local anesthesia improves hemostasis. Myectomy is often combined with other lid procedures, such as repair of brow ptosis, dermatochalasis, levator aponeurosis dehiscence, or lateral canthal tendon laxity, since many patients with essential blepharospasm have significant eyelid abnormalities resulting from constant manual elevation of the eyelids.

Elliptical incisions are made superior to the eyebrow and are carried down to the periosteum, excising a full-thickness wedge of tissue. A dissection plane is next developed under the brow between the skin and orbicularis and continued to slightly superior to the lashline. It is then extended between the eyes and over the bridge of the nose to include the corrugator and procerus muscles, and also extended laterally to obtain the lateral one-third of the lower eyelid orbicularis. The superior orbicularis is grasped with forceps and excised with small scissors. We are careful not to damage the orbital septum, levator aponeurosis, or tarsus. Similarly, the corrugator, procerus, and adjacent orbicularis are excised. Any blepharoplasty, levator aponeurosis

repair, or canthal repairs are performed at this time. Drains are placed after the brow is closed in layers. If needed, a subcilary incision is made and a similar procedure is performed on the inferomedial orbicularis. The complications are similar to overtreatment with botulinum or facial nerve avulsion, and are caused by paralysis of the eyelids and facial muscles. If an undereffect occurs, supplemental treatment with botulinum toxin or a repeat surgical procedure is possible.

Acupuncture and biofeedback behavior modification techniques have been used with limited success in some patients with blepharospasm. Alcohol injections of the junction of the facial nerve and orbicularis and chemical or thermal ablation of the peripheral facial nerve have also been used, but with poor results. At present, the safest and most predictable treatment is botulinum injection.

ACKNOWLEDGMENTS

Dr. Striph is a 1989–1990 Heed Ophthalmic Foundation Fellow. This work was supported in part by a grant from the Martin Foundation to Fight for Sight, Inc., New York City, in honor of Charles A. Perera, M.D.

SUGGESTED READING

Bosniak SL, Smith BC, eds. Advances in ophthalmic plastic and reconstructive surgery: blepharospasm. Vol. 4. New York: Pergamon Press, 1985.

Botulinum toxin injection for ocular muscle disorders. Med Lett Drugs Ther 1987; 29:101–102.

Dutton JJ, Buckley EG. Botulinum toxin in the management of blepharospasm. Arch Neurol 1986; 43:380–382.

Frueh BR, Nelson CC, Kapustiak JF, et al. The effect of omitting botulinum toxin from the lower eyelid in blepharospasm treatment. Am J Ophthalmol 1988; 106:45–47.

Mauriello JA, Jr. Blepharospasm, Meige syndrome, and hemifacial spasm: treatment with botulinum toxin. Neurology 1985; 35:1499–1500.

PATIENT RESOURCES

Benign Essential Blepharospasm Research Foundation, Inc.
755 Howell Street
Beaumont, Texas 77706
Telephone: (409) 892-1339

A list of physicians currently employing botulinum on an investigational basis may be obtained from:

Smith-Kettlewell Eye Research Foundation
2232 Webster Street
San Francisco, California 94115

HEMIFACIAL SPASM

STANLEY FAHN, M.D.
PAUL GREENE, M.D.

Hemifacial spasm is a syndrome involving repetitive contractions of muscles of one side of the face. The twitching usually begins in the periorbital muscles and gradually spreads to involve those muscles of the lower face innervated by the seventh cranial (facial) nerve. The twitching may be intermittent initially, but with time it often becomes constant; it may be present during sleep. Eventually, prolonged spasms may appear. Attempts to voluntarily use any muscles of the affected side of the face will trigger twitching in all muscles on that side of the face that are innervated by the seventh nerve. An occasional patient may have bilateral hemifacial spasm. The spasms are socially disabling and annoying. Periorbital spasms may result in sustained eyelid closure, which can interfere with vision. Rarely, patients will have pain associated with the spasms.

Observations at the time of neurosurgery indicate that in many patients, hemifacial spasm is associated with compression of the root exit zone of the facial nerve by a loop of blood vessel. Electrophysiologic studies have shown evidence of abnormal electrical transmission between different fibers of the facial nerve (ephaptic transmission or "cross talk"). Other physiologic studies implicate a central mechanism, which is also suggested by the observation that the frequency of spasms changes with sleep and is affected by the patient's emotional state. Currently the consensus is that the symptoms of hemifacial spasm are produced by an interaction between peripheral nerve damage and central mechanisms.

The main problem in diagnosing this condition is distinguishing "idiopathic" hemifacial spasm (compression by an aberrant blood vessel) from compression by a mass in the cerebellopontine angle (e.g., tumor, aneurysm, draining vein from an arteriovenous malformation, or other masses). This can be accomplished with magnetic resonance imaging (MRI) or a computed tomographic (CT) scan of the posterior fossa. Occasionally patients with epilepsia partialis continua have hemifacial twitching identical in appearance to typical hemifacial spasm. Most of these patients have an abnormal electroencephalogram (EEG). Other conditions that may produce facial twitching include cranial dystonia, tardive dyskinesia, myokymia, and motor tics. None of these have synchronous movements in multiple facial muscles. As a Bell's palsy heals, some patients develop innervation of multiple muscles by a single nerve fiber (synkinesis). These patients have contractions in multiple facial muscles when they attempt to make a single movement. They do not experience spontaneous twitching, although some patients may develop hemifacial spasm after a Bell's palsy.

BOTULINUM TOXIN TREATMENT

We believe that botulinum toxin type A (Botox) injections are the best treatment for hemifacial spasm. Botox interferes with the release of acetylcholine from cholinergic nerve terminals, resulting in long-lasting but temporary muscle weakness. Botox (a total of 15 to 25 U of toxin activity) is injected subcutaneously in four to six sites around the eye. Twitching muscles in the lower face can be injected intramuscularly through a hollow core electromyogram (EMG) needle using EMG guidance to verify needle placement. Muscles in the lower face typically require 2.5 to 7.5 U of Botox to relieve the spasms without creating excess weakness. More than 90 percent of patients improve substantially after receiving Botox injections. Benefit from the injections lasts for 4 to 6 months, at which time patients can receive reinjections. Patients with symptomatic hemifacial spasm also improve after receiving Botox injections.

Side effects of Botox injections are short-lived and include ptosis (from the spread of the toxin to the levator palpebrae), ecchymoses, excess tearing, and facial drooping (when lower facial muscles are injected with an excessive dose of Botox). Ptosis, the most serious common side effect of Botox injections, can be minimized by placing the injections in the pretarsal component of the orbicularis oculi far from the insertions of the levator palpebrae. Antibody formation to Botox has not occurred after injections using these low doses. Relative contraindications to the use of Botox include pregnancy, anticoagulation, myasthenia gravis, and prior existence of antibotulinum toxin antibodies.

MEDICAL TREATMENT

Patients who fail to benefit from Botox injections or who refuse injections may be treated with anticonvulsants such as clonazepam, valproate sodium, and carbamazepine. Although most patients fail to improve with the use of these agents, some patients have dramatic benefit. Since the response seems to be dose related, the dose can be increased until adverse effects appear while the blood levels are monitored.

SURGICAL TREATMENT

For the rare patient who fails to improve with Botox injections or anticonvulsants, posterior fossa craniotomy provides a possibility for relief. In sur-

gical series, decompression of the root exit zone of the facial nerve provides partial or total relief of spasms in the majority of patients. The benefit has been long-lasting in most cases, although some patients have required repeat operations. The reported mortality and serious morbidity rates of this operation are low, although some patients have developed hearing loss or facial weakness postoperatively. Because this surgical procedure conveys an operative risk, we recommend it only if the more conservative approaches mentioned above fail to provide relief.

SUGGESTED READING

Alexander G, Moses H. Carbamazepine for hemifacial spasm. Neurology 1982; 32:286–287.

Jannetta P. Hemifacial spasm. Neurol Neurosurg 1982; 3:1–7.

Tolosa E, Marti MJ, Kulisevsky J. Botulinum toxin injection therapy for hemifacial spasm. Adv Neurol 1988; 49:479–491.

TORTICOLLIS

GARRETT E. ALEXANDER, M.D., Ph.D.
STEPHEN G. REICH, M.D.
MAHLON R. DeLONG, M.D.

Torticollis (often referred to as "spasmodic torticollis") is characterized by involuntary phasic (clonic) and/or tonic deviation of the head and neck from intended postures. While generally recognized as an organic condition, torticollis continues to be defined phenomenologically (based on its characteristic symptomatology), as the etiology has remained elusive. Most commonly, a rotational component is predominant, with the chin deviated toward the shoulder. Added to this may be elements of lateral deviation ("laterocollis") and anteroflexion or retroflexion ("anterocollis" or "retrocollis"). Less frequently, laterocollis, anterocollis, or retrocollis may occur in the absence of a significant rotational component. Torticollis is the most prevalent of the focal dystonias, which include blepharospasm, oromandibular dystonia, and limb dystonia. It is not unusual for torticollis to coexist with one or more of these other conditions, and its association with essential tremor is also well established.

NATURAL HISTORY

Torticollis may be congenital or acquired, with the latter separated into childhood-onset and adult-onset presentations. Many of the congenital and childhood cases are considered "symptomatic" when associated with lesions or anomalies of the neck musculature, cervical spine, craniovertebral junction, spinal cord, or posterior fossa. By contrast, isolated torticollis presenting in adults is seldom associated with underlying structural or metabolic disease.

The adult-onset variety, whether isolated or occurring in the context of other dystonic movements, is frequently heralded by a transient phase during which the patient notices brief, phasic rotational jerking of the head and neck to one side. The symptoms are usually unprovoked, although occasionally patients associate them with a previous episode of trauma. In some patients, the initial phasic symptoms resolve spontaneously after a period of months, only to recur in subsequent years. In others, there is an insidious progression to a stable state of tonic deviation of the head and neck. This is the typical, chronic form of torticollis, and it is usually accompanied by intermittent phasic or "spasmodic" jerking of the head and neck in the direction of the deviant posture. While spontaneous remissions have been reported, most were described as occurring in young patients early in the course of the disease and were not accompanied by long-term follow-up. Thus, the incidence of permanent remissions remains uncertain, but may be less than the published estimates of 10 to 15 percent.

Although torticollis is not life-threatening and generally remains static after several years of early progression, many patients report that pain and embarrassment are two important factors during the chronic stages of the disease. Like other movement disorders, torticollis is exacerbated by emotional stress, improves with relaxation, and disappears during sleep. These features are commonly misinterpreted by friends and family members as indicating that the disorder is under voluntary control. Most patients discover sensory "tricks" that can temporarily suppress the abnormal motor activity. These include counterpressure against the chin, face, or occiput, and various postural maneuvers, such as reclining.

ETIOLOGY AND PATHOPHYSIOLOGY

The etiology of torticollis remains obscure. It is generally assumed that torticollis is of central origin, although the pathophysiologic substrates are unknown. This assumption is based on several lines of evidence, including (1) that "symptomatic" torticollis may arise after an episode of encephalitis, (2) that

animal models of torticollis have been produced through the creation of lesions of central motor pathways, (3) that torticollis may be seen in certain symptomatic, generalized dystonias (e.g., Wilson's disease), and (4) that stereotaxic thalamotomy has proven beneficial in some patients. Nevertheless, there have been no published cases of focal brain pathology associated with isolated torticollis. This has led some to argue that torticollis may result from peripheral factors such as irritation of cervical roots, although direct evidence for this view is also lacking.

DIAGNOSTIC EVALUATION

Because of the rare association of torticollis with craniovertebral abnormalities, we usually obtain cervical spine films in new patients with torticollis. When torticollis is part of a more generalized dystonic state, and especially in cases with associated hemidystonia, we obtain a computed tomographic (CT) scan or magnetic resonance image (MRI) of the brain to exclude focal neostriatal or thalamic lesions that may be associated with these other conditions. Further diagnostic studies are seldom indicated in adults, although in relatively young patients we also screen for Wilson's disease with serum ceruloplasmin and slit-lamp examination.

PHARMACOLOGIC TREATMENT

Medical therapy for torticollis is of limited benefit in the majority of patients, a fact that is worth stressing to patients from the outset in order to minimize future disappointment. As with all forms of dystonia, medical treatment of torticollis is empiric, but some patients do benefit from this approach. We generally begin with anticholinergic therapy, unless there are contraindications such as narrow-angle glaucoma, urinary retention, or pre-existing cognitive dysfunction. Patients receive either trihexyphenidyl hydrochloride (Artane) or ethopropazine hydrochloride (Parsidol) initially at very low dose (Table 1), which is slowly increased over a period of weeks to months as tolerated. Common side effects such as dry mouth, constipation, and visual blurring are generally tolerable, and the latter, if severe, can be managed with pilocarpine eye drops. The most frequent limiting side effects are cognitive and memory disturbances, and urinary retention, which are much more likely to occur in the elderly.

If symptoms of torticollis persist at the maximum tolerated dose of anticholinergic therapy, we generally add or substitute one of the benzodiazepines. Our first choice is usually clonazepam (Klonopin). Although somnolence is an early side effect, it tends to disappear with prolonged use. Other benzodiazepines are likewise effective in the treatment of torticollis, with the choice being based mainly on relative safety rather than demonstrable differences in efficacy.

Most patients receive some benefit from an anticholinergic agent or clonazepam, used alone or in combination. In some cases, however, no improvement is seen with either type of drug before the occurrence of unacceptable side effects. For these patients, we generally attempt a series of different agents which have been found useful in a smaller proportion of cases. These include levodopa/carbidopa (Sinemet), bromocriptine (Parlodel), baclofen (Lioresal), carbamazepine (Tegretol), and propranolol (Inderal). Although some have advo-

Table 1 Pharmacologic Treatment of Torticollis

Drug	Starting Dose	Maintenance Dose	Major Side Effects
Anticholinergics			
Trihexyphenidyl hydrochloride (Artane)	2 mg, b.i.d.	10–40 mg/day*	Confusion, memory loss, blurred vision, urinary retention, anhydrosis
Ethopropazine hydrochloride (Parsidol)	50 mg, b.i.d.	200–600 mg/day*	Confusion, memory loss, blurred vision, urinary retention, anhydrosis
Benzodiazepines			
Clonazepam (Klonopin)	0.5 mg, q.h.s.	4–16 mg/day*	Drowsiness, confusion
Diazepam (Valium)	5 mg, b.i.d.	20–60 mg/day*	Drowsiness, confusion
Miscellaneous			
Levodopa/Carbidopa (Sinemet)	25/100 mg, b.i.d.	75/300–75/750 mg/day*	Confusion, hypotension, nausea
Bromocriptine (Parlodel)	1.25 mg, b.i.d.	5–15 mg/day*	Hypotension, confusion
Baclofen (Lioresal)	10 mg, b.i.d.	50–100 mg/day*	Weakness, confusion
Carbamazepine (Tegretol)	100 mg, b.i.d.	600–1,200 mg/day*	Dizziness, confusion, leukopenia
Propranolol (Inderal)	20 mg, tid	160–320 mg/day*	Hypotension
Botulinum A toxin (Oculinum)	50–200 U IM†	100–200 U q3–4mos.	Local discomfort

* In 3–4 divided doses.
† 50 U/muscle/session.

cated the use of haloperidol and other dopamine receptor blockers, we have not found them to be sufficiently effective or well tolerated to justify the risk of inducing tardive dyskinesia.

In addition to the abnormal head movements and postures, most patients with torticollis also experience significant degrees of chronic pain. This is frequently localized to the posterior cervical muscles on the side opposite the direction of head rotation. Such pain can often be managed effectively with nonsteroidal anti-inflammatory drugs. We have also found tricyclic antidepressants to be useful, particularly when pain is associated with insomnia or depression. We begin with nortriptyline (Pamelor), 10 to 25 mg every hour of sleep, gradually increasing the dose until a therapeutic blood level is reached. Narcotics are to be strictly avoided in the management of this type of chronic pain.

BOTULINUM TOXIN INJECTIONS

In contrast to the limited effectiveness of oral medications, local intramuscular injections of botulinum A toxin have been shown to offer significant relief of both the muscle spasms and pain associated with torticollis. Since the original report on this agent in 1985, more than a dozen studies have confirmed that this form of treatment is effective, and to date there have been no reports of clinically significant side effects. The toxin exerts its effect by irreversibly binding to the presynaptic membrane at the neuromuscular junction and preventing the release of acetylcholine. The clinical reversibility of this effect is related to the sprouting of new nerve terminals that eventually form contacts with the postsynaptic motor end-plate.

We use clinical observation (visual inspection, palpation) to select the most active cervical muscles for injection. Others have employed surface electromyographic (EMG) recordings, but whether the added complexity of this approach is justified by enhanced therapeutic results has yet to be determined. Only the superficial neck muscles are selected, typically including the sternocleidomastoid, splenius capitus, cervical paraspinous, and trapezius. Muscles are chosen for injection based on their apparent involvement in generating the abnormal postures and neck movements, or as loci of spasm-induced pain and tenderness. The toxin is reconstituted with sterile saline to a concentration of 50 mouse units per milliliter. (One mouse unit is the dose [approximately 20 ng] that kills one-half of 18 to 20 female Swiss-Webster mice.) Patients then receive a total of 50 to 200 U per session, divided among two to four muscles. The percutaneous injections are performed with tuberculin syringes and 25-gauge needles. Although some patients tempo-

rarily experience mild local discomfort, this has not proven to be a significant limitation.

Patients begin to notice improvement in neck movements or posture, or a reduction in pain, within 4 to 10 days after receiving the injections. The beneficial effects typically last from 3 to 4 months, after which reinjection is necessary. Occasionally, after experiencing transient improvement, patients return with a new pattern of muscle involvement. In these patients, it is common to find the expected flaccid paresis of muscles that were previously injected superimposed on palpable overactivity of the deeper, uninjected muscles. Several of our patients who failed to improve after the first series of injections have experienced benefit after subsequent sessions in which additional muscles were injected.

At present, botulinum A toxin is available only on an experimental basis at a limited number of referral centers. With further experience and continued demonstration of its long-term effectiveness and safety, it may well become the first-line treatment for torticollis. Nevertheless, many patients require a combination of oral medications and botulinum toxin injections to achieve optimal therapeutic results.

SURGICAL TREATMENT

Since the advent of botulinum toxin therapy, we rarely find it necessary to recommend surgical intervention for patients with torticollis. Several surgical approaches have been advocated, including anterior cervical rhizotomy, selective peripheral denervation, and stereotaxic thalamotomy.

Anterior rhizotomy involves opening the spinal canal and meninges to expose the anterior roots of C1-3 which are then sectioned under direct visualization. Although some patients have experienced relief with this procedure, it carries the risk of inadvertent damage to the spinal cord or to lower cervical segments supplying the phrenic nerve, and has the added disadvantage of nonselectively denervating muscle groups that may not be involved in the clinical expression of torticollis.

In some centers, selective denervation of specific branches supplying the sternocleidomastoid or posterior muscles is the procedure of choice, replacing anterior cervical rhizotomy. The benefits of this procedure include selective weakening of only those muscles that are implicated in the abnormal movements. In addition, with this approach it is possible to determine in advance the pattern of weakness that will result from the final denervation procedure, by performing a preliminary, reversible block with percutaneous injections of a local anesthetic.

Stereotaxic ventrolateral thalamotomy has also been employed in the treatment of torticollis. Unfortunately, fewer than one-half of the patients treated with this procedure have shown significant improvement, and in many cases the effects were short-lived. More prolonged effects were achieved occasionally by the creation of bilateral lesions, but the well known side effects of dysphonia and hypophonia generally preclude this approach. We do not recommend stereotaxic thalamotomy for the treatment of torticollis.

MISCELLANEOUS FORMS OF TREATMENT

Some patients experience significant relief of pain through physical therapy, but in our experience, this has not been associated with a reduction in the abnormal movements of torticollis. Similarly, a small proportion of patients, specifically those who experience relief of spasms with counterpressure applied to the neck, may experience some relief by wearing a hard cervical collar. We do not routinely recommend either of these approaches, although in selected patients they may prove beneficial.

SUGGESTED READING

Friedman A, Fahn S. Spontaneous remissions in spasmodic torticollis. Neurology 1986; 36:398–400.
Lowenstine DH, Aminoff MJ. The clinical course of spasmodic torticollis. Neurology 1988; 38:530–532.
Suchowersky O, Calne DB. Non-dystonic causes of torticollis. In: Fahn S, Marsden CD, Calne DB, eds. Dystonia 2 (Advances in Neurology, Vol. 50). New York: Raven Press, 1988:501.
Tsui JK, Eisen A, Stoessl J, et al. Double-blind study of botulinum toxin in spasmodic torticollis. Lancet 1986; 2:245–247.

PATIENT RESOURCES

National Spasmodic Torticollis Association, Inc.
P.O. Box 873
Royal Oak, Michigan 48068-0873
Telephone: (313) 647-2280

Dystonia Foundation
8383 Wilshire Boulevard
Suite 800
Beverly Hills, California 90211
Telephone: (213) 852-1630

TOURETTE'S SYNDROME

GERALD ERENBERG, M.D.

Tics are the most common form of movement disorder in childhood. They are sudden, rapid, recurrent, purposeless, nonrhythmic, stereotyped motor movements or vocalizations. The diagnosis of tics is clinical, and no biological markers for the condition are known. There is a spectrum of tic disorders, and the terminology used to describe tics is based on the types of tics as well as on their duration. Tics usually begin before the age of 21 years, are more common in males, and occur many times a day. Most persons with tics have a single motor or vocal tic that lasts for less than 1 year. Chronic tic disorders consist of one form of either motor or vocal tics (but not both) and last for more than 1 year.

Tourette's syndrome is defined as multiple motor and vocal tics that range from mild to severe and last for more than 1 year. Most patients become symptomatic between the ages of 5 and 10 years. The current concept is that Tourette's syndrome has an organic basis. This has been supported by recent clinical, biochemical, and genetic investigations. Yet despite these findings, no consistent abnormal biological feature has been determined. In the past, the involuntary tics of Tourette's syndrome were believed to be of psychiatric or emotional origin. In part, this determination was based on the observation that many patients with Tourette's syndrome have behavioral or learning problems. Commonly associated behavioral difficulties include attention deficit disorder with or without hyperactivity, high levels of anxiety, emotional lability, and obsessive-compulsive behaviors. It is now believed that these associated behavioral problems are not the cause of but rather are an integral part of the disorder. A dopaminergic hypothesis for Tourette's syndrome has been suggested by the often dramatic symptomatic response of this disorder to dopamine receptor–blocking drugs.

NONMEDICAL THERAPY

Education

It is important that information on Tourette's syndrome and its various manifestations be provided to the patient's family, his or her school personnel or employers, and to any others who might be involved in the patient's everyday life. Even though Tourette's syndrome has become more widely known during the past decade, many people have not heard of this disorder. To them, the motor and vocal tics with their pattern of waxing and waning can be difficult to understand. All children with this disorder have, at least at some point, been accused of acting in this "mysterious" manner voluntarily. The involuntary nature of the tics must be stressed to such people so that they may have a better understanding of the patient's behavior. The potential problems that result from the short attention span, hyperactivity, impulsiveness, or learning disabilities must be brought to the attention of school personnel. Special arrangements may be necessary in the classroom to help overcome a child's problem with poor handwriting or difficulty with taking timed tests.

Coping and Adapting

Patients or their parents react to the diagnosis in a manner that reflects their personalities, their abilities to cope with uncertainty and stress, and the availability of social and medical support. Much help is necessary to deal with the anxiety, shame, anger, and guilt that may be engendered. If a patient is to be referred for counseling, the provider must be knowledgeable about Tourette's syndrome. In helping a patient adapt to and cope with their disorder, one must remember that the manifestations of Tourette's syndrome may vary greatly. One patient may have only mild vocal and motor tics, while another may have the same symptoms in a more severe and obtrusive form. In addition to the tics, some patients have no associated learning or behavioral problems, whereas others may be attempting to cope with the additional burdens of severe behavioral problems as well as significant learning disabilities.

Fortunately, all concerned can be helped through the services provided by the Tourette Syndrome Association, an active public support group with a national office as well as many regional offices. They can share in the education of families by speaking with them directly as well as by sharing the many fine publications that they have written in their attempt to educate both the public at large as well as affected individuals and their families.

MEDICAL TREATMENT

All available medications provide only symptomatic relief and are not curative. There is no evidence that early treatment with these agents leads to any alteration in the long-term prognosis. Initially, most diagnosed cases of Tourette's syndrome have had the severe form of this disorder. It was therefore felt that all patients with Tourette's syndrome should be treated as soon as the diagnosis was made. In recent years, however, it has been recognized that many patients have a mild form of the disorder.

In my own experience, 50 percent of patients with Tourette's syndrome have symptoms that can be tolerated without the use of medication. Because of the side effects of medications, I believe that patients with milder cases fare better if they do not receive pharmacologic treatment. Some patients, however, suffer psychological damage if their disruptive tics are not modified by symptomatic medication. Because the ability to tolerate tics varies from family to family, families and patients should become part of the decision making process and each case should be assessed individually. Once the family decides that medication is necessary, the physician usually finds that this is the correct decision and should begin the medication program at that time.

Neuroleptic Drugs

Haloperidol

This dopamine-blocking agent has been used the longest in the treatment of Tourette's syndrome. All other neuroleptics have the same general potential for symptomatic relief as well as the same possible side effects. The choice of a specific neuroleptic agent is based on the user's familiarity with that agent as well as on the fact that certain neuroleptics have somewhat fewer side effects.

Haloperidol is able to reduce tics in 70 percent of treated patients, but more than 50 percent of patients complain of side effects. Only 25 percent of patients receiving neuroleptic agents report significant improvement without any side effects. Because therapeutic and toxic dosages are so close, it is best to keep the total dosage at an amount that will decrease symptoms by approximately 75 percent.

The dosage required for the treatment of patients with Tourette's syndrome is considerably less than that used to treat psychotic patients. Neuroleptic agents such as haloperidol have a long half-life and tend to accumulate in the body until a steady state is reached within approximately 4 days. Increases in medication are therefore made approximately every week so that the impact of the most recent change can be fully evaluated.

Haloperidol comes in a variety of tablet strengths, and the lowest available preparation contains 0.5 mg per tablet. In all age groups, therapy is begun with only 0.25 mg given each evening for the 1st week. The dosage is then increased every week, if necessary, by 0.25 mg per day. Most patients can be successfully treated through the use of a twice-daily regimen (with equal doses given in the morning and evening). The treatment program is based on balancing the beneficial response against the incidence of side effects, and it is important to tell patients that they do not need to continue increasing the dosage if a sufficient degree of relief has been obtained. In my experience, the usual patient receives only 1.5 to 2.5 mg per day. There are exceptions, of course, with some patients receiving as little as 0.5 mg per day or more than 10 mg per day.

Acute extrapyramidal reactions are usually avoidable if medication is introduced in a low dosage and if further adjustments are made slowly. If they do occur, treatment with antihistamines or anticholinergic medications is able to rapidly reverse this reaction. Families are told to watch the patient for excessive sedation, depression, school- or work-phobia, or rapid weight gain caused by an increase in appetite. More subtle side effects may include cognitive blunting or apathetic, listless behavior.

Chronic parkinsonlike side effects may generally be avoided by careful attention to dosage. If such side effects occur even with minimal amounts of medication, the patient may be treated with the concomitant administration of anticholinergic medications such as benztropine mesylate at 0.5 mg per day. Few patients require the use of these agents, and there is no proven benefit in providing them routinely.

In my experience, other potential side effects have been unusual. These could include anticholinergic effects such as dry mouth, mydriasis, blurred vision, and constipation. Photosensitivity with increased reactions to sunlight exposure has also been reported. Impairment of liver function is extremely uncommon, and I have not found it necessary to routinely monitor liver function tests.

Although relatively low doses are used, treatment is often maintained for several years. Such prolonged use raises concerns regarding the development of tardive dyskinesia. Fortunately, the appearance of tardive dyskinesia with the use of haloperidol appears to be a rare phenomenon; although several cases have been reported, in each instance, the symptoms disappeared after discontinuation of the drug. Nevertheless, all patients should be warned of this potential complication. Also of concern is the withdrawal emergent syndrome. In this syndrome, symptoms appear after discontinuation or reduction of neuroleptic agents. The symptoms are characterized by choreoathetoid and myoclonic movements of the trunk, extremities, and orofacial region. They generally occur only when there has been the sudden withdrawal of relatively high doses of medication. The involuntary movements are self-limited and disappear spontaneously within weeks to months. The occurrence of the withdrawal emergent syndrome can usually be avoided by lowering the dosage of medication slowly on a weekly basis.

Untreated tic disorders spontaneously go through periods of exacerbation and improvement, and this pattern is not altered by the use of medication. There must be close monitoring of symptoms so that the dosage can be decreased when the tics have entered a phase during which they are less obvious. Although there cannot be a strict policy regarding drug "holidays," it is best to attempt to lower and even discontinue the medication when patients have entered into a situation in which their tics are under better control. On the other hand, there will be other times when the dosage should be temporarily increased to help the patient cope with an increase in tics.

Pimozide

Because of the high incidence of side effects with haloperidol, other neuroleptic agents have been developed that might provide the same beneficial response with a lower occurrence of adverse reactions. Pimozide is an alternative neuroleptic drug that has been used in other countries for many years, but it was approved for use in the United States only as recently as 1984. The manufacturer and the Food and Drug Administration continue to caution against the use of pimozide in children younger than 12 years of age because of the lack of documentation of its safety and efficacy in this age group. This is a common situation with relatively new medications, but several studies have shown that pimozide can be used in young children with the same safety and efficacy as in adults.

While pimozide and haloperidol may have different effects on neurotransmitters, in the clinical setting, both medications work in approximately the same fashion. My experience has been that although pimozide is as effective as haloperidol in reducing tics, it tends to have fewer side effects such as sedation. When adverse reactions occur, they are exactly the same as those seen in patients using haloperidol.

Pimozide is available in 2-mg tablets. In terms of potency, 2.5 mg of pimozide is equivalent in action to 1 mg of haloperidol. I begin treatment with 1 mg of pimozide given daily at bedtime. The dosage is increased once per week by 1 mg per day until symptom relief is obtained or intolerable side effects intervene. The current recommendation is that children not receive more than 10 mg of pimozide per day. Adolescents and adults may receive a maximum of 20 mg per day. Considerably higher doses have been associated rarely with death. There has been concern that pimozide has adverse cardiac effects and will prolong the Q-T interval. I have performed serial electrocardiograms (ECGs) in children receiving pimozide and have not been able to document any significant alteration in the Q-T interval. At this time, I am therefore not performing routine follow-up ECGs or other safety studies in patients receiving pimozide, although the manufacturer still recommends that this be done.

Others

Early reports indicated that not all neuroleptic agents were capable of modifying tics, even though they share the ability to block dopamine receptors. The apparent lack of efficacy may have resulted from insufficient dosages of these medications. Other neuroleptic agents that can be used include trifluoperazine and fluphenazine. Fluphenazine is the best studied of the alternative agents, and 4 mg of fluphenazine appears to be equal in potency to 3 mg of haloperidol. In general, fluphenazine seems to be similar to pimozide in both its efficacy as well as its potential for causing side effects.

Other Drugs

Clonidine

Clonidine has been used in the treatment of Tourette's syndrome since 1979. Clonidine is more easy to use than the neuroleptic drugs and is relatively free of serious side effects. The most frequent side effect is sedation. Higher dosages may also be associated with orthostatic hypotension and dizziness, but tardive dyskinesia has not been reported. In addition to reducing tics, clonidine produces favorable responses in associated behavioral problems. The potential of this agent to alleviate behavioral problems along with suppressing tic activity is important, since many patients with Tourette's syndrome have both problems. In general, the neuroleptics do not improve behavior.

Unfortunately, the reported effectiveness of clonidine has varied from study to study. In my experience, clonidine is not as potent an anti-tic medication as the neuroleptic agents. Approximately 30 percent of my patients have found clonidine to be preferable to neuroleptics.

Clonidine is available as 0.1-mg tablets. Treatment is started with 0.05 mg given both at breakfast and at bedtime. The response to clonidine is not immediate, and several weeks may pass before improvement is noted. If the initial dosage is tolerated, it is increased after 2 weeks to 0.05 mg taken 3 times per day. After an additional 2 weeks, the daily dosage is increased by 0.05 mg per day on a weekly basis. Some patients cannot tolerate more than 0.05 mg per dose. For these patients, the dosage can be given as often as every 2 hours. The dose is increased until the patient experiences sedation or dizziness. A transdermal patch is available in different strengths. They have been formulated to deliver the equivalent of 0.1 mg, 0.2 mg, or 0.3 mg per day. Each patch will deliver medication for an average of 1 week. Although the patch may be tried in those patients who cannot tolerate high dosages or who need to take their medication frequently, many persons develop a dermatitis to the patch. If treatment with clonidine is unsuccessful, the medication should be gradually tapered over a minimum of 2 weeks.

Clonazepam

This benzodiazepine is an approved antiepileptic agent. Some patients with Tourette's syndrome have responded well to this medication. Side effects are relatively uncommon and include personality changes and sedation. My own experience has confirmed reports of the relatively low incidence of side effects, but I have not found clonazepam as a sole agent to be highly effective. I currently use clonazepam as an adjunct to either clonidine or a neuroleptic agent in patients for whom monotherapy does not lead to the desired response. The lowest-strength tablet available is 0.5 mg, and therapy is started with a dose of 0.25 mg per day. The daily dose is then increased once per week by 0.25 per day until there is a clinical response or until the patient experiences side effects.

Stimulant Drugs

Several reports have suggested that the use of psychostimulant medication in patients with an attention deficit disorder may precipitate Tourette's syndrome or may increase the number of tics in individual patients. This property is shared by all of the available psychostimulants, including methylphenidate, dextroamphetamine, and pemoline. Whether the stimulant medications cause Tourette's syndrome, or rather, precipitate tics in persons who are otherwise predisposed to this disorder is an unresolved issue. Because more than 50 percent of patients with Tourette's syndrome have symptoms of attention deficit disorder, this remains an important issue. In general, most children with Tourette's syndrome experience the onset of their restless, poor attentive behavior before the onset of their tics.

I believe that psychostimulant drugs can increase or induce tics in some (but not all) individuals who are already destined to have Tourette's syndrome. If a patient receiving such a drug develops tics, every attempt must be made to discontinue the medication. Unfortunately, the discontinuing of the stimulants often leads to a major deterioration in the child's adjustment to school and home. If the tics remain mild in severity, I continue to administer the stimulant drugs after informing the parents that the tics may worsen. If the level of tic activity is high or worsens, I discontinue the stimulant agent and offer a trial with clonidine or a tricyclic antidepressant as treatment for the attention deficit disorder. The tricyclic antidepressants generally do not cause a further increase in tics, and there is a large body of experience indicating their potential for improving attention span and behavior. My personal choice is nortriptyline which is somewhat less sedating than imipramine hydrochloride. The dose range for both agents is the same. Nortriptyline is available in capsule and liquid form, and I generally give patients an initial dose of 10 mg at breakfast and dinnertime. The dosage necessary for improving attentional difficulties is much less than the dosage necessary when the agent is used as an antidepressant. I do not increase the dosage to more than 30 to 40 mg per day, and this low dosage has not been associated with any ECG arrhythmias. If alternative drugs do not help the attentional problem, however, I treat some patients with a combination of a stimulant drug such as methylphenidate along with clonidine or a neuroleptic agent.

RECOMMENDATION

No medications available to the physician can be relied on to help in all cases of Tourette's syndrome without the risk of significant side effects. Patients with milder cases do not need to be treated with pharmacotherapy. Treatment of patients with Tourette's syndrome is both an art and a science. It is imperative that the physician educate the family and patient regarding the disorder and help them cope with the difficulties associated with it.

When deciding that treatment is in the best interest of the patient, it is important to first determine if it is more important to decrease tics or to improve the associated behavioral difficulties. In some cases, it is necessary to decrease tics and to improve behavior simultaneously.

Figure 1 outlines the general program for treating patients whose tics are mild but who have significant behavior problems. In this case, my first suggestion is treatment with a tricyclic antidepressant such as nortriptyline. If this is unsuccessful, I discontinue the nortriptyline and begin a program of treatment with clonidine. If the patient shows no improvement with this treatment, I discontinue the clonidine and begin treatment with methylpheni-

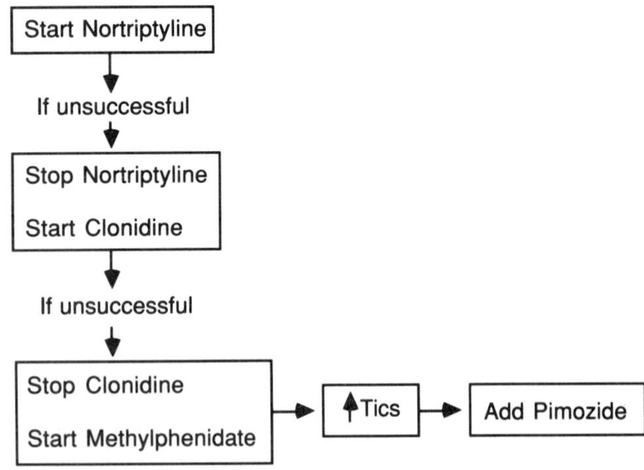

Figure 1 Treatment of patient with minor tic problem and major attentional problem.

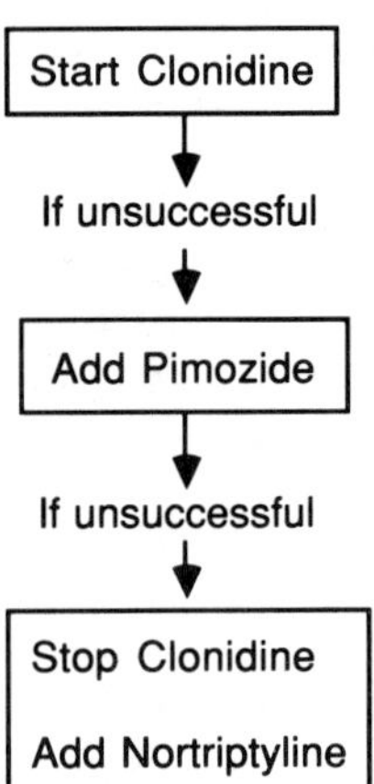

Figure 2 Treatment of patient with moderate or severe tic problem and major attention problem.

date. The methylphenidate can be used by itself, but pimozide is added if the stimulant drug is associated with a major increase in tics.

Figure 2 is the plan for treating patients with both moderate or severe tics as well as major behavior problems. My first suggestion is a trial of monotherapy with clonidine. If there is insufficient improvement, pimozide is added to the clonidine. If this combination does not relieve symptoms or causes significant side effects, the next plan is to discontinue the clonidine and to add nortriptyline to the pimozide. If the behavior improves but the tics do not, the sequence outlined in Figure 3 can be followed.

Figure 3 illustrates the plan of treatment for patients with moderate or severe tics but no associated behavioral difficulties. The first treatment to be used is a trial of monotherapy with pimozide. If this is unsuccessful, the patient is treated with a combination of pimozide and clonidine. For those who are resistant to this combination, the clonidine is discontinued, and the patient is treated with a combination of pimozide and clonazepam. For those patients unresponsive even to this regimen, the next program is to discontinue all previous medications and to begin sequential monotherapy with other neuroleptics. Such alternatives may include haloperidol or fluphenazine. Some patients respond better to one neuroleptic than to another. For those whose response is short-lived, a program of alternating neuroleptic drugs can be instituted.

Even after medication has provided symptomatic improvement, it remains necessary to closely monitor the patient's progress. Because of the natural tendency for tic symptoms to wax and wane, alterations in dosage will periodically be necessary. For school-age patients, summer vacations are often used as a time to attempt decreasing the dose or even

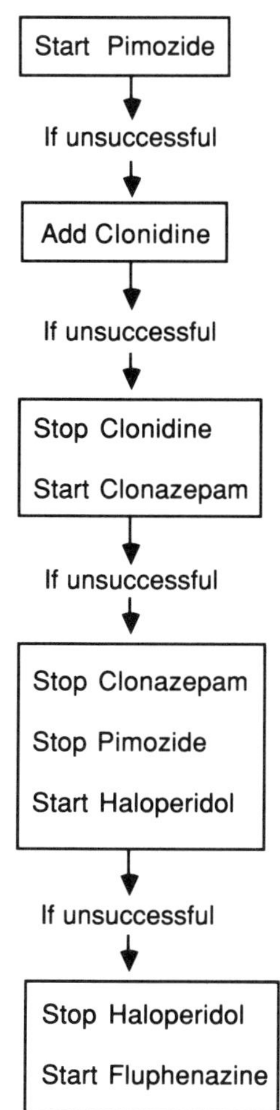

Figure 3 Treatment of patient with moderate or severe tics and no attentional problem.

discontinuing the medication altogether, if this is considered feasible.

It is hoped that future reports on the treatment of tic disorders will include a larger number of effective and safe medications. Even when treated by the most experienced of physicians, approximately one-third of patients with significant tic disorders do not benefit from currently available medications. This is in addition to the patients whose major problems are caused by their associated behavioral difficulties and not by their actual tics. It is hoped that future research will clarify the situation and allow the practitioner to treat this potentially disabling condition more effectively.

SUGGESTED READING

Cohen DJ, Bruun RD, Leckman JF, eds. Tourette's syndrome and tic disorders: clinical understanding and treatment. New York: John Wiley and Sons, 1988.
Shapiro AK, Shapiro ES, Young JG, Feinberg TE. Gilles de la Tourette syndrome. 2nd ed. New York: Raven Press, 1988.

PATIENT RESOURCE

Tourette Syndrome Association
42-40 Bell Boulevard
Bayside, New York 11361-9596
Telephone: (718) 224-2999

HYPERACTIVITY IN CHILDREN: ATTENTION-DEFICIT HYPERACTIVITY DISORDER

HARVEY S. SINGER, M.D.

Defining the term ''hyperactivity'' or the broader concept of attention-deficit hyperactivity disorder is a difficult task made more onerous by the lack of a confirmatory diagnostic procedure. The diagnosis of hyperactivity is subjective and imprecise; excess motor activity may be appropriate in a normal 3-year-old boy but is certainly counterproductive in a 7-year-old who has difficulty remaining seated or twists and wiggles in his classroom seat. In addition, as with many behavioral problems, the extent to which the hyperactivity is accepted depends on the tolerance of the child's teacher or parent.

Nevertheless, hyperactivity is a common symptom in individuals with a variety of impairment disorders, such as mental retardation, brain damage, emotional disturbance, and hearing loss. Together with inattention and impulsivity, it is also one of the primary components of the neurobehavioral problem currently termed attention-deficit hyperactivity disorder (ADHD). This chapter focuses on ADHD because of its potential to interfere with a child's ability to adjust throughout his/her life.

When ADHD is properly diagnosed, educational intervention, behavior management, and pharmacotherapy have been shown to be extremely beneficial. However, what appears at first glance to be a simple therapeutic issue is, in fact, a highly controversial topic in both medical and lay publications. Factors leading to this dispute include questions about nosology, diagnostic factors, different degrees of tolerance toward childhood behavior, and concerns about drug usage. Understanding each of these issues should permit the physician to design a rational approach to treatment of attention problems and hyperactivity.

NOSOLOGY

Because symptoms such as hyperactivity, inattention, distractibility, aggressiveness, restlessness, and impulsivity can appear after an insult to the brain (e.g., trauma, infection), these behaviors were initially believed to be secondary to minimal brain damage. Thirty years ago, the term "minimal brain dysfunction" was adopted to reflect a lack of any anatomic change. Subsequently, in an attempt to improve diagnostic distinctions, behavioral components such as hyperactivity, inattention, and impulsivity were selected and emphasized in the Diagnostic and Statistical Manual of Mental Disorders (third edition) (DSM-III, 1980). More specifically, two subtypes were defined based on the presence or absence of hyperactivity: attention-deficit disorder (ADD) with hyperactivity and ADD without hyperactivity. In the more recent revised third edition (DSM-III-R, 1987), the nomenclature has been arbitrarily changed combining, without any conceptual or operational improvement, the symptoms of hyperactivity, inattention, and impulsivity into the term ADHD. Children with developmentally inappropriate and marked inattention who have no symptoms of hyperactivity, previously labeled ADD without hyperactivity in DSM-III, are now placed in a residual category called "undifferentiated attention-deficit disorder." The confounding of attentional problems and hyperactivity in the DSM-III-R has been criticized and may be revised yet again.

DIAGNOSIS

The essential components of ADHD are "developmentally inappropriate" degrees of inattention, impulsiveness, and hyperactivity. At present, the most widely used diagnostic scheme for ADHD is under the heading of "disruptive behavior disorders" in the DSM-III-R. The diagnosis of ADHD should be considered if eight or more of the 14 symptoms listed in Table 1 are present for at least 6 months, if they began before the age of 7 years, and if the child does not have a disorder for which there are other conditions that may present with similar symptoms (e.g., pervasive developmental disorder, mental retardation, mood disorder, age-appropriate overactivity, or behavioral problems resulting from an inadequate, disorganized, chaotic environment). As a classification system, the Diagnostic and Statistical Manual of Mental Disorders clearly emphasizes the attentional component rather than focuses on hyperactivity.

To aid the diagnosis of behavioral disorders and to systematize information from other sources, several child rating instruments have been developed, including the Conners Parent and Teacher Rating Scales, Achenbach and Edelbrock's Child Behavior Checklist (CBCL), Yale Children's Inventory (YCI) and the Aggregate Neurobehavioral Student Health and Educational Review (ANSER) System. Although most widely used in studies of hyperactivity,

Table 1 Diagnostic Criteria for Attention-Deficit Hyperactivity Disorder

A. A disturbance of at least 6 months during which the child has at least eight of the following symptoms:
  1. Often fidgets with hands or feet or squirms in seat (in adolescents, may be limited to subjective feelings of restlessness)
  2. Has difficulty remaining seated when required to do so
  3. Is easily distracted by extraneous stimuli
  4. Has difficulty awaiting turn in games or group situations
  5. Often blurts out answers to questions before they have been completed
  6. Has difficulty following through on instructions from others (not due to oppositional behavior or failure of comprehension)—e.g., fails to finish chores
  7. Has difficulty sustaining attention in tasks or play activities
  8. Often shifts from one uncompleted activity to another
  9. Has difficulty playing quietly
  10. Often talks excessively
  11. Often interrupts or intrudes on others—e.g., butts into other children's games
  12. Often does not seem to listen to what is being said to him or her
  13. Often loses things necessary for tasks or activities at school or at home (e.g., toys, pencils, books, assignments)
  14. Often engages in physically dangerous activities without considering possible consequences (not for the purpose of thrill-seeking)—e.g., runs into street without looking
B. Onset before age 7 years.
C. Does not meet the criteria for Pervasive Developmental Disorder, mental retardation, mood disorder, age-appropriate overactivity, or come from an inadequate, disorganized, chaotic home environment.

the Conners scale has no independent attention scales consistent with the DSM criteria. Additional studies are necessary to determine the validity of these techniques as relevant tools in assisting the clinician in diagnosing ADHD. Until then, the diagnosis of ADHD is most appropriately made by a physician who is aware of the inclusion and exclusion criteria and who has obtained a careful and complete interdisciplinary evaluation.

BACKGROUND

The prevalence of ADHD in preadolescents is approximately 3 percent, and the disorder is four to six times more common in males than in females. Symptoms usually appear before the age of 4 years, although frequently they are not identified until the child enters school. Behavioral problems tend to be age-related: in infants, they are irritability, colic, and sleep problems; in toddlers, temper tantrums and gross motor hyperactivity; in children, restlessness, inattentiveness, distractibility, and impulsiveness; and in teenagers, less obvious hyperactivity but persistent attentional deficits that result in rebellious and antisocial behavior. About one-third of children with ADHD have some symptoms that persist into adulthood. Learning disabilities in the ADHD population are substantial, occurring in an estimated 9 to 20 percent of patients, and failure in school is common. Recent etiologic evidence supports the importance of a genetic component, although several environmental, behavioral, and biological factors have also been linked to ADHD. Pharmacologic and biochemical studies have suggested a catecholaminergic abnormality, both a dopaminergic and noradrenergic mechanism have been proposed.

EVALUATION

Establishing an accurate diagnosis involves obtaining historical information on factors such as the patient's birth, development, family, and academic achievement, as well as on medical and psychosocial issues. A history of tics in the patient or his or her family is a relative contraindication to the use of stimulant medications. Observation of the child in a variety of settings (home, school, play) is essential. A routine physical and neurologic examination usually yields normal results; the significance of minor congenital anomalies is controversial. The neuromaturational examination, which may identify minor (soft) signs, such as mirror movements, is not diagnostic.

Psychometric testing, used to assess ability and achievement, is valuable in separating the effects of attentional deficits from cognitive ability and scholastic achievement. For the school-age child, the Wechsler Intelligence Scales for Children-Revised (WISC-R) provides a test of both verbal and performance skills; children with ADHD generally show poor scores on the subtests of Arithmetic, Coding, Information, and Digit span. Various other measures are available (e.g., Woodcock-Johnson Psychoeducational Battery, Wide Range Achievement Test, Beery Developmental Test of Visual Motor Integration), and a formal referral for psychometric testing should be made when appropriate. The need for additional laboratory testing (e.g., thyroid function tests, lead levels, metabolic screening tests, chromosomal analysis, electroencephalography [EEG], magnetic resonance imaging [MRI]) should be determined on an individual basis based on the history and pertinent findings on physical examination.

TREATMENT

After establishing the diagnosis of ADHD, the physician has an important and pivotal role in discussing with the patient, the patient's family, and the school personnel the implications of this disorder and its proposed management. The physician should emphasize to the child that ADHD is not secondary to a lack of motivation or intelligence and that he or she has an active role in its control. The parents should be made aware of its possible genesis, age-dependent symptomatology, chronicity, and treatment strategy. The school teacher requires information on the importance of educational intervention and interdisciplinary cooperation. It is essential to convey to all involved persons that the management of ADHD is multimodal; educational intervention and behavior management training are employed first, and for those who fail to respond to these initial approaches and continue to have symptoms that either significantly affect academic performance or are associated with a serious behavior disorder, pharmacotherapy should be initiated.

Educational Intervention

In formulating an educational program designed to deal with behavioral difficulties, poor academic performance, and specific learning disabilities, it is often beneficial to have the input of a team of trained professionals (e.g., teachers, psychologists, educators). The physician should recognize the importance of educational assessment and tracking; of the child's placement in small, self-contained class or resource room; of flexible educational programs that emphasize individual attention and enhance motivation; and of structured environments and predictable routines that reduce distractions and reinforce appropriate behavior. It is recommended that the effect of the aforementioned educational interventions be monitored through the use of formalized rating instruments (e.g., Conners parent and teacher rating scales, CBCL, YCI, or continuous performance tasks.

Behavior Management

A major factor in the improvement of a child's behavior is the strengthening of the management skills of the parents. Trained professionals should instruct the family on the establishment of consistent management, the setting of household rules that specifically define acceptable behavior, the reinforcement of behavior that is appropriate, and the use of negative reinforcement for inappropriate behavior. Behavioral modification has been shown to improve parent-child interaction, reduce parental frustration and depression, and enhance the child's self-esteem. As such, behavioral therapy is a valuable adjunct to educational intervention and pharmacotherapy in the management of ADHD. Individual psychotherapy should be considered if the child has additional psychiatric diagnoses, significant emotional problems, or if there is a chaotic home environment.

Pharmacotherapy

Pharmacotherapy should be considered only after an adequate trial of prescriptive teaching, environmental modification, and behavior therapy. Stimulants (methylphenidate, dextroamphetamine, pemoline) for the treatment of ADHD are effective in 70 to 80 percent of affected children. These agents reduce hyperactivity as well as improve attention span, impulse control, restlessness, and the ability to complete assignments. Hyperactivity alone usually does not require drug treatment. Similarly, stimulants are not a panacea for all school difficulties, and their effects on academic achievement and cognitive function remain controversial. Those individuals who do not respond to stimulants or in whom these agents may be contraindicated (e.g., those with Tourette's syndrome) may be aided by alternative pharmacotherapy such as the use of antidepressants (imipramine hydrochloride, desipramine hydrochloride) or the alpha-adrenergic agonist clonidine.

Once a medication is selected, possible side effects and realistic expectations of the therapy should be explained to the patient and his or her parents. Specific target symptoms that are most troublesome need to be identified and monitored by teacher and parent reports, through the use of standardized qualitative weekly rating scales. A double-blind crossover trial comparing medication with placebo has the intrinsic value of identifying a placebo effect and providing the physician with reliable objective means by which to identify drug responders. Some investigators advocate evaluating the child's response to two different doses of medication and placebo.

Stimulants

Methylphenidate Hydrochloride (Ritalin Hydrochloride). The starting dose of methylphenidate hydrochloride is 0.3 mg per kilogram given in the morning before the child leaves for school. After 1 week of treatment, if the desired therapeutic effect has not been achieved, the dose should be increased to 0.6 to 0.8 mg per kilogram. If symptoms persist after 2 weeks, the medication should be changed or the patient should be re-evaluated. In those instances in which ADHD symptoms become worse in the afternoon, an additional dose of 0.3 mg per kilogram may be administered 3 hours after the first dose. Several investigators have shown that there is no advantage to the use of the sustained-release formulation. Whether medications should be withheld on weekends, holidays, and vacations is controversial. As a general rule, although I recognize the need for individualization, I prescribe stimulants to be taken every day during the school year, but omit them during long holidays and summer vacation. The requirement for reinitiation of medication is assessed at the beginning of each academic year. Treatment is continued for as long as is necessary to control socially maladaptive behaviors.

The adverse effects of stimulants include insomnia, which is usually transient, anorexia, and abdominal pain. Growth suppression is dose dependent; discontinuing treatment during vacations should therefore permit the patient to "catch-up" in height and weight. Other less frequent side effects include headaches, dizziness, dry mouth, nausea, and constipation. The appearance of irritability, tearfulness, fatigue, withdrawal, or depression necessitates reduction of the dose and sometimes discontinuation of medication. The use of stimulants in children with ADHD does not enhance their risk for substance abuse as teenagers or adults. Seizures are not a contraindication to the use of stimulants.

Stimulants may provoke the appearance of motor and phonic tics and have been shown to exacerbate tic symptoms in individuals with Tourette's syndrome (TS). Hence, in patients with ADHD who also have either TS, chronic multiple (motor or vocal) tics, a family history of tics, or in whom tics appear after treatment with stimulants, I recommend clonidine or desipramine hydrochloride as an alternative medication. If the symptoms of ADHD in these patients do not respond to treatment with clonidine or desipramine, the patient is given a brief trial with a central stimulant. If the child improves and tics are not exacerbated, the drug is maintained. If, however, the symptoms of ADHD improve but tics worsen, the drug is discontinued, a trial with another stimulant is begun, and the patient is closely observed. In the rare instance in which a psychostimulant is required for the patient to attend school and tics remain constant, stimulants and tic-suppressing medications are used concurrently.

Dextroamphetamine (Dexedrine). The use of dextroamphetamine is similar to that of methylphenidate hydrochloride except for the dosage schedule. The recommended dextroamphetamine dose (0.15 to 0.4 mg per kilogram) is approximately one-half that of methylphenidate hydrochloride, and treatment is initiated with a dose of 0.15 mg per kilogram. Although both stimulants have comparable beneficial effects, dextroamphetamine may have more adverse reactions.

Pemoline (Cylert). In comparative studies, results are similar for the use of methylphenidate hydrochloride, dextroamphetamine, and pemoline in the treatment of ADHD, although beneficial effects may be delayed for several days with the use of pemoline. Pemoline, with a half-life of approximately 12 hours, is administered in a once-daily morning dose. In children 6 years of age and older, the starting dose is 37.5 mg per day, which is then incrementally increased by 18.75 mg, as necessary, to attain the usual effective range of 56.25 to 75 mg per day. The side effects associated with this drug are similar to those seen with the use of other stimulants. Hepatic dysfunction also occurs in some patients.

Tricyclic Antidepressants

Overall, tricyclics are not as effective as stimulants in the treatment of ADHD, and side effects may be more prominent with the use of these agents. They are, however, superior in the treatment of the child with ADHD who is depressed or highly anxious. Moreover, tricyclics are appropriate drugs of choice for the individual who does not respond to stimulants or in whom stimulants are contraindicated.

Imipramine Hydrochloride (Tofranil). Imipramine hydrochloride is administered in an initial dose of 10 mg twice per day, and the therapeutic range is 20 to 100 mg per day. The use of this drug is limited by dose-dependent negative effects on heart rate and measures of motor speed and motor pursuit. Other factors limiting its usefulness include cardiovascular effects, severe toxicity with overdose, and the development of tolerance to its therapeutic action.

Desipramine Hydrochloride (Norpramin). Desipramine is a metabolite of imipramine with less pronounced sedative and anticholinergic actions than those of the parent compound. Several recent studies have confirmed the clinical efficacy of desipramine hydrochloride for the control of hyperactivity, impulsivity, and inappropriate classroom behavior in children. Reported side effects include increased heart rate and blood pressure. Our starting dosage is 25 mg per day, which is increased incrementally every week as needed until a maximum of 100 mg per day (in divided doses) is achieved.

Clonidine

Clonidine (Catapres) is an alpha-adrenergic agonist that preferentially acts on presynaptic alpha$_2$ neurons to inhibit noradrenergic activity. In several studies, clonidine significantly improved the overall behavior ratings for hyperactivity, impulsiveness, and inattentiveness in children with ADHD. A dosage of 4 to 5 μg per kilogram per day administered in divided doses (average of 0.05 mg four times daily) is usually effective, with sedation being the major side effect. The initial dose is 0.05 mg per day with increases of 0.05 mg every 5 to 7 days as needed.

Other Medications

In general, the use of drugs in this category is reserved for hyperactive children who have mental retardation, autism, or a pervasive developmental disability, and who do not respond to treatment with stimulants. The neuroleptic drugs, including thioridazine (Mellaril), haloperidol (Haldol), and chlorpromazine hydrochloride (Thorazine), have all been used to treat hyperactivity. Because these drugs also cause sedation, reduce attention span, and interfere with learning, they are rarely appropriate in the treatment of ADHD. Lithium has been used in hyperactive children who are experiencing mood swings and who have a positive family history for manic-depressive illness.

Other Approaches

A variety of other approaches, including the use of vitamins, minerals, caffeine, and dietary manipulations, have been touted for the treatment of hyperactivity. None of these, however, has withstood the test of strict scientific scrutiny. The Feingold diet proposes that avoiding foods containing natural salicylates, sugar, food colors, and other additives is beneficial in controlling hyperactivity. Well-controlled studies have not substantiated this claim. Similarly, studies do not support that sucrose has an adverse effect on hyperkinetic children. Proponents of megavitamin therapy claim that central nervous system dysfunction can be treated with extremely large doses of vitamins. Other than in the rare individual with a specific inborn error of metabolism, this approach is not only ineffective but can be potentially toxic and should be discouraged. In conclusion, physicians should maintain a degree of skepticism and insist on scientific evidence before accepting new therapies.

SUGGESTED READING

Committee on Children with Disabilities and Committee on Drugs: medication for children with an attention deficit disorder. Pediatrics 1987; 80:758–760.

McBride MC. An individual double-blind crossover trial for assessing methylphenidate response in children with attention deficit disorder. J Pediatr 1988; 113:137–145.

Shaywitz SE, Shaywitz BA. Evaluation and treatment of children with attention deficit disorders. Pediatr Rev 1984; 6:99–109.

Shaywitz SE, Shaywitz BA. Attention deficit disorder: current perspectives. In: Kavanagh JF, Truss TJ, eds. Learning disabilities: proceedings of the National Conference. Washington, D.C., U.S. Government Printing Office (in press).

Zametkin AJ, Rapoport JL. Neurobiology of attention deficit disorder with hyperactivity: where have we come in 50 years? J Am Acad Child Adolesc Psychiatry 1987; 26:676–686.

DEGENERATIVE DISEASE

DEMENTIA

PETER V. RABINS, M.D., Ph.D.

EVALUATION

The treatment of dementia begins with the evaluation. Between 2 and 5 percent of individuals presenting for an assessment of memory complaints suffer from a potentially reversible disorder, and perhaps half of these experience a full recovery upon treatment. Thus at the initial assessment, the physician should explain to the family and patient that a full evaluation for treatable causes of dementia is appropriate but that there is little likelihood that a reversible condition will be found. Clinical experience suggests that the clinician can usually identify those patients with reversible dementias from the information gained during the history and physical examination; these patients have signs and symptoms of depression, thyroid disease, focal central nervous system lesions, or hydrocephalus or a history of head trauma, medication misuse, or alcoholism.

According to the recent National Institute of Health (NIH) Consensus Conference on Dementia, the evaluation for reversible dementia should include a complete blood count, electrolyte panel, screening metabolic panel, thyroid functions, vitamin B_{12}, folate, Venereal Disease Research Laboratory (VDRL), urinalysis, electrocardiogram, and chest x-ray examination. Most clinicians would include computed tomography (CT) of the head on this list. Many clinicians obtain electroencephalograms (EEGs) in all patients, although I do so only when symptoms have been present for less than 2 years, when the case is atypical, or if I have concerns about the possibility of seizures or a metabolic etiology. The EEG is useful in cases in which the etiology of the dementia is unclear and is most informative when the clinical picture and EEG are disparate. For example, marked diffuse slowing in mildly impaired individuals suggests a metabolic or toxic etiology. Conversely, a normal EEG in a person with definite cognitive impairment should prompt one to focus attention on searching for depression or other psychiatric etiologies. However, the EEG may be normal in patients with early Alzheimer's disease and other degenerative dementias.

A lumbar puncture should also be considered in the assessment of all patients with dementia. My practice is to recommend a lumbar puncture when the dementia has been present for less than 2 to 3 years. In more chronic cases, infectious etiology is unlikely.

Human immunodeficiency virus (HIV) testing should be considered in all patients with dementia; permission for testing should be sought in individuals with high-risk behaviors or exposures, in patients with signs and symptoms compatable with the acquired immunodeficiency syndrome (AIDS) spectrum, and in any patient in whom the cognitive and behavioral changes have been present for less than 6 months. Screening for other unusual causes of dementia depends on the patient's history and the clinical findings. The presence of movement disorders should raise the possibility of Wilson's disease or Huntington's disease. The presence of a neuropathy suggests a toxic or metabolic cause, and specific tests such as heavy metal screens and tests for deficiency diseases should be considered.

The role of magnetic resonance imaging (MRI) in the treatment of dementia is still under debate. In the elderly, MRI often presents information that is more confusing than helpful. I limit the use of MRI to patients for whom there is a high suspicion of focal lesion (including vascular disease) and those younger than 65 years of age, or if a condition is suspected for which the MRI is more specific than a CT scan (e.g., AIDS or multiple sclerosis).

The evaluation of dementia may well disclose other untreated or insufficiently treated medical conditions, and their proper management may improve cognition or prevent progression of the dementia, although it will not cure it. Patients with a vascular dementia caused by emboli should be assessed for a cardiac or extracranial carotid source and treated appropriately. Recent research suggests that patients with vascular dementia may benefit from the use of aspirin or other antiplatelet aggregation therapies.

Identification of Treatable Symptoms in Irreversible Dementia

After the diagnosis of an irreversible dementing disorder has been made, the next step is to identify comorbid medical, behavioral, or mood symptoms that might respond to treatment. The evaluation for reversible causes of dementia may disclose coexisting conditions such as heart failure, the treatment for which can improve the function of the patient. If a referring or family physician is involved, drawing his or her attention to these issues might be the most appropriate intervention.

Behavior disorder is common in dementias of various etiologies. Sleep disorder, hallucinations, delusions, and agitation are common. Some of these symptoms are clearly induced by the environment or by unrealistic expectations of the patient's family, friends, or treating institutions. For example, the behaviors resulting from apraxias, agnosias, perseveration, and apathy are often perceived of as willful refusal. Identifying these symptoms and the accompanying behaviors as arising from the brain disease can redirect caregivers to find ways to minimize their impact. Sometimes the most appropriate ''treatment'' is for the patient's family members or the staff of the treating institution to modify their expectations.

Some behavioral symptoms that arise from the brain disorder are upsetting, but because of the risk of drug side effects, pharmacotherapy is not justified. For example, if the demented patient accuses people of stealing money, the first intervention should be to help the family or nursing home to accept the fact that this symptom arises from the brain disease. However, if symptoms such as accusations cause significant distress to the patient or lead to dangerous behaviors such as striking others, then a cautious trial of a neuroleptic drug is indicated. No one neuroleptic drug is indicated over another, and the extrapyramidal side effects and orthostatic hypotension they commonly induce are often more troublesome than the behavior for which they are prescribed. However, some patients do respond to low doses of the neuroleptics and a time-limited trial (3 to 6 weeks) aimed at relieving a specific target symptom is sometimes appropriate.

A neuroleptic is chosen by determining which agent is least contraindicated based on its side effect profile. In patients for whom orthostasis is a serious risk or who are already receiving antihypertensive treatment, a high-potency, low-milligram neuroleptic such as haloperidol (starting dose of 0.5 to 1 mg twice daily), thiothixene (starting dose of 1 to 2 mg twice daily), or fluphenazine (starting dose of 1 mg twice daily) should be considered. For patients with frequent agitation in whom sedation would be desirable, thioridazine (starting dose of 10 to 20 mg three times daily or at bedtime) might first be tried. All neuroleptics may induce extrapyramidal symptoms that are often debilitating. However, when used judiciously (and in patients for whom nondrug treatments have failed or are unavailable), these medications can diminish severe behavior disorders.

Sleep disorder is common in many dementing illnesses. Behavioral interventions rarely seem to work in patients with this condition, and if the sleep disorder is not troublesome, it may be best not to treat it pharmacologically. However, sleep disorder can place the patient in danger of falling in a darkened home or cause extreme distress to an elderly family caregiver who cannot sleep at night because of it. In such cases, a judicious trial of chloral hydrate (500 to 1,500 mg at bedtime) or, in patients with sleep disorder who also have behavioral problems for which neuroleptics are indicated, a prescription of neuroleptics taken at night only might help.

Fifteen to 20 percent of patients with dementia of the Alzheimer type and vascular dementia suffer from depression. Patients who have been experiencing weight loss, frequent crying, behavioral disorder, and sleep disturbance should be considered for treatment with an antidepressant. Drugs with low anticholinergic side effect profiles such as nortriptyline (starting dose of 10 to 20 mg at bedtime) or desipramine hydrochloride (starting dose of 25 mg) are useful. If the patient is experiencing sleep disruption, this may be the only necessary treatment.

ASSESSMENT OF SUDDEN BEHAVIORAL CHANGE IN PATIENTS WITH DEMENTIA

Suddenly changing cognition and behavior in an individual with dementia suggests that the patient has suffered a new central nervous system insult, developed a new medical or psychiatric comorbidity (e.g., a new urinary tract infection, upper respiratory infection, or depression), or become delirious from a medication that has been added during the past month. Patients who undergo a change in behavior should therefore be assessed for each of these conditions. In the elderly, it may take as long as 30 days for a drug to accomplish the five half-lives necessary for it to reach steady state; thus medication changes during the previous 30 days should be reviewed when subacute or acute changes in conditions occur.

INVOLVEMENT OF THE FAMILY

Family members are usually involved at all stages of the patient's management. Often it is the family rather than the patient who initiates the assessment, and indeed, early on, patients often deny that there are problems. A clear, accurate diagnosis should be relayed to the family in such instances. When there are several diagnostic possibilities, the family should be informed of these and of their prognostic significance. Some families find that they are greatly benefited by referral to such organizations as the Alzheimer's Disease Association or the Huntington's Disease Association. They provide emotional support for the family and specific information about legal, social, and long-term health care resources.

LEGAL, SOCIAL, AND FINANCIAL ISSUES

Patients with early dementia may be able to drive an automobile safely, but no accurate means exists for identifying when driving becomes dangerous for these patients. In cases where motor impairment is prominent, visuospatial or perceptual abnormalities are significant, or judgment is impaired, the patient and family should be instructed that he or she must discontinue driving. The decision to notify the motor vehicle bureau rests on the clinician's judgment that the situation is indeed dangerous. One alternative is to suggest that the patient take a driving test at a local driving education agency. Because state requirements for notification vary, the clinician should be aware of the law in his or her locality.

Families also need to seek financial, legal, and social advice from individuals skilled in the practice of these disciplines, and physicians can make an important contribution by encouraging them to seek such counsel. Because of changing laws, it is important that families do so early. This is particularly important if the family and patient desire a durable power of attorney. This allows a competent person to appoint a person who can make major decisions for him if he becomes demented, without needing a judicial process to declare him incompetent. Once a demented person becomes incompetent, however, it is no longer possible to obtain such a document. Some families benefit from talking to a knowledgeable financial counselor.

Because nursing home placement is a difficult subject for many patients and families, recommending that they seek social work advice before placement becomes a necessity may prevent the complications that arise from last-minute decisions. Thus occasional office visits over time that identify new symptoms, treat behavioral comorbidity, and direct the family to needed social interventions can contribute to the well-being of the patient and his or her family, even in the face of progressive dementing illnesses.

SUGGESTED READING

Cummings J, Bensen DF. Dementia: a clinical approach. Stoneham, MA: Butterworth, 1984.
Drachman DA. Who may drive? Who may not? Who shall decide? Ann Neurol 1988; 24:787–788.

PATIENT RESOURCES

Literature
Mace NL, Rabins PV. The 36-hour day: a family guide to caring for persons with Alzheimer's disease, related dementing illnesses, and memory loss in later life. Baltimore: Johns Hopkins University Press, 1981.

Associations
Alzheimer's Disease and Related Disorders Association (ADRDA)
70 East Lake Street
Chicago, Illinois 60601
Telephone: 1-800-621-0379

Huntington's Disease Society of America (HDSA)
140 West 22nd Street
New York, New York 10011
Telephone: (212)242-1968

AMYOTROPHIC LATERAL SCLEROSIS

RALPH W. KUNCL, M.D., Ph.D.
LORA L. CLAWSON, R.N., B.S.N.

The work of the neurologist who *cares* for the ALS patient is to dissuade both the patient and himself from the idea that the patient is untreatable. In a recent article in the New England Journal of Medicine, Drs. Bulkin and Lukashok make the following observation on physicians' approach to the incurably ill.

Physicians are trained to investigate, diagnose, prolong life, and cure. When these goals are no longer relevant, physicians often feel they have no skills to offer and distance themselves from the patient. Some turn the patient over to other care givers. Many, like the physician in Tolstoi's *Death of Ivan Ilyich*, continue to prescribe cures in an effort to hide the reality that the patient is dying. The family is then placed in the position of Ilyich's wife, insisting that the patient adhere to the doctor's protocol and refusing to acknowledge the truth. Thus, the patient's final act of living is denied validity, and the patient and family are deprived of the opportunity to come to terms with it and with each other. All are left with the perception that there is some sort of shame attached to being incurably ill, and the patient is left with a sense of having been abandoned at the time of greatest crisis. Yet in truth, there remains much that the physician can offer the patient when curing skills are no longer required.

Few patients are as needy as those with amyotrophic lateral sclerosis (ALS). Paradoxically, there are few patients for whom neurologists provide worse continuing care. Many patients with ALS—perhaps most—leave their doctor's office with the idea that they ("the average patient") will die in 3 years, and that ALS is "untreatable." Thus this chapter might be subtitled, "What to do when there is nothing to do," or "Treating the untreatable."

WHAT ALS PATIENTS SAY THEIR DOCTORS NEED TO KNOW

It is because of the sense of having been abandoned that ALS patients experience and the psychosocial problems that arise that we began an ALS support group in the early 1980s in Baltimore, with the collaboration of the Muscular Dystrophy Association. What the pressing needs of ALS patients are, which solutions work best, what unspoken questions patients harbor—these things we have learned best by simply listening to members of the support group, in a setting away from the formality of the office. When asked, "What is the worst part about having ALS," patients' answers have included the following: "I was in the dark for 6 months without a diagnosis." "Not being told about the MDA." "Nothing ever truly helps; things only become temporarily more tolerable." "The fear of the respirator—not being *on* it, but the machine itself, sort of like the fear some people have of using a computer. But it was much easier than I'd ever anticipated."

When asked "What are the most important things you learned and who did you learn them from?" patients answered as follows: "No physician can help." "We improvise—it's a matter of living with it . . . self-discovery." "I found out I was too afraid of the gastrostomy; it was no big deal." "I handled each symptom as it came up, through the support group and my doctor and my therapist." "Doctors need to learn how to talk to patients with ALS."

Talking to Patients With ALS

There seem to be two extremes in how doctors talk to patients with ALS. The first extreme is avoidance, whether active or unconscious. It naturally evolves from the doctor's feeling of helplessness about the disease. It leads to withdrawal from the patient, curtness, obfuscation concerning the diagnosis, a concentration on documenting the inevitable neuromuscular decline without discussing solutions to the problems of everyday living, and even to the formal discharge of the patient to the care of other previously unengaged specialists such as pulmonary physicians or internists. Of course, it often works in reverse. The patient may withdraw from the doctor in a sense of embarrassment or anger about the diagnosis or the way in which it was given or received. This combination of avoidance behaviors no doubt explains the common switching of doctors that occurs with this disease early in its course.

The opposite extreme is the physician who actively engages the patient, transmitting his or her great experience with the natural history of the disease or its multiple symptoms and treatments by launching into a nonstop treatise on every conceivable outcome. Such speeches are seldom heard during the clinician's first encounter with the patient, and if they are, they are probably very frightening. The advice of experienced ALS clinicians is always to schedule a second visit after a short time for reflection, in order to discuss the prognosis and its meaning regarding activities of daily living. It is then important to take the occupational therapists' approach and attempt to "fix" only what the patient perceives as "broken." To do otherwise leads to overload and a feeling of hopelessness. Thus, for example, extensive conversations or demonstrations about communication problems and the many devices available to aid communication are rarely of value to patients who have no trouble speaking. Despite our best intentions to prepare people well in advance for any contingency, human nature is such that most of us will not prepare for future risks. Inundating patients with information about their illness is to be avoided in favor of focusing on a single or a few distinct current problems.

A final point on talking to patients with ALS is that it pays to kneel or sit whenever talking to a patient in a wheelchair. This brings the doctor and patient eye to eye, removing the patient's need to strain his weak cervical paraspinal muscles while craning the neck during conversation, and removes the position-of-authority body language.

DIAGNOSIS

The diagnosis of ALS is usually straightforward. *Progressive* weakness accompanied by other lower motor neuron signs such as atrophy or fasciculation must be present. It is important to note that fasciculation is a lower motor neuron sign that accompanies many disorders and is *not* in and of itself pathognomonic of ALS. Further, although the tongue is always examined, it is only denervated in one-fourth of patients at the time of diagnosis. The definite diagnosis of ALS requires the presence of *widespread* denervation (Lambert's criteria) that is not explainable by neuropathy or radiculopathy and which occurs in the presence of upper motor neuron signs but in the absence of significant sensory, bowel, or bladder abnormalities. Although easy to recognize in approximately 80 percent of cases, ALS remains a diagnosis of exclusion. This requires the exclusion of disorders that may mimic it, such as cervical and lumbar spondylotic myeloradiculopathy, multifocal motor neuropathy with conduction block and antiganglioside antibodies, plasma cell dyscrasias, lead intoxication, adult hexosaminidase deficiency, hyperthyroidism, hyperparathyroidism, polymyositis, chronic inflammatory demyelinating polyneuropathy, and other primarily motor neuromuscular diseases. A few patients with ALS present with breathing difficulty from diaphragmatic paralysis as their first symptom. This is an important differential diagnostic point because few neuromuscular diseases present with predominant respiratory weakness. These include myasthenia gravis, polymyositis, adult acid maltase deficiency, amyloid myopathy, and ALS. Rarely are unusual presentations of multiple sclerosis or Parkinson's disease misdiagnosed as ALS.

THERAPEUTIC APPROACHES TO FOUR COMMON PROBLEM AREAS IN ALS

Weakness

The rule in treating weakness associated with ALS is that autonomy equals therapy. Weakness is only functionally important insofar as it prevents a particular activity. This is the premise of the occupational therapist who inquires about activities of daily living. One will never know that the patient needs a prescription for a raised toilet seat until the patient is asked whether he or she can rise from it and about his or her feelings of helplessness. One will never know that the patient needs a card-holding device until he or she is asked about hobbies and it is discovered that the patient's whole social life circles around the game of bridge. One will never know that the patient needs a wrist splint until it is learned that he can no longer shave by himself and that this depresses him. These basic but essential problems are not likely to be addressed in the course of a half-hour return visit to the hurried but compulsive

Table 1 Most Useful Adaptive Aids for Weakness in ALS

Personal Hygiene	**Feeding**
Long-handled sponge	Mobile arm support, ball-bearing feeder
Wash mitt	Non-skid foam (DYCEM)
Soap on a rope	Plate guard
Lightweight built-up handles for toothbrush, comb, razor, nail file	Rocker knife
Electric toothbrush with suction brush device	Lightweight built-up silverware (tubular foam)
Electric razor	Lightweight mugs with easy grip handles
Hand-held shower head	
Raised toilet seat	
Dressing	**Meal Preparation**
Button hook	Long-lever jar opener with adaptive turning knob
Zipper ring, hook, loop	Lap tray (bean bag; bed tray/table)
Dressing stick	Lightweight built-up handles for cooking utensils, pots
Long-handled shoehorn	Adapted paring board
Velcro clothing closures	Twist off bottle opener
Suspenders	Milk carton holder
Positioning	**Other**
Ankle-foot orthosis (AFO)	Lamp extension switch
Cock-up wrist splint	Triangular pencil grip
Transfer board	Book holder
Foam wedge cushion (bed)	Card holder
Cervical collars: open Kydex frame collar with Plastozote padding; Philadelphia collar; soft collar	Page turner (hand-held, mouth-held)
Head strap	Rubber thimble
Cervical pillow	Speaker phone with automatic dialing
	Operator headset
	Lightweight reachers
	Adapted built-up key holder
	Doorknob extension lever
	Self-opening scissors
	Antiembolism stockings (Ted)

Table 2 Durable Medical Equipment

Four-prong cane
Forearm crutches
Upright rolling walker (adapt with forearm supports, vertical
  grip handles, and basket)
Manual wheelchair—measured and fitted by physical therapist
  (best choice is lightweight, portable, with removable
  armrests and swing-away removable leg supports; add high-
  density foam cushion and sheepskin)
High-back recliner electric wheelchair—measured and fitted by
  physical therapist (should be adapted with changeable
  control switch—i.e., joystick, suck/blow controls—and with
  space under seat for respirator or computer as weakness
  progresses; should have removable armrests, swing-away
  removable leg supports, and cushion and sheepskin as
  above)
Portable suction machine, with Yankar oral/tonsil adaptor
Fracture bedpan/urinal
Hand rails/safety bars for tub or shower and toilet
Hospital bed (electric preferred; with high-density eggcrate
  mattress and sheepskin)
Overbed table with tilting top
Mechanical patient lift (portable preferred) with full body sling
  (e.g., Hoyer)
Drop-arm bedside commode
Accessible shower stall with rolling shower/commode chair (or
  tub chair)
Electric reclining seat-lift chair
Outdoor ramps
Stairway glide
Van adapted with electric hydrolic lift for wheelchair passenger

neurologist who is busy documenting semeiologically how the patient's muscles have worsened since the last visit. The number of devices that can aid patients suffering from symptomatic weakness are as legion as the number of activities that can be impaired in this disease. The breadth of the problem and what we and our patients have found to be the most helpful solutions are shown in Tables 1 and 2. However, a picture is worth a thousand words. It is a good idea to lend your patient a catalogue of self help aids (such as that by Sammons) to thumb through at home, and to keep a copy as an office reference. The issue of excercise is discussed separately later in this chapter.

Swallowing

Conservative measures and helpful eating strategies (Table 3) go a long way towards improving swallowing and preventing aspiration. When swallowing is first jeopardized and aspiration is a risk, patients and their families should be trained in the Heimlich maneuver and cardiopulmonary resuscitation. They should obtain a portable suction machine to help clear secretions and retrieve from the posterior larynx boluses that cannot be expectorated and which jeopardize the airway. With the conservative measures outlined, many patients are surprisingly able to eat (though with great caution) despite severe corticobulbar dysfunction and severe impairment as measured by cine-esophagogram.

When the patient's intake of food provides inadequate nutrition, some form of tube feeding must be considered in consultation with a trained nutritionist. Patients may mistakenly think about feeding tubes in the same category as all tubes, including an endotracheal tube, as if it were a "heroic" measure. This can be demystified by demonstrating the devices or referring the patient to another patient using the device. There are many options. Simple nasogastric tubes are often the easiest solution. Keough tubes have the advantage of smaller size and greater flexibility and comfort, but with chronic use they frequently become occluded. The most easily tolerated surgical procedure seems to be feeding gastrostomy, rather than cervical esophagostomy or feeding pharyngotomy with cricopharyngeal myotomy. One should emphasize the current best option, which is endoscopically guided gastrostomy performed with the patient under local anesthesia.

Sialorrhea is a difficult and humiliating problem. The problem with all treatments for drooling is that an excessively dry mouth may in fact make swallowing *more* difficult. We have only occasionally found permanent procedures such as parotid gland irradiation or tympanic neurectomy helpful. Unfortunately, such procedures may make residual saliva tenacious and difficult to expectorate or even inspissated—a cure worse than the original symptom. Most patients end up using a suction apparatus or a cloth in the mouth as the most practical solution. Over-the-counter antihistamines may be tried. Amitriptyline has the advantage of being a very

Table 3 Swallowing: Helpful Strategies

Position	Sit upright at a 45- to 90-degree angle (high-Fowlers), with head bent slightly forward.
Attention	Concentrate on swallowing; avoid communication and other distractions at mealtime and eat in a comfortable, unhurried setting.
Adjustment of taste, texture, and temperature	Avoid excessively sweet or sour foods as they increase saliva production; avoid bitter and salty foods as they increase thirst.
	Use soft, cooked, moist foods and gelled, pureed, strained foods; add sauces.
	Avoid extremes of temperature.
Common sense	Have frequent, small feedings—six per day.
	Cut foods into small bite-size pieces.
	If adjustment of food texture limits nutrition, use high-calorie, high-protein supplements.
	Patient and family should be instructed in Heimlich maneuver.

potent anticholinergic agent for sialorrhea, as well as an antidepressant and hypnotic agent (although the drug is not indicated for sole use as a hypnotic over the long-term). There are, of course, many atropinic agents, but the most convenient is the scopolamine patch. Its convenience is its relatively constant therapeutic effect without the patient's needing to swallow anything, but its chief disadvantage, as with all atropinic agents, is potentiation of glaucoma, urinary retention, or adverse central nervous system (CNS) effects. The chief advantage of glycopyrrolate, a quaternary anticholinergic agent, is that it does not cross the blood-brain barrier.

Communication

Rarely is the low volume of the voice the only problem, so that amplification devices are rarely or briefly usable. For some patients with limited use of certain fingers, portable hand-held print-out devices such as the Canon Communicator are quick ways to produce a written output. For those with few recognizable spoken words and weakness of the hands there are still numerous strategies for communication (Table 4). Speed is the most frustrating aspect. ETRAN display boards are an old standard. Letters, phrases, or words can be indicated using eye movements or pointing. The pointer can be as simple as a soda straw held in the mouth if lip muscles or neck muscles are strong enough. A clear Lucite communication board is an ideal way to improve eye contact between the "speaker" and interpreter. Simple eye-blink (yes/no) strategies cost nothing and rely on the inventiveness of the patient and family in developing the quickest strategies for scanning the alphabet or developing codes. The disadvantages of such systems are that they become idiosyncratic and do not transfer to friends or multiple therapists. Personal computers have the potential for speed and permanent printout. Input can be linked to any residual movement (eyebrow, finger

flicker, eye movement) via microswitch. Many kinds of software exist, and a popular one in our clinic is Words Plus. The more complex the algorithm of the software, such as the ability to predict the next letter or word from known common spelling patterns or rules of grammar and rhetoric, the more speedy the output. Inefficiency and slowness of certain scanning programs make patients put their computers back in boxes and revert to simpler eye-blink and alphabet board strategies. An advantage of computers is the fact that the output can be linked to a speech synthesizer to add a human speech quality to communication, to printers to allow for correspondence, and to modems to allow telephone interaction. An important new national volunteer agency, Volunteers for Medical Engineering, is able to help provide and train handicapped patients with such devices. One should not forget that the old-fashioned pencil and note pad or the 29-cent magic slate are communication tools far superior to all the other "high tech" devices if the patient can use his or her hands.

Some speaking habits that caregivers develop are particularly irritating to ALS patients. These include speaking to family members rather than directly to the patient, speaking without eye-to-eye contact with the patient, standing far above the patient when addressing him or her, speaking loudly as if the patient were deaf, pretending to understand speech that is not understandable, completing patient's sentences and thoughts, or speaking in a manner or tone of voice as if one were speaking to a child.

Breathing

Respiratory impairment is the most serious sign in ALS. To the physician, the patient, and the family members it may appear to represent the beginning of the end. Pneumonia or aspiration, as secondary complications of severely weakened respiratory and bulbar muscles, are the usual causes of death.

Assessment

The two most important measurements for assessing neuromuscular respiratory impairment are vital capacity (VC) and negative inspiratory force (NIF). VC is the single-most important measurement, since it can be easily measured by spirometry (a hand-held Wright's spirometer is convenient). As a global indicator of lung function, VC should direct the physician's care in dealing with impending respiratory insufficiency. NIF begins to decline into a useful measurable range when the VC falls below 1.5 L or half of the patient's predicted baseline. It is a useful indicator of respiratory *muscle* status (with contributions from intercostals, diaphragm, and accessory muscles of respiration), exclusive of paren-

Table 4 Communication Aids

Note pad
Magic slate
Call device (dinner bell, clicker, intercom system, Speak and
   Spell)
Letterboards (ETRAN, letter cuff [alphabet list worn on
   forearm])
Electric typewriter
Hand-held computers with print-out device (Canon
   Communicator)
Personal computer (desk top)
Computer augmentation devices
   Specific software capabilities adapted to patient needs such
     as Words Plus
   Voice synthesizer
   Switches adaptable to head movement, eye blink, or suck/
     blow

chymal lung disease. Arterial blood gas evaluations are rarely useful, since serious changes are only late indicators of respiratory muscle failure in ALS. PaO_2 levels remain well preserved until late in the course of the disease. CO_2 retention to levels greater than 45 mm Hg is a poor prognostic sign, common in patients presenting with severe respiratory failure (Fig. 1).

Symptomatic Care

Treatment should be directed toward maintaining and improving the patient's ventilation by instruction of family members in chest physiotherapy, nasopharyngeal suctioning, assistive cough techniques (Heimlich maneuver used synchronously with the patient's cough attempt), and use of intermittent positive pressure breathing (IPPB). Episodes of acute respiratory difficulty should not be automatically attributed to the progression of ALS but be properly diagnosed by examination of sputum, temperature, respiratory rate and effort, and by chest x-ray examination. Acute upper respiratory infection, aspiration, or dehydration should be treated early with intravenous fluids and/or antibiotics, as they further compromise an already poor respiratory status. Bronchodilators, such as metaproterenol sulfate or albuterol (preferably administered by a nebulizer), may be given if indicated by bronchospasm associated with mucus plugging. Long-acting theophylline compounds are used as well because of their putative direct effects on muscle to relieve respiratory muscle fatigue. Adequate hydration and nutrition to liquify secretions and maintain strength should be emphasized.

Mechanical Ventilation

The issue of mechanical ventilation should be openly and supportively discussed with the patient and the patient's family as soon as the involvement of respiratory muscle is observed. While symptomatic treatments may alleviate the initial symptoms, the underlying problem of respiratory muscle fatigue and eventual paralysis will not be solved until the decision regarding the use or refusal of mechanical ventilation is made. Although this decision is difficult, most patients and family members have difficulty grasping the consequences of their choices and are grateful to the physician for the opportunity to discuss them. There is no simple way to direct such a discussion other than to adopt an unhurried, honest approach. Discussion of a living will may be a catalyst in this conversation. The living will outlines in writing one's decision whether or not to use mechanical ventilation to sustain life. Many states have adopted the living will as a legal right; however, the patient should investigate if it is legal in his or her state. These documents can be obtained easily through a lawyer or directly from the Society for the Right to Die. The patient should understand that the decision does not have to be made immediately and is revocable.

The optimal family situation for home ventilator use requires many resources. Close proximity to an acute care hospital, supportive care by a dedicated nurse and physician, a home health agency, insurance coverage, financial support for that family member who will become the primary caretaker, respite care, emotional support for the patient and family members, and equipment and necessary electrical adaptations of the home are a few of the tangible and intangible resources necessary to improve the transition to total ventilator support. Most insurance companies assist financially with the cost of nursing care and respiratory therapy to allow the patient to remain in the home. Some agencies such as Muscular Dystrophy Association assist in the purchase of electric wheelchairs that, when modified, can include space for a portable ventilator to allow the patient mobility. After some initial adjustment, many patients can be weaned from the ventilator for several hours during the day. Travel to areas of interest is made possible by a wheelchair-accessible van equipped with a hydraulic lift. While the picture is not entirely rosy, it is not the same picture that one may envision of the patient attached to a large, noisy respirator in a socially isolated hospital ward. The patient can live a life of quality, albeit increasingly vicarious, if the appropriate support is available.

Tracheostomy by itself is an option for the patient whose problem with aspiration of food or secretions predominates over respiratory impairment. This procedure can be performed relatively easily and can increase comfort when the airway is jeopardized by aspiration. After a period of time, the patient can have a talking tracheostomy tube inserted, or in some cases, may be able to speak simply by deflating the tracheostomy cuff.

For the patient with moderate to severe respiratory difficulty who decides against using mechanical ventilation, other supportive measures can still be used (see Fig. 1). Negative pressure ventilation, although only a short-term solution, is possible with cuirass devices (chest shell or poncho style) that use a cage through which a vacuum motor provides negative pressure to the chest wall, thus enabling the patient's chest to rise and fall. Continuous positive airway pressure (CPAP) administered by a nasal mask or face mask, as recently used in the treatment of sleep apnea, can be successfully used in the ALS patient as well. In patients with otherwise marginal respiration, ventilation can be maintained for long periods, using CPAP at night and a continuous IPPB apparatus during the day to force otherwise atelectatic airways open. Low-flow oxygen (1 to 3 L per minute via nasal cannula) can be used, particularly

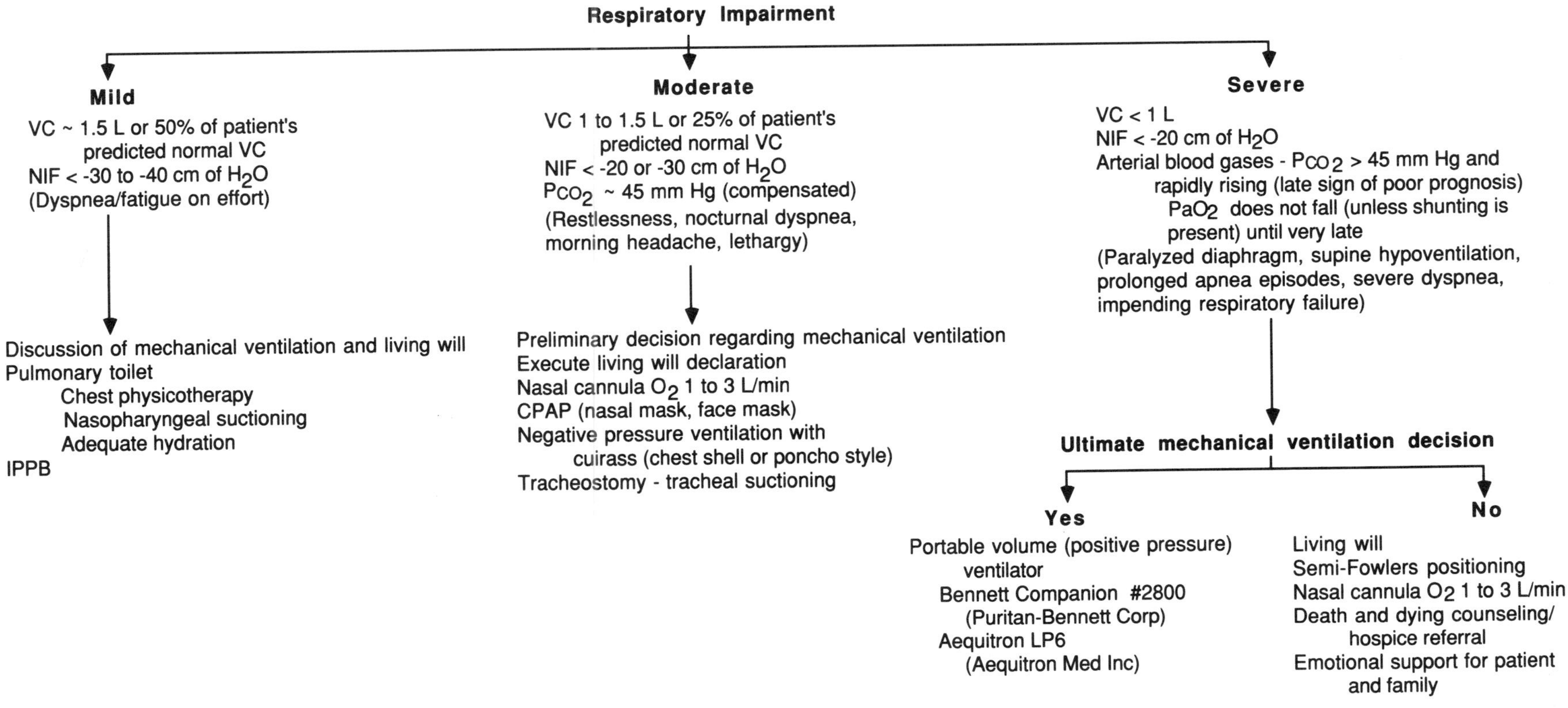

Figure 1 Treatment of respiratory impairment. The severity of respiratory impairment is determined by symptoms, signs, and the key measurements of vital capacity and negative inspiratory force, as listed across the top of the figure. Suggested treatment options follow below for each phase of severity.

VC = vital capacity; NIF = negative inspiratory force; IPPB = intermittent positive pressure breathing; ABG = arterial blood gas; CPAP = continuous positive airway pressure.

at night to combat the typical supine hypoventilation that causes eventual hypoxia. Patients should sleep in a semi-Fowler's position (30 to 45 degrees) to aid in ventilation.

Sleeplessness and Breathing

In the context of respiratory insufficiency, sleeplessness may become a more significant problem. It can easily be treated with low-dose triazolam or flurazepam hydrochloride, but these should be used for a short time intermittently. Anxiety symptoms may be helped by these or other benzodiazepine derivatives when administered in low doses. If cough is the problem, short-term codeine also promotes rest. Alcohol or over-the-counter antihistamines should not be used routinely as hypnotics, since they are less effective, are prone to suppress rapid eye movement (REM) sleep, and cause adverse side effects when taken in overdose. In the moribund patient, administration of morphine—with the full knowledge of the potential for further respiratory suppression that exists with the use of all anxiolytics and hypnotics—allows patients partial mental detachment from their situation. However, at this stage of the disease, the majority of patients may be already naturally sedated or lethargic from CO_2 narcosis, and usually die quietly in their sleep. Referral to a local hospice agency long before this may provide much needed support for the patient and family members. The professional counseling and physical and emotional support that this multidisciplinary team can provide are invaluable resources for patients at this stage of ALS.

Any ALS patient has the right to change the decision regarding mechanical ventilation at any time. Whatever decision the patient makes, the physician should seek to understand it from the patient's perspective. In fact, the physician needs to become the student of the patient. Openness, flexibility, and most of all *caring* are essential in treating all aspects of this disease, but especially when treating the respiratory insufficiency that eventually progresses to respiratory failure.

QUESTIONS ALS PATIENTS ASK

"What Do I Have?"

The answer to this question should be simply "ALS." It is now the name that the lay public knows and uses in North America. A more generic and unfamiliar (e.g., British) term like "motor neuron disease" is often used as a form of medical obfuscation. Such a term should be reserved for truly atypical cases that fail to meet the criteria for the diagnosis of ALS. If a more specific form of motor neuron disease can be diagnosed, the specific correct term

(e.g., progressive bulbar palsy, spinal muscular atrophy, primary lateral sclerosis, multifocal motor neuropathy) should be used and explained to the patient. To prevent common confusion, explicitly distinguish ALS from Alzheimer's disease (the other "A" disease), multiple sclerosis (the other "sclerosis"), and muscular dystrophy.

One should be honest when discussing the diagnosis and then let the patient limit the discussion during the first visit. One should allow an unhurried hour for this discussion. In explaining the meaning of ALS, avoid the impulse to say, "That's what Lou Gehrig had." Everyone is familiar with the picture of a stooped, tearful Lou Gehrig in his uniform. It evokes a sense of hopelessness, early retirement, and early death. Nowadays it is much more helpful to say something like "it's what Senator Jacob Javits had," since this evokes a sense of hopefulness, visibility, acceptance, and continued productivity.

"How Long Do I Have to Live?"

The wrong answer is "God only knows when *any* of us will die. We could be hit on the highway tomorrow by a truck. The average patient dies in 3 years." To someone who is assured of his death, it is not comforting to be told that they may be hit by a truck as well, and such a comment immediately conveys to the patient that the doctor does not really understand the dilemma. Further, quoting a specific time of survival is always wrong, since the patient can only assume that he is like the "average patient" spoken of. A much better answer evokes hope: "Half of the patients who come to us are alive 3 years after the onset of the disease, and many live for a much longer time—even for as long as 10 years or more." One may convincingly add at that point, "And all along the way there will be many treatments we can offer you for every problem that might arise." Such hopefulness is quite a different message to receive than the more typical 3-year "death sentence" that many patients end up hearing.

"Should I Exercise?"

One should resist the urge to answer in a scholarly way, "There is really no research on it, but if you do exercise, don't do too much—don't exert yourself to the point of fatigue." We see a surprising number of patients with ALS who have been forbidden by their physicians to exercise, even warned to quit active exercise programs to which they were previously accustomed, out ot some unspoken fear of the harmfulness of fatigue or an unfounded idea about motor units wearing out. Telling a patient to exercise but not to exert himself to the point of fatigue is like telling a child to have fun swimming but not to go near the water. ALS is in fact marked by reinnervation of muscle, as evidenced by electromyography and muscle biopsy. One should capitalize on this. Motor units *need* usage in order to prevent atrophy of innervated muscle fibers. Movement of joints is essential to prevent both disuse and contracture. The simplest of all reasons to prescribe exercise is that exercise *feels* good. It can produce a sense of euphoria and encourages hopefulness. Of course, there are no new converts to exercise; a sedentary person unaccustomed to exercising is unlikely to take up the challenge of a new way of coping with the diagnosis of ALS. Passive stretching exercises should certainly be encouraged. This is particularly important for families to learn in order to prevent contracture of shoulder joints, which, aside from being painful, can make such simple activities as dressing difficult.

When active exercise programs are undertaken, they should be designed and supervised by a physiotherapist or physiatrist who specializes in exercise evaluation and prescription. One common formula for a resistance exercise program begins by determining for the target muscle what the maximum resistance is for ten repetitions of an exercise. Prescribed exercise then consists of a series of graded efforts as follows: five to ten repetitions each at 50 percent maximum resistance, at 75 percent, and then 100 percent, with each cycle interspersed with 2 minutes of rest. Such programs, targeted at particular muscles that are functionally important for the individual patient, can be combined with cardiac fitness exercise programs using swimming, stationary bicycling, or other sustained activity, depending on the abilities of the patient at that stage of his illness. Overexertion can be prevented by using some fairly liberal rules of thumb, so that the level of exercise is reduced if any of the following occur: (1) tachycardia greater than two times the baseline heart rate, (2) persistent tachycardia of greater than 10 beats per minute over baseline heart rate at 10 minutes after exercise has ceased, (3) dyspnea for more than "a few" minutes, (4) angina, or (5) excessive pain and fatigue on the day *after* exercise.

"What Do I Do Now?"

Resources

In response to this question, the first advice one should give is to contact the Muscular Dystrophy Association, which is the single largest provider of money for research and patient services for this disease in the world. It is surprising how few patients are referred early to the Muscular Dystrophy Association or to the ALS Association (a fund-raising and educationally oriented association). Given the gravity of the diagnosis, the second piece of advice should be to obtain a responsible second opinion. One should then suggest that the entire family join a

support group for ALS patients and families. Such support groups are now offered by every major clinic supported by the Muscular Dystrophy Association or the ALS Association. Support groups offer a place to vent anger and frustration, share common solutions to vexing problems (such as coping with insurance companies or determining which of the many available orthopedic and occupational aids are truly useful), deal with the sense of abandonment by physicians or friends or family, discuss the problem of respite care, and provide a forum where psychological needs can be heeded to carry patients and their families through phases of depression. In addition, probably the most important function such groups serve is that of creating a network that provides the most practical education about the disease and which provides friends with an understanding of what it feels like to have ALS.

Clinical Trials

The final prescription may be to encourage patients to participate in valid clinical research. One should strongly resist the urge to provide placebo therapy in the hope that it "might help keep the disease from progressing." The extensive menu of such placebos (from bee pollen to pancreatic enzymes) changes with time, but they are always used with the misguided rationale that "at least they won't do any harm." Expensive quack treatments like snake venom and transfer factor injections have been truly harmful by virtue of their expense alone. Placebo responses last from weeks to months. Their eventual failure leads to withdrawal of patients from health professionals and to hopelessness; they do not encourage attendance at clinic, nor do they provide the psychological support often intended. Rather, regular visits to a specialized multidisciplinary clinic that offers the services of social worker, patient service coordinator, nurse clinician, physician, occupational therapist, orthopedist, physiotherapist, speech therapist, and dietician offer infinitely better therapy and psychological support than all the prescribed cures of Ivan Ilyich's doctor.

A valid, controlled clinical trial is a real expression of hope. More than half of patients with ALS will want to participate in a clinical trial at least once. The physician's work is to be an advocate and to help the patient evaluate the validity of a particular trial. Quackery abounds with this disease as much as it does with cancer. Besides advocating participation in valid research, the physician needs to be a resource to help patients screen out quackery. The following can be offered to ALS families as obvious "red-flags" that should evoke their strong caution: (1) treatments that are good for many seemingly unrelated diseases, (2) treatments for which no formal protocol can be produced, (3) a rationale or an experimental trial that is neither written nor explainable to the referring physician, (4) the absence of controls, (5) supporting literature that relies on testimonials, (6) nonsponsored research that has not undergone some form of peer review, (7) high costs that are *all* borne by the patient. Any of these should evoke caution, but the presence of several should be indicative of quackery.

Current clinical research available to participants with ALS in the United States include trials of immunomodulators such as cyclophosphamide and neurotransmitter or neuropeptide modulators such as thyrotropin-releasing hormone, branched-chain amino acids, and N-methyl-d-aspartate receptor antagonists.

FINAL SUGGESTIONS

1. When you make the diagnosis of ALS, plan two sessions: first to give conclusions, and secondly to lay out your plans.
2. Know and connect the patient with essential public resources such as the Muscular Dystrophy Association.
3. Do not discuss all possible outcomes and available devices at an early stage. This only leads to information overload and feelings of helplessness.
4. Prescribe exercise. It is invigorating and encourages hopefulness. It prevents the development of frozen joints and subsequent pain, capitalizes on the potential for reinnervation of muscle, and is not harmful if certain rules of thumb regarding limits are followed.
5. Be knowledgeable about aids for activities of daily living; buy a Sammons catalogue or its equivalent. Read it and discuss it with a knowledgeable occupational therapist. Question patients on their needs and abilities, and when particular needs arise, have them try occupational aids. Use occupational therapists, nurse clinicians, or other professionals *experienced* and *interested* in ALS.
6. Start a support group for ALS patients and their families. Use other patients with ALS as a resource. You will learn everything that will be useful to you in treating these patients from the patients and families themselves.
7. Encourage the patient to participate in valid research. This fulfills altruistic motives and is morally rewarding for the patient to do at least once. It is an activity that inspires hopefulness. Become an active advocate to help patients screen various research opportunities.

ACKNOWLEDGMENTS

We gratefully acknowledge the dedicated assistance of Blair Ertel. Our ALS research and patient care have been generously supported by the Jay Slotkin Fund for Neuromuscular Research, the Baltimore Relief Foundation, and the Muscular Dystrophy Association. We are indebted to our colleagues in the Neuromuscular Division, and most of all to the many members of the Baltimore ALS Support Group and our ALS patients whose courage, patience, and guidance contributed greatly to the contents of this chapter.

SUGGESTED READING

Caroscio JT, ed. ALS: a guide to patient care. New York: Thieme, 1986.
Brooks BR, ed. Amyotrophic lateral sclerosis. Neurol Clin 1987; 5(1):1–195, 5(2):197–290.

PATIENT RESOURCES

Associations

The Muscular Dystrophy Association is a nonprofit national organization (information and referral agency) whose main focus is to provide funds for medical care, equipment, education, support groups, research, coordination, and financing of clinics for many neuromuscular diseases including ALS.

Muscular Dystrophy Association
810 Seventh Avenue
New York, New York 10019
Telephone: (212) 586–0808

The Amyotrophic Lateral Sclerosis Association is a nonprofit national organization (information and referral agency) whose main focus is to provide funds for education and research, and to sponsor chapter groups for patients with ALS.

Amyotrophic Lateral Sclerosis Association
21021 Ventura Boulevard Suite 321
Woodland Hills, California 91364
Telephone: (800) 782–4747

The Volunteers for Medical Engineering is a nonprofit national organization of engineers who donate equipment, time, and ingenuity to solving specific problems of the disabled.

Volunteers for Medical Engineering
The Good Samaritan Hospital
5601 Loch Raven Boulevard, 3 East 329
Baltimore, Maryland 21239
Telephone: (301) 532–4360

The Society for the Right to Die provides literature and documents related to living wills.

Society for the Right to Die
250 West 57th Street
New York, New York 10107
Telephone: (212) 246–6973

Literature

Appel V, Callender M, Sunter S. ALS: maintaining mobility—a guide to physical therapy and occupational therapy. MDA, Houston, Texas, 1988.
ALS Association: Five Manual Series. Manual I: Finding Help; Manual II: Muscular Weakness; Manual III: Swallowing Difficulty; Manual IV: Breathing Difficulty; Manual V: Communication Difficulty. Woodland Hills, California: ALS Association, 1986.
Fred Sammons Catalogue. 145 Tower Drive, Dept. #423, Burr Ridge, Illinois 60521-9842. Telephone: (312) 325-1700.
Sears & Roebuck Co. Catalogue.

NEUROGENIC DYSPHAGIA

DAVID W. BUCHHOLZ, M.D.

Although dysphagia caused by neurologic disease is common, it is underappreciated, and even when it is appreciated, it is undertreated. The evaluation and therapy of neurogenic dysphagia have developed exponentially during this past decade but remain unfamiliar to many neurologists.

Swallowing consists of three phases: oral, pharyngeal, and esophageal. The oral phase is under voluntary, cortical control and ends when a bolus passes from the oral cavity into the oropharynx. There the pharyngeal phase, governed by involuntary mechanisms in the brain stem, is automatically triggered. The esophageal phase, beginning when a bolus passes through the pharyngoesophageal sphincter (the cricopharyngeal muscle), is under brain stem and intrinsic neural control. Neurologic disease causing dysphagia usually does so by impairing muscle performance during the oral and pharyngeal phases of swallowing. Esophageal phase impairment may occur but is less likely to be problematic.

A wide array of neurologic diseases can cause dysphagia, and most are diseases of the central nervous system (CNS), most notably stroke. Conventional wisdom holds that stroke must cause brain stem or *bilateral* corticobulbar tract damage to produce dysphagia, because each corticobulbar tract connects with bilateral bulbar nuclei and the brain stem "swallowing center," which collectively mediate swallowing. Recent evidence, however, suggests that mild to moderate dysphagia can result from isolated, unilateral hemispheric stroke. Other CNS diseases can cause dysphagia through the disruption of corticobulbar and/or bulbar function, such as head trauma, multiple sclerosis, motor neuron disease, neoplasm, poliomyelitis, and a myriad of degenerative diseases, most commonly Alzheimer's disease and Parkinson's disease.

Outside the CNS, neurologic diseases may lead to dysphagia by affecting lower cranial nerves (as in Guillain-Barré syndrome, neoplastic meningitis, and skull base tumors), neuromuscular junctions (as in myasthenia gravis), and muscles of the pharynx, larynx, tongue, and face (as in polymyositis, muscular dystrophy, mitochondrial myopathy, sarcoid myopathy, and thyroid disease). Occasionally, neurologic disease interacts with otherwise clinically inapparent, non-neurologic disease in causing dysphagia. For instance, pre-existing otolaryngologic problems such as pharyngeal webs or diverticula and gastroenterologic problems such as gastroesophageal reflux, esophageal dysmotility, or esophageal stricture may become symptomatically manifest when the addition of neurologic disease further compromises pharyngoesophageal function and undermines compensatory mechanisms. It is important to be alert to this interplay, because the non-neurologic disease may be treatable, whereas the neurologic disease may not.

DIAGNOSIS

The first step in treating any problem is to become aware of it. Surprisingly, the symptoms of neurogenic dysphagia may be relatively obscure before the development of either insidious complications such as malnutrition and dehydration or abrupt complications such as aspiration pneumonia and asphyxia. The known presence of any neurologic disease that can affect pharyngeal and laryngeal function should prompt one to consider the possibility of dysphagia, but sometimes dysphagia is a primary presenting symptom, occurring before neurologic disease has been diagnosed, especially in the case of motor neuron disease, multiple small subcortical strokes, and late-onset muscular dystrophy.

History

When dysphagia develops insidiously, patients may inexplicably lose weight or gradually modify dietary and feeding habits while escaping overt symptoms such as cough/choke episodes (indicating laryngeal penetration) and retarded food passage (indicating oral or pharyngeal retention). Initially, dysphagia symptoms may present only in provocative situations, such as nasal regurgitation while bending over to drink water from a fountain or nocturnal awakening due to choking on accumulated secretions during sleep. Sentinel events such as aspiration pneumonia and the need for a Heimlich maneuver must be explored as to their cause. One should search for nondysphagia symptoms of pharyngeal and laryngeal impairment (such as dysarthria), symptoms of potentially interacting diseases (such as gastroesophageal reflux), and medication usage. Any drug that depresses CNS function may add to neurogenic pharyngeal compromise; especially noteworthy are sedative-hypnotics, anticholinergics, muscle relaxants, and topical anesthetics.

Neurogenic dysphagia is often relatively *silent* until presenting as catastrophe. The symptom most often drawing attention is coughing or choking episodes during feeding, but this may not occur if the cough reflex to laryngeal penetration is diminished. It may be diminished as a consequence of sensory impairment of the larynx, but it is much more often *suppressed* as a result of habituation in the face of chronic, recurrent laryngeal penetration. Patients with neurogenic dysphagia may pour material into their airway every time they swallow without realizing and reporting it. The index of suspicion for occult dysphagia must be high in the presence of neurologic disease, despite the absence of overt symptoms of dysphagia.

Physical Examination

Signs of malnutrition and dehydration are usually obvious but are too often casually ascribed to nonspecific cachexia rather than carefully considered as being caused by dysphagia. During the interview with the patient, a thoughtful examiner may notice that the patient frequently clears his throat and shows other signs of difficulty managing secretions, such as drooling, coughing, and a "wet" voice. A box of tissues sitting in the patient's lap is not to be ignored. Mentation should be assessed, because not only can dementia cause dysphagia by impairing voluntary oral feeding, it also interferes with treatment of dysphagia by impeding rehabilitation efforts. Emotional lability may be a clue to pseudobulbar palsy. Special attention should be directed to voluntary and involuntary movements of the face, tongue, and palate. Too much reliance is placed on the gag reflex as a measure of swallowing function. The gag reflex does nothing to facilitate swallowing; in fact, it is inhibited during swallowing. It may be abnormally increased or decreased as a consequence of neurologic disease with or without coincident dysphagia. One cannot predict a patient's swallowing ability based on one's observation of his or her gag reflex.

It is most helpful to observe the patient directly while he or she is drinking and feeding. You should listen for gurgling and a wet voice and note dietary preference, food preparation on the plate, bolus sizing and delivery to the mouth, mastication, head and neck posture, and any difficulty initiating swallowing. The patient may demonstrate unmistakable symptoms of dysphagia such as cough/choke episodes and nasal regurgitation before your eyes, or he may evidence more subtle clues of compensated dysphagia such as double swallowing or using liquids to wash down solids.

EVALUATION

Radiologic Studies

Every patient with suspected neurogenic dysphagia should undergo videofluoroscopy or cineradiography of oral, pharyngeal, and esophageal performance during swallowing of barium boluses of varying volumes and consistencies. A routine barium swallow is inadequate in the setting of neurogenic dysphagia, because it cannot image the rapid-sequence events of the mouth and pharynx, where

neurologic disease is most likely to strike. The study should be performed by a well-trained radiologist, ideally acting in concert with a knowledgeable speech-language pathologist or other swallowing specialist who can manipulate factors such as the bolus, head and neck posture, and feeding techniques during the study to provide information of not only diagnostic but also therapeutic usefulness. The study should be conducted without the use of an indwelling nasogastric feeding tube, if possible. Every attempt should be made to duplicate the patient's normal feeding circumstances. It is sometimes useful and generally safe to add provocative measures to the routine study in a case where the standard procedure fails to demonstrate swallowing impairment that is clinically suspected. Such maneuvers may include large-volume and repetitive swallowing and placing the patient into a potentially compromising (but for him, usual) feeding position. Too often a swallowing study is aborted when minor airway contamination by barium is seen, even though similar problems are likely occurring with food at every meal without serious immediate consequence, and even though much more information could be safely gained by continuing the study.

Chest x-ray examination is useful for assessing complications of acute and chronic aspiration. Newer methods of pharyngeal evaluation such as magnetic resonance imaging, ultrasonography, and radionuclide imaging are experimental and not generally applicable.

Other Studies

Measurement of daily weight, fluid and caloric intake, and blood markers of nutrition and hydration status can help assess the impact of dysphagia and determine the need for supplemental feeding. Otolaryngologic and gastroenterologic consultation can exclude coincident structural lesions, esophageal dysmotility, and gastroesophageal reflux, treatment of which in the setting of neurogenic dysphagia may at least provide partial symptomatic relief. Pharyngoesophageal endoscopy and manometry and esophageal pH probe testing may be useful diagnostic measures.

TREATMENT

General Measures

Medications should be reviewed, and drugs that depress the CNS or otherwise compromise swallowing should be reduced or eliminated, if possible. Coincident diseases such as pharyngeal webs, esophageal stricture, esophageal dysmotility, and gastroesophageal reflux may deserve treatment if symptomatic interplay with neurogenic dysphagia is suspected. Dental appliances should be checked; often they need to be refitted in the setting of neurologic disease affecting the mouth and throat.

Using anticholinergic or antihistaminic medication to decrease salivary volume and thereby relieve retention of secretions is often counterproductive. Such medication can make secretions thick, tenacious, and more difficult to manage. A trial of medication may be worthwhile, but I actively discourage *irreversible* measures such as salivary gland irradiation for the purpose of secretion management.

If the neurologic disease causing dysphagia is treatable, needless to say, treat. You may wish, for example, to schedule anti-parkinsonian medication to achieve peak effect at mealtimes.

I emphatically urge that the services of swallowing therapists (usually speech-language pathologists or occupational therapists), rehabilitation medicine specialists, and dieticians be utilized. If properly trained, these individuals can assist patients with mild to moderate dysphagia in maximizing oral intake, minimizing complications, and avoiding tube feeding. Their treatment is often best guided by information obtained from x-ray studies of swallowing during which factors such as the bolus and head and neck posture are intentionally manipulated. Diet can be modified to enhance sensory appeal and promote the ease, safety, and nutritional value of the oral feeding. As a general rule, patients with neurogenic dysphagia do best with mechanically soft or pureed solids and thickened liquids.

Swallowing therapists can coach patients to avoid conversation and other distractions while eating and may arrange for cognitively or physically dependent patients to have trained feeding supervision. Attention is given to food preparation in the kitchen and on the plate, bolus delivery to the mouth, and bolus management within the oral cavity. Tools such as special spoons and tableware may be helpful, and some severely impaired patients derive benefit from suckle-feeding devices. Therapists can advise patients as to optimal body, head, and neck positioning at mealtimes. If the patient has difficulty initiating swallowing, he or she may be trained to displace food manually into the oropharynx or use techniques such as cold thermal stimulation of the oropharynx to help trigger swallowing. Techniques such as double swallowing each bolus or routinely taking a deep breath, holding it, swallowing, and then coughing can help minimize complications of pharyngeal retention. It is very important that you enlist the help of a trained swallowing therapist in treating patients with neurogenic dysphagia.

Intravenous Feeding

For short-term purposes, intravenous administration of crystalloid, colloid, and hyperalimentation solutions may be indicated either to provide a temporary boost to a patient's volume and nutritional status or to buy time until a more permanent solution to the feeding problem can be established. Although patients can be treated with long-term total parenteral nutrition, that is rarely necessary or desirable for patients with neurogenic dysphagia, since they tend to have functional enteral tracts.

Enteral Tube Feeding

A temporary or permanent enteral feeding tube is indicated when oral intake is either inadequate for maintenance of hydration and nutrition or unsafe, posing risk of aspiration pneumonia and asphyxia. Feeding adequacy is assessed by following body weight, fluid intake, calorie counts, and appropriate blood studies. The issue of safety can be evaluated based on evidence of airway penetration (such as a history of or chest x-ray findings of aspiration pneumonia), the need for Heimlich maneuver, and x-ray study findings of swallowing. As long as it is mild, the finding of laryngeal penetration by barium during a swallowing study does not necessarily mandate avoidance of oral feeding and need for tube feeding, especially if swallowing therapy is available. Pulmonary clearance and defense mechanisms are remarkably effective. However, the occurrence of clinical complications of laryngeal penetration or the radiographic demonstration of moderate to severe laryngeal penetration should discourage oral feeding and encourage tube feeding.

Despite my reluctance to recommend tube feeding to patients and their families, I have found that for many it is a welcome relief from the effort, time, and concern that have been devoted to arduous oral feeding. Moreover, patients with neurogenic dysphagia may globally improve after switching from oral to tube feeding simply because they become well nourished and hydrated for the first time in months.

If a patient with neurogenic dysphagia is expected to improve (such as following a mild brain stem stroke) or is not expected to live long, a small-bore, flexible nasogastric or nasoduodenal tube is preferable to gastrostomy, assuming patient tolerance. A nasoduodenal tube has the advantage of minimizing the risk of gastroesophagopharyngeal reflux and consequent aspiration. To further minimize this risk, any patient being tube-fed should be seated as upright as possible during and shortly after the process. A dietician should be involved in determining the type and volume of liquid food. Feeding should be regulated by a pump to reduce the risk of gastric overload leading to reflux, discomfort, and diarrhea. The feeding schedule should be individually adjusted according to the patient's tolerance and activities.

A permanent feeding tube is best when the patient is not expected to improve but is expected to live more than a few months. The tube of choice is gastrostomy, ideally placed by percutaneous endoscopic route. Jejunostomy is sometimes necessary and is less likely to be associated with reflux, although it is more likely to become occluded. Generally there is much greater disadvantage than advantage to the use of feeding tubes at other sites such as pharyngostomy and cervical esophagostomy.

Other Surgical Procedures

During swallowing, tracheostomy does not, as a rule, protect the airway of a patient with neurogenic dysphagia. An uncuffed tracheostomy allows room around the tube for material to pass down the trachea and into the lungs once the material has entered the larynx from the pharynx. The tube can exacerbate laryngeal penetration by interfering with laryngeal elevation, which is a major laryngeal protective mechanism during swallowing. Tracheostomy compromises the ability to clear the larynx by coughing after swallowing, unless the tracheostomy is occluded. In short, tracheostomy may be necessary in a patient with neurogenic dysphagia but should not be thought of as alleviating the potential complications of oral feeding.

Injection of the vocal cords with Gelfoam or Teflon is sometimes advocated as a measure to promote vocal cord closure in the setting of vocal cord dysfunction, thereby protecting the airways. It may work, but I am unaware of any controlled study indicating that it does, and I am doubtful. Laryngeal protection is primarily achieved by elevation of the larynx and down-tilting of the epiglottis, and apposition of the vocal cords is a relatively weak barrier. As evidence of the limited role of vocal cord closure in laryngeal protection, one should note the *infrequency* with which patients with isolated unilateral vocal cord paralysis (and, therefore, incomplete vocal cord closure) encounter symptoms or complications of laryngeal penetration.

Feeding a patient entirely through an enteral tube unburdens the pharynx and larynx of food but not of secretions and refluxed gastric material. Patients may therefore still suffer aspiration pneumonia and asphyxia. Suctioning may help, but full protection is achieved only by permanent laryngeal closure. This is sometimes indicated but necessitates tracheostomy and obliterating laryngeal speech. These may have already ensued, however, in which case there is little to lose by performing laryngeal closure.

Cricopharyngeal (C-P) myotomy is a popular but unproved method for surgical treatment of neurogenic dysphagia that is believed to promote pharyngeal clearance and relieve symptoms and complications of retained material. Myotomy is often performed based on the assumption that the cricopharyngeal segment is "spastic" as determined by its appearance during an x-ray study of swallowing. In fact, manometric studies indicate that radiographically prominent C-P segments in the setting of pharyngeal paresis rarely generate high pressure and are therefore not spastic. The prominent appearance of the C-P segment in patients with neurogenic dysphagia is usually a result of failure of C-P segment opening, which is normally achieved by anterior traction on the relaxed C-P segment by the suprahyoid (strap) muscles. When the pharyngeal muscles are weak, the suprahyoid muscles are often also weak, and consequently the C-P segment is not pulled open and therefore appears "tight" even though it is flaccid. In such a circumstance, the C-P segment does not represent an obstacle to pharyngeal clearance, despite its prominent radiographic appearance, and cutting the muscle offers no benefit. As long as pharyngeal constrictors are weak, pharyngeal clearance will be impaired, with or without C-P myotomy. In fact, most of the retained material in a weak pharynx tends to be held in the valleculae and piriform recesses, not directly above the C-P segment, further undermining potential benefit from C-P myotomy.

One should be cautious of the radiographic diagnosis of "cricopharyngeal spasm" or "cricopharyngeal achalasia." These terms are often applied to the observation of C-P prominence, usually without the appreciation of coincident pharyngeal and suprahyoid muscle weakness that constitute the real problem. Indeed, such radiographic diagnoses should prompt a search for neurologic disease causing pharyngeal impairment. Having argued against C-P myotomy as a widely useful procedure for neurogenic dysphagia, I must add that some patients may benefit from this procedure. Unfortunately, controlled trials to define the selection criteria for and the efficacy of this treatment are lacking. For now, one should be especially cautious of offering C-P myotomy to patients with coincident gastroesophageal reflux and pharyngeal paresis, because such patients may be dangerously predisposed to aspiration of refluxed gastric contents postoperatively, after the C-P barrier to reflux has been surgically broken down.

SUGGESTED READING

Groher ME, ed. Dysphagia: diagnosis and management. Boston: Butterworths, 1984.

Robbins JA, Sufit R, Rosenbek J, et al. A modification of the modified barium swallow. Dysphagia 1987; 2:83–86.

Sitzmann JV, Mueller R. Enteral and parenteral feeding in the dysphagic patient. Dysphagia 1988; 3:38–45.

Weg AL, Miskovitz PF. Percutaneous endoscopic gastrostomy (PEG): a critical appraisal. Dysphagia 1987; 1:227–231.

NORMAL-PRESSURE HYDROCEPHALUS

DANIEL F. HANLEY, M.D.
CECIL O. BOREL, M.D.
SUSAN HERDMAN, Ph.D.

Originally described by Hakim and Adams, normal-pressure hydrocephalus is a neurologic syndrome that has eluded precise clinical and biological definition. A working definition is the presence of clinical signs of dementia, gait instability, and incontinence associated with ventricular enlargement on cerebral imaging studies, and the absence of elevated intracranial pressure with lumbar puncture. The apparent paradox between an anatomic picture of communicating hydrocephalus and a physiologic measurement of normal intracranial pressures is yet to be completely resolved. Clinically and functionally, however, it is empirically known that this group of patients frequently improves with diversion of cerebrospinal fluid (CSF) from the cranial cavity to another part of the body such as the peritoneum or the venous circulation.

CLINICAL PRESENTATION

The initial complaints of individuals with this syndrome fall into three categories: (1) altered mentation, (2) unsteadiness or falling spells, and (3) isolated ventricular enlargement. The majority of patients present during the seventh, eighth, and ninth decades of life with complaints of unsteadiness when walking, particularly on turning, or when changing position from the seated to standing position. These complaints eventually progress to falling spells, and finally, the inability to ambulate. Alternatively, the patient may initially present with mild cognitive impairment, such as disinterest in previous avocations or difficulty in dealing with complex activities of day-to-day living (e.g., making financial or travel arrangements). Short-term memory is often found to be impaired on clinical questioning. Language, judgment, and affect tend not to be impaired. With progression of the disease, the cognitive impairment causes the patient to have increasing difficulty in dealing with the activities of daily living, as well as disinterest and apathy. In some individuals, urinary urgency characterized by the inability to inhibit bladder contractions is either a complaint at the time of presentation or can be elicited on careful review of systems. With progression of the disease, complete incontinence of urine and stool occurs. Because the individuals who develop this syndrome are predominantly elderly and at risk for Alzheimer's disease and other forms of senile dementia, symptoms often progress without medical attention. These changes are often accepted as signs of aging. We encourage early evaluation of symptoms associated with the normal-pressure hydrocephalus syndrome because treatment appears to be more effective when initiated before dementia, gait apraxia, or incontinence becomes established.

The neurologic examination of the patient with fully developed normal-pressure hydrocephalus syndrome is characterized by a significant dementia with mild to severe short-term memory loss. Complete anterograde amnesia is not uncommon. Comprehension and naming skills are usually intact, as is judgment. Affect is usually not altered from its premorbid condition. The motor examination is remarkable for symmetric bulk, increased voluntary tone with the inability to produce voluntary relaxation. Most often both agonist and antagonist muscle groups show simultaneous increases in tone. Tremor is usually not observed in this group of patients. Reflexes are symmetric and Babinski's sign is usually absent. Often there is a disparity between lower extremity tone/motor performance and upper extremity capabilities. Precise and rapid movements of the lower extremities are difficult for the patient to perform when standing or seated, but are performed more easily when the patient is in the lying position. Gait is remarkable for retropulsion, which is usually obvious when the patient turns rapidly and when he or she changes position from the seated to the standing position. Most often, the patient takes small steps, shuffling the foot along the floor rather than taking normal strides. The patient's station is usually wide, with axial instability and retropulsion induced by either a narrow stance or a tandem stance. A positive physical examination or a history consistent with the normal-pressure hydrocephalus syndrome should be used as an indication for further evaluation.

DIAGNOSTIC EVALUATION

Detailed testing has at least two goals: (1) the elimination of other causes of dementia, gait instability, and incontinence, and (2) the objective measurement of the degree of impairment. Results of these investigations assist in decision making with regard to when to offer treatment and in evaluating the efficacy of treatment. Several useful diagnostic tests should be included in routine evaluation for normal-pressure hydrocephalus syndrome. These include (1) computed tomography (CT) or magnetic resonance imaging (MRI) of the brain, ventricles, and CSF pathways, (2) lumbar puncture, (3) radioisotope cisternography, (4) formal cognitive functioning, (5) posturography or video gait analysis, (6) urography, and (7) invasive monitoring (24-hour intracranial pressure monitoring, CSF absorption studies, and/or a continuous trial of CSF drainage).

Brain imaging is an important factor in making the diagnosis of normal-pressure hydrocephalus syndrome. The demonstration of enlarged ventricles with periventricular lucency is central to the presumed pathophysiology of this illness. Either CT scanning or MRI can be used for this purpose. At present, there are no precise correlations of ventricular enlargement and clinical symptomatology, but improvement in symptomatology can occur without normalization of ventricular size. Contrast should be administered with either CT scan or MRI if focal lesions are apparent or if tumor is suggested by either the imaging study or history. The presence of concurrent pathology such as multiple infarcts with ventricular enlargement makes the diagnosis less likely. The size of cerebral sulci has been suggested as a qualitative indicator of increased cortical mantle pressure and thus of normal-pressure hydrocephalus. We have not found this to be a good discriminator, and furthermore, this is a difficult finding to objectify. Thus, all patients who have enlarged ventricles (including the fourth ventricle) in a pattern of communicating hydrocephalus are suspected of having normal-pressure hydrocephalus. We perform radiolabeled cysternography in this group of patients to confirm the presence of communicating hydrocephalus and to define any delay in CSF reabsorption. The presence of isotope in the cerebral ventricular system at 24 hours is considered a positive indicator of communicating hydrocephalus with isotope reflux and slowed CSF resorption. We measure the lumbar CSF pressure at the time of radioisotope installation. If this pressure is greater than 200 cm of water, the patient is suspected of having CSF diversion. If the pressure is less than 200 cm of water, definition of the risks and benefits of a shunt is indicated.

We usually perform detailed cognitive function testing, including a personality assessment, measurements of the level of consciousness affect, and tests of language and naming skills, short-term memory, visual-spatial function, and the patient's use of reasoning and logic. These tests are used to develop a cognitive profile and a replicable measurement of performance.

Quantitative posturography is helpful in the mildly impaired patient who can stand and walk on his own but who is complaining of performance limitations. With this assessment, repetitive tests of postural stability are performed with the patient using visual, proprioceptive, and vestibular cues to maintain balance. This testing is then repeated to determine the relative contribution of these sensory cues to the ability of the patient to maintain balance. In this way, physiologic dysfunction of visual proprioceptive and vestibular systems can be elimi-

nated. The position of the center of body mass in the AP plane is also determined. The latency of the patient's automatic balance responses to sudden translational or rotational movements of the support surface are recorded. Posturography can be repeated after diagnostic lumbar puncture or diagnostic short-term removal of cerebral spinal fluid has a test of potential long-term therapeutic efficacy.

Diagnostic urography should be performed. A structural assessment of the urethra and bladder are helpful in defining alternative or coexisting etiologies for incontinence. Where no anatomic explanation for incontinence exists, infusion cystometrography is helpful. This test often shows the inability of spontaneous bladder contractions to be inhibited at low bladder volumes. In the absence of spinal cord lesions, this pattern of abnormalities is consistent with a spastic bladder of intracranial etiology. In some situations, evaluation for other medical problems is pertinent. If the patient has visual impairment, an opthalmologic evaluation for both acuity and cataracts can be helpful. Similarly, if the patient has proprioceptive impairment, a detailed neurologic evaluation for peripheral neuropathy should be performed. Finally, in the presence of lower motor neuron or upper motor neuron deficits, myelography may be indicated to better define the presence of either lumbar stenosis or cervical stenosis. Both conditions occur frequently in patients in this age group.

For the patient who presents with the clinical triad of normal-pressure hydrocephalus plus an anatomic picture of obstructive hydrocephalus but has a low intracranial pressure as demonstrated by lumbar puncture, we believe that a diagnostic test of CSF drainage is particularly helpful (Table 1). We therefore advocate performing either intermittent or continuous removal of CSF. We believe that this is most helpful when coupled with a repeat of the testing of cognitive function, posturography/gait testing, or urography, as well as with daily clinical evaluations of mental state and gait.

Table 1 Diagnostic Criteria for Normal-Pressure Hydrocephalus

History
Dementia
Gait disorder
Incontinence
Clinical Examination
Short-term memory deficit
Gait apraxia
Impaired use of vestibular cues to maintain balance
Diagnostic Testing
Enlarged ventricles
Delayed CSF absorption
Impaired cognitive function
Postural vestibular deficits
Trial CSF drainage

CSF Drainage

We recommend some form of a therapeutic trial of CSF drainage if the clinical and diagnostic picture suggests normal-pressure hydrocephalus. Depending on the availability of individuals skilled in placing lumbar catheters and nursing services capable of maintaining these catheters without infection, system disconnection, or uncontrolled CSF drainage, two different strategies can be used: (1) repeat lumbar puncture, or (2) continuous lumbar drainage. If the clinician has little experience with these systems, we recommend a trial of intermittent lumbar puncture with removal of 30 to 50 ml of CSF. Lumbar puncture can be performed as an outpatient procedure with serial revisits to the physician's office, or it may be performed on an inpatient basis, through which the patient's gait, posture, and cognition can be monitored more closely. A lumbar puncture can be repeated with withdrawal of CSF for several days in a sequential manner. Repeated withdrawal of CSF may be necessary to confirm equivocal signs of clinical improvement. This removal of CSF often results in improved gait and some change in cognitive state, which is often noted by persons familiar with the patient, such as the patient's spouse or children. For this reason, regardless of whether the test is performed in the physician's office or at the hospital, questioning of the patient's family members should be undertaken as part of the assessment for beneficial effects.

Since on our service, CSF drainage is frequently performed continuously, we usually opt for the second strategy. Drainage is undertaken through the lumbar space usually at L3-4 or L2-3 after sterile placement of a 16-gauge lumbar drain into the lumbar subarachnoid space (Fig. 1). The drain site and proximal skin are kept sterile with an occlusive dressing. The drain tubing is then attached to the skin in the midaxillary line with sutures. Sterile, pressurized tubing is passed anteriorly over the patient's shoulder and further secured at the shoulder with tape. The system is then attached to an airfiltered drainage bag, which can be set at any number of heights with respect to the patient's lumbar drain site. The relationship between the height of the drainage bag and the position of the patient's lumbar spine is kept fixed until a uniform rate of CSF drainage can be established. This rate is approximately 10 to 20 ml of CSF per hour. When this rate is established, we allow the patient to ambulate ad lib, maintaining a relatively constant rate of CSF drainage by altering the height of the drainage bag with relationship to patient position. The overall goal is to achieve about 240 ml of CSF drainage per day.

This system allows for essentially continuous CSF drainage and effectively produces a greater amount of drainage than does intermittent lumbar punctures. Additionally, if a stable rate of drainage can be achieved, this situation best simulates that of a permanent low-resistance shunt. We do not perform continous drainage in patients who are taking anticoagulants or antiplatelet agents. The physician may also wish to prescribe bedrest for the patient if the patient is thought to be at high risk for the accumulation of subdural hematomas on the basis of age, ventriculomegoly, or prior subdural hematoma. We

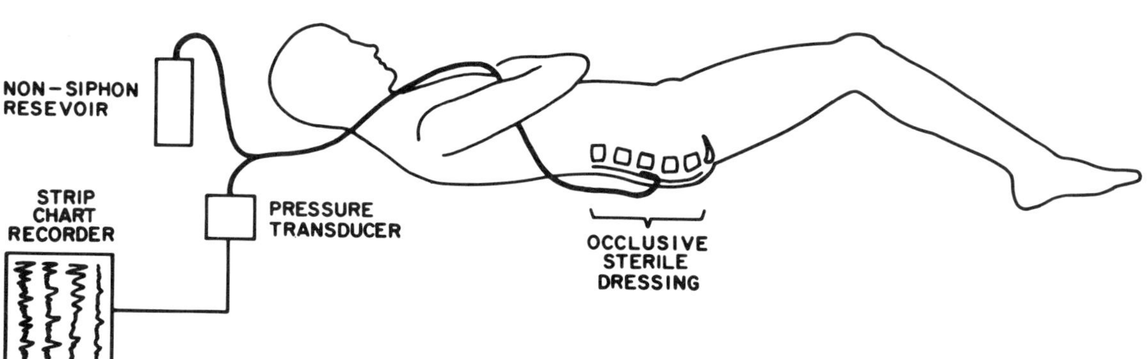

Figure 1 CFS pressure monitoring and continuous drainage system.

occlude the drainage system if the patient is to leave the general area of nursing observation for other diagnostic testing. We find that doing this decreases the likelihood of excessive CSF drainage. Similarly, we occlude the system if low-pressure headache occurs. The usual symptomatic presentation of this complication is position-dependent headache that is frequently located in the occiput and high neck regions. In order to avoid infection, the drainage period is kept as short as possible (2 to 5 days). Drainage is terminated when a clear-cut clinical improvement is demonstrated, particularly if it can be confirmed with some other diagnostic test such as posturography, gait assessment, or diagnostic urography. Similarly, temporary lumbar drainage is always discontinued if the patient develops fever or if inadvertent disconnection of the system occurs.

Pressure Monitoring

When the results of temporary CSF drainage are equivocal or when the value of a low-resistance shunting system is not clear, we recommend continuous evaluation of CSF pressure. This type of evaluation is performed in a monitoring environment where physicians and nurses are familiar with the maintenance and interpretation of intracranial pressure data. CSF pressure is monitored from either the cranial subarachnoid space or the lumbar subarachnoid space. In both situations, the dynamics of CSF pressure and its absolute magnitude are carefully validated before the period of monitoring. The absolute pressure is verified with a sterile, biologic calibration of the isovolumetric pressure transducer used for monitoring. After this calibration, in vivo recording of the CSF pulsatile wave form is performed. A dynamic response to cough and valsalva is demonstrated, and the Queckenstedt test is performed to demonstrate the elevation of cranial vault pressure with jugular venous compression. This maneuver assures that fluid coupling of the cranial CSF spaces and the lumbar space exists. These specific biologic maneuvers are repeated at the end of the monitoring period, as is the direct calibration of the pressure transducer. Thus the interpreter of the tracing can account for any system drift and/or catheter changes occurring over the monitored period that might alter interpretation of the data set.

The patient is then kept at bedrest but allowed to perform all regular activities of daily living from bed. The pressure transducer is maintained level with the head, using the external auditory meatus as a landmark. Simultaneous recording of chest wall motion and heart rate can be helpful in detecting artifactual changes in intracranial pressure. Pulse oximetry may be useful in identifying patients with sleep apnea. Careful attention is paid to the nocturnal record, and careful nursing annotation of the patient's sleeping behavior is made with the record. This trac-

ing is produced for every 24 hours that the patient is monitored. The recording can then be evaluated for intracranial pressure elevations, their frequency of occurrence, their duration, and the absolute magnitude of these elevations. This physiologic information is often highly useful to the neurosurgeon who must weigh the need to correct a low-pressure hydrocephalus against the risk of cerebral spinal fluid hypotension–induced complications such as low-pressure headache syndrome and subdural hematoma.

CSF Infusion Studies

CSF infusion studies can be performed with the use of a lumbar arachnoid catheter. These studies are performed by measuring the effect of continuous infusion of sterile saline on CSF pressure. A derived measure of CSF outflow resistance can be calculated and used as confirmatory evidence in favor of a CSF resorptive block. CSF outflow studies have the drawback of requiring infusion into the subarachnoid space with a concomitant increased likelihood of infection. However, unlike a test with more descriptive capabilities, such as cysternography, these studies do quantitate CSF resistance. Although we do not presently advocate infusion studies, some experienced clinicians find this information helpful for defining the nature of the hydrocephalic process.

SURGICAL DECISION

We recommend shunting for all individuals who show a clear history and examination consistent with normal-pressure hydrocephalus as well as evidence of the syndrome on anatomic and physiologic testing (Table 2). Our final criterion for recommending shunting is demonstrated improvement when the patient is receiving some form of temporary CSF drainage. Although we also perform shunting in individuals who have only historical and examination evidence of normal-pressure hydrocephalus, we believe that the addition of testing and a trial of drainage add significant certainty to this procedure for any individual patient. We believe that this degree of certainty is important, since shunt failure and shunt complications are, unfortunately, common events. We find it helpful in achieving patient and family cooperation when repeat surgery or

Table 2 Criteria for CSF Shunting

Positive history and examination
Communicating hydrocephalus
Impaired CSF flow
Improvement with trial lumbar drainage

revision of the surgical shunt is required. In these cases, prior demonstration of deficits that remitted with temporary drainage is helpful to all those involved in the decision making process. We believe that, in this setting, the optimal therapeutic result is more easily achieved.

Several different types of shunts can be used to achieve the same beneficial result. For patients with clear-cut elevations of intracranial pressure to 20 to 35 mm Hg, either a ventriculo-peritoneal or lumbo-peritoneal shunt can be used effectively. When CSF pressure is only moderately elevated to 15 to 20 mm Hg, the lumbo-peritoneal shunt may not be effective. The efficacy of this shunting system probably depends in part on the total amount of time the patient spends in the upright position, as CSF drainage is greatly improved when the patient maintains this position. For individuals with no elevation of CSF pressure or rare intermittent elevations in CSF pressure but who also have clear-cut improvement with trial CSF drainage, a ventriculo-peritoneal shunt with low outflow resistance is the shunting technique of preference.

SUGGESTED READING

Adams RD, Fisher CM, Hakim S, et al. Symptomatic occult hydrocephalus with "normal" cerebrospinal fluid pressure. N Engl J Med 1965; 273(3):117–126.

Black PMcL. Idiopathic normal-pressure hydrocephalus: results of shunting in 62 patients. J Neurosurg 1980; 52:371–377.

Graff-Radford NR, Godersky JC, Jones MP. Variables predicting surgical outcome in symptomatic hydrocephalus in the elderly. Neurology 1989; 39:1601–1604.

Haan J, Thomeer RTWM. Predictive value of temporary external lumbar drainage in normal pressure hydrocephalus. Neurosurgery 1988; 22:388–391.

Thomsen AM, Borgesen SE, Bruhn P, Gjerris F. Prognosis of dementia in normal pressure hydrocephalus after a shunt operation. Ann Neurol 1986; 20:304–310.

TOXIC DISEASE

ALCOHOL INTOXICATION AND WITHDRAWAL

ROBERT H. DAILEY, M.D.
IVAN DIAMOND, M.D., Ph.D.

ACUTE INTOXICATION

Ethanol is readily absorbed from the gastrointestinal tract and distributed throughout the body. There is no blood-brain barrier to ethanol, and uptake into the brain is limited only by blood flow and capillary perfusion. Therefore, within a short period after drinking, the concentration of alcohol in the brain is nearly identical to the level of ethanol in the blood. In nonalcoholics, symptoms of acute alcohol intoxication occur at blood levels ranging from 50 mg to 150 mg per 100 ml. The symptoms and signs of intoxication are easily recognized. Most individuals usually feel euphoric, lose social inhibitions, and exhibit expansive, sometimes garrulous behavior, while others become tearful, hostile, or even assaultive. Neurologic signs include slurred speech, mild truncal ataxia, increased reflexes, nystagmus, and impaired motor coordination and cognitive function. Signs of increased sympathetic activity include mydriasis, tachycardia, and skin flushing. Findings of central nervous system depression predominate at blood alcohol levels of 250 to 500 mg per 100 ml. With increasing intoxication, patients become lethargic with bradycardia, reduced blood pressure, and diminished respirations, sometimes complicated by vomiting and pulmonary aspiration. In nonalcoholics, fatalities are encountered at blood alcohol levels of approximately 500 mg per 100 ml, and are usually associated with hypotension and respiratory depression with ventilatory acidosis. In chronic alcoholics, however, the magnitude of increased tolerance to ethanol is not often appreciated, and the symptoms and signs of intoxication develop at higher blood alcohol levels. Indeed, some chronic alcoholics can even be sober at blood alcohol concentrations that are lethal in nonalcoholics.

Evaluation and Treatment

The extent of acute intoxication with alcohol depends not only on the quantity of alcohol consumed, but also on the rate of drinking, the amount of food in the stomach, gastric emptying, use of other drugs, and the underlying mental status of the patient. Therefore, appropriate evaluation of the intoxicated patient requires information regarding the degree of intoxication, complicating medical and psychiatric disorders, and the patient's social history. After medical examination, ambulatory patients with mild intoxication who are otherwise well may be discharged if accompanied by a reliable adult. However, patients with a history of repeated alcohol abuse or alcoholism require more complete medical and social evaluation and appropriate referral for follow-up care.

Severe alcohol intoxication is an indication for immediate medical attention. The stuporous patient, unable to ambulate safely, should be examined in an acute care facility, and a standardized approach should be followed. First, the patient's airway patency, adequacy of ventilation, and ability to handle secretions must be assessed. Marked hypoventilation, inability to handle secretions, and coma are all indications for endotracheal intubation with assisted ventilation and immediate admission to an intensive care unit. If vital signs are judged to be adequate, the patient is undressed completely, gowned, and a waist belt restraint applied to prevent falls. Pulse, blood pressure, respirations, and rectal temperature are measured, and a careful head-to-toe examination is performed to search for common associated abnormalities and to rule out lateralizing neurologic signs. The physician must observe the patient for symmetrical spontaneous motor activity, evaluate muscle tone and deep tendon reflexes, and determine plantar responses. The scalp must be inspected meticulously for abrasions and contusions, the pupils observed for inequalities and abnormal reactivity, extraocular movements must be observed, and the ears must be examined for hemotympanum. If focal abnormalities suggest serious intracranial injury, a computed tomographic (CT) scan should be done immediately to search for a subdural hematoma or other conditions constituting a neurosurgical emergency. The routine use of CT scans for patients with alcohol intoxication without other clinical indications is costly and not warranted.

If vital signs are normal, level of consciousness acceptable, and significant closed head injury ruled out by clinical examination, medical evaluation can proceed in a more leisurely manner. A complete physical examination should be performed, followed by an immediate effort to obtain information about the patient from other sources, including the patient's friends, relatives, personal physician, and hospital records. If reliable information is obtained quickly and there are no associated or complicating medical problems, the patient should be kept under observation until normal mental status returns as ethanol is metabolized. However, if the information obtained is inadequate, it is necessary to rule out or treat common conditions associated with acute alcohol intoxication and the complications of chronic alcohol abuse. A complete blood count and determinations of blood glucose, electrolytes, magnesium, phosphate, urea nitrogen, and arterial blood gases should be obtained. Hypokalemia, hypophosphatemia, and hypomagnesemia are commonly found. A serum ammonia can be measured if hepatic encephalopathy is a possibility. A bedside blood glucose (Visidex or Dextrostix) immediately rules out alcoholic hypoglycemia. Alternatively, 12.5 to 25 g of glucose ($\frac{1}{2}$ to 1 ampule of 50 ml of 50 percent glucose) may be given intravenously while one is awaiting the results of the blood glucose measurement. An intravenous infusion of 5 percent dextrose in $\frac{1}{2}$ normal saline ameliorates alcoholic ketoacidosis, and 100 mg thiamine must be given by intravenous "push" to prevent or treat acute Wernicke's encephalopathy.

If ethanol-induced coma is caused by massive proximate ingestion of alcohol, gastric lavage is indicated after endotracheal intubation. Charcoal does not absorb ethanol but may be useful for concomitant drug ingestion. Fructose and caffeine have little clinical value in the management of acute alcohol intoxication. Determining the blood alcohol level is useful if it is too low to account for the patient's obtundation. In that case, the physician must search for other causes of stupor. If obtundation presumed secondary to alcohol intoxication does not clear as expected, a CT scan and a toxic/metabolic evaluation is mandatory. Hemodialysis may be lifesaving if other toxins such as methanol are involved.

Chronic alcoholics who present with acute alcohol intoxication should be evaluated for commonly associated neurologic conditions, including seizures, dementia, Wernicke's disease, Korsakoff's disease, cerebellar degeneration, neuropathy, and alcoholic myopathy and cardiomyopathy. Usually such evaluation can be completed only when the patient has regained normal mental status and is able to walk without assistance. In addition, other medical complications such as gastritis, pancreatitis, alcohol hepatitis and cirrhosis, upper gastrointestinal bleeding, multiple vitamin and mineral deficiencies, and extracellular volume depletion also require medical attention. Hospitalization is necessary for any acute complication that cannot be resolved within a few hours in the emergency department. The disagreeable appearance and behavior of chronic alcoholics must not cause the physician to overlook serious medical disorders associated with alcohol abuse. These patients must not be prematurely discharged from acute care, and appropriate follow-up referrals to medical and social facilities must be arranged.

ALCOHOL WITHDRAWAL

Chronic alcoholics are physically dependent on ethanol and develop symptoms of ethanol withdrawal after a sudden decrease in drinking. It is clinically useful to divide the alcohol withdrawal syndrome into minor and major stages, and to consider alcohol withdrawal seizures separately.

Minor Alcohol Withdrawal Syndrome

The minor withdrawal syndrome develops approximately 5 to 8 hours after the last drink, often the morning after overnight abstinence ("morning shakes"). Tremulousness is the most characteristic early symptom, becoming most intense within 24 to 36 hours. Alcohol withdrawal tremor resembles an accentuated physiologic tremor and is generalized, coarse, and rapid. It is accompanied by signs of sympathetic autonomic hyperactivity including anxiety, arousal, sweating, facial flushing, mydriasis, tachycardia, and mild hypertension.

"Self-treatment" commonly consists of taking a "stiff drink" on arising in the morning, whereas medical management is aimed at controlling the manifestations of sympathetic nervous system hyperactivity. A variety of drugs used successfully include benzodiazepines, barbiturates, clonidine, chlormethiazole, carbamazepine, beta-adrenergic blockers, and calcium channel blockers. Benzodiazepines are the most widely used agents, and the frequency, amount, and route of administration is adjusted to the severity of symptoms. Mild tremulousness with few associated symptoms is treated with oral diazepam, 5 to 10 mg every 4 to 6 hours, as needed. If symptoms are severe enough to warrant parenteral treatment, 5 to 10 mg of diazepam is injected into the tubing of a rapidly infusing intravenous line over 1 to 2 minutes, and repeated at 3- to 5-minute intervals until adequate sedation is achieved. Unfortunately, diazepam is short-acting and must be given repeatedly; it should not be given intramuscularly because of poor absorption. Phenobarbital is also quite effective in controlling symptoms of minor withdrawal. Initially, 260 mg of phenobarbital is given intravenously over 1 to 2 minutes; 130 mg is then given at 15- to 30-minute intervals thereafter until relief of symptoms is achieved. Because phenobarbital has a longer half-life, patients who receive this drug do not need oral medication after leaving the acute care facility. Since patients undergoing alcohol withdrawal are markedly resistant to treatment with sedatives, frequent and high doses are often required to calm these patients. The physician should be comforted by the knowledge that oversedation and respiratory depression are dangerous complications only if drugs continue to be given *after* adequate relief of symptoms has been achieved. Thus the sometimes astronomically high doses that would ordinarily be dangerous in nonalcoholics are safe in alcoholics undergoing withdrawal. Vital sign or electrocardiographic monitoring is not necessary when mild sedation is used as an end-point of treatment.

Alcohol Withdrawal Seizures

Alcohol withdrawal seizures are estimated to occur in 5 to 33 percent of alcoholics. They are usually associated with a history of daily alcohol consumption, but 5 to 7 days of binge drinking may also end with convulsions. Generalized tonic-clonic seizures usually occur within 12 to 24 hours after cessation or reduction of ethanol consumption. Seizures are frequently multiple (1 to 6 in number), and 85 percent occur within the first 6 hours. Focal seizures occur in less than 5 percent of patients and should suggest an etiology other than alcohol withdrawal. Status epilepticus occurs in approximately 3 percent of patients, but alcohol withdrawal may account for approximately 15 percent of all patients who present with status epilepticus. The development of alcohol withdrawal seizures is often patient-specific; patients who have had seizures during alcohol withdrawal once are likely to have seizures again during another occurrence of alcohol withdrawal.

Most alcohol withdrawal seizures are brief and self-limited and do not require specific anticonvulsant therapy. Although some clinicians advocate the use of phenytoin, there is no evidence that phenytoin prevents withdrawal seizures. However, uncontrolled clinical experience suggests that phenobarbital or diazepam may be of value in treating the minor symptoms of alcohol withdrawal and alcohol withdrawal seizures. Status epilepticus caused by alcohol withdrawal is, of course, a medical emergency and should be treated with anticonvulsants in the same manner as status epilepticus of any other etiology. When chronic alcoholics present with either generalized seizures or status epilepticus, it is necessary to consider other treatable conditions for convulsions, such as meningitis, hypoglycemia, hyponatremia, other drug ingestions, and occult head trauma. While one is awaiting laboratory results, administering intravenous treatment with 100 mg of thiamine, 25 g of dextrose, and multivitamins is sensible.

Major Alcohol Withdrawal Syndrome (Delirium Tremens)

The presence of delirium tremens (DTs) is the most important feature of the major alcohol withdrawal syndrome and requires vigorous emergency treatment and hospitalization. Premonitory symptoms include insomnia, unpleasant dreams, and dysphoria. Approximately 16 percent of alcoholics become delirious within 2 to 5 days after alcohol withdrawal, and about one-third of these develop the syndrome of DTs. Widespread signs of autonomic sympathetic hyperactivity may persist but usually resolve within 72 hours after alcohol withdrawal. Patients exhibit global confusion and disorientation, distorted perceptions, disagreeable and threatening visual and auditory hallucinations, mumbling, and/or incoherent speech, tremor, agitated arousal, and restlessness with constant pulling at bedclothes and intravenous lines. These patients are terrified by their hallucinations and can be combative, destructive, and highly dangerous. They must have an intravenous line secured with multiple circumferential tapings of the looped intravenous tubing so that persistent aggressive attempts at its removal are thwarted. When delirium and hallucinations occur without sympathetic hyperactivity, it can be difficult to distinguish DTs from acute psychosis. However, in a chronic alcoholic undergoing withdrawal, the diagnosis is usually suggested by the evolution of symptoms. DTs must be differentiated from alcoholic hypoglycemia, overdose with anticholinergic agents, and intoxication with amphetamines, cocaine, and PCP. Other important conditions in the differential diagnosis include encephalitis, meningitis, thyrotoxicosis, and withdrawal from other sedatives. In these patients, the major threats to life include associated illness or injuries, hyperthermia, and dehydration with circulatory collapse.

The delirium and accompanying sympathetic manifestations of DTs are often quite severe and require vigorous treatment. A variety of sedatives, neuroleptics, and sympatholytic drugs have been administered to patients with DTs, usually in uncontrolled trials. Today the mainstay of therapy is benzodiazepines. We usually administer 5 to 10 mg of diazepam intravenously every 5 to 10 minutes until the patient is calm, then follow this with 5 to 10 mg every 1 to 2 hours as needed to control delirium and agitation. Special care must be taken to maintain fluid and electrolyte balance. Volume depletion accompanying DTs may cause circulatory collapse, and fluid losses may require replacement of 4 to 10 L during the first 24 hours.

WERNICKE'S ENCEPHALOPATHY

Acute Wernicke's encephalopathy is a complication of thiamine deficiency that occurs most commonly in alcoholics. The clinical syndrome includes ophthalmoplegia, ataxia, and a confusional state. Gaze-evoked horizontal nystagmus is the most frequent oculomotor abnormality, but many patients have bilateral asymmetric lateral rectus palsy. The gait disorder probably represents a combination of cerebellar ataxia, vestibular paresis, and peripheral neuropathy. The majority of patients have a global confusion marked by profound disorientation, indifference, and inattentiveness. Most patients are alert with impaired memory. A depressed level of consciousness occurs in less than 5 percent of patients.

Thiamine is the only effective agent for the treatment of Wernicke's disease. Patients should be hospitalized and treated intravenously with 100 mg thiamine daily for several days. Recovery usually begins promptly. Ophthalmoplegia begins to resolve during the 1st day; nystagmus, gait ataxia, and the global confusional state first show improvement within days to weeks.

LONG-TERM CONSIDERATIONS

Alcoholism cannot be treated in isolation from the patients' medical, behavioral, and socioeconomic problems, and patients must be referred to appropriate inpatient and outpatient detoxification and rehabilitation programs. Successful treatment usually requires the active participation of family members, friends, and peer group support. In addition, many patients and families find Alcoholics Anonymous and Al-Anon to be helpful.

SUGGESTED READING

Adinoff B, Bone GHA, Linnoila M. Acute ethanol poisoning and the ethanol withdrawal syndrome. Med Toxicol Adverse Drug Exp 1988; 3:172–196.

Diamond I, Charness ME. Alcohol toxicity. In: Diseases of the nervous system. Asbury AK, McKhann GM, McDonald WI, eds. Philadelphia: WB Saunders, 1986:1324.

Porter R, Mattson R, Cramer J, Diamond I, eds. Alcohol and seizures: basic mechanisms and clinical concepts. Philadelphia: FA Davis, (in press).

PATIENT RESOURCES

Literature

Hart S. Rehabilitation. New York: Harper & Row, 1988. (A comprehensive guide to recommended drug and alcohol treatment centers in the United States.)

Associations

Alcoholics Anonymous World Service (for alcoholics)
Al-Anon (for family members)
(Local chapters are usually listed in the White Pages of the phone book.)

DRUG OVERDOSE AND WITHDRAWAL

WALTER ROYAL III, M.D.

The use of addictive substances for recreational or therapeutic purposes frequently results in the development of drug tolerance, the requirement of higher doses to achieve a desired effect, or drug dependence, the occurrence of undesirable physical or psychological symptoms after withdrawal from the substance. Drug abuse has been defined as the use of a chemical substance for more than 1 month resulting in impairment of social or occupational functioning or both. This chapter discusses the various classes of sedative, stimulant, and hallucinogenic agents and the recognition and treatment of the associated toxic and withdrawal syndromes.

OPIATES

The opiod (or narcotic analgesic) drugs include morphine, its semisynthetic derivatives, and structurally distinct classes of synthetic drugs with morphinelike pharmacologic properties. The opiods possess tremendous addictive potential. Their extensive use in medical therapy often leads to variable degrees of physical and psychological dependence. In the general population overt abuse may occur with any of these medications. Heroin is the mainstay of illegal street drug trafficking predominantly in urban areas. It is generally mixed with quinine or sugars such as lactose and mannose, and this results in variability of the final concentration of active drug. Individual use may vary from occasional small doses resulting in mild intoxication to large amounts used several times daily. It is therefore difficult to estimate an individual's tolerance and the amount of heroin used by an addict.

The signs of opiod intoxication include hypotension, bradycardia, slurred speech, miosis, and respiratory depression. Seizures may occur secondary to the use of meperidine hydrochloride, despite significant tolerance, and they may be caused by the severe anoxia induced by overdose of this drug. The signs of overdose include pinpoint pupils that are nevertheless reactive, respiratory depression, and coma; pulmonary edema may also occur. Treatment consists of prompt administration of naloxone and appropriate support of respiration and circulatory function. Naloxone is most effective when administered intravenously at a dose of 0.4 mg every 3 to 10 minutes until there is a clinical response. It may also be administered intramuscularly or subcutaneously, thus increasing the duration of its action. Repeated doses are often necessary and continuous infusions occasionally required to prevent recurrence of symptoms of overdose since the half-life of naloxone is less than that of both heroin and methadone. Ventricular arrhythmias associated with naloxone administration have been reported, and caution should therefore be exercised in treating patients with cardiac disease. The most frequent side effect, however, is the precipitation of withdrawal symptoms in addicts and reversal of analgesia in individuals with a history of a pain syndrome.

With the possible exception of meperidine-related seizures, the opiod withdrawal syndrome, although dramatic, is not life-threatening. The approximate time of onset of abstinence symptoms after the last dose of an opiate drug has been taken is as follows: 2 to 4 hours for meperidine, 4 to 8 hours for heroin, and 12 to 48 hours for methadone. Early symptoms include drug craving, anxiety, anorexia, and insomnia with muscular irritability, diaphoresis, rhinorrhea, lacrimation, dilated pupils, and piloerection. Abdominal cramping, diarrhea, nausea, vomiting, fever, hypertension, tachycardia, and tachypnea may develop later.

The symptoms of the abstinence syndrome may be attenuated with methadone in an initial dose of 10 to 20 mg and thereafter in doses of 5 to 10 mg administered as often as four times per day, as needed. After stabilization has been achieved, the dose may be reduced by 10 to 25 percent daily, with the clinician continuing to follow signs of withdrawal. Although it is difficult to achieve this in practice, the duration of methadone treatment should be equal to the time usually taken for abstinence symptoms to abate (7 to 10 days for heroin and as long as 3 weeks for morphine).

Clonidine (0.1 to 0.2 mg twice per day) has also been used for treatment of acute symptoms of opiate withdrawal, although it may not be as effective as methadone in relieving insomnia and lacrimation. Bradycardia and hallucinations may develop with clonidine treatment, and abrupt discontinuation may precipitate hypomania. Clonidine should be used cautiously in patients who have been receiving tricyclic antidepressants chronically. The metha-

done congener L-alpha acetyl methadol (methadyl acetate, LAAM) may also be effective in the treatment of opiate withdrawal. Buprenorphine is a mixed agonist antagonist that may be as effective as methadone for treating abstinence, but with lower toxicity and abuse potential.

SEDATIVES AND HYPNOTICS

This group of drugs includes the barbiturates, the nonbarbiturate sedative-hypnotics, and the benzodiazepines. These drugs are cross-tolerant within the group and with ethanol. The signs of sedative-hypnotic overdose and withdrawal are also similar to those seen with ethanol, with the shorter-acting drugs causing more severe withdrawal symptoms. Except in the case of withdrawal from the benzodiazepines, fatalities due to respiratory depression caused by the withdrawal from sedatives and hypnotics are common. Mild intoxication may be associated with drowsiness, nystagmus, slurred speech, and ataxia. Hyporeflexia, respiratory depression, hypotension, confusion, stupor, and coma may be seen in patients with moderate to severe intoxication. In patients with acute intoxication, electroencephalography initially shows diffuse fast activity. With progression to coma, the fast activity may be followed by generalized slowing and intermittent or sustained isoelectric periods.

Several unique signs and symptoms may be caused by the nonbarbiturate sedative-hypnotics, including seizures (caused by methaqualone and glutethimide), pupillary abnormalities (dilated, unreactive pupils with glutethimide, pinpoint pupils with chloral hydrate), psychosis and myoclonus (caused by methaqualone), cardiovascular collapse (caused by methaqualone, methyprylon, ethchlorvynol), metabolic acidosis, gastric bleeding, and pulmonary damage (caused by paraldehyde), and muscle spasm, ileus, and bladder atony (caused by glutethimide).

Treatment consists of respiratory and circulatory support and removal of unabsorbed drug. Emesis may be induced if the patient is conscious, while one observes closely for progressive drowsiness and aspiration. Unabsorbed gastrointestinal contents should be removed by performing gastric lavage and administering a cathartic and activated charcoal. Excretion or removal of the drug may be accomplished with urinary alkalinization and forced diuresis or dialysis. Because of its effect on urinary output, dopamine is the preferred pressor when poisoning is the result of ingestion of medium or long-acting barbiturates. Central stimulants may precipitate seizures and should therefore be avoided.

The abstinence syndrome associated with the use of barbiturates may occur after either total drug withdrawal or reduction of the usual dose. It is the most lethal of all withdrawal syndromes, with the most severe abstinence syndromes occurring with the shorter-acting drugs. Tremulousness, weakness, nausea, vomiting, agitation, insomnia, anorexia, pupillary dilatation, tachycardia, tachypnea, and orthostatic hypotension may develop within hours after the last dose of a short-acting barbiturate is taken. Seizures may occur after 24 to 72 hours and are generally brief single or multiple episodes, and less frequently, may be status epilepticus. A syndrome similar to delirium tremens may appear after 2 to 5 days, with agitation, confusion, delusions, hallucinations and formication, hyperthermia, and circulatory collapse.

Mild withdrawal symptoms caused by discontinuation of any of the barbiturate and nonbarbiturate sedative-hypnotics may be treated with pentobarbital. If the administration of 200 mg of pentobarbital does not lead to signs of intoxication, then significant tolerance to the drug is likely. The occurrence of mild ataxia and nystagmus 1 hour after the 200-mg dose suggests a daily tolerance to 600 mg of pentobarbital. In general, for patients who are physically dependent on sedative-hypnotics, withdrawal symptoms may be controlled with a dose of 200 to 400 mg of pentobarbital administered every 4 to 6 hours, with the drug withheld to watch for signs of intoxication. After 2 or 3 days, the drug may be tapered by 100 mg per day or in decrements of 10 percent of the initial dose or as tolerated.

Pentobarbital may also be used to treat hallucinations and delirium tremens. The latter is a medical emergency, and patients should be treated aggressively to control fever (exclude infection), fluid and electrolyte balance, and cardiac and renal status. Withdrawal seizures may be treated acutely with benzodiazepines such as diazepam (5 to 10 mg) or lorazepam (2 to 4 mg) while the clinician carefully monitors for hypotension and respiratory depression. It may be necessary to treat severe seizures with more than 1 g of phenobarbital.

Withdrawal of antianxiety doses of benzodiazepines has been associated with increased anxiety, depersonalization, visual disturbances, tinnitus, paresthesias, and muscle twitching. Disorientation and psychotic reactions as well as seizures have occurred after discontinuation of high doses of these drugs.

STIMULANTS

In cases of acute overdose of stimulants, there is a marked clinical presentation of prominent stimulatory effects on both the central and peripheral nervous systems, which these drugs produce. Included in this category of drugs are several sympathomimetics, such as amphetamine (Benzedrine), dextroamphetamine (Dexedrine), methamphetamine (Desoxyn or "speed"), and phenmetrazine (Preludin), as well as cocaine and its alkaloid derivative, "crack." All of these drugs produce an intense "rush" when used intravenously. The amphetamines are also taken orally. Cocaine is ineffective when taken orally but is effective when used intranasally, intravenously, or smoked ("free-based"). Crack is also smoked and has a profound effect that occurs within seconds, lasts for a few minutes, and is followed by a rapid and extremely unpleasant "crash." This results in an intense craving and is the reason for remarkably high addictive potential that is associated with crack.

The symptoms of amphetamine intoxication include a sense of well-being, elation, agitation, and occasionally aggressive, violent behavior. These symptoms may occur in association with hypertension, tachycardia, mydriasis, anorexia, insomnia, nausea, and vomiting. Stereotyped and repetitive movements may be seen as well. Severe overdose may be associated with cardiac arrythmia, high fever, delirium, hallucinations, seizures, coma, and death. Similar symptoms may also occur with cocaine intoxication, as may cardiac arrhythmias, myocardial infarction, and potentially fatal seizures.

Agitation caused by mild to moderate intoxication may be managed by the administration of benzodiazepines. Haloperidol may be administered in doses of 5 to 10 mg for patients with more severe overdose; however, it may also lower the seizure threshold. Because of the violent behavior sometimes induced by overdose of these drugs, patients may need to be restrained. To enhance excretion of the drug, the urine should be acidified to maintain a pH of 4 to 5.

Prolonged parenteral administration of large doses of stimulant or "runs" may be followed by sleep that may last for several days and severe depression, which may respond to treatment with antidepressants.

HALLUCINOGENS

Hallucinogens cause a wide range of effects, ranging from a mild euphoric state to marked modification of perception. Included in this category of drugs are lysergic acid diethylamide (LSD), dimethyltryptamine (DMT), 2,5-dimethoxy-4-methlyamphetamine (DOM or STP), trimethoxytryptamine (TMA), psilocybin, mescaline, phencyclidine (PCP), thiocyclodine (TCP) delta-9-tetrahydrocannabinol (THC), and marijuana (cannabis). The effects of these drugs begin several minutes to 1 hour after these substances have been taken, with individuals experiencing a euphoric or an altered perceptual state. Variable degrees of tolerance occur with the use of these drugs. With the exception of cannabis, which contains the active ingredient delta-

9-tetrahydrocannabinol, the drugs of this class have been associated with marked alteration of states of consciousness and behavior.

LSD, DOM, DMT, TMA, mescaline, and psilocybin may cause marked perceptual distortion, tachycardia, dilated and reactive pupils, tremor, hyperreflexia, piloerection, and incoordination. Acute intoxication may be managed by "talking down" (i.e., calming) the patient or with benzodiazepines or haloperidol. Overdoses are not known to be directly fatal. Slight tolerance may develop, and after abstaining from taking the drug, persistent anxiety, depression, or delusions may occur and persist for variable lengths of time. "Flashbacks," or brief hallucinations, may occur for weeks to years after a period of drug use.

PCP in low doses causes a sensation of numbness, emotional lability, and euphoria or dysphoria. High doses cause symptoms ranging from anxiety, confusion, and distorted perception and sensations, to rigidity, paranoid psychosis, a catatonic-like state, seizures, coma, and death. Toxicity may also result in hepatic necrosis, myoglobinuria, and severe hypertension that develops several days after the use of the drug. Treatment consists of continuous gastric suctioning, blood pressure control, and in the absence of myoglobinuria, urine acidification. If necessary, agitation may be acutely controlled with haloperidol, using caution since this may precipitate the neuroleptic malignant syndrome. Benzodiazepines may be subsequently administered intravenously. Patients should be placed in an environment with minimal external stimulation. The symptoms of acute toxicity usually clear within 3 to 6 hours, although the psychosis may last for weeks. In some cases, long-term abnormalities of speech and memory may occur.

THC may be smoked or ingested and commonly causes dry mouth, increased appetite, conjunctival injection, and tachycardia. Individuals using this drug may complain of significant anxiety or depression, a psychosis may occur at high doses. A significant degree of tolerance may develop. No specific abstinence syndrome has been identified for this drug.

INHALANTS

A common practice among older children and adolescents is the inhalation of vapors of various substances. Among the substances abused in this manner are glues, plastic and rubber cements, fingernail polish remover, furniture polish, lacquers, enamels, cleaning fluid, and gasoline. The symptoms commonly include mild euphoria, confusion, disorientation, and ataxia but may progress to develop into delirious or psychotic behavior, seizures, and coma. In general, the effects of acute intoxication resolve after several hours to days. However, damage may occur to the kidney, liver, and bone marrow which, in addition to cardiac arrhythmias, aspiration, and asphyxia, may result in death. There has been no abstinence syndrome associated with inhalant abuse.

Treatment consists of appropriate supportive measures to control impulsive behavior or neurologic or cardiac complications. A hematologic profile, determinations of electrolytes, blood urea nitrogen (BUN), creatinine, and urinary sediment, chest x-ray examination, and electrocardiography should be performed to search for specific organ damage.

SUGGESTED READING

Gossop M. Clonidine and the treatment of opiate withdrawal syndrome. Drug Alcohol Depend 1988; 21:253–259.
Millman RB. Evaluation and clinical management of cocaine abusers. Clin Psychiatry 1989; 49:27–33.

PATIENT RESOURCES

For information about drugs, drug use, and abuse:

National Clearing-House for Alcohol and Drug Information
P.O. Box 2345
Rockville, Maryland 20852
Telephone: (301) 468-2600

For information concerning treatment centers located throughout the United States:

National Institute on Drug Abuse
Treatment and Referral Hotline
1-800-662-HELP

NEUROLEPTIC TOXICITY

JOSEPH H. FRIEDMAN, M.D.

The term "neuroleptic" is generally used to refer to antipsychotic drugs. These medications, which include haloperidol (Haldol), chlorpromazine hydrochloride (Thorazine), thioridazine (Mellaril), trifluoperazine hydrochloride (Stelazine), are among the most prescribed drugs in the United States. They are useful in controlling most psychotic behavior disorders, including schizophrenia, organic mental syndromes, and mania, among others. These drugs all share the similar pharmacologic mechanism of blocking dopamine receptors. Because the neuroleptic complications of these drugs are shared by medications that block dopamine receptors but which lack antipsychotic properties, such as the gastrointestinal motility drug metoclopramide and the antiemetics prochlorperazine and droperidol, this chapter discusses all dopamine-blocking drugs.

Certain adverse effects of these drugs are not usually considered "neurologic" problems and therefore will only be mentioned. These include the elevation of prolactin levels causing gynecomastia, galactorrhea, and irregular menses; sleepiness; dry mouth; miosis, mydriasis; and orthostatic hypotension.

These drugs have a very wide spectrum of neurologic adverse effects. The easiest way to categorize these effects is to divide them into the following three groups, based on the time of their onset: (1) those occurring within minutes to a few days, (2) those occurring after a few days, and (3) those occurring after 3 months or more. Within this broad classification, there is overlap, so that reactions usually seen early may occur after several months. It is important to keep in mind that virtually all neuroleptic-induced disorders were described in psychiatric patients long before the medications were developed. It is also crucial to recall that most patients require the antipsychotic drugs that they are prescribed. Clinical interpretations and decision making are frequently complicated by the patient's mental status. Patients are occasionally caught in the middle between the neurologist who wants to discontinue a drug and the psychiatrist who believes the patient requires the neuroleptic for psychosis control.

The first side effects to occur are usually akathisia and acute dystonia.

ACUTE DYSTONIA

Acute dystonia generally occurs within the first hours to days of use of a neuroleptic but may occur after long-term drug use, generally following a dose increase or a change from one drug to another. These patients are not commonly seen by neurologists as they are either treated by a psychiatrist or are seen in the emergency room. To the physician without prior experience with acute dystonia, the syndrome may seem bizarre. To the patient, the syndrome is extremely uncomfortable and embarrassing.

There is a wide range of acute dystonic reactions. Most patients experience involuntary jaw and tongue movements. Oculogyric crisis, a syndrome in which the eyes are forced up and (usually) to one side, is also common. Acute torticollis and axial and limb dystonias are less common but may occur. Jaw and tongue dystonia may interfere with speech. I have seen an elderly man with severe generalized stiffness as an acute dystonic reaction, but believe that this is rare.

Patients frequently overcome the dystonia and eye movement disorder with effort, but as their concentration wanes, the dystonia returns. Although the movements may be merely painful or simply uncomfortable, they are often extremely threatening to the patient suffering from acute dystonia for the first time. This is especially true if it occurs in the context of treatment for acute psychosis.

My personal experience has involved mainly those patients who do not have psychiatric disorders. Some have experimented with a friend's pills (or perhaps bought them on the street) and some have taken anti-emetics or metoclopramide. Significantly, these patients often adamantly deny having taken any pills at all until finally they admit having taken the medication of a friend or relative to ease some somatic complaint. When prescribing anti-emetics and metoclopramide, physicians often fail to warn patients of this potential side effect.

Treatment of acute dystonia is uniformly excellent. Diphenhydramine (Benadryl) in a dose of 50 mg administered intravenously usually aborts the syndrome completely within 2 to 5 minutes. Benztropine in a dose of 1 mg administered intravenously works equally well and is less sedating. Benztropine may also be given intramuscularly when the intravenous route is unavailable, but the response will be delayed. The decision of whether to continue treatment after the first episode of acute dystonia depends on the continued use of the offending agent. If the neuroleptic drug is needed, the patient should receive benztropine, 1 to 2 mg by mouth three times daily, for a few weeks. The anticholinergic should then be tapered and discontinued. If the offending drug can be safely discontinued, I recommend treating the patient with an oral preparation of whichever medication was successful when given intravenously. Thus if diphenhydramine was given intravenously, I would treat the patient with 25 mg by mouth three times daily for 2 to 3 days. Obviously, if a depot neuroleptic was given, prophylactic treatment of acute dystonia should be maintained longer.

AKATHISIA

The term "akathisia" stems from the Greek phrase meaning "not to sit." It refers to a syndrome of restlessness that, when severe, makes it uncomfortable for an affected individual to remain seated for more than a few seconds. It is occasionally present in Parkinson's disease but most commonly occurs with neuroleptic use. Because it is so dysphoric, it is believed to be a major reason for drug noncompliance. It usually begins within minutes to a few days of either the initiation of treatment using a neuroleptic or a dose increase. The patient feels a subjective restlessness that forces him to move and to remain moving. It is unpleasant and described as a foreign, irresistible force taking over one's body. It is difficult to interpret the signs and symptoms of this syndrome if the patient is also psychotic or confused.

Two examples at opposite ends of the spectrum illustrate the condition. A 20-year-old man was hospitalized after a suicide attempt. He was initially believed to be psychotic and was treated with a major neuroleptic. Within a few days, his psychosis resolved but he became restless, unable to remain seated during ward meetings or while watching television programs. He carried a towel with him during the day to wipe off the sweat produced by his constant pacing, jumping jacks, and other calisthenics. His psychiatrist thought he was "acting out" to gain attention. The patient told me he could not sleep and was losing weight because he could not stop moving. His examination revealed very mild parkinsonism, yet he could not sit still. While talking he would stand up, sit down, stand, and do jumping jacks, while apologizing for his abnormal conduct. He was treated with benztropine, 2 mg three times daily; within 2 days his condition improved and he was discharged.

The second patient was a 75-year-old man who had been hospitalized for abdominal pain. The first night he became mildly confused and was given haloperidol. Shortly thereafter he became mildly agitated, was given more haloperidol, and eventually was prescribed a standing haloperidol order because of persistent restlessness that had not been present on admission. His abdominal pain resolved for unexplained reasons, and he was sent home and continued to receive the neuroleptic. When I saw him 3 months later, he had moderate parkinsonism and severe restlessness that was making him and his family miserable. He needed to stand every minute or so while I interviewed him, and he apologized profusely for his inability to control his bizarre behavior. His haloperidol was discontinued. Benztropine, 2 mg three times daily, was begun and within a few days he felt considerably better. Within 2 weeks he was virtually normal. Eventually the benztropine was discontinued as well.

Akathisia can be difficult to recognize, especially in the context of severe psychosis. The hallmark of acute akathisia is the inability to stand in one place. Patients tend to march in place or constantly shift weight from one foot to another. When seated, they tend to cross their legs one way and then the other, tap their feet and lift themselves off the chair. Like most syndromes, akathisia has a wide clinical spectrum so that the observer has to be alert for these signs. The patient may complain of a restlessness that arises in the legs rather than in the mind and a compulsion to move. Moving, however, provides relief only during the act of moving so that the compulsion to move recurs immediately on resting. When the patient is severely psychotic and agitated, interpretation of a hyperactive state must depend on an assessment of the change in the patient's level of activity since the introduction of the new drug. When an antipsychotic agent has produced the paradoxical response of heightened rather than lessened activity, akathisia should be strongly considered.

Unfortunately, akathisia is not always easy to treat. When it arises early during drug treatment (late onset akathisia is discussed later in this chapter, in the section on Tardive Syndromes), discontinuing the offending agent cures the akathisia, although there may be a lag time of 2 to 4 weeks. More commonly, the neuroleptic cannot be discontinued. In these cases, I recommend that the neuroleptic be switched from one class of antipsychotics to another—e.g., from a butyrophenone to a phenothiazine or thioxanthene. In addition, the patient should begin receiving symptomatic therapy for the akathisia. Recent literature suggests that propanolol is the drug of choice when administered in low doses (propanolol, 20 mg three times daily). My own experience with propanolol has been limited but disappointing. When akathitic patients have signs of parkinsonism, anticholinergic agents such as benztropine, 1 to 2 mg three times daily, and trihexyphenidyl hydrochloride, 2 to 5 mg three times daily, are very effective. These should be continued at the maximum dosage for at least 1 week before the treatment can be called a failure and a new medication tried. If the anticholinergic is successful, it should be continued while the neuroleptic is continued. After the patient has been clinically stable for several weeks, the anticholinergic may be tapered and discontinued. When parkinsonism is not present, treatment is often unsatisfactory. I generally start treatment with benztropine (2 mg three times daily for a young patient and 1 mg three times daily in an older patient). In an older patient, I increase the dose to 2 mg three times daily after 1 to 2 days. I continue to administer this dose for 1 week and then switch to propanolol, 20 mg three times daily, if treatment with the anticholinergic fails. If propanolol, 20 mg three times daily, is not helpful after 1 day of its use, it should be increased to 120 mg daily (one dose of the long-acting form or 40 mg three times daily). After 3 to 5 days I would discontinue the propanolol and try first amantadine hydrochloride, 100 mg twice daily for 3 to 5 days and then diphenhydramine hydrochloride, 50 mg three times daily. As interventions fail, strong consideration should be given to discontinuing the use of the offending neuroleptic.

NEUROLEPTIC MALIGNANT SYNDROME

The neuroleptic malignant syndrome (NMS) is certainly the worst of the possible toxic effects of neuroleptics and is quite accurately named. The onset of NMS varies from days to months after the initiation of treatment using a neuroleptic, but has been reported to occur from minutes to years after drug inception. In any patient receiving a neuroleptic this diagnosis must be considered when fever, stiffness, or mental status changes are present. Making a confident diagnosis, however, may be difficult. The syndrome is most easily recognized when fullblown, at which time symptoms of high fever (temperatures greater than 104°F being common), severe rigidity, autonomic instability, and mental status impairment are seen. Supporting features are an elevated creatine phosphokinase (CPK) levels (in the absence of trauma), severe tachypnea (without lung or cardiac disease), and a leukocytosis. The problem with diagnosis, however, is the marked variability of the signs. The fever may be mild (around 101°F), there may be other extrapyramidal signs such as dystonia or tremor (usually in addition to rigidity), and the mental impairment ranges from mild confusion to obtundation. In addition, not all of the features are necessarily present. The common belief that CPK must be elevated is incorrect, as is the belief that an elevated CPK level in a patient treated with neuroleptics is tantamount to a diagnosis. The cardinal features of the NMS are fever, severe extrapyramidal signs, and autonomic instability for which there are no other explanations in a patient treated with neuroleptics.

In young, healthy patients, these changes, which develop over hours, are easier to recognize than they are in debilitated and confused nursing home patients. The problems arising in diagnosis are major. Fever may be caused by infection that can cause diaphoresis and tachypnea in any individual, young or old. Because the patient is receiving a neuroleptic to treat a mental derangement, assessment of mental status is difficult, especially if the patient has not been evaluated previously. Obtundation or total indifference might simply be due to high fever or other systemic "toxicity"; stiffness

might be caused by drug-induced parkinsonism or acute dystonia, especially in the elderly, who are quite sensitive to these drugs. Even the supportive laboratory data of an elevated CPK level may be caused by unrecorded intramuscular injections or trauma. Mildly elevated CPK has been a common finding in psychotic patients who have no evidence of NMS. A leukocytosis is usually present in patients who have bacterial infections or who are under extreme stress.

Two cases I saw recently illustrate the pitfalls in diagnosis. A 75-year-old man with known mild dementia taking thioridazine was seen in the emergency room with severe stiffness, a temperature of 101°F, worsened mental status, elevated blood pressure, and mild tachypnea. NMS was strongly entertained, but the possibility of infection and a generalized acute dystonic reaction was also considered. An intravenous push of 1 mg of benztropine produced improvement of the rigidity within minutes, and pneumonia was found when the patient was able to cooperate enough to undergo a chest x-ray examination. A second case involved a 27-year-old man with advanced Huntington's disease who had a seizure disorder and in whom haloperidol had been discontinued. At the nursing home he developed a temperature of 107°F with severe stiffness, diaphoresis, tachypnea, and bilateral muscle jerks without loss of consciousness. His baseline severe dysarthria made mental evaluation difficult. At the time of his arrival in the emergency room, he was found to have myoclonic seizures (rather than rigors), which later generalized. These findings explained his fever, stiffness, and elevated CPK level.

The essential point is that NMS must be considered in the differential diagnosis of any patient treated with neuroleptics who has stiffness, fever, and an altered mental status. Because NMS is rare, the diagnosis is ultimately infection in most cases. It must be pointed out, however, that untreated NMS is frequently fatal. The treatment of choice is bromocriptine administered in a dose of 5 to 15 mg three times daily and increased as needed. Unfortunately, because this drug must be administered orally, a nasogastric tube may be necessary. A combination of carbidopa and levodopa (Sinemet) has also been found to be effective, but there is less experience with this medication than with bromocriptine. Concerns regarding an increase in psychosis with the use of bromocriptine have not been substantiated in practice. Mental state improves as the physical signs of NMS improve. Dantrolene appears to be less effective because it works peripherally by interfering with muscle contraction and not in the brain, where the problem is. Patients have been reported who remain febrile or confused when treated with dantrolene alone. Bromocriptine doses should be decreased slowly, as tolerated, several days after returning to the baseline and then discontinued. Too rapid a taper may result in recurrence of the NMS. The initial dosing of bromocriptine depends on the severity of the condition. In severely ill patients, a high dose of 15 mg three times daily can be given. Since the action of the drug is slow and improvement may take several hours or more, attention must be given to other potential explanations of the febrile syndrome, particularly infection. Appropriate evaluation and treatment must be administered for these as well.

Fulminant NMS can occur over hours with such severe stiffness that respiration is compromised. Rhabdomyolosis occurs with fulminant NMS and may cause renal failure. Temperatures can be high enough to cause heat stroke. For patients with this syndrome, I recommend very early paralyzation and simultaneous treatment with bromocriptine. Paralysis allows easy ventilation and aborts the stiffness, thus reducing the fever which was generated by the muscle contraction.

PARKINSONISM

Drug-induced parkinsonism generally occurs days or weeks after the patient begins treatment with a neuroleptic. While certain medications, such as thioridazine and molindone are less prone to cause this than higher-potency drugs such as haloperidol, all neuroleptics can cause this syndrome. In evaluating any individual with parkinsonism who is taking a neuroleptic, one must strongly consider the diagnosis of the reversible, drug-induced syndrome, rather than the idiopathic variety of parkinsonism. In elderly patients receiving a low dose of a neuroleptic, idiopathic Parkinson's disease may be unmasked prematurely. In this case, the patient's condition improves when the drug is discontinued, only to worsen several months later as the idiopathic Parkinson's disease progresses.

There are three major facts that one must bear in mind in approaching drug-induced parkinsonism. The first is that neuroleptic-induced parkinsonism is always reversible. Unlike the postencephalitic and MPTP-induced syndromes, which cause neuronal death, neuroleptic-induced parkinsonism arises as a result of temporary, albeit long-lived, dopamine receptor blockade. Thus drug-induced parkinsonism always resolves when the offending agent is discontinued. The second fact to keep in mind is that neuroleptic drugs are extremely lipophilic and last much longer in the brain than is reflected by their serum half-lives. Once the drug is discontinued, the duration of the parkinsonism depends on the total dose, the nature of the drug (i.e., long-acting depot versus oral preparations), and the age of the patient. Parkinsonism may persist for as long as 18 months after the last dose of neuroleptic. Finally one must note that despite the theory that schizophrenia represents

a dopamine excess condition and parkinsonism represents a dopamine-depleted state, neither disease offers protection against the development of the other. Presumably the dopaminergic lesions are in different brain locations.

The clinical appearance of neuroleptic parkinsonism cannot be distinguished from the idiopathic variety of parkinsonism. Patients generally become akinetic, with a stooped posture and reduced armswing when walking. Resting tremor and rigidity are common. In general, the severity of neuroleptic parkinsonism is less than that of idiopathic parkinsonism, but this simply reflects the younger age of most of the patients with neuroleptic parkinsonism as well as the dose of the drug. As in idiopathic Parkinson's disease, tremor may or may not be present and is variably responsive to medication. Manifestations may be asymmetric. When used in high doses, neuroleptics can cause severe, debilitating parkinsonism. This can be a diagnostic challenge for the physician faced with a psychotic individual who has received high doses of a neuroleptic at one or more institutions and then was evaluated at yet another institution for possible catatonia. Often one can make the diagnosis by talking to the patient. If the patient is still highly psychotic or mute, however, one may be forced to treat empirically. Because parkinsonism responds more easily than catatonia, it should be treated first.

Most patients with neuroleptic-induced parkinsonism respond well to anticholinergic drugs such as benztropine, trihexiphenidyl hydrochloride, and procyclidine, or they may respond well to amantadine. For young patients, I recommend administering trihexiphenidyl hydrochloride in an initial dose of 2 mg three times daily or benztropine in an initial dose of 1 mg three times daily, and then if required after a few days, increasing the dose to 5 mg three times daily (trihexiphenidyl) or to 2 mg three times daily (benztropine). When these higher doses are inadequate, I add amantadine, 100 mg twice daily. These medications are much better tolerated in the young psychiatric population than in the older population with idiopathic Parkinson's disease. There is little problem with associated confusion or hallucinations. Usually there is no difficulty in continuing to administer the neuroleptic while these medications are added. However, if the parkinsonism is debilitating, the neuroleptic must be discontinued. On rare occasions, Sinemet or bromocriptine needs to be added. Because few patients are treated with both a neuroleptic and Sinemet or bromocriptine, little is known about it. My personal experience is that these medications can be helpful in treating parkinsonism.

In the elderly demented patient with drug-induced parkinsonism, the risks of anticholinergic side effects and the adverse effects of amantadine are significant. Sometimes the parkinsonism may need to be tolerated in order for behavior to be controlled. Obviously drugs such as thioridazine hydrochloride and molindone (which are associated with the least risk of induced parkinsonism) should be used whenever possible.

TARDIVE SYNDROMES

Although tardive dyskinesia is a well-known syndrome, physicians often do not realize that the classic oral-facial-lingual-buccal dyskinetic movements represent only one of several different syndromes associated with chronic exposure to dopamine-blocking drugs. The duration of drug exposure required to produce a tardive syndrome is unclear. Authors in the field generally consider 3 months as the minimum, but this is mainly for purposes of definition in performing clinical studies.

Tardive dyskinesia generally involves the structures in and around the mouth (tongue, lips, jaw) and, to a lesser extent, the face. Its onset is insidious and is generally masked by the very drugs that originally caused the syndrome. The movements may involve any collection of writhing tongue movements, lip puckering (the "bon-bon" sign), and various jaw movements (lateral, chewing, thrusting), blinking, frowning, and eyebrow raising, among others. Tardive dyskinesia is not limited to the face. Hands, feet, and axial structures may also be involved, but this is less common. It is also easier for patients to mask the appendicular movements by incorporating involuntary arm movements into voluntary gestures such as stroking one's hair or rubbing one's face. As with most involuntary movement disorders, severity worsens with stress, improves with relaxation, and resolves during sleep.

Although there are many speculations in the literature on risk factors for tardive dyskinesia, such as age, sex, type of drug used, duration of drug exposure, neurologic impairment, and psychiatric diagnosis, only two facts need to be recalled. Anyone can develop tardive dyskinesia and it can be permanent. Older individuals are more susceptible and are less likely to go into remission when the drug is withdrawn. Approximately 60 percent of older patients and 40 percent of younger patients receiving chronic neuroleptics develop tardive dyskinesia, and of these, approximately half appear to have this on a permanent basis. The permanency of the tardive dyskinesia may depend on the duration of drug exposure and the duration of the tardive dyskinesia prior to drug discontinuation.

Few cases of tardive dyskinesia require therapy. In fact, in most instances, patients are unaware of involuntary movements. When tardive dyskinesia requires intervention, reserpine is my first choice. This agent acts by depleting catecholamines, thus masking the movements, but unlike the neurolep-

tics, does not itself cause tardive dyskinesia. Reserpine therefore is used for symptomatic purposes, while the tardive dyskinesia either resolves on its own or persists, masked in part by this drug, but is not worsened during the therapy.

Tardive akathisia is a form of restlessness whose time course is similar to that of other forms of tardive dyskinesia. It may be a persistent form of an akathisia that appeared early in treatment, or it may arise later in the course of drug treatment. It is usually associated with a choreoathetoid movement disorder. Deciding whether movements of the legs are adventitious or an akathitic response to an inner sense of restlessness is difficult if the patient is not compensated enough mentally to provide reliable information. The treatment of tardive akathisia with slowly increasing doses of reserpine is generally quite effective. My own experience has been that beta-blockers and anticholinergics are not useful in the treatment of this disorder. I recommend administering reserpine in an initial dose of 0.1 mg three times daily and increasing this dose by 0.1 mg every 3 to 5 days while monitoring symptoms of hypotension.

Tardive dystonia is a persistent form of dystonia arising after months or years of neuroleptic use. Although initial reports described this syndrome as unresponsive to therapy, this probably reflected the severity of the cases recognized. The persistent form of dystonia, unlike the acute form, does not involve oculogyric crises, but does usually involve the neck, causing some form of torticollis. Limbs may also be involved. Blepharospasm may occur, as may even action-induced dystonia. I consider dystonia a much more ominous sign than oral-facial dyskinesias. Patients are aware of their dystonia and are troubled by it. Secondly, it may become debilitating. In this case, I attempt discontinuing neuroleptics, if at all possible, or reducing the dosage. The usual treatment consisting of a slow titration upward of an anticholinergic is then begun. Sometimes simply discontinuing the neuroleptic improves the patient's condition. When treatment is unsuccessful or if neuroleptic use is probably going to be required for a long time, patients should be treated with clozapine. The "atypical neuroleptics" are not associated with extrapyramidal side effects and thus do not cause worsening of the dystonia.

Other movement disorders that may occur with chronic neuroleptic use include, among others, tics and Gilles de La Tourette syndrome. Not infrequently, patients have complex mixtures of these syndromes (e.g., a combination of choreoathetosis, dystonia, akathisia, and tics). Treatment approaches should be aimed at the symptoms that bother the patient most, and as always, attempts should be made to discontinue the neuroleptic. It is sometimes helpful to counsel other treating physicians and medical personnel that these movements are both involuntary and iatrogenic. Occasionally patients with unusual movement disorders are believed to be "acting out" and performing their repertoire of adventitious movements deliberately. These patients are then doubly punished; they suffer from an iatrogenic problem and then are blamed for it.

SUGGESTED READING

Fahn S. A therapeutic approach to tardive dyskinesia. J Clin Psychiatry 1985; 46:19–24.
Mueller PS. Neuroleptic malignant syndrome. Psychosomatics 1985; 26:654–662.
Fahn S, Marsden CD. The treatment of dystonia. In: Marsden CD, Fahn S, eds. Movement disorders. Vol. 2. Boston: Butterworth Publishers, 1987:359.
Hardie RJ, Lees AJ. Neuroleptic-induced Parkinson's syndrome: clinical features and results of treatment with levodopa. J Neurol Neurosurg Psychiatry 1988; 51:850–854.

PATIENT RESOURCES

A tardive dyskinesia and tardive dystonic foundation is being established in Seattle, Washington but is not yet organized.

Dystonia Clinical Research Center
Box 22
710 West 168th Street
New York, New York 10032

National Mental Health Association
1021 Prince Street
Alexandria, Virginia 22314-2971
Telephone: (703) 684-7722

National Association of Protection and Advocacy Systems
220 I Street N.E.
Suite 150
Washington, DC 20001
Telephone: (202) 546-8202

METABOLIC DISEASE

INHERITED NEURODEGENERATIVE DISEASES OF CHILDHOOD

SAKKUBAI NAIDU, M.B., B.S.

Because of the rapid advances in the recognition, genetics, and treatment of inborn errors of metabolism, it is essential that practicing physicians be able to recognize these diseases. The significance of a precise diagnosis cannot be overemphasized. Some of these disorders are becoming medically treatable, and mental retardation may be reduced or prevented by simple means such as the use of dietary restriction in phenylketonuria (PKU) and galactosemia. Moreover, carrier detection and prenatal diagnosis are now often feasible. Unfortunately, different metabolic conditions can present with similar clinical manifestations because common neuroanatomic areas are involved. For example, the metabolic disorders homocystinuria and Marfan syndrome with ectopia lentis may show the same clinical manifestations despite their having different biochemical defects, or similar chemical abnormalities may manifest as totally different phenotypes (e.g., elevated very long chain fatty acids [VLCFA] in patients with generalized peroxisomal diseases and the X-linked form of adrenoleukodystrophy). The clinician must first ascertain the presence of a progressive neurologic or dementing disease and then consider the biochemical, radiologic, or neurophysiologic tests that are most appropriate. New diseases and variants of known diseases are reported at a faster rate than can be assimilated. In my own experience, I have been surprised by positive test results when they were least expected.

The clinical manifestations can be protean, particularly in the neonate, where poor feeding and lethargy, for example, are often mistaken for neonatal sepsis. Infants with metabolic disease may become debilitated and develop infection. Metabolic diseases can be ruled out by laboratory tests. Sometimes simple screening tests will suffice; other disorders require a complex search for specific enzymes and products of impaired metabolism that can only be checked by specialized laboratories.

In certain disorders, the signs and symptoms are highly specific, and the physician should therefore be aware of the constellation of symptoms in such disease entities. Age of onset is an important diagnostic clue, but may be difficult to assess when the course is insidious, particularly in the case of disorders with early infantile onset or slow progression. Often such a course is interpreted as delayed development caused by birth trauma or a static encephalopathy of developmental origin. The choice of a laboratory test or tests is based on the suspected disorder and is dictated by the age of onset, presenting symptoms and signs, and the type of brain and peripheral nerve involvement.

Therefore for this group of disorders, I suggest a logical progression of tests until, through the process of elimination, the less likely possibilities prevail. It is necessary to pursue the biochemical workup vigorously to establish the diagnosis and to provide a reasonable prognosis as well as genetic counseling for the parents and siblings. The success rate of diagnosis is limited only by the current state of medical knowledge and the clinician's perseverance. A working guide is provided in Figure 1. Because eye changes reflect important associated abnormalities of the central nervous system, these are elaborated in Table 1. The biochemical abnormalities and mode of inheritance of a few of the neurodegenerative disorders are listed in Table 2. There are probably hundreds of neurodegenerative disorders, but only those with definitive treatment or treatment approaches are considered here. Because certain disorders occur early and are associated with rapid progression and death, newborns and young infants are distinguished from those manifesting illness later in life. Also, the medical management of the associated complications differs for the two groups.

NEWBORN PERIOD AND EARLY INFANCY

Infants with inherited neurodegenerative diseases share common manifestations, which may in-

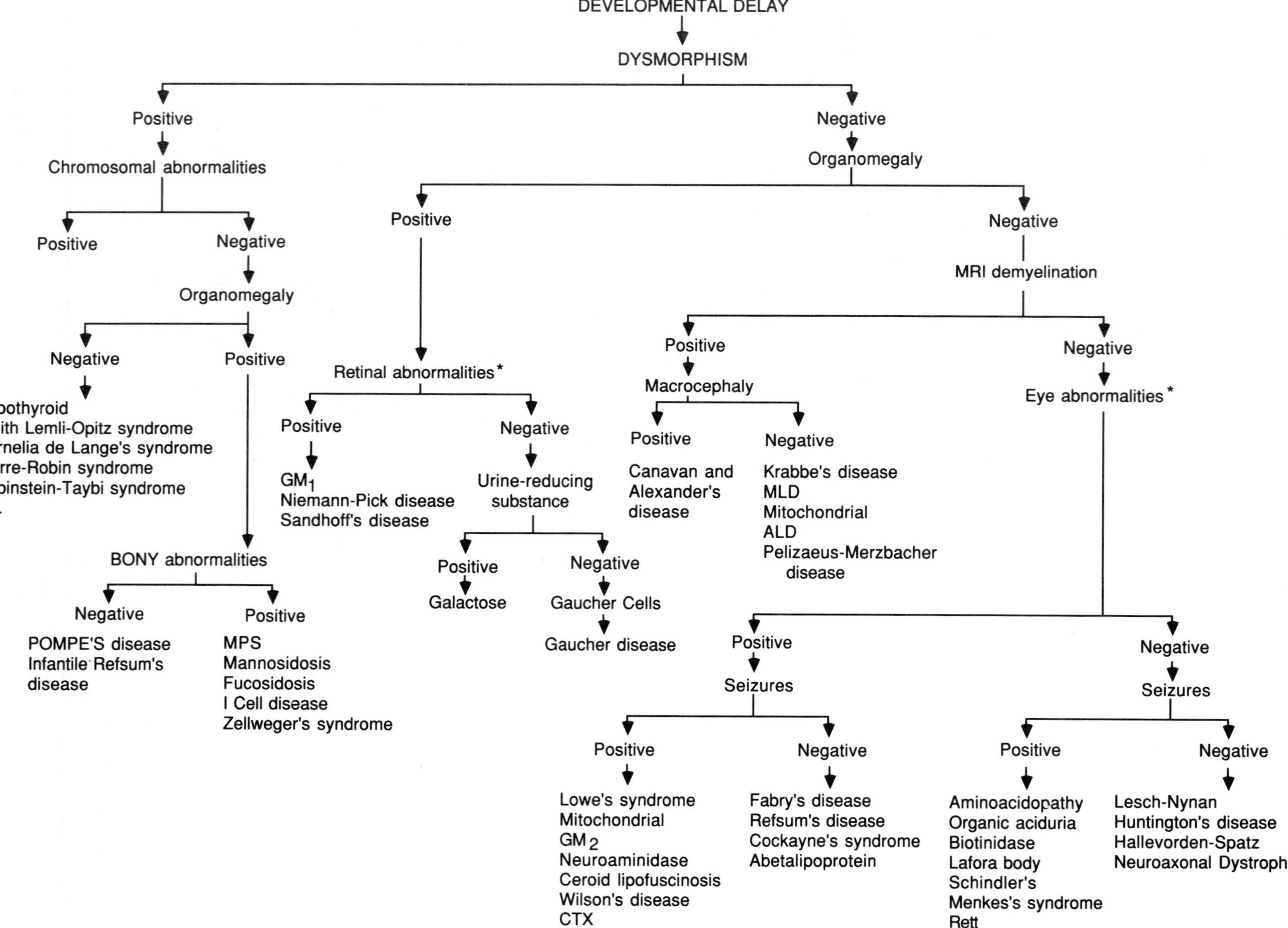

Figure 1 Diagnosis of inherited neurodegenerative diseases of childhood.
* Table 2 details eye and retinal abnormalities, with and without organomegaly.

Table 1 Eye Abnormalities and Associated Abnormalities of the Central Nervous System

Eye Abnormalities	Neurologic Disorders
Kaiser Fleischer ring	Wilson's disease
Corneal opacity	Fabry's disease Zellweger's syndrome MPS Lowe's syndrome Juvenile Gaucher GM_1 gangliosidosis
Cataracts	Galactosemia Zellweger's syndrome Lowe's syndrome Cerebrotendinous xanthomatosis Fabry's disease
Retinal pigmentary degeneration	Refsum's disease Mitochondrial abnormalities Zellweger's syndrome, NALD, infantile Refsum's disease Cockayne's syndrome Abetalipoproteinemia
Cherry red spot	GM_2 gangliosidosis GM_1 gangliosidosis Sandhoff's disease Neuraminidase deficiency with myoclonus Niemann-Pick disease
Macular degeneration	Ceroid lipofuscinosis
Optic atrophy	Leber optic atrophy MLD, Krabbe's disease, X-linked ALD Canavan's disease and Alexander's disease Pelizaeus-Merzbacher disease Neuroaxonal dystrophy
Glaucoma	Zellweger's syndrome Lowe's syndrome Homocystinuria

MLD = metachromatic leukodystrophy; ALD = adrenoleukodystrophy.

clude significant apathy, alteration in muscle tone, seizures, apnea, and respiratory distress. The following features provide initial guidelines for identification of a few of the disorders.

Poor Feeding. This results from lethargy and reduced muscle tone, which is common to many disorders, including aminoacidopathies, organic acidurias, lysosomal disorders, mitochondrial diseases with severe lactic acidosis, and peroxisomal diseases.

Vomiting. Vomiting is often persistent, particularly in patients with conditions associated with protein intolerance after regular feeding, as well as in those with hyperammonemic syndromes, organic

acidurias, galactosemia, PKU, Menkes's kinky hair disease, and Lesch-Nyhan syndrome.

Dysmorphism. Although this can be a feature of inherited neurodegenerative disease, chromosomal aberrations and other known dysmorphic syndromes must be ruled out in making the diagnosis. In patients with the peroxisomal disorders, in particular Zellweger's syndrome, dysmorphic features are the rule. Others include mucopolysaccharidosis (MPS), GM_1 gangliosidosis, I cell disese, and the oligosaccharidoses (mannosidosis, fucosidosis).

Macroglossia. This is seen in patients with Pompe's disease and has also been described to occur in GM_1 gangliosidosis, I cell disease, hypothyroidism, and MPS.

Organomegaly. Organomegaly is not usually evident in most newborns with lysosomal disorders, although hepatomegaly may be present in severe forms of GM_1 gangliosidosis and Wolman's disease (acid lipase deficiency). In other disorders, including glycogen storage disorders (types 1, 3, and 4,) and, most consistently, peroxisomal diseases and disorders such as methylmalonic aciduria, argininosuccinic aciduria, alpha$_1$-trypsin deficiency, tyrosinemia, hereditary fructose intolerance, and galactosemia, significant liver enlargement and abnormalities of liver function are demonstrable, including jaundice. As these disorders are also common features in intrauterine infections, these should be excluded by appropriate assay of blood titers (toxoplasmosis, rubella, cytomegalovirus, and herpes simplex).

Eye Examination. An eye examination performed to establish evidence of chorioretinitis in support of intrauterine infection is essential. Cataracts are present in galactosemia, Lowe's disease, and sometimes in Zellweger's syndrome. Glaucoma is present in Zellweger's and Lowe's syndrome.

Abnormal Hair. This is a tell-tale sign of inherited neurodegenerative disease. The hair is sparse as well as kinky in Menkes's disease, rather pale and friable in argininosuccinic aciduria, and underpigmented in untreated PKU. Alopecia is noted in multiple carboxylase deficiency.

Hypoglycemia. Hypoglycemia is a feature of some glycogen storage disorders but may be a concurrent abnormality of maple syrup disease, tyrosinemia, hypermethioninemia, methylmalonic acidemia, or congenital lactic acidosis.

Metabolic Acidosis. This feature of inherited neurodegenerative disease has a distressing generalized adverse effect on multiple systems and should prompt a search for organic acidurias, lactic acidosis, and glycogen storage diseases, including those with renal and respiratory causes.

Seizures. Seizures are the most blatant evidence of central nervous system injury. Their occurrence is often overestimated in the newborn. Once hypoxia and an electrolyte imbalance have been

Table 2 The Biochemical Abnormalities and Mode of Inheritance of Neurodegenerative Disorders

Disease	Defect	Mode of Inheritance
GM$_1$ gangliosidosis		Autosomal recessive
Type 1 (infantile)		
2 (juvenile)	Beta-galactosidase	Autosomal recessive
3 (adult)		
GM$_2$ gangliosidosis		Autosomal recessive
Type 1 (Tay-Sachs)	Hexosaminidase A	
2 (Sandhoff)	Hexosaminidase A and B	
3 (juvenile)	Hexosaminidase A (partial)	
4 (adult)	Hexosaminidase A	
Niemann-Pick		Autosomal recessive
Type 1 (previous A and B)	Sphingomyelinase	
Type 2 (previous C, D, E, and with sea blue		
histiocytes)	Primary defect uncertain	
	Secondary sphingomyelin storage	
Metachromatic leukodystrophy		Autosomal recessive
Late infantile		
Juvenile	Arylsulfatase A	
Adult		
Activator deficiency	Sphingolipid activator protein I	Autosomal recessive
Pseudodeficiency	Structural alteration of arylsulfatase A	
Gaucher's disease		Autosomal recessive
Infantile		
Adult	Beta-glucosidase	
Juvenile		
Krabbe's disease		Autosomal recessive
Infantile	Galactocerebroside beta-galactosidase	
Juvenile		
Adult		
Fabry's disease	Alpha-galactosidase	X-linked
Farber's disease	Acid ceramidase	Autosomal recessive
Glycoproteinosis		Autosomal recessive
Mannosidosis	Alpha-mannosidase	
Fucosidase	Alpha-fucosidase	
Aspartylglycosaminuria	Amidase	
Mucolipidosis I (cherry red spot myoclonus)	Neuraminidase	
Mucolipidosis II (I cell disease)	N-acetyl glucosaminyl phosphotransferase	
Glycogenosis		Autosomal recessive
Type II (Pompe's disease)	Alpha-glucosidase	
X-linked ALD	VLCFA	X-linked
Disorders of Peroxisome biogenesis (e.g.,	VLCFA, plasmalogen synthesis, phytanic acid,	Autosomal recessive
Zellweger's syndrome)	bile acid intermediates	
Canavan	N-acetyl aspartic acid	Autosomal recessive
	Aspartoacylase	
Schindler's	Alpha-N-acetyl	
	Galactosaminidase	
Galactosemia	Galactose transferase	Autosomal recessive
	Galactose kinase	Autosomal recessive
Lesch-Nyhan	Hypoxanthine-guanine	X-linked
	Phosphoribosyl transferase	

eliminated and seizures become persistent, other metabolic causes such as the aminoacidopathies, organic acidurias, and peroxisomal diseases should be strongly considered, as they often present with early seizures. It is important to identify pyridoxine dependency–induced seizures, primarily because they are treatable. They may have a later onset of seizure-free intervals even in the absence of supplementation with pyridoxine.

Treatment

The first step in the management of an infant suspected of having a metabolic process is to establish its cause so that appropriate treatment may be instituted. The management of the hyperammonemic disorders, aminoacidopathies such as maple syrup disease, PKU, organic acidurias, and mitochondrial disorders are beyond the scope of this chapter.

Acute Symptomatic

Hypoglycemia should be treated with 25 percent dextrose, 0.5 to 1 g per kilogram of body weight administered intravenously, and maintained at 0.5 g per kilogram per hour.

Seizures are controlled with phenobarbital, 20 mg per kilogram of body weight administered intravenously over 10 minutes, and if seizures persist, one should maintain at 3 to 4 mg per kilogram divided into doses taken intravenously, intramuscularly, and orally. Phenobarbital has an age-dependent half-life of 100 hours by 14 days and of 20 hours by 28 days. The therapeutic range is 20 to 40 μg per milliliter, and if the blood level is 40 μg or more, there is no therapeutic value in continuing phenobarbital. If seizures persist, phenytoin (Dilantin) may be added to the regimen in a dose of 20 mg per kilogram of body weight administered intravenously at a rate of 1 mg per kilogram per minute followed by 3 to 4 mg per kilogram per day. Early in the neonatal period, the age-dependent half-life is 104 hours and 2 to 7 hours during the subsequent weeks. The therapeutic range is 15 to 20 μg milliliter. If seizures are still not controlled, diazepam may be added at 0.25 mg per kilogram administered intravenously slowly over a 2-minute period and repeated as often as necessary. The half-life is 25 hours for preterm infants and 31 hours for term infants. Paraldehyde may be added in cases of status epilepticus in a single dose of 400 mg per kilogram administered intravenously or at 200 mg per kilogram per hour in 5 percent dextrose; it can be maintained at 20 to 50 mg per kilogram per hour. The half-life is 18 hours, with a therapeutic level of 100 to 200 μg per milliliter. As the half-life of these drugs is prolonged, repeated administration is often unnecessary. Blood levels should be followed as a possible guide for further use in the event of continued seizures, or to search for additional causes of coma.

Pyridoxine deficiency or dependency is established by giving 50 to 100 mg of pyridoxine intravenously during the electroencephalographic (EEG) recording. If the EEG shows background activity to return to normal, pyridoxine must be continued at 50 to 100 mg per day. If intrauterine seizures are suspected, the mother is given a vitamin B_6 supplement of 100 mg per day.

Seizures and peculiar kinky and sparse hair are the key clinical features of Menkes's disease, which results from a lack of copper absorption from the gut and copper transport in various tissues. It is an X-linked disease. No effective treatment is available, but according to Edwin Myer (personal communication, June 1989), attempts to increase copper with copper histidine (500 μg per milliliter) in a dose of 0.5 ml given subcutaneously daily, beginning when the infant is 2.5 months of age, have resulted in increased serum copper levels. When the infant is 10 months of age hair color and quantity have been shown to improve, although without neurologic improvement. Possibly many of the neurologic adverse effects are established in utero. Prenatal testing is attempted in only a few laboratories because of the strict cell culture conditions required to assess labeled copper retention in amniotic cells after 24 hours.

Hyperbilirubinemia in excess of 20 mg, or less in the presence of acidosis and prematurity, requires an exchange transfusion. When levels of bilirubin appear to be rising early in the course of the illness, fluorescent lights alone may be beneficial.

Life support in the form of ventilation and intravenous fluids administered with a close watch on acid-base balance and renal status is essential.

Long-Term

For most patients with inherited neurodegenerative disease, long-term care consists of supportive care and palliation. In some patients, anticonvulsants may be required on a continuing basis. Poor swallowing requires nasogastric feeding, to be followed by gastrostomy with the Nissen's plication procedure if necessary. In the absence of specific therapies, the main management requirements are supportive care, genetic counseling, and prenatal testing. Symptoms of irritability and poor sleep require treatment with sedatives such as chloral hydrate (10 to 50 mg per kilogram), pentobarbital (5 mg per kilogram), or diphenhydramine (2 to 3 mg per kilogram). When spasticity interferes with adaptive function or contributes to contractures, diazepam in doses of 0.5 to 10 mg may be given every 6 hours. Baclofen may be given alone or in conjunction with diazepam to alter muscle tone. Baclofen has the advantage of not having sedative effects. It is added in gradually increasing doses of 5 to 25 mg every 6 hours. Dantrolene sodium in increasing doses of 12.5 mg twice daily to 25 mg every 6 hours has occasionally been helpful. Muscle spasms, which occur often in the leukodystrophies, can sometimes be blocked by bromocriptine in a dose of 1.25 mg twice daily to 5 mg every 4 hours, particularly if dystonia is an associated complication. Levodopa/carbidopa 100/25 in a dose of half-tablet per day to 1 tablet every 6 hours or trihexyphenidyl in a dose of 2 mg twice daily to higher levels of 20 mg per day (depending on tolerance or effectiveness) have been tried with some success. Drug interactions with anticonvulsants and sedative, gastrointestinal, and respiratory side effects should be monitored.

LATER-ONSET NEURODEGENERATIVE DISEASES

It is easier to recognize a progressive disease in older patients (>24 months of age), and with increasing age, the course is often less fulminant. Although most neurodegenerative diseases are incurable at present, many of the patients remain in a stable condition for prolonged periods and require supportive care (as described earlier for neonates and infants). Relief must be provided for symptoms such as seizures, poor feeding with malnutrition, dental problems, and spasticity. The identification of heterozygotes is essential for counseling parents on the risk of neurodegenerative disease in future offspring. Identifying heterozygotes has been particularly effective in Tay-Sachs disease. If a pregnancy is at risk, prenatal diagnosis by chorionic villus biopsy or amniocentesis is becoming available for an increasing number of disorders. For many of the diseases, parent support groups are available (names of some pertinent organizations are provided at the end of this chapter).

Lysosomal Diseases

Neufeld and her collaborators observed correction of the enzyme defect in mucopolysaccharidosis when skin fibroblasts from patients with this disorder were cocultured with normal skin fibroblasts. This triggered attempts to extend the in vitro observation to treatment of patients with various lysosomal disorders. These ventures included the use of infusions of unfractionated plasma or white blood cells, and the use of injections of purified enzymes from plasma, placenta, or the spleen. Subcutaneous implantation of fibroblasts and amniotic cells and organ transplants of the spleen, liver, and kidney have also been attempted. Most of these procedures were not successful. Liver and kidney transplants have corrected failing function of these organs, but in most instances have not had an impact on overall metabolism. However, there is preliminary evidence that bone marrow transplantation (BMT) is of benefit for at least some of these disorders.

The aim of BMT is to provide normal white blood cells that will carry the required enzyme to the central nervous system. The technical problems of this procedure, the difficulty of obtaining an HLA-matched donor, and the inherent risks of immunosuppression raise practical and ethical issues. This mode of treatment has been successful in two patients with Wiskott-Aldrich's syndrome. Hobbs reported that two patients with mucopolysaccharidosis demonstrated clearing of corneal clouding and of liver and spleen enlargement, but showed no improvement in bony abnormalities. BMT was extended to patients with metachromatic leukodystrophy and to a few with Krabbe disease. In patients with other conditions such as the Norrbottnian variant of Gaucher's disease, Niemann-Pick's disease, Farber's disease, Lesch-Nyhan's disease, glycogen storage disorder type 11 (Pompe's disease), and adrenoleukodystrophy, BMT has been attempted with varying results, and the complications of transplantation have been distressing in advanced cases. The patients with the best outcome appear to be those children in whom the procedure is performed early in the course of the illness and who have the least involvement of the central nervous system. Even with HLA-matched donors, the procedure has a 30 percent mortality rate and its effectiveness in improving neurologic function still needs to be established. It is hoped that advances in immunology will reduce the morbidity rate as well as the mortality rate associated with this procedure. BMT may be viewed as a prelude to gene therapy. If a continuously increased level of enzyme, caused by BMT, could be shown to result in clinical improvement, this would provide strong impetus for new techniques that introduce the missing gene into the patient's own bone marrow–derived cells.

Of great practical value is the study of animal models that have lysosomal storage disease comparable to that of humans. The twitcher mouse is a model of the galactosylceramidase deficiency in Krabbe's disease. The transplantation of bone marrow from a normal animal into the twitcher mouse has resulted in prolonged survival, increased levels of the enzyme in visceral organs and the brain, and reduced levels of psychosin, the presumed toxic substance that accumulates in the brain. Globoid cells, which are the pathologic hallmark of the disease, gradually disappear and foamy macrophages of donor origin are present in the brain, accompanied by extensive remyelination. Such favorable results are most encouraging and will undoubtedly provide new insights as regards the therapy of human disease states.

Peroxisomal Diseases

The generalized peroxisomal diseases (Zellweger's syndrome, neonatal adrenoleukodystrophy (NALD), and infantile Refsum's disease) are autosomal recessive and have a neonatal and early infantile onset with variable clinical progression. The X-linked form of adrenoleukodystrophy (ALD) first manifests after the age 3 years or even during adulthood. The diagnosis is based on clinical symptoms, the time of their first appearance, the mode of inheritance, and the demonstration of elevated levels of plasma very long chain fatty acids (VLCFAs). There is no established treatment or cure. In an attempt to ameliorate symptoms and prevent progression of illness, a dietary treatment that normalizes plasma levels of VLCFA is currently being tested. In cultured skin fibroblasts from ALD patients, the synthesis of VLCFAs was inhibited when the medium was rich in oleic acid. When ALD patients were tested with restricted intake of the VLCFAs and increased intake of oleic acid to provide 60 to 75 percent of fat calories, plasma

VLCFAs were reduced 50 percent, although without significant clinical improvement. A new approach is being attempted with the addition of erucic acid to the diet mentioned above. This oil has a more powerful effect on fatty acid metabolism and has been shown to normalize plasma VLCFAs. Whether this will alleviate symptoms or prevent progression remains to be seen.

Phytanic acid is also elevated in the generalized peroxisomal diseases. As dietary restriction of phytanic acid results in considerable improvement in patients with Refsum's disease, this has also been attempted in some infants with NALD and infantile Refsum's disease, and may help to stabilize the clinical status in some of the more mildly affected patients.

Ceroid Lipofuscinoses

This group of disorders manifests in various forms. The *infantile* form (Infantile Neuroal Ceroid Lipofuscinosis [INCL]- Haltia-Santavouri form) often becomes symptomatic during the 1st year of life with microcephaly, hypotonia, myoclonic seizures, visual loss with macular degeneration, and ataxia. The diagnosis is based on a low-amplitude EEG and electroretinogram (ERG) and on the demonstration of granular membrane-bound inclusions on electron microscopy of skin. In the *late infantile* form (Late Infantile Neuroal Ceroid Lipofuscinosis [LINCL]-Jansky-Bielschowsky form), onset usually occurs at the age of 2 to 3.5 years. Tonic-clonic and myoclonic seizures predominate, with visual failure, macular degeneration, retinal pigmentary changes, speech disturbance, and ataxia. Cortical atrophy on computed axial tomographic (CAT) scans, low-amplitude ERG, and intracytoplasmic curvilinear bodies aid diagnosis. The *juvenile* form (Juvenile Infantile Neuroal Ceroid Lipofuscinosis [JNCL]-Spielmeyer-Vogt form) begins at 5 to 6 years of age, with visual loss and clumping of retinal pigment, and macular degeneration. A few years later there is insidious onset of behavior problems, mental retardation, and seizures, followed by loss of speech, ataxia, and gait disturbance. Progressive deterioration of EEG and cortical atrophy occur. Diagnosis is established on the basis of an abnormal ERG and intracytoplasmic vacuoles with membane-bound fingerprint-patterned inclusions in skin or rectal biopsy. All of the above diseases are transmitted in an autosomal recessive manner. The *adult-onset* form (Kuf), however, has been reported as having autosomal recessive and autosomal dominant forms and may be mistaken for Huntington's disease or Creutzfeld-Jakob disease because of the occurrence of behavioral disturbance, dementia, extrapyramidal signs, and in some patients, seizures. Considerable cortical atrophy is observed on CAT scans; diagnosis is established by skin biopsy and demonstration of ceroid lipofuscin accumulation in the cells. In a study done by MacLeod, prenatal testing on amniocytes at 16 weeks' gestation showed typical inclusions in two of six cases. Despite these positive results, because of the use of uncultured cells, the technique presents difficulties that may be accompanied by nonviable cells and debris.

Various treatments have been ineffective in curing the disease; however, improved seizure control has been obtained with the use of antioxidants. The largest experience is reported by Santavouri and Westermark, who found that the best results were obtained in patients with the juvenile form of the disorder. The patients were noted to have lowered levels of erythrocyte glutathione peroxidase, which contains selenium as selenocysteine at its active site. In conjunction with other antioxidants such as vitamin E glutathione peroxidase protects the cell against damage from oxidants by reducing the accumulation of lipid hydroperoxides. In an attempt to enhance the activity of glutathione peroxidase, Santavouri and Westermark have administered sodium selenite, 0.05 to 0.1 mg per selenium per kilogram of body weight to be taken orally, and vitamin E as alpha-tocopherol acetate, 0.014 to 0.05 g per kilogram of body weight. Subsequently, vitamin B_2 (0.75 to 3 mg daily) and vitamin B_6 (10 to 60 mg daily) were included. While the antioxidants did not benefit vision or prolong ambulation, they did appear to improve seizure control and the progression of neurologic dysfunction. Selenium levels in excess of $4~\mu$M per liter appear to be toxic. Side effects include a garlic odor to the breath, brittleness and white spotting of fingernails, hair loss, skin irritation, pain, paresthesia, and polyneuropathy in chronic overdose.

Wilson's Disease

Wilson's disease, or hepatolenticular degeneration, is transmitted as an autosomal recessive trait and is characterized by reduced plasma ceruloplasmin and excessive copper deposition in tissues, notably in brain and liver. It first manifests between the ages of 3 to 12 years with a slowly progressive dementia and early Parkinsonianlike features, including tremor or cerebellar signs. Choreiform movements may lead one to confuse this disease with Sydenham chorea. Ocular motility may be affected and seizures are common in the childhood-onset forms. Treatment is discussed elsewhere in this text.

Cerebrotendinous Xanthomatosis

This is a form of normolipidemic xanthomatosis associated with dementia, pyramidal tract signs, cerebellar dysfunction, peripheral neuropathy, and tendon xanthomas. Seizures occur in a few patients. Menkes and associates reported the accumulation of cholestanol in the brain tissue of patients with this disorder. Salen reported that chenodeoxycholic acid excretion in bile was greatly reduced. The increased rate of synthesis of cholesterol precursors in bile and elevated tissue sterol concentrations are believed to be secondary to a block in chenodeoxycholic acid production with consequent loss of feedback inhibition. These authors therefore treated patients with chenodeoxycholic acid in a dose of 750 mg per day, and demonstrated remarkable improvement in cognitive function and pyramidal and cerebellar signs. Peripheral neuropathy was no longer detected, the EEG and brain stem auditory–evoked response (BAER) became normal, and CAT scans improved. Plasma cholestanol levels declined, and abnormal bile acid synthesis was suppressed. In addition, the concentration of sterol and apolipoprotein A-I and B in cerebrospinal fluid declined.

Refsum's Disease

This is a rare disease inherited as an autosomal recessive disorder. An unusual 20-carbon, branched-chain fatty acid—phytanic acid which is of purely exogenous origin—accumulates in blood and other tissues, owing to a deficiency of phytanic acid alpha-hydroxylase. The clinical features are cerebellar ataxia, peripheral neuropathy, retinitis pigmentosa, ichthyosis, nerve deafness, and nonspecific electrocardiographic changes.

Treatment consists of a diet low in phytanic acid. If carried out consistently, this can normalize plasma phytanic acid levels in 6 months. Excessively high levels of phytanic acid can cause quadriparesis due to peripheral nerve involvement or cardiac arrhythmia. Under these circumstances, plasma exchange can bring about rapid improvement. Hearing and retinal pigmentary changes are stabilized.

Abetalipoproteinemia

This is a lipoprotein deficiency inherited as an autosomal recessive trait. Apolipoprotein B, which is present in chylomicrons and very low–density lipoproteins, is involved in the transport of triglycerides. In this disorder, apolipoprotein B is absent or markedly reduced. Abetalipoproteinemia is characterized by acanthocytosis, a striking abnormality in the shape of red blood cells. Retinitis pigmentosa, sensory ataxia, and neuropathy develop gradually. An associated fat malabsorption is present almost from birth and gives rise to steatorrhea. It is believed that this leads to a deficiency of vitamin E, which has been convincingly linked to the acquired neuromuscular abnormalities.

Treatment consists of restricting dietary intake of triglycerides, especially those containing long-chain fatty acids (C16–C24), and substituting the calories with protein and carbohydrate. Supplements of fat-soluble vitamins A and K are necessary for improved vision and coagulation. Vitamin E in doses of 100 mg per kilogram per day as a water-miscible or fat-soluble form over a prolonged period of time is reported to prevent progression of neuromuscular and retinal degeneration.

Multiple Carboxylase Deficiency

This disorder can be caused by a dietary insufficiency of biotin, an abnormality of the biotin-recycling enzyme, biotinidase, or by a deficiency of the holocarboxylase synthetase apoenzyme. The brain normally does not recycle biotin and is dependent on a continued supply from across the blood-brain barrier. Children with the disorder involving reduced activity of biotinidase suffer from an inability to liberate and recycle biotin during holocarboxylase turn-over. An abnormality of holocarboxylase synthetase apoenzyme may also cause the disorder. In both conditions, symptoms begin by the second half of the 1st year of life and include seizures, ataxia, hypotonia, deafness, developmental delay, skin rash, and alopecia. It may be associated with metabolic acidosis and variable organic aciduria. In some patients, seizures may be the only presenting feature. Both enzyme deficiencies respond to biotin supplementation.

Isolated deficiencies of the mitochondrial biotin-containing carboxylases also occur. A decrease in brain pyruvate carboxylase results in a severe accumulation of lactate, early neurologic manifestations, and death. Other forms of isolated individual carboxylase deficiencies are proprionicacidemia, caused by a deficiency of propionyl-CoA carboxylase, and 3-methylcrotonyl-glycinuria (cat-urine odor), caused by 3-methylcrotonyl-CoA carboxylase deficiency. These three disorders usually do not respond to biotin supplementation. However, protein restriction, avoidance of fasting, and general supportive measures during periods of metabolic stress are beneficial.

Normal levels of plasma biotin are 0.8 to 3 nM. Treatment consists of 10 mg of biotin per day, which is 200 times the daily requirement.

SUGGESTED READING

Adams R, Lyon G. Neurology of inherited metabolic diseases of children. New York: McGraw Hill, 1982.

Opitz JM, Pullarkat RK, Reynolds JF, et al, eds. Ceroid lipofuscinosis: Batten disease and allied disorders. Supplement 5. New York: Liss, 1988.

Scriver CR, Beaudot AL, Sly WS, Valle D, eds. The metabolic basis of inherited disease. Vols. 1 and 2. New York: McGraw-Hill, 1989.

AMINOACIDEMIA

REBECCA S. WAPPNER, M.D.

Inborn errors of amino acid and organic acid metabolism are inherited abnormalities of the body's biochemistry in which a metabolic pathway is blocked at a specific step. Compounds that accumulate before the block, along with metabolites and other precursors of the block, lead to the clinical symptoms of these disorders. A deficiency of products that result from the reaction may also contribute to the pathophysiology. The disorders are usually caused by single gene defects that involve the enzyme or cofactor for the specific biochemical step involved. Defects at the molecular level have recently been described for many of the disorders.

The disorders vary in clinical severity and mode of presentation, depending upon the degree of toxicity of the compounds and abnormal metabolites involved. The disorders may present in critically ill neonates or infants with massive acidosis or hyperammonemia, or they may be so indolent that they present only as unexplained mental retardation. In many patients, these disorders can be detected by newborn screening programs that have been established to identify cases of phenylketonuria (PKU), maple syrup urine disease (MSUD), homocystinuria, and biotinidase deficiency, among others. The findings of developmental disability, mental and motor retardation, neurologic abnormalities such as those suggestive of interference with myelin formation, unusual odors, cyclic or persistent vomiting or lethargy, or a family history of unexplained infant deaths or of similarly affected individuals should make one consider an inborn error of amino acid or organic acid metabolism.

For all inborn errors of metabolism it is important that an exact biochemical diagnosis be established, not just for accurate therapy, but for use in genetic counseling and prenatal testing when requested by family members of affected individuals. Most of the disorders can be diagnosed on the basis of blood and urine metabolic findings, but an exact enzymatic diagnosis should be established if possible. For many of the disorders, molecular genetic techniques using restriction-fragment-length polymorphisms (RFLP) are also available for carrier detection and prenatal diagnosis.

The number of disorders involving amino acid and organic acid metabolism has grown rapidly over recent years, paralleling the expansion of knowledge about and the availability of diagnostic techniques for these disorders. It is for this reason that comments concerning diagnosis are included along with therapies in this chapter.

ACUTE METABOLIC DISEASE IN NEONATES AND YOUNG INFANTS

Most patients appear to be asymptomatic for the first days of life. Thereafter, usually by 2 weeks of age, there is the onset of poor feeding, behavioral changes, irritability, vomiting, lethargy, and seizures which may progress to coma, and on occasion, circulatory collapse or cardiorespiratory arrest. If a metabolic disorder is suspected, all protein food sources should be discontinued. General supportive measures should be given as indicated, including supportive respiration. Because infections may precipitate an acute episode of an underlying metabolic disorder, cultures should be obtained and appropriate antibiotics given until culture results are known. Initial laboratory testing should include determinations of blood electrolytes, pH, ammonia, and a general chemistry screening panel. It is important to obtain both blood and urine samples for diagnostic testing at the time of the initial presentation, when the patient is most symptomatic. In addition, samples of heparinized plasma (1 ml) and urine (20 ml) should be stored frozen, since additional studies may be needed to clarify the diagnosis.

With all of the disorders, initial management should include special attention to caloric and fluid requirements. Caloric needs may be given initially with intravenous 10 percent glucose-electrolyte solutions and lipids. Modified intravenous hyperalimentation without protein or with selected special amino acid mixtures, such as Hepatamine, may be indicated. Oral or nasogastric feedings with protein-free supplements, such as Mead-Johnson's Protein Free Diet Powder, may be given if the patient's condition allows. Young infants with acute metabolic disease frequently require 120 to 150 kcals per kilogram per day during acute episodes to prevent protein mobilization and achieve control of their disorder. Special attention should be paid to hydration since many of the patients have had either decreased intake or vomiting as part of their symptomatology. Volume expanders and vasopressors may be indicated. In patients with significant hyperammonemia, however, secondary cerebral edema may occur and restriction of fluid intake and intracranial pressure monitoring may be needed.

Acidosis

For patients who present with profound acidosis, with or without hyperammonemia, an organic acidemia should be the presumptive diagnosis. Blood should be obtained to test for quantitative amino acids, short-chain fatty acids, lactate, and pyruvate. Urine should be obtained for organic acids. Ketonuria may be present, which is an unusual finding in neonates. Additional samples should be stored frozen in anticipation of further studies. While one is awaiting these studies, the acidosis should be treated initially with hydration, administration of nonprotein calories, and sodium bicarbonate (in a dose of 1 to 4 mEq per kilogram per body weight). If large amounts of sodium bicarbonate are needed, sodium bicarbonate may be placed in the intravenous hydrating solution instead of sodium chloride. Many patients also require one and one-half to two times the daily maintenance fluid requirements. If this approach does not show improvement in the acidotic state, hemodialysis or peritoneal dialysis should be considered. The hyperammonemia that is seen in patients with organic acidemias is secondary and due to the inhibition of the initial step of the urea cycle by the organic acids. This secondary hyperammonemia usually improves fairly rapidly as the acidosis is corrected, and it is reflective of the degree of control of the organic acidemia.

Organic acidemias that present with overwhelming acidosis in young infants include MSUD, propionicacidemia (PA), methylmalonic acidemia (MMA), and primary lactic acidosis (LA). Abnormalities in plasma amino acids, short-chain fatty acids, and urine organic acid determinations demonstrate the abnormal patterns that confirm the diagnosis. Because many patients with organic acidemias are cofactor-responsive and the cofactors do not appear to be toxic at the doses used, it is not unreasonable to give high doses of the cofactors to an acutely ill child with a presumptive diagnosis of an organic acidemia before the exact diagnosis has been established. The cofactors and initial doses (with related disease) are as follows: thiamine, 100 to 300 mg daily (MSUD, LA), biotin, 10 mg daily (PA), and hydroxocobalamin, 500 to 1,000 μg administered intramuscularly daily (MMA). This dosage should be adjusted once the exact diagnosis is established. For many of the disorders, specialized nutritional products are available that contain lowered amounts of or no specific amino acid precursors for the pathways affected. These products may be used for initial enteral management. Once the patient is stabilized and the acidosis controlled, small amounts of the specific amino acids involved and natural protein may be introduced to promote adequate growth. The nutritional prescriptions must be individualized for each child and monitoring and adjustments made frequently to allow optimal growth and control of the disorder.

Supplemental L-carnitine therapy may also be of benefit in that these patients often develop a secondary total and free carnitine deficiency state with increased plasma levels and urinary loss of acylcarnitines which are esterified with the organic acids. The initial dosage of L-carnitine is 25 mg per kilogram per day in divided doses. This may be slowly increased to 100 mg per kilogram per day in divided doses, if indicated. Supplemental L-glycine (250 mg per kilogram per day) has also been shown to be of benefit in the treatment of isovalericacidemia in that the isovalery-glycine formed is nontoxic and rapidly excreted.

Acute Hyperammonemia

For patients who present with acute hyperammonemia without acidosis, the presumptive diagnosis should be that of an inborn error involving the urea cycle. Blood should be sent for quantitative amino acids. Urine should be sent for quantitative determinations of amino acids and orotic acid, a metabolite in the pyrimidine pathway that is increased as a result of carbamyl phosphate accumulation in some of the urea cycle defects. The pattern of abnormalities demonstrated by this testing usually indicates a specific defect in the urea cycle. Because some of the organic acidemias may present with hyperammonemia as the initial major problem, urine should also be collected for organic acid determination. Intravenous 10 percent glucose-electrolyte solutions and lipids, as well as enteral nonprotein feedings (if tolerated) should be given to prevent protein catabolism. Reduction of markedly elevated plasma ammonia levels (>350 μM) is accomplished most effectively by hemodialysis. However, this is often technically difficult to perform in small infants. Alternatively, peritoneal dialysis may be used. Exchange transfusion, which is the least effective means of reducing plasma ammonia levels, may be done if there is a delay in starting dialysis. Drugs that provide alternate pathways for waste nitrogen excretion, sodium benzoate and sodium phenylacetate, may be used intravenously for mild to moderate primary hyperammonemia ($<350\ \mu$M). These drugs are also used enterally to maintain acceptable plasma ammonia levels after acute episodes in patients with the more severe forms of the urea cycle disorders. Sodium phenylbutyrate is also available for enteral use only. Supplemental L-citrulline or L-arginine is usually needed, initially by intravenous administration, and later as part of enteral feedings, to help "prime" the urea cycle by supplying what has become an essential amino acid due to the specific enzymatic block. As with the organic acidemias, acute hyperammonemia requires nonprotein caloric supplements to prevent catabolism. Folic acid and pyridoxine may be given to promote transamination. In addition, supplements of essential amino acids mixtures (0.72 g per kilogram per day) and limited amounts of natural protein (0.4 to 1.5 mg per kilogram per day) are usually required to maintain control of the disease. The nutritional prescriptions must be individualized for each child and frequently monitored to achieve optimum growth and control of the disorders.

Even with prompt and aggressive therapy, many of the patients who present with massive acidosis or massive hyperammonemia during the first 2 weeks of life do not survive. Of those who do survive, the majority have significant neurologic deficits and psychomotor retardation. Seizure disorders, cortical atrophy, and spastic quadriplegia are also common. The patients are at risk for subsequent intercurrent episodes of exacerbations of their disease, which may also lead to further neurologic sequelae or death. The families of these children need intensive social as well as medical supportive services. The children should be referred for rehabilitative services, such as occupational therapy, physical therapy, and special preschool programs.

For most of the disorders, the exact biochemical enzyme deficiency can be documented in cultured skin fibroblasts. For this reason, a skin fibroblast culture is recommended at the time of initial presentation. Skin biopsy may be obtained at the time of catheter placement for dialysis or by punch biopsy, usually of the forearm. However, the disorders of the urea cycle that involve mitochondrial enzymes require that a liver biopsy be done to demonstrate the enzymatic defect. Because many of the infants that survive their initial presentation require feeding gastrostomies because of their neurologic impairment, liver biopsy may be obtained at the time of this surgical procedure. Alternatively, punch or open liver biopsy may be obtained with careful clinical preparation of the patient, or for those who do not survive, during the immediate postmortem period. With all specialized metabolic testing, it is important that the laboratories that perform the testing be contacted before samples are obtained to ensure that proper collection and shipment techniques are used.

Milder forms of both the organic acidemias and hyperammonemias have been reported in older children and young adults. Patients with these disorders may present with an acute episode similar to that seen in younger children, or they may have a history of repeated episodes of cyclic vomiting, lethargy, or ataxia. Treatment is similar to that used for younger children.

Dicarboxylic Acidurias

The dicarboxylic acidurias are associated with faulty beta-oxidation of fatty acids and named after the unusual organic acid pattern noted in patients during acute exacerbations of their disease. Short-chain, medium-chain, and long-chain acyl-CoA dehydrogenases are needed for beta-oxidation of fatty acids, and deficiencies of all three types of dehydrogenases are known to produce significant clinical illnesses. Medium-chain acyl-CoA dehydrogenase (MCAD) deficiency, the most common form, is estimated to occur in as many as one in 10,000 persons and is associated with Reye's-like episodes of vomiting, lethargy, hypoglycemia, mild hyperammonemia, and acidosis, which may proceed to coma and death. Most patients present as young children between the ages of 15 months and 4 years. During episodes, patients have a characteristic urinary organic acid pattern which may be normal between episodes as demonstrated by conventional gas chromatography and mass spectrometry. However, measurement of urinary acyl-carnitine profiles with fast-atom bombardment or measurement of urinary acyl-glycine profiles demonstrate the disorder *between* episodes. Once recognized, the disorder is easily treated, with therapy based on the avoidance of fasting and the avoidance of utilization of fats to satisfy caloric needs. A diet that is high in carbohydrates, relatively low in fat, and based on a frequent-feeding schedule is recommended. Medium-chain triglyceride supplements and formulas should be avoided. Some patients respond to riboflavin at a dosage of between 50 and 750 mg daily. As with other organic acidemias, supplemental L-carnitine therapy may also be of benefit for this disorder. Intercurrent episodes should be promptly treated with intravenous glucose-electrolyte hydration. Once the disorder is recognized and promptly treated, many patients do well, in contrast to patients with other types of organic acidemias. Despite this fact, approximately 25 percent of patients have been reported to have died during their first episode before recognition of the disease, and many of the cases of affected siblings were thought to have been caused by sudden infant death syndrome. Other disorders of fatty acid oxidation may present with similar clinical features and require treatment similar to that used for MCAD deficiency.

OTHER AMINO ACID AND ORGANIC ACID DISORDERS

Certain disorders of amino acid metabolism have characteristic features that suggest their diagnosis, such as the marfanoid habitus and dislocated lens of homocystinuria, gyrate atrophy of the retina associated with ornithine aminotransferase deficiency, and wooly or kinky hair associated with argininosuccinicaciduria. Some organic acidemias have characteristic odors such as the "sweaty-sock" odor of isovaleric acidemia. More often, patients are suspected of having an amino acid or organic acid disorder on the basis of common clinical findings such as seizures, unexplained psychomotor retardation, episodic vomiting and lethargy, or pigment dilution when compared with family members. Many laboratories offer a metabolic screening urine panel that includes spot testing for ketoacids and sulfur-containing amino acids as well as one-dimensional amino acid electrophoresis. The most inclusive testing, however, includes determinations of plasma ammonia, quantitative amino acids, urinary quantitative amino acids, and organic acid testing.

Newborn Screening Programs

Newborn screening programs have been established throughout the United States for the detection of PKU and hypothyroidism. In addition, in many states, screening is done for other inborn errors of metabolism such as galactosemia, MSUD, homocystinuria, and biotinidase deficiency. Early detection and treatment allows the children optimum outcomes for their disorders.

Treatment

Specific therapies are available for many of the disorders. For each child, a nutritional prescription is made to limit the intake of offending amino acids or amino acid precursors to that needed for control of the disorder, while providing adequate sources of the specific amino acids and other amino acids for body maintenance and growth. Commercial protein formulations, in crystalline or powder form, which limit certain amino acids are available for many of the individual disorders. Often these formulas also contain essential nutrients such as calories, vitamins, and minerals. Limited amounts of natural protein sources are given as tolerated in the form of breast milk (especially for patients with PKU), standard infant formulas, or measured amounts of cow's milk or table foods. It is important that the families be educated and involved in the planning and daily

Table 1 Vitamin Therapy in Amino and Organic Acidemias

Vitamin	Daily Dosage	Disorder
Thiamine	10 mg/kg 100–300 mg or more in divided doses	MSUD Pyruvate dehydrogenase complex deficiency
Riboflavin	50–750 mg in divided doses	Dicarboxylic acidurias Glutaric acidemia II
Pyridoxine	300–900 mg in divided doses	Homocystinuria Hyperoxaluria Ornithine aminotransferase deficiency
Hydroxocobalamin	500–1,000 μg IM q 1–7 d	MMA Cobalamin activation defects, (homocystinuria plus MMA)
Folic acid	1 to 15 mg	Homocystinuria, classic and remethylation defects
Nicotinamide	40–200 mg	Hartnup's Disease

D-Biotin	10–50 mg	Biotinidase deficiency
		Carboxylase deficiencies
		    Propionyl-CoA carboxylase
		    Methylcrotonyl-CoA carboxylase
		    Pyruvate carboxylase
		    Multiple carboxylases

monitoring of their child's protein intake. Resources are available that list the protein and individual amino acid content of common foods. Lowered-protein recipes and cookbooks, prepared lowered-protein foods, and specialized low-protein food products are also available. Nonprotein caloric needs may be supplied by the special formulas mentioned earlier in this chapter, Mead Johnson's Protein-Free Diet Powder or natural foods. Other essential nutrients, vitamins, and minerals are supplemented when indicated. Vitamin therapies that may be indicated for certain disorders are listed in Table 1. Other adjunct therapies for specific disorders include the use of L-glycine in patients with isovaleric acidemia, betaine in patients with homocystinuria (promotes remethylation of homocystine to methionine), L-cystine in patients with homocystinuria (becomes an essential amino acid because of the site of the metabolic block), D-penicillamine or its analogs in patients with cystinuria (increases urinary solubility of cystine), L-carnitine in patients with organic acidemia (discussed earlier in this chapter), and agents that provide alternate means of waste nitrogen excretion (discussed earlier in this chapter) in patients with hyperammonemia. The patients must be monitored frequently for growth parameters, dietary intake of nutrients, and blood and urinary levels of metabolites. Dietary adjustments must be made frequently to achieve optimum control and outcome. Frequently, intercurrent illness with the demand for more calories causes the disorder to be uncontrolled. Despite adequate therapy, some disorders are not able to be managed with currently available medical and nutritional therapy. Liver transplantation may be indicated in refractory cases of hereditary tyrosinemia and in certain cases of carbamyl phosphate synthesis and ornithine transcarbamoylase deficiencies of the urea cycle.

It is recommended that children with inborn errors of amino acid and organic acid metabolism be referred to a specialized treatment program. These patients will require some form of specialized dietary therapy for life, as well as nutritional and medical education, genetic counseling, and psychosocial support for their families, which is best given by multidisciplinary teams who have specialized expertise in this area.

SUGGESTED READING

Holton JB. The inherited metabolic diseases. New York: Churchill-Livingstone, 1987.

Nyhan WL. Abnormalities in amino acid metabolism in clinical medicine. Norwalk, CT: Appleton-Century-Crofts, 1984.

Scriver CR, Rosenberg LE. Amino acid metabolism and its disorders. Philadelphia: WB Saunders, 1973.

Stanbury JB, Wyngaarden JB, Fredrickson DS, et al. The metabolic basis of inherited disease. 5th ed. New York: McGraw-Hill, 1983.

PATIENT RESOURCES

Dietary Information

The following list is not all-inclusive, and families should be advised by their clinics as to which listings and foods are appropriate.

Food listings:

Pennington JAT, Church HN. Bowes and Church's food values of portions commonly used. 14th ed. Philadelphia: JB Lippincott, 1985.

Roberts RS, Meyer BA. Lo-Pro diet guide. 3rd ed. 1987. (Copies available from the Metabolism Office, Riley Hospital, Room A-36, Indianapolis, Indiana 46202-5225; telephone: (317)274-3966; price: $15.00 each.)

Cookbooks:

Schuett VE. Low protein cookery for phenylketonuria. 2nd ed. (revised and expanded), 1988. (Copies available from the University of Wisconsin Press, 114 North Murray Street, Madison, Wisconsin 53715; telephone: (608)262-8782; price: $35.00 for hard cover, $13.75 for spiral notebook.)

Low-protein food products:

Dietary Specialties, Inc.
P.O. Box 227
Rochester, New York 14601
Telephone: (716)263–2787 (New York only)
or
1-800-544-0099

Ener-G-Foods, Inc.
5960 First Avenue South
P.O. Box 84487
Seattle, Washington 98124-5787
Telephone: 1-800-331-5222
or
1-800-325-9788
(Washington State only)

Med-Diet, Inc.
1409 Fairfield Road South
Minnetonka, Minnesota 55343
Telephone: (612)546-3285
or
1-800-633-3438

Associations

National PKU News, Inc.
7760 Ridge Drive, N.E.
Seattle, Washington 98115

Research Trust for Metabolic Diseases in Children (RTMDC)
53 Beam Street
Nantwick, Cheshire, CW5 5NF
United Kingdom

The Organic Acidemia Association, Inc.
1532 S. 87th Street
Kansas City, Kansas 66111
Telephone: (913)422-7080

Maple Syrup Urine Disease Family Support Group
R.R. 2, Box 24A
Flemingsburg, Kentucky 41041
Telephone: (606)849-4679

National Organization for Rare Disorders (NORD)
P.O. Box 8923
New Fairfield, Connecticut 06812
Telephone: (203)746-6518

ACUTE HEPATIC PORPHYRIA

LINDA M. FAMIGLIO, M.D.

Rarely is the neurologist the first or only physician to care for the patient with acute hepatic porphyria. The varied symptoms often lead the patient to multiple medical specialists. First, the hepatic porphyrias are not common, especially in the United States. Second, symptomatic patients present with a variety of difficult problems, including labile hypertension, gastric and intestinal ileus, photosensitivity and skin ulcerations in some forms, psychosis, as well as cranial nerve, autonomic, and peripheral neuropathies. The severity of symptoms ranges from subtle and difficult to diagnose to life-threatening.

The porphyrias are a group of disorders of hepatic and erythrocytic origin that result in accumulation of porphyrins and porphyrin precursors in the blood and tissues. Specific enzyme defects in the pathway of heme biosynthesis are responsible for different varieties of porphyria. Only three of the well-known porphyrias—acute intermittent porphyria, variegate porphyria, and hereditary coproporphyria—all of which are hepatic, have neurologic consequences and drug-induced attacks. The acute hepatic porphyrias are inherited in an autosomal dominant pattern with variable phenotypic expression. The most common form, acute intermittent porphyria, is linked to a deficiency in uroporphyrinogen I synthetase (also known as porphobilinogen [PBG] deaminase). It occurs in all races, but is most common in Scandinavians and Anglo-Saxons. Variegate porphyria occurs in South African whites with an incidence of one per 1,000 whites. Hereditary coproporphyria is the least common form.

The clinical course is one of acute attacks triggered by drugs, malnutrition, menses, or illness, followed by latent phases. Treatment during a severe, acute attack of polyradiculoneuropathy is challenging. If treatment is delayed, the mortality rate may reach 50 percent during the first episode and rises to nearly 100 percent with a second acute attack. Although recovery can be complete, severe episodes are more likely to result in a residual motor neuropathy requiring months of rehabilitation. Some patients may be entirely asymptomatic, but biochemical evidence of a deficiency of one or more of the enzymes in the pathway of heme biosynthesis can be demonstrated during any phase of the disease. An acute episode of porphyria before puberty is rare. Two-thirds of initial attacks occur during the second or third decades. Less than 10 percent of patients with porphyria have a first attack after the age of 50 years.

RATIONALE FOR THERAPY

The most successful therapy is directed towards altering the biochemical events which precipitate and perpetuate an attack (Fig. 1). The synthesis of heme begins with the formation of delta-aminolevulinic acid (ALA), catalyzed by ALA synthase, the rate-limiting enzyme in heme production. Exogenous or endogenous factors may induce ALA synthase, resulting in increased production of ALA and PBG, the porphyrin precursors. These precursors and subsequent intermediates build up behind points of partial enzyme deficiency. The precise nature of drug-induced attacks is not well understood. Inciting drugs may act by depleting hepatic cytochromes, particularly the P-450 system during drug detoxification. Evidence exists that some drugs (e.g., carbamazepine) may act directly to decrease the activity of an already abnormal enzyme in the pathway. Heme normally controls ALA synthase activity via a negative feedback loop. In acute porphyric attacks, decreased heme production results in loss of feedback inhibition and a spiraling increase in intermediates that overwhelm the partially deficient enzyme.

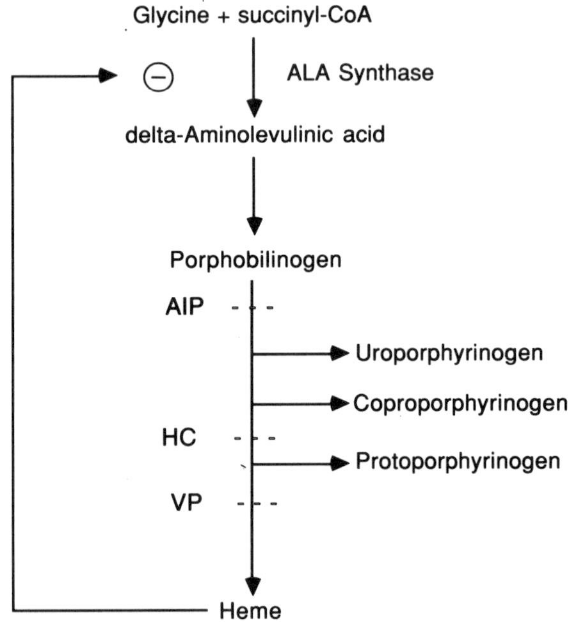

Figure 1 Simplified scheme of heme biosynthesis. ALA synthase is the rate-limiting enzyme. Partial enzyme blocks are indicated in relation to other blocks and the excess intermediates excreted. Heme regulates its own metabolism by negative feedback to ALA synthase. AIP = acute intermittent porphyria; HC = hereditary coproporphyria; VP = variegate porphyria.

THE ACUTE ATTACK

Treatment of the acute attack has two major components: (1) suppression of the induced ALA synthase and (2) monitoring and treatment of the secondary phenomenon (Fig. 2). As soon as there is clinical suspicion of an acute attack, potentially harmful drugs must be discontinued. More than 100 drugs listed in the International Review of Drugs in Acute Porphyria—1980 have been implicated in precipitating attacks, including barbiturates, most anticonvulsants, sulfonamides, and ethanol (Table 1). Not only is it essential to discontinue provocative drugs immediately, but it is prudent to avoid the use of any medications unless specifically indicated. As soon as possible, either a simple "window sill" test, or a Watson-Schwartz reaction for urinary PBG should be done. The "window sill" test exposes fresh urine to sunlight, which turns urinary PBG a dark red color. The Watson-Schwartz test relies on the reaction between Erlich's aldehyde in acid solution and urine PBG to result in a pink color. This qualitative assay can detect urinary PBG at a concentration of 9 mg per liter or more. Acute attacks of porphyria causing neurologic dysfunction consistently present with a urinary PBG of 30 mg per 24 hours, well above the level of reliable detection. There is no reason to wait for confirmatory tests. If the preliminary tests are negative, the diagnosis should be reconsidered.

Starvation, which may occur in the setting of binge drinking (itself a precipitant) or hyperemesis gravidarum, can also initiate an episode of acute attack. Conversely, administration of a high-carbohydrate load represses ALA synthase and reduces the excretion of porphyrin precursors. Attacks can be aborted by glucose in a dosage of 400 to 500 g per day or 20 g per hour. Both the intravenous and oral routes are suitable although the latter may be limited by diarrhea. Hyperglycemia should be treated with sliding scale doses of regular insulin.

Symptomatic and biochemical improvement can be obtained with intravenous administration of hematin, also known as hemin (Panhematin). Like heme, it represses ALA synthase and presumably produces therapeutic effects by decreasing the production of porphyrins and precursors. Hematin is an orphan drug that must be obtained directly from the pharmaceutical company. It is shipped in a lyophilized form that must remain refrigerated. Once it is reconstituted in an alkaline solution, it must be used immediately. The half-life of the solution at room temperature is approximately 4 hours. The breakdown products of hematin do not appear effective in suppressing ALA synthase. More importantly, the expired drug solutions may be responsible for treatment failures and significant side effects. The side effects include coagulopathies, transient renal failure, and cardiovascular collapse. A dosage of 3 to 4 mg per kilogram once or twice daily should result in decreased excretion of porphyrin precursors within 3 to 4 days. The dose must be infused via a normal saline-flushed intravenous system over a 15-minute period. If the patient remains symptomatically improved, doses can be withheld while the patient is monitored closely for any increase in uri-

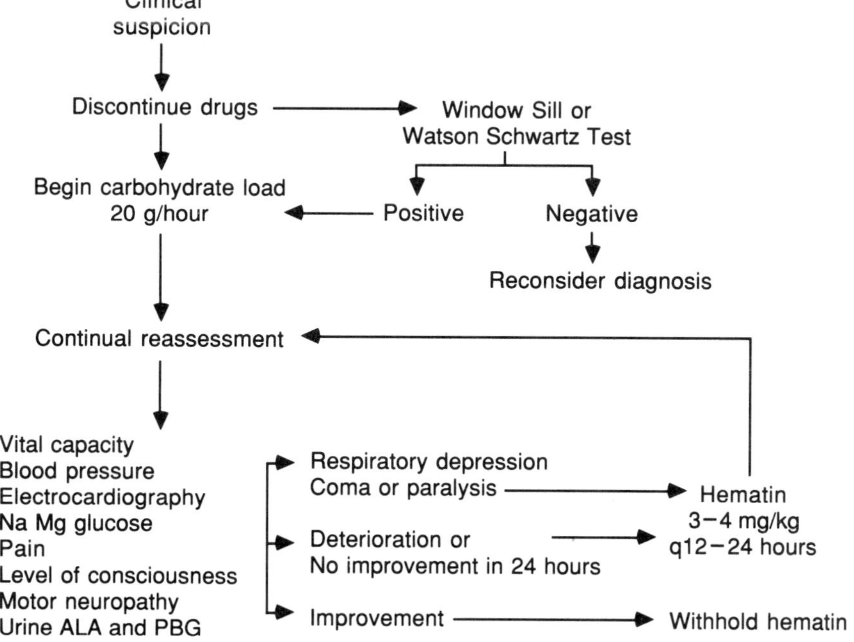

Figure 2   Management of acute porphyric episode.

Table 1 Drug Choices in the Treatment of Acute Hepatic Porphyrias

Drugs to be Avoided	Drugs Believed to be Safe
Alcohol	Ampicillin
Amphetamines	Aspirin
Barbiturates	Atropine
Carbamazepine	Bromides
Chloramphenicol	Cephalosporins
Chlordiazepoxide	Chloral hydrate
Danazol	Chlorpromazine
Ergots	Cloxacillin
Estrogens	Codeine
Furosemide	Diazepam
Griseofulvin	Digoxin
Imipramine hydrochloride	Diphenhydramine
Meprobamate	Fentanyl
Methyldopa	Heparin
Pentazocine	Insulin
Phenytoin	Meperidine hydrochloride
Sulfonamides	Morphine
Tetracycline	Nitrofurantoin
Theophylline	Nitrous oxide
Tolbutamide	Penicillin
Valproic acid	Prochlorperazine
	Propranolol
	Streptomycin
	Succinylcholine chloride

nary porphobilinogens. Symptomatic relief may lag behind biochemical improvement for days, especially in severe cases. No therapy has been found to be effective in the treatment of residual or chronic neuropathy; hematin has been used without improvement in symptoms. There have been anecdotal reports that other therapies, including plasmapheresis, charcoal hemoperfusion, and oral folic acid have a beneficial effect in the treatment of an acute attack of porphyria, but these cannot be considered standard treatment. Heme arginate is a new compound found to be effective in decreasing urinary excretion of porphyrins and inhibiting ALA synthase. Whether it has any advantages over hematin therapy has not yet been demonstrated.

Successful control of the biochemical aspects of the disease does not ensure that the patient will recover. Severely affected individuals can be more fragile than patients with severe Guillain-Barré syndrome. The motor and autonomic neuropathy threaten cardiovascular function. Continuous cardiac monitoring is essential when autonomic symptoms are present. Sudden death is more likely to be caused by a cardiac arrhythmia than by respiratory failure. Labile hypertension and tachycardia are common; if treatment is necessary, propranolol can be used without further inducing ALA synthase. However, no drug with an autonomic mechanism of action or side effect should be prescribed without serious consideration. Parasympathetic dysfunction has been described to occur even during remission and in patients with latent porphyria.

Respiratory function must be monitored closely using frequent vital capacities and conservative criteria (e.g., vital capacity < 15 ml per kilogram) for elective intubation in the deteriorating patient. Bulbar dysfunction compromises airway protection, and prevents adequate oral nutrition unless nasogastric feeding is used. Severe constipation and ileus can result from the autonomic neuropathy. Electrolyte management is complicated by hyponatremia, partly because of the syndrome of inappropriate antidiuretic hormone (SIADH), and by hypomagnesemia. Pain and dyesthesias can be severe enough to require the use of meperidine or morphine. Agitation, hallucinations and other signs of psychosis can be treated with chlorpromazine. Seizures are not common in acute attacks of porphyria, but pose a difficult management problem. Diazepam can be used safely, but most other anticonvulsants have been reported to trigger attacks. Bromides may be used for chronic seizure management.

LATENT AND SUBACUTE PORPHYRIA

Prevention of acute episodes is the best treatment for acute hepatic porphyria. Only through screening of family members at risk for the disease can avoidance of provocative factors and early treatment be successful. In the patient with a remote history of mild symptoms or a positive family history of the disease, a more leisurely diagnostic work-up can be pursued. Twenty-four–hour samples of stool and urine should be collected in light-protected containers. The porphyrins and their precursors are excreted in the urine and stool according to their degree of water solubility. The more distal the enzyme defect, the more lipophilic are the accumulating intermediates. The lipophilic porphyrins are excreted in the stool. Various patterns of urine and stool porphyrin excretion are characteristic of the subtypes of porphyria even in the latent phase of the disease (Table 2). Quantification of

Table 2 Pattern of Porphyrin and Precursor Excretion in Acute Hepatic Porphyria

Specimen	AIP	HC	VP
Urine	ALA	ALA	ALA
	PBG	PBG	PBG
		COPRO	COPRO
			URO
Stool	NONE	COPRO	PROTO
			COPRO
Enzyme assay	RBC uroporphyrinogen I synthetase	Limited availability	

AIP = acute intermittent porphyria; HC = hereditary coproporphyria; VP = variegate porphyria; ALA = delta-aminolevulinic acid; PBG = porphobilinogen; COPRO = coproporphyrinogen; URO = uroporphyrinogen; PROTO = protoporphyrinogen.

urine and stool porphyrins should indicate the specific diagnosis. Assays of enzyme activities other than uroporphorinogen I synthetase associated with acute intermittent porphyria are not readily available in the United States. When acute intermittent porphyria is suggested by excretion studies, or if a relative of the patient is known to have the disease, assay of the specific enzyme can confirm the diagnosis. Analysis may find more than one defective enzyme. These disorders usually present in the heterozygous state. Levels of enzyme activity are therefore approximately 50 percent of the normal levels.

Skin ulcerations and photosensitivity are caused by porphyrin deposition in skin. Porphyrin precursors alone are not photosensitizers. Variegate porphyria and hereditary coproporphyria, both of which are caused by more distal enzyme deficiencies, do accumulate porphyrins in the skin and are thus associated with skin lesions.

In those unusual instances of recurrent premenstrual exacerbations, suppression of cyclic ovarian hormone secretion may prevent the attacks. Hormonal suppression therapy avoids the hospitalization and thrombophlebitis associated with frequent hematin infusions. A long-acting agonist of luteinizing hormone-releasing hormone (LH-RH) has been used successfully for this purpose.

Patient education and the prevention and prompt recognition of induced attacks are the keys to successful management of acute hepatic porphyrias. Milder cases can be diagnosed before the pain, psychosis, and paralysis become advanced if simple urine screens are performed. Once recognized, the acute attack must be treated urgently in order to prevent the high morbidity and mortality rates associated with these diseases.

SUGGESTED READING

Anderson E, Spitz M, Sassa S, et al. Medical intelligence: prevention of cyclical attacks of acute intermittent porphyria with a long-acting agonist of luteinizing hormone-releasing hormone. N Eng J Med 1984; 311:643–645.

Goetsch C, Bissell D. Medical intelligence: instability of hematin used in the treatment of acute hepatic porphyria. N Eng J Med 1986; 315:235–238.

Moore MR. International review of drugs in acute porphyria—1980. Int J Biochem 1980; 12:1089–1097.

PATIENT RESOURCES

The American Porphyria Foundation
P.O. Box 11163
Montgomery, Alabama 36111

Abbott Laboratories
For information on administration of hematin, call collect: (312)937-7302
To obtain hematin:
Monday–Friday 7AM–6:30PM (central time): 1–800–255–5162
For after-hours emergencies, call collect 1–312–937–7970

WILSON'S DISEASE

ANNE B. YOUNG, M.D., Ph.D.
GEORGE J. BREWER, M.D.

Wilson's disease is a rare autosomal recessive inherited disorder of copper metabolism. Although rare, the disease can be treated immediately, and it is therefore of the utmost importance to recognize it early in its course. The primary lesion in Wilson's disease is still unknown. The protein in blood that binds copper, ceruloplasmin, is decreased in patients with Wilson's disease, but the properties of the ceruloplasmin itself are normal. Futhermore, the ceruloplasmin structural gene is not responsible for Wilson's disease since it lies on chromosome 3, whereas the Wilson's disease gene has been recently located on the long arm of chromosome 13 in five Middle-Eastern and nine North American families. Thus, the Wilson's disease gene is likely to affect the regulation or processing of ceruloplasmin and thereby interfere with the secretion of ceruloplasmin into the blood and the excretion of copper into the bile. Approximately one in 100 individuals are carriers, and the risk of Wilson's disease in the general population is one in 40,000. For the offspring of affected patients, the risk is approximately one in 200. At greatest risk for the disease are siblings of affected persons; for these individuals, the risk is one in four. Therefore once a patient with Wilson's disease is identified, it is important to screen the siblings and nonsibling relatives of that patient to identify other affected individuals.

CLINICAL PRESENTATION AND DIAGNOSIS

The most important aspect of diagnosing Wilson's disease is to suspect it. Wilson's disease can present with a wide variety of clinical symptoms, including psychiatric, neurologic, hepatic, and hematologic symptoms. Recently we identified a young woman who was admitted to the pulmonary service with a bronchial mass. The mass was found to be an enlarged lymph node secondary to frequent aspiration caused by dysphagia. The patient had minimal neurologic complaints at the time of diagnosis. If the disease is not recognized early and treated promptly, however, the results can be disastrous. Most patients present during the second or third decade of life, although patients have presented as early as the first decade or as late as the sixth decade.

The most common presenting neurologic signs are dysarthria, dysphagia, poor fine motor coordination, tremor, and rigidity. Occasionally, patients present with chorea, dystonia, or cerebellar ataxia. Behavioral and personality changes, depression, and emotional lability are common. Another interesting case from our institution was a young woman who presented to the neuromuscular clinic with the complaint of difficulty speaking and swallowing. The examination at the time showed weakness of voluntary tongue movements, slowed rapid alternating movements of the tongue, and poor elevation of the palate. A brain stem lesion was suspected, and the patient was evaluated with magnetic resonance imaging (MRI). Because of the large number of cases of Wilson's disease that we have followed at this institution, the radiologists were quite sensitive to the MRI changes in Wilson's disease. On completing the scan, the radiologist called the neurologist to indicate that the patient had no evidence of a brain stem lesion but, rather, had probable Wilson's disease which had caused signal changes in the basal ganglia. Subsequent examination of the patient documented clear Kayser-Fleischer rings. It is likely that this diagnosis would have been missed if either the MRI was not carried out or if the radiologist had not seen prior cases of Wilson's disease. In interviewing a patient with suspected Wilson's disease, an accurate medical history is important to obtain because patients sometimes have had episodes of unexplained hepatitis or hemolytic anemia. The diagnosis should be considered in all patients with movement disorders and dysarthria with or without psychiatric complaints.

Therapy

Once a diagnosis is established, the siblings of the patient should be screened, since each has a 25 percent risk of homozygosity for the gene. In any identified individual, prophylactic therapy should be instituted to prevent the onset of symptoms.

Three major therapies are currently available for the treatment of Wilson's disease: D-penicillamine, triethylenetetramine dihydrochloride (Trien), and zinc (Table 1). Regardless of the type of therapy

Table 1 Treatment Regimens for Wilson's Disease

Treatment	Initial Regimen	Maintenance Therapy	Advantages	Disadvantages
Penicillamine	1 g/day in 2–4 divided doses (adults) 30 min. before or 2 hours after meals 25 mg pyridoxine daily Monitor: 24-hour urine copper, free serum copper, blood and platelet count, serum chemistries, urinalysis weekly for 6 weeks, then less frequently.	1 g/day in 2–4 divided doses (adults) 25 mg pyridoxine Monitor: 24-hour urine copper, free serum copper, blood count, serum chemistry, urinalysis every 3–12 mos.	Generally effective, greatest experience	Long list of toxicities (early and late) Syndrome of initial neurologic worsening
Triethylenetetramine hydrochloride (Trien)	1 g/day in divided doses (adults) 25 mg pyridoxine Monitor: Same as for penicillamine	Same as for penicillamine Monitor: same as for penicillamine	Generally effective	Knowledge of toxicity and long-term experience limited
Zinc	50 mg zinc acetate three times per day for presymptomatic patients Monitor: 24-hour urine copper and zinc, free serum copper every 3 to 12 months. Oral ^{64}Cu uptake after 6 weeks of therapy, then as needed, if available.	50 mg zinc acetate three times per day Monitor: 24-hour urine copper and zinc, free serum copper every 3 to 12 months. Oral ^{64}Cu uptake after 6 weeks of therapy, then as needed, if available.	Generally effective Very low toxicity	Not drug of choice and experience limited for symptomatic patients. Long-term experience limited.

used, certain measures should be monitored repeatedly. It is especially important to monitor copper status so that inadequate therapy and continued copper accumulation can be identified before the onset of increased symptomatology and toxicity. Twenty-four–hour urine collections for copper and plasma samples of nonceruloplasmin copper are the primary variables to be monitored. It is the nonceruloplasmin–bound copper (i.e., free serum copper) that is potentially toxic to various organ systems. In untreated patients with Wilson's disease, these levels are 50 μg per deciliter or more whereas in normal subjects, these levels are about 10 μg per deciliter. The objective of therapy is to reduce the free serum copper to 20 μg per deciliter or less. After the initial diagnosis, clinical monitoring should also be carried out weekly or monthly to assess the possibility of worsening. We carry out semiquantitative neurologic examinations, video recordings, and handwriting samples as part of the monitoring process. Slit-lamp examinations can be used to assess semiquantitatively the amount of copper in the cornea. For patients with liver disease, bilirubin and serum enzymes of liver origin should be measured frequently. It is also important to follow the complete blood count including platelets. Many patients with Wilson's disease have subclinical cirrhosis and hypersplenism or both.

It is probably not necessary to follow as rigorous a low copper diet as has previously been suggested. Many of the older estimates of food copper were inaccurate. Several studies have found that the average human diet contains approximately 1 mg of copper per day, with the range being approximately 0.6 to 1.4 mg. In the initial phases of therapy, it is wise to avoid liver and shellfish, two types of food with very high copper content. Later, during maintenance therapy, these foods may be eaten safely once per week. Occasional individuals have high copper concentrations in their drinking water. One of our patients had a copper content in his drinking water, which resulted in up to 3 mg per day of copper being ingested. Another patient was taking a mineral supplement that had high copper content. Patients should therefore be carefully interviewed before therapy to ascertain potential sources of high copper intake. It should be emphasized to the patient that all of the therapies for Wilson's disease should be taken separately from food or drink. These medications are most effective when taken with water only. They should not be taken with snacks or juices. It is also important to impress upon the patient the gravity of their disease and of the consequences of failure to comply with therapy.

D-Penicillamine

For adults and older children, the usual recommended dosage of penicillamine for the initial de-coppering therapy is 250 mg four times daily given either 30 minutes before or 2 hours after meals. In children 5 years of age or younger, the recommended daily dose is 0.02 g penicillamine per kilogram of body weight, which may be rounded to the nearest multiple of 250 mg. In addition, penicillamine has antipyridoxine effects, and patients should take 25 mg pyridoxine daily. Neurologic deterioration has been observed in approximately one-third of patients during initial therapy, and although the cause for this worsening is unknown, we have become concerned about vigorous initial decoppering. We often titrate the dose of penicillamine during initial therapy while monitoring the 24-hour urine copper. We aim for a dose of penicillamine that results in the urinary excretion of 1.5 to 3 mg copper per day. If excretion is higher than that (and some patients can excrete as much as 10 mg per day when taking 1 g of penicillamine), we lower the dose of penicillamine. For the initial month of therapy, we examine patients at least weekly to monitor for side effects of penicillamine. The side effects include fever, rash, leukopenia, thrombocytopenia, and proteinuria. Blood counts and urinalyses should be done three times per week for the 1st week, twice a week for the 2nd week, and finally weekly for the next 6 weeks. If no problems emerge, the frequency of blood and urinalysis testing can be decreased to every 3 months. Urine copper and free plasma copper should be followed weekly during the initial phases of the disease, and then less frequently at monthly intervals during the 1st year.

As the patient becomes decoppered, the excretion of copper in the urine decreases, so that by the time maintenance therapy is reached, the patient may be excreting only 0.5 mg of copper in the urine per day. If therapy is proceeding effectively, the free serum copper should decrease to 20 μg per deciliter. Under the best of circumstances, patients gradually improve in terms of their neurologic and hepatic function. Most patients, however, are left with some degree of cirrhosis. Some patients have more extensive liver disease and must be maintained on a low-protein diet in order to control blood ammonia and hepatic encephalopathy. The movement disorder in neurologically affected patients often deteriorates in the presence of mild hepatic encephalopathy. Esophageal or gastric varices may develop and may ultimately cause severe bleeding. Liver transplants have been successfully performed in patients with Wilson's disease.

As mentioned above, some patients either fail to improve neurologically or deteriorate neurologically during initial penicillamine therapy. The mechanism for this deterioration is not known, but it may involve initial redistribution of the large hepatic store of copper to the brain. Ultimately, other forms of therapy may prove most useful in the initial decoppering process to prevent this sudden redistribution of copper. By monitoring the free serum and 24-hour urine copper, we hope to minimize any potential distribution problems. Once the 24-hour urine copper has stabilized at less than 1 mg of copper excreted per day and the free plasma copper is decreased to less than 20 μg per deciliter, the patient can be considered to be on maintenance therapy. For the 1st year, 24-hour urine copper and free plasma copper should be monitored at 3-month intervals and subsequently at 6- to 12-month intervals. If the free plasma copper begins to increase, patient compliance with the therapeutic regimen should be questioned.

Side Effects

Approximately 20 percent of patients develop serious side effects when receiving penicillamine therapy. These include urticaria, skin rash, fever, or lymphadenopathy. If serious reactions occur, three options are open to the physician. The first option is to use alternative drugs such as Trien or zinc. The second option is to discontinue penicillamine until the side effects disappear. Penicillamine can then be reinstituted at a very low dosage of perhaps 25 mg per day with a gradual increase over several weeks back to the therapeutic dose. As a third option, the penicillamine can be discontinued until the side effects resolve, and then 20 to 30 mg of prednisone can be given for 2 to 3 days before the reinstitution of penicillamine. After several weeks, the steroid may be tapered and subsequently discontinued. Additional side effects to penicillamine include thrombocytopenia, leukopenia, lupus-like syndromes, and stomatitis. Some of these side effects cannot be managed without switching the patient to another drug.

Trien

Triethylenetetramine dihydrochloride (Trien) was approved for use in the treatment of Wilson's disease in 1986. For adults, the recommended dosage for initial decoppering and maintenance therapy is 1 g per day in divided doses, with each dose taken at least 1 hour before or 2 hours after meals. For children younger than 10 years of age, 0.5 g per day in divided doses is the recommended dosage. Experience with Trien is limited, but in trials that have been carried out, the drug has proved quite useful. Monitoring should be done as with the use of D-penicillamine. Renal, bone marrow, and dermatologic toxicity are most common.

Zinc

Zinc has been used by two groups independently in the treatment of Wilson's disease. It is well tolerated with no identified serious toxicities. Our group has used zinc acetate. Zinc acetate appears to cause less gastric irritation than zinc sulfate. Zinc acts as a decoppering agent by inducing metallothionein in the intestinal cell. The metallothionein has a high affinity for copper and blocks copper absorption into the blood. Copper bound to metallothionein is lost in the stool. The usual dosage of zinc is 50 mg three times per day, taken either 1 hour before or 2 hours after the meals. Zinc is an excellent maintenance therapy for symptomatic patients with Wilson's disease who have already been decoppered, or for treating the presymptomatic patient from the beginning. From the theoretical standpoint, it is also excellent for the pregnant patient. For the initial treatment of the symptomatic patient, zinc is somewhat slow in its onset of action, at least as a sole anticopper therapy. Monitoring of zinc therapy is carried out with 24-hour urine copper and free serum copper as with the other therapies. Since zinc does not promote urinary excretion of copper, the 24-hour urine copper becomes a reflection of the body status of copper. It goes down gradually with decoppering. The aim of therapy is to reduce the 24-hour urine copper to 125 μg or less and keep it there. In addition, zinc blocks gastrointestinal uptake of copper, and this can be monitored with ^{64}Cu uptake. The uptake of copper is dramatically suppressed by zinc therapy. In patients who do not have blockade of uptake, compliance with the medical regimen should be questioned. The 24-hour urine and plasma zinc are also useful monitoring tools. Patients taking this dose of zinc should excrete a minimum of 2.5 mg of zinc in the urine per 24 hours, and plasma zinc should range from 150 to 300 μg per deciliter.

The Pregnant Patient

Penicillamine and trien are teratogenic in animals. Limited information in humans is available, but a 2 to 5 percent risk of fetal abnormalities has been estimated for pregnant women taking penicillamine. Little data are available on the effects of trien and zinc on pregnancy. We have treated two pregnant women with zinc and both had normal babies.

Prognosis with Long-Term Therapy

In patients presenting with liver failure, there is a significant risk of initial mortality. Once past the initial phases of therapy, however, patients often do very well despite little reserve hepatic function. Reversal of neurologic/psychiatric symptoms is much more variable. Some patients have remarkable recovery from quite severe deficits, whereas others with less severe disease can continue to progress even during initial therapy. Usually, once copper toxicity is controlled, improvement is complete within 1 year. Occasionally a patient continues to regain function for as long as 2 years. Once a patient is on maintenance therapy, any worsening should suggest poor compliance.

SUGGESTED READING

Bowcock AM, Farrer LA, Cavalli-Sforza LL, et al. Mapping the Wilson's disease locus to a cluster of linked polymorphic markers on chromosome 13. Am J Hum Genet 1987; 41:27–35.

Brewer GJ, Hill GM, Prasad AS, et al. Oral zinc therapy for Wilson's disease. Ann Intern Med 1983; 99:314–320.

Brewer GJ, Yuzbasiyan-Gurkan V, Young AB. Treatment of Wilson's disease. Semin Neurol 1987; 7:209–220.

Hill GM, Brewer GJ, Juni JE, et al. Treatment of Wilson's disease with zinc II. Validation of oral ^{64}copper with copper balance. Am J Med Sci 1986; 292:344–349.

Hoogenraad TU, Van Hattum J, Van den Hamer CJA. Management of Wilson's disease with zinc sulphate: experience in a series of 27 patients. J Neurol Sci 1987; 77:137–146.

Iyengar V, Brewer GJ, Dick RD, Owyang C. Studies of cholecystokinin-stimulated biliary secretions reveal a high molecular weight copper-binding substance in normal subjects that is absent in patients with Wilson's disease. J Lab Clin Med 1988; 111:267–274.

Scheinberg IH, Sternlieb I. Wilson's disease. Philadelphia: WB Saunders, 1984.

Walsche JM, Dixon AK. Dangers of non-compliance in Wilson's disease. Lancet 1986; 1:845–847.

Yuzbasiyan-Gurkan V, Brewer GJ, Boerwinkle E, Venta PJ. Linkage of the Wilson disease gene to chromosome 13 in North American pedigrees. Am J Hum Genet 1988; 42:825–839.

PATIENT RESOURCE

Wilson's Disease Association
P.O. Box 75324
Washington, D.C. 20013
Telephone: (703) 636-3003
or
(703) 636-3014

REYE'S SYNDROME

DARRYL C. De VIVO, M.D.

Although the annual incidence of Reye's syndrome (RS) has declined sharply in recent years, sporadic cases continue to appear in the pediatric and adult populations. The reason for this decline in incidence seems to be linked to the decreased use of salicylate-containing products by patients who are acutely ill with a viral illness. Other factors may ultimately prove to be more important, but at the moment, public attention is riveted on the widely publicized association between RS and aspirin.

In the past, the annual incidence of RS ranged from 0.3 to 6.5 cases per 100,000 children at risk. Sporadic cases were often associated with varicella, and epidemic outbreaks coincided with the prevalence of influenza in the community. To date, approximately 25 cases have also been reported in adults. About half of these patients reportedly took aspirin during the acute illness.

I use the term RS to describe an acute illness that affects the brain and liver primarily. It is initiated by a systemic viral infection and followed by a potentially life-threatening encephalopathy. The conscious state is altered and the intracranial pressure elevated. Liver dysfunction coexists, but there is no jaundice. If the patient survives, there are no further attacks. This distinction sets RS apart from a host of other diseases that are genetically determined metabolic errors. These cases produce a recurrent RS-like illness that requires thorough investigation to document the predisposing biochemical defect. Inherited defects of fatty acid oxidation most closely mimic RS. These conditions produce a primary or secondary alteration of carnitine metabolism. Medium-chain acyl-CoA dehydrogenase deficiency and 3-hydroxy-3-methyl glutaryl-CoA lyase deficiency are two notable examples of inborn metabolic errors that produce an RS-like syndrome. Inborn errors that involve the urea cycle, gluconeogenic pathway, and the respiratory chain may also mimic RS. In addition, the RS phenotype may be associated with various environmental intoxicants, including salicylates, tetracyclines, valproic acid, disulfiram, phenformin, margosa oil, chlordane, pyrrolizidine, camphor, methylbromides, and lead.

The etiology of RS appears to be the antecedent viral illness. No study has demonstrated a biochemical or immunogenetic predisposition, and the pathogenesis is debated. All available information indicates that the mitochondrion is the primary site of intracellular injury. Mitochondrial abnormalities affect multiple organ systems and result in a generalized alteration of cellular energy metabolism.

The typical patient develops clinical symptoms of a viral illness. Pernicious vomiting develops several days later and may continue for hours or days. At this point, there is evidence of a generalized metabolic derangement. The patient manifests a diffuse encephalopathy, and the liver function tests are abnormal. The most immediate threat to life is the development of cytotoxic cerebral edema and increased intracranial pressure. Treatment is designed to provide maximal fuel for glycolysis and oxidative metabolism and to mitigate the intracranial hypertension. As such, hypertonic solutions of glucose and mannitol are central to the treatment of patients with this syndrome. Parenthetically, a similar treatment paradigm is employed in the management of patients who are acutely ill with a RS-like syndrome.

DIAGNOSIS

In most cases, the clinical and laboratory profiles are distinctive and the diagnosis is obvious, particularly if the physician has had previous experience with the syndrome. The diagnostic criteria are based on the following clinical and laboratory observations:

1. The presence of an antecedent viral infection.
2. A latent interval of 4 to 7 days before the onset of pernicious vomiting.
3. The development of a metabolic encephalopathy.
4. The lack of any other obvious explanation for the encephalopathy.
5. A three-fold or greater elevation of the serum transaminase activities.
6. Prolongation of the prothrombin time.
7. Hyperammonemia.
8. Normal cerebrospinal fluid (CSF) examination except for possible elevated opening pressure and decreased glucose associated with hypoglycemia.

Clinicians have debated the advisability of a lumbar puncture in patients with this illness, but it has been my practice to perform this procedure as part of the initial assessment. Unexpected CSF findings such as a pleocytosis, red blood cells, or the elevation of the protein concentration should lead one to consider other diagnostic possibilities. These possibilities include bacterial meningitis, viral encephalitis, subarachnoid hemorrhage, and child abuse. Deferring a lumbar puncture until later in the course of illness may delay these diagnoses. Also, there appears to be an increased likelihood of central herniation if the lumbar puncture is performed after the illness has evolved and treatment has been started.

A brain imaging procedure, computed tomography (CT) or magnetic resonance imaging (MRI), is of limited value in RS. One only expects to see correlates of cerebral edema, such as the compression of the cerebral sulci and ventricles and effacement of the gray and white matter. The greater value of the study is that it can yield an unexpected finding such as a mass lesion or blood that would indicate another condition simulating RS. Depending on the certainty of the clinical diagnosis, CT scanning is an optional procedure.

A liver biopsy is also an optional procedure. The diagnosis may be difficult to make in infants, and the liver biopsy findings may be valuable. Microvesicular steatosis is a common finding and is not specific for RS. Ultrastructural studies must be done to justify the risk of this procedure. Any existing coagulopathy must be corrected before the biopsy is performed.

Admission blood studies should include a total hematologic and chemical profile, coagulation studies, and determinations of ammonia, osmolality, and lactate concentration. I repeat these studies every 24 hours and obtain repeat glucose, lactate, osmolality, pH, PaO_2, and $PaCO_2$ every 4 hours. These measurements gauge the metabolic progress of the patient. Typically, a low serum phosphorus concentration is present, which will decrease after administration of hypertonic glucose. It is therefore important to maintain adequate amounts of phosphate in the intravenous solution. A decreasing serum calcium concentration may indicate pancreatic involvement. This complication, usually associated with the use of corticosteroids, is potentially devastating. In fact, there is no clear indication for the use of steroids in managing patients with RS.

TREATMENT

The medical management of patients with RS has been standardized over the years and relies on the basic principles of intensive medical support. Treatment is determined by the neurologic condition of the patient at the time of admission to hospital.

The therapeutic goal is to achieve a metabolic steady state during which time the patient will gradually recover from the illness. Relatively few adjustments are necessary once the patient's condition has been stabilized. It is important to minimize environmental stimuli that will arouse the patient. I have seen dramatic fluctuations of the intracranial pressure occur when the patient is stimulated. Repeated neurologic examinations are unnecessary. Rather, serial observations of the patient's posturing, the size and reactivity of the pupils, and the positioning of the eyes provides enough information to gauge the clinical course.

All patients with RS need to be hospitalized immediately. Early vigorous treatment probably limits the progression of the illness and increases the likelihood of a satisfactory outcome. Children with stage 1 disease exhibit subtle behavioral disturbances such as inattention, inappropriateness, lethargy, somnolence, confusion, or mild irritability. These patients are managed by intravenous hydration with a 10 percent hypertonic glucose-multielectrolyte solution. The fluids are administered at a rate of 1,600 to 1,800 ml per m² per day. Vitamin K is administered intravenously (1 mg) or intramuscularly (5 mg), and this dose is repeated every 24 hours.

Children in stages II through IV of the disease and those children whose conditions have deteriorated from stage I after admission to hospital should be transferred to the intensive care unit. The patient with stage II disease is disoriented or demonstrates agitated delirium, stupor, or coma associated with decorticate posturing. The sympathetic nervous system overactivity is evident through tachycardia, systemic hypertension, hyperthermia, hyperpnea, diaphoresis, and dilated pupils. The patient with stage III coma demonstrates decerebrate posturing of limbs and trunk. The eyes may be forced into a down-gaze indicative of midbrain dysfunction. Further neurologic deterioration results in loss of brain stem function (stage IV). The patient then develops tachycardia, hypotension, apnea, pulmonary congestion, and nonreactive dilated pupils. Several procedures should be carried out while the patient is anesthetized and paralyzed with sodium thiopental (Pentothal, 4 mg per kilogram IV) and succinylcholine (Anectine, 1 mg per kilogram IV), and a servocontrolled cooling blanket should be placed on the bed to counteract hyperthermia. The procedures include placement of a nasotracheal tube, radial artery catheter, central venous catheter, nasogastric tube, and urinary catheter. These procedures should be carried out as quickly as possible, and sodium thiopental and succinylcholine should be repeated, as necessary, until these studies are completed. It is important to hyperventilate the patient at this point, maintaining an arterial carbon dioxide tension of approximately 25 torr. I prefer to place the central venous catheter through the superficial saphenous vein into the inferior vena cava for delivery of hypertonic solutions of glucose and mannitol. Placement of the central venous catheter through the subclavian vein necessitates placing the patient in the Trendelenburg position, which may aggravate coexisting intracranial hypertension. Hypertonic glucose solution can be infused continuously through the central venous catheter, and hypertonic mannitol can be piggy-backed through this line when necessary.

The hypertonic glucose solution used to treat patients in stages II through IV of the disease contains 200 g of glucose, 40 mEq of sodium chloride, 15 mEq of potassium acetate, and 15 mEq of potassium phosphate per liter. One ampule of multiple vitamins is added per liter of solution, and the solution is infused at a daily rate of 1,600 to 1,800 ml per m^2. This rate of infusion provides approximately 500 mg of glucose per kilogram of body weight per hour. Also, the fluid volume allows for gradual rehydration of the dehydrated patient. We expect that the patient will remain hyperglycemic with blood glucose concentrations ranging from 250 to 350 mg per deciliter. Less compromised patients metabolize the glucose more efficiently and maintain lower blood concentrations. Blood glucose concentrations exceeding 400 mg per deciliter may occur in the more compromised patients who are desperately ill. The glucose concentration in the IV solution may be decreased to 15 or 10 percent as necessary while still maintaining a constant fluid rate. Glucose concentrations in the range of 300 mg per deciliter decreases the need for mannitol and provides more optimal circulating concentrations of glucose to support glycolysis. It is assumed, but not proven, that the brain glucose requirements are increased in RS when the mitochondrial systems are compromised. Readjustments of the fluid rate should be discouraged because continual fluctuations of the glucose concentration seem to be associated with clinical and metabolic instability. It is imperative that the continuous infusion of glucose not be interrupted, otherwise the blood glucose concentration and the serum osmolality will decrease.

Cerebral edema is managed by the administration of hypertonic mannitol. I favor early placement of an epidural monitor to assess the moment-to-moment need for mannitol. All patients in stages II - IV of the disease should have an epidural monitor placed through a burr hole overlying the right frontal cortex. This procedure is carried out by a neurosurgeon in the intensive care unit using local anesthesia. Intravenous boluses of hypertonic mannitol (0.25 g per kilogram) are often sufficient to control the intracranial hypertension. Mannitol is administered through the central venous catheter over 3 to 5 minutes without interrupting the continuous infusion of hypertonic glucose. Mannitol may be given in repeat doses as frequently as necessary. Higher doses of mannitol ranging from 0.5 to 2 g per kilogram may be administered if necessary and should be infused over longer periods of time (10 to 30 minutes). Daily mannitol doses of 4 to 6 g per kilogram have been sufficient to control cerebral edema in RS patients who are managed with this hypertonic glucose regimen. Smaller daily doses of mannitol are often sufficient. We believe that the induced hyperglycemia decreases the daily requirement of mannitol in these patients. As a result, hyperosmolality is seldom encountered with this treatment regimen. It is unusual to see serum osmolalities in excess of 320 mOsm per liter, and most patients who receive this treatment maintain a serum osmolality of 290 to 310 mOsm per liter. Maintenance of the head and neck in a neutral midline position and elevation of the head of the bed by 20 to 30 degrees facilitate venous drainage and are helpful simple maneuvers in managing intracranial hypertension.

Pentobarbital may be used to control intracranial hypertension if frequent doses of mannitol are ineffective. Pentobarbital doses of 1 to 5 mg per kg IV may be repeated every 4 to 8 hours to achieve serum concentrations of 30 to 50 mg per liter. These doses are adequate to control intracranial hypertension. However, complications resulting from the pentobarbital regimen include impaired cardiac output, systemic hypotension, and hypoventilation. Mechanical ventilation is necessary as the patient is further depressed by the administration of the barbiturate. Fortunately, mannitol is sufficient to control the intracranial hypertension in most cases. Seizures, when they do occur, also may be managed with pentobarbital.

I generally allow the patient to breathe independently, while a state of mild hyperoxia and hypocapnea with PaO_2 values of 100 to 150 torr and $PaCO_2$ values of 20 to 27 torr is maintained. Most patients in the earlier stages of coma maintain these arterial values spontaneously while breathing humidified oxygen through a T-tube adapted to the nasotracheal tube. Elective nasotracheal intubation is recommended for all patients admitted to the intensive care unit. If necessary, ventilatory assistance in the intermittent mandatory ventilation (IMV) mode may be necessary, particularly if there is evidence of altered respiratory pattern, hypoventilation, or periodic breathing. Suctioning of the airway should be carried out carefully and coordinated with the administration of mannitol or after the administration of thiopental and succinylcholine. Excessive suctioning of the patient under other circumstances may be associated with marked elevations of the intracranial pressure.

Patients with RS often develop fever during the period of treatment. Elevations of body temperature are managed by a cooling blanket and acetaminophen suppositories. I make no effort to lower the body temperature below normal. Although gastric contents often contain small amounts of blood, no specific treatment is necessary since fewer than 10 percent of patients with RS develop clinically significant hemorrhage. Infusion of freshly frozen plasma or fresh whole blood may be necessary when significant hemorrhage occurs.

Most patients demonstrate clinical or laboratory improvement within 1 to 3 days after admission. Approximately 90 percent of children with stage I disease at the time of admission remain stable and recover uneventfully. The remaining 10 percent of patients with stage I disease worsen initially and require intensive medical support before making a full recovery. An equally good outcome is expected from patients who are admitted with stage II or stage III disease, but patients admitted with stage IV disease are at high risk for dying or recovering with neurologic disability.

Once the patient has regained consciousness, the glucose concentration in the RS solution is tapered by 25 percent decrements every 8 hours and the patient is extubated. Patients may usually take liquids by mouth within 24 hours of regaining consciousness, at which time the remaining catheters can be removed.

A complete recovery is the expected outcome for most patients with RS. The neurologic or psychological sequelae associated with RS probably result from attendant complications such as hypoglycemia, systemic hypotension, hypoxia, and uncontrolled intracranial hypertension. These potentially devastating complications are usually avoided if the diagnosis of RS is made early and intensive medical support is instituted without delay.

SUGGESTED READING

Corkey BE, Hale DE, Glennon MC, et al. Relationship between unusual hepatic acyl-Coenzyme A profiles and the pathogenesis of Reye syndrome. J Clin Invest 1988; 82:782–788.
Hurwitz ES, Barrett MJ, Bregman D, Public Health Service Study of Reye's syndrome and medications. JAMA 1987; 257:1905–1911.
Meythalar GM, Varma RR. Reye's syndrome in adults: diagnostic considerations. Arch Intern Med 1987; 147:61–64.
Wood C. Reye's syndrome. Oxford: Royal Society of Medicine Services, Ltd. 1988.

PATIENT RESOURCE

National Reye's Syndrome Foundation, Inc.
426 North Lewis
Bryan, Ohio 43506
Telephone: (419) 636-2679

DISTURBANCES OF SODIUM AND OSMOLALITY

MICHAEL N. DIRINGER, M.D.
JEFFREY R. KIRSCH, M.D.

A large number of neurologic patients develop disturbances of sodium and osmolality. Often these disturbances are first recognized as an abnormal serum sodium concentration; however, they may present with altered mental status, seizures, or dehydration. Through proper managment, these complications can be avoided or limited. Appropriate evaluation facilitates recognition of the type of dysfunction and determines the direction of therapy, while familiarity with the natural history guides the nature and timing of therapeutic interventions.

ASSESSMENT

In the evaluation of patients with an abnormal serum sodium concentration, it is important to consider the clinical situation, the integrity of sodium and water regulation, and possible confounding factors. The diagnostic and therapeutic approach is often dictated by the clinical situation. For example, after pituitary tumor surgery, high urine output is often caused by an insufficient amount of circulating antidiuretic hormone (ADH); however, it may also represent an appropriate diuresis caused by intraoperative administration of mannitol or fluids. Hyponatremia following subarachnoid hemorrhage is usually associated with volume contraction and negative sodium balance, but may be due to the syndrome of inappropriate secretion of antidiuretic hormone (SIADH). Brain tumor patients may present with hyponatremia caused by SIADH, diuretic use, or (rarely) salt wasting.

The initial investigation of an abnormal serum sodium concentration should begin with collection of a data base. Historical data should be reviewed to determine if there is a history of heart failure, cirrhosis, renal disease, endocrinopathy, diuretic use, diarrhea, vomiting, or recent surgery or trauma. Oral fluid intake and the quantity and type of intravenous fluids administered to the patient should be ascertained. Comparison of measured and calculated serum osmolality detects pseudohyponatremia caused by the presence of additional osmoles in the blood such as mannitol or ethanol. Urinary osmolality represents the end point of osmoregulation and reflects, in normal kidneys, the level of plasma ADH. Urine sodium content gives an indication of sodium excretion, which is best interpreted in relation to intravascular volume. Measurement of central venous pressure (CVP), pulmonary capillary wedge pressure (PCWP), and orthostatic blood pressure changes can be used to estimate vascular volume. Direct measurement of plasma volume with the tracer dilution method using labeled albumin may provide a more sensitive indicator of volume status and is easily obtained.

This data base usually provides sufficient information to exclude hypernatremia or hyponatremia resulting from cardiovascular, liver, renal, or endocrine causes. If doubt remains, further evaluation may be indicated. Renal function can be assessed through determination of the creatinine clearance. Hypoaldosteronism is suggested by hyponatremia, hyperkalemia, and dehydration, and can be confirmed by measurements of the circulating aldosterone. Morning cortisol levels and free thyroxine index help evaluate for possible adrenal insufficiency or hypothyroidism. Once these possible etiologies have been eliminated, the disturbance can be attributed to altered central nervous system (CNS) function.

An appreciation of the time course of the change in sodium concentration is important in the evaluation of patients and in planning their therapy. The severity of symptoms, and thus the urgency of intervention, is directly related to the rate of change in serum sodium. A sodium of 120 mEq per liter that has developed over several weeks is most often asymptomatic and can be managed conservatively. On the other hand, the same sodium concentration that has developed over several hours can be life-threatening and requires aggressive intervention.

The remainder of this chapter focuses on the evaluation and treatment of the disturbances of sodium and osmolality most often seen in neurologic patients. These disturbances result from altered CNS function and thus may fluctuate with the patient's neurologic condition. They can usually be distinguished on the basis of serum and urine sodium concentrations and osmolality and intravascular volume. These relationships are summarized in Table 1.

Table 1 Characteristics of Primary CNS Disturbances of Sodium and Volume

Disturbances of Sodium and Volume	Serum Sodium	Urine Sodium	Urine Osmolality	Vascular Volume
DI	$\leftrightarrow$ or $\uparrow$	$\leftrightarrow$	$\downarrow$	$\leftrightarrow$ or $\downarrow$
SIADH	$\downarrow$	$\leftrightarrow$ ($\uparrow$)	$\uparrow$	$\leftrightarrow$ or $\uparrow$
SAH (salt wasting)	$\leftrightarrow$ or $\downarrow$	$\uparrow$	$\leftrightarrow$ or $\uparrow$	$\downarrow$

SYNDROME OF INAPPROPRIATE SECRETION OF ANTIDIURETIC HORMONE (SIADH)

SIADH is a disorder of osmoregulation without a primary disturbance of sodium or volume regulation. It is usually caused by inappropriate secretion of ADH, which results in free water retention and a dilutional hyponatremia. Urinary concentration, as determined by the urine to plasma osmolal ratio, is inappropriate for the serum osmolality and/or circulating blood volume. Thus, once hyponatremia occurs, there is either normal or modestly elevated intravascular and extracellular volume. CNS disorders including head trauma, infections, tumors and Guillain-Barré syndrome are associated with hyponatremia caused by SIADH. The diagnostic criteria for SIADH include (1) hyponatremia with hypoosmolal serum, (2) inappropriately concentrated urine, (3) continued sodium excretion (urinary sodium of >25 mEq per liter), and the exclusion of renal or endocrine disease. There must also be an absence of stimuli that produce nonosmotic release of ADH, such as hypovolemia, hypotension, pain, stress, and nausea. Medications that can produce this syndrome include oral hypoglycemia agents, opiates, and carbamazepine.

The primary treatment of SIADH is volume restriction (1,000 to 1,500 ml per day) and maintenance of adequate salt intake. This treatment requires that total renal and insensible water losses exceed intake. Correction of hyponatremia is gradual, rarely exceeding 6 mEq per liter per day. Some have advocated the use of osmotic diuretics such as glycerol (two to three doses of 80 to 120 g each) or mannitol (one to two doses of 25 g each). Severe hyponatremia (<120 mEq per liter) is often associated with confusion, lethargy, and seizures, especially if the decrease in sodium concentration has been rapid (i.e., occurring over several hours). In patients with underlying brain lesions, these complications represent particularly serious conditions. They are best prevented by aggressive treatment of the hyponatremic patient. Most experienced clinicians recommend that severe hyponatremia in symptomatic patients be treated aggressively for 12 to 24 hours with a target serum sodium of 125 to 130 mEq per liter. This can be achieved by administering 100 ml aliquots of 3 percent saline over 1- to 2-hour intervals. Alternatively, the patient's extracellular volume can be estimated (weight in kilograms × 0.6), and the rate at which 3 percent saline is to be infused can then be determined so that the sodium concentration is corrected to a target value within 12 to 24 hours. For example, a 70-kg patient with a serum sodium of 120 mEq per liter requires approximately 420 mEq of sodium to reach a serum sodium of approximately 130 [(70 × 0.6) × (130−120)]. This could be accomplished in 24 hours by infusing 3 percent saline at a rate of 34 ml per hour. When a serum sodium concentration of 125 to 130 mEq per liter is achieved, a regimen of water restriction (1 to 1.5 L per day) can be established that leads to further correction of hyponatremia. Hypertonic solutions should only be administered via a catheter in a central vein and frequent reassessment (every other hour) of serum sodium concentration is necessary. Congestive heart failure occasionally complicates this therapy and is best avoided by monitoring of CVP or PCWP. The administration of diuretics (e.g., furosemide) prevents precipitating heart failure and also aids in free water clearance.

An association between severe hyponatremia (110 mEq per liter) and central pontine myelinolysis has been described. Predisposing factors may include concurrent malnutrition and liver disease associated with rapid (>2 mEq per liter per hour) correction of sodium concentration. However, there is recent evidence that overcorrection (i.e., hypernatremia) or the occurrence of a hyperosmolar state from any cause (i.e., hyperglycemia) is more directly related to the development of central pontine myelinolysis. Until the controversy is resolved, we recommend that the serum sodium concentration not be corrected more rapidly than 2 mEq per liter per hour and that overcorrection be avoided.

SIADH can be a transient phenomena not requiring prolonged therapy. In other situations, when chronic inappropriate secretion of ADH continues, blockade of the renal effects of the hormone by use of demeclocycline (600 to 1,200 mg per day) or lithium (900 mg per day) may be helpful.

HYPONATREMIA IN SUBARACHNOID HEMORRHAGE: CEREBRAL SALT WASTING

Aneurysmal subarachnoid hemorrhage (SAH) is frequently complicated by hyponatremia. In earlier reports, hyponatremia was often attributed to SIADH since the patients had hypo-osmolar serum and inappropriately concentrated urine. However, measurements of CVP, PCWP, and body weight suggested that these patients were hypovolemic, a finding that is inconsistent with SIADH. In fact, direct measurements of blood volume confirmed this clinical observation, and sodium balance studies demonstrated an excessive renal loss. Thus, although in some patients hyponatremia may be caused by SIADH, in the majority it appears to be the result of sodium and volume loss rather than water excess. It has been proposed that this sodium and volume loss may be caused by a natriuretic hormone or altered neural input to the kidneys. A further study suggested that volume restriction of patients with SAH produced an increased incidence of cerebral infarction from vasospasm. A more physiologically appropriate treatment for this syndrome is replacement of sodium and volume losses.

This therapy also improves central venous and arterial pressures and thus has the additional benefit of potentially improving perfusion to areas rendered ischemic from vasospasm.

Current management of hyponatremia after SAH focuses on the administration of adequate amounts of fluid and sodium in order to maintain normal intravascular volume. This strategy parallels the development of a physiologic approach to the treatment of vasospasm. The ability of volume expansion to reverse ischemic deficits caused by vasospasm underscores the importance of maintaining vascular volume after SAH. Because hyponatremia and vasospasm often occur simultaneously, careful attention to volume status is essential.

From the time of the initial presentation, management of intravenous fluids after acute aneurysmal SAH should be directed toward maintenance of vascular volume. This serves to preclude the development of hypovolemia and potentially prevents

vasospasm from becoming symptomatic. The administration of 2.5 to 3.5 L per day of normal saline is recommended for all patients presenting with SAH. Volume status should be closely monitored with daily weights and meticulous recording of fluid balance (input versus output). Whenever possible, CVP or PCWP should be recorded several times per day. A persistently negative fluid balance or a decrease in body weight, CVP, or PCWP may indicate a volume loss that usually precedes hyponatremia. If signs of persistent volume depletion occur, the patient should be transferred to an intensive care unit. In addition to monitoring of fluid balance and daily weights, monitoring should include CVP or PCWP and daily serum sodium measurements. Serial neurologic examinations are necessary to monitor for signs of vasospasm, which often accompanies and is exacerbated by volume depletion. Initial attempts to replete intravascular volume should employ administration of a large amount of normal (0.9 percent)

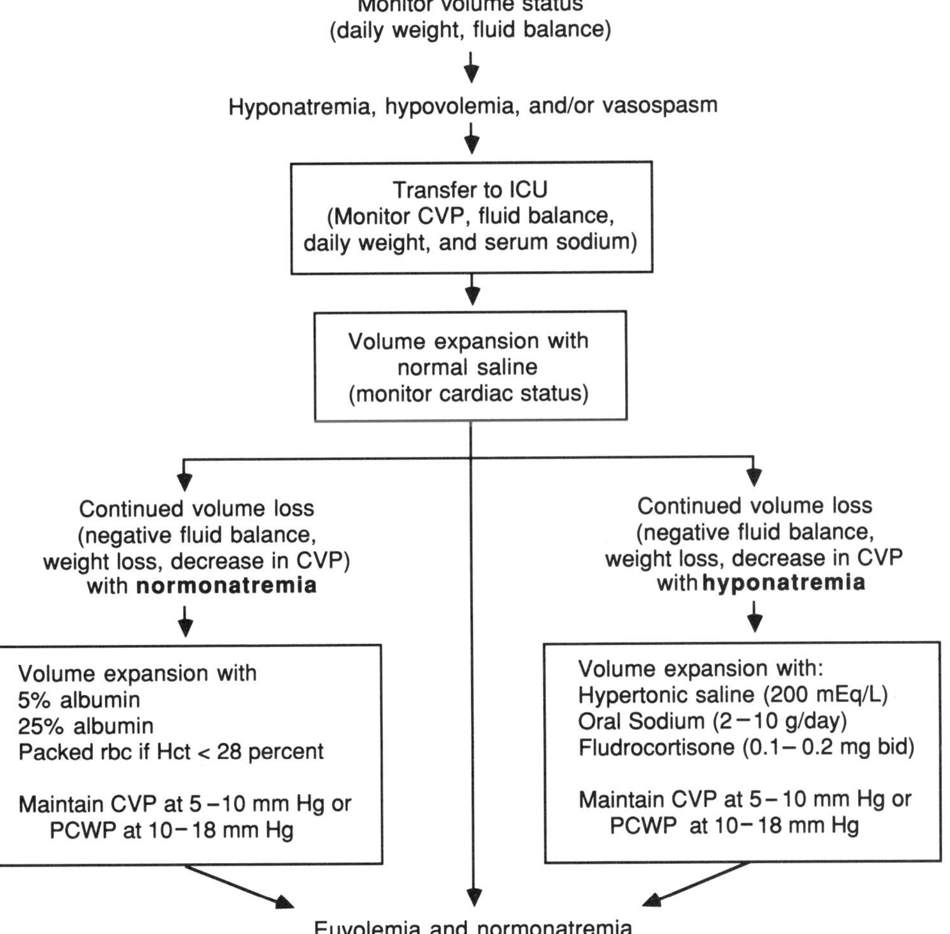

Figure 1 Management scheme for sodium and volume administration after subarachnoid hemorrhage. Treatment should begin with normal saline (2.5 to 3.5 L per day) and monitoring of volume status. Management of volume contraction with and without hyponatremia is presented.

saline, beginning with 10 to 15 ml per kilogram over 1 hour. Occasionally, infusion rates of as much as 1 L per hour may be necessary to correct deficit and "keep up" with losses. If there is continued evidence of volume loss and serum sodium is stable, colloids such as 5 or 25 pecent albumin should be administered. If the hematocrit is less than 28 percent, we administer packed red blood cells. In an attempt to limit blood viscosity, we do not raise the hematocrit to more than 35 percent. If the volume loss is accompanied by a decrease in serum sodium, greater amounts of both fluid and sodium should be administered. This can be accomplished with mildly hypertonic saline (200 mEq per liter) or oral sodium chloride (2 to 10 g per day administered every 4 to 6 hours). Fludrocortisone, an oral halogenated derivative of cortisol with potent mineralocorticoid and moderate glucocorticoid effects, may be employed to aid in both fluid and sodium retention. Administration should begin with a dose of 0.1 to 0.2 mg administered orally or intravenously twice per day, which can then be increased every 24 to 48 hours. Care must be employed in increasing the dose since a response may not be seen for 24 to 72 hours. Once stable intravascular volume and serum sodium have been achieved, the therapy should be maintained for several days. The duration of the defect is unknown, as are the clinical predictors of its end. Withdrawal of therapy should therefore be gradual, and volume status and serum sodium should be monitored. Once supplemental therapies have been withdrawn, patients should be maintained on moderate rates (100 to 200 ml per hour) of normal saline infusion for up to 1 additional week. Figure 1 is a flow diagram for the management of patients after subarachnoid hemorrhage.

This therapy is not without complications. Patients with heart disease are at risk for ischemia or development of congestive heart failure. Invasive cardiovascular monitoring with a Swan-Ganz catheter and monitoring of daily electrocardiograms is recommended in these patients. In addition, because of excessive urinary loss, there is potential for the development of hypokalemia, hypomagnesemia, and hypophosphatemia. Serum potassium, magnesium, and phosphate should be monitored daily. Some patients may require continuous replacement of these electrolytes.

Cerebral salt wasting does not appear to be unique to SAH patients. While the majority of patients with intracranial disease who develop hyponatremia will have SIADH, some patients develop hyponatremia with associated volume contraction. This has been reported to occur in patients with brain tumors, carcinomatous meningitis, and head trauma. On initial presentation, cerebral salt wasting may be difficult to distinguish from SIADH. The most important distinguishing feature is volume status (Table 1), a property that can be difficult to quan-

titate clinically. If there is doubt regarding vascular volume, it should be measured with the tracer dilution method. In a hyponatremic patient who has not suffered a SAH and who appears euvolemic, initial treatment should be for SIADH. The response to therapy should be carefully monitored by following serum sodium, body weight, and vascular pressures. A continued decrease in serum sodium, weight loss of more than 1 kg per day, or the development of signs of dehydration should not occur if the primary disturbance is the result of SIADH. If these signs develop, therapy should be altered to provide ample sodium and volume replacement with careful monitoring of the response.

DIABETES INSIPIDUS

In central diabetes insipidus (DI), excessive renal free water excretion results from a relative deficiency of circulating ADH. It is usually a manifestation of CNS diseases in the region of the optic chiasm or pituitary gland. Etiologies include mass lesions (tumors, vascular malformation), basilar inflammation (meningitis, sarcoidosis), and brain death. Ethanol or phenytoin can produce DI by inhibiting the release of ADH. Clinically these patients produce hypotonic urine (specific gravity as low as 1.001) with a high output ranging from 3 to 15 L per day. Individuals who have intact osmoreceptive mechanisms experience feelings of thirst and drink large volumes of water to compensate for losses. If they are denied water or if they become obtunded, failure to replace water losses can result in severe hypernatremia and hyperosmolality. This may also occur if the mass extends into the anterior hypothalamus and directly impairs thirst mechanisms. Signs and symptoms of hyperosmolality include restlessness, irritability, lethargy, coma, and seizures.

Surgical exploration of chiasmal tumors is a common cause of DI. Disruption of ADH secretion is often transient, and polyuria lasts 12 to 24 hours with a subsequent return to normal osmoregulation. Rarely the infundibular stalk has been sectioned or severely contused with cessation of ADH release. However, 1 to 5 days postoperatively, cell bodies die, which frequently leads to excessive release of ADH. The result is a period of high urine output caused by the initial absence of ADH release, followed by a period of water retention and hyponatremia due to abrupt and unregulated release of large amounts of ADH from degenerating perikarya. Persistent excessive volume replacement or prior hormonal replacement with long-acting ADH preparation can complicate the management of these patients and should be avoided.

Before one may conclude that DI is the cause of high urine output, other etiologies should be excluded (Fig. 2). These include the administration of

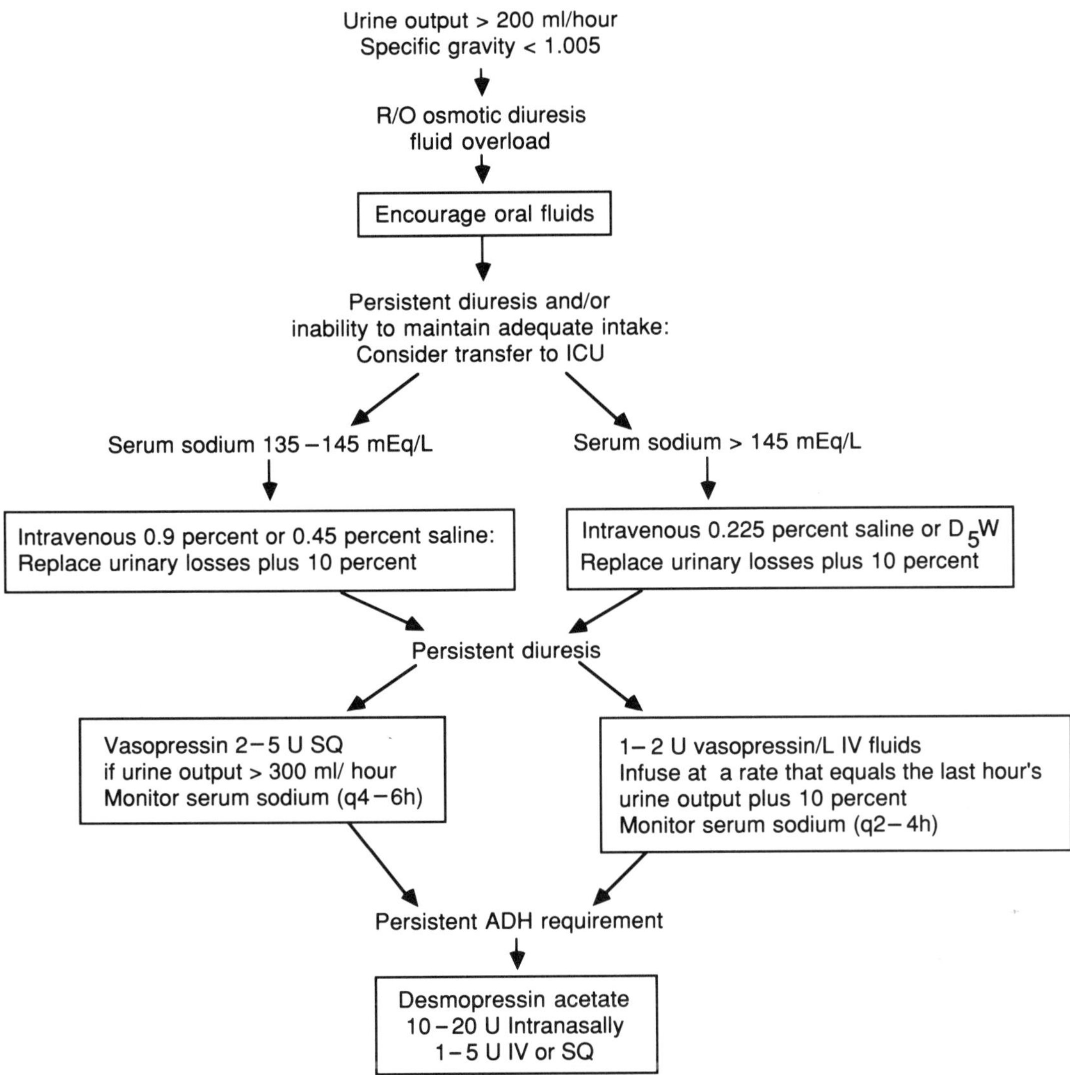

Figure 2 Evaluation and treatment of DI. Once DI has been established as the cause of high urine output, treatment should begin with oral fluid administration. Persistent diuresis or poor intake is treated with intravenous fluids. Fluid choice is based on the serum sodium concentration. Persistent diuresis can be treated with ADH supplementation by subcutaneous or intravenous routes. Long-acting agents (desmopressin acetate) should be administered only after a persistent requirement for ADH has been demonstrated.

large volumes of fluid and osmotic diuresis caused by mannitol or hyperglycemia. Initial treatment of DI should begin with oral or intravenous fluid replacement. If the serum sodium concentration is elevated, the intravenous fluid should be hypotonic (i.e., D_5W or $D_5\frac{1}{4}$ normal saline). If easy control is not achieved, ADH should be replaced with short-acting agents. For example, 2 to 5 U of ADH can be given subcutaneously every few hours. The dosing interval is best determined by monitoring urine output and repeating the dose when output exceeds 300 ml per hour. The response to therapy should be monitored with serial measurements (every 4 to 6 hours) of urine specific gravity and serum sodium. A useful alternative is to dilute 1 to 2 U of aqueous vasopressin in 1 L of intravenous fluid (choice of fluid depends on plasma sodium concentration) and infuse the solution at a rate that equals the urine output of the previous hour plus 10 percent. This method is especially useful in patients who have a fluctuating requirement for ADH replacement, and it requires close monitoring (every 2 hours) of serum sodium until stable requirements for fluid and ADH are achieved. Long-term replacement is necessary for patients with complete or near complete destruction of the neurohypophysis and should only be started after several days of consistently impaired water regulation. Desmopressin acetate in a dose of 10 to 20 μg administered intranasally or 1 to 5 μg administered intravenously or subcutaneously produces water retention for 12 to 24 hours. Intramuscular vasopressin tannate in oil (2 to 5 U) can produce antidiuretic activity for as long as 72 hours but its absorption is less predictable and therefore is not recommended.

SUGGESTED READING

Schrier RW. Renal and electrolyte disorders. Boston: Little, Brown and Company, 1986.
Lester MC, Nelson PB. Neurological aspects of vasopressin release and the syndrome of inappropriate secretion of antidiuretic hormone. Neurosurgery 1981; 8:735–740.
Robertson GL, Aycinea P, Zerbe RL. Neurogenic disorders of osmoregulation. Am J Med 1982; 72:339–353.
Wijdicks EFM, Vermeulen M, Hijdra A, van Gijn J. Hyponatremia and cerebral infarction in patients with ruptured intracranial aneurysms: is fluid restriction harmful? Ann Neurol 1985; 17:137–140.

HEPATIC ENCEPHALOPATHY

JEFFREY D. ROTHSTEIN, M.D., Ph.D.
GUY M. McKHANN, M.D.

Hepatic encephalopathy is a neuropsychiatric syndrome that complicates both acute and chronic liver disease. It is often seen in children with congenital urea cycle enzyme defects. Subtypes of this disorder are classified by the rate of progression and nature of the underlying hepatic disease. Fulminant hepatic failure results in hepatic encephalopathy within 8 weeks of the onset of liver injury and is associated with a high mortality rate. Subacute or chronic hepatic encephalopathy, which is associated with chronic hepatocellular disease, is episodic and milder.

Hepatic encephalopathy may be caused by potentially reversible metabolic abnormalities. Although the pathogenesis of hepatic encephalopathy remains obscure, it reflects direct or indirect central nervous system (CNS) exposure to substances not cleared by the liver.

CLINICAL AND LABORATORY FEATURES

The typical clinical course of hepatic encephalopathy is characterized by (1) alterations in behavior including inattention to personal hygiene and appearance and impairment of consciousness (delirium, coma); (2) alterations in motor tone and posture (tremor, paratonia, asterixis, hyperactive muscle stretch reflexes); (3) slowing of the electroencephalogram (EEG) ("triphasic" slow waves); and (4) characteristic elevations in fasting plasma ammonia and cerebrospinal fluid (CSF) glutamine concentrations. These signs and symptoms may vary, depending on the subtype of the hepatic encephalopathy.

Staging

Although manifestations of hepatic encephalopathy are protean, they are generally grouped into four clinical stages based on the severity of encephalopathy (Table 1). Signs and symptoms may vary within each stage. This staging may help in following patients and assessing the efficacy of therapy. Early hepatic encephalopathy, stage I or "incipient" encephalopathy, may be overlooked because of stable symptoms, such as reversal of sleep patterns or personality changes.

Asterixis and a worsening of mental status are seen in patients with stage II hepatic encephalopathy. Asterixis is a transient loss of postural tone of the extensors or the wrist when the hands are out-

Table 1 Signs and Symptoms of Hepatic Encephalopathy

Stage	Mental status and behavior	Motor/Reflexes
I	Diminished attention	Fine postural tremor
	Mild confusion	Slowed coordination
	Anxiety	
	Irritability	
	Agitation	
	Diminished attention	
	Impaired serial 7's	
	Altered sleep patterns	
	Depression	
II	Drowsiness	Asterixis
	Lethargy	Dysarthria
	Gross personality changes	Primitive reflexes
	Disorientation (time)	(sucking, grasping)
	Poor recall	Paratonia
	Inappropriate behavior	Ataxia
III	Profound confusion	Hyperreflexia
	Paranoia	Seizures
	Disorientation of time and place	Babinski's sign
		Hyperventilation
	Incomprehensible speech	Incontinence
	Somnolent but arousable	Hypothermia
		Myoclonus
IV	Coma	Decerebrate posturing
		Brisk oculocephalic reflexes

stretched. It is not specific for hepatic encephalopathy and may be seen in patients with uremia, pulmonary disease, malnutrition, and polycythemia rubra vera.

Stage III of the disease heralds more profound and serious neurologic abnormalities. Focal or generalized seizures may develop. The patient may become somnolent or incontinent. Rapid, deep respirations may accompany hyperreflexia with extensor plantar reflexes. With stage IV coma, a diminished response to pain with decerebrate and decorticate posturing is seen. Unlike other diseases, with hepatic encephalopathy this posturing is reversible.

Establishing the Diagnosis

It is relatively easy to recognize encephalopathy in a patient with fulminant hepatic failure. When hepatic disease is not clinically obvious, however, the nonspecific characteristics of early hepatic encephalopathy make diagnosis more difficult. Abnormal laboratory tests of hepatic function may establish the presence of liver disease. An elevated plasma ammonia level may be useful in confirming the diagnosis of hepatic encephalopathy, but a normal plasma ammonia concentration does not exclude this diagnosis. Furthermore, the degree of elevation of plasma or cerebrospinal fluid (CSF) ammonia levels does not correlate with the severity of encephalopathy. An elevation in CSF glutamine concentration is the most specific and sensitive laboratory test for this disease and correlates well with the degree of hepatic encephalopathy. Unfortunately, glutamine assays are not performed in some clinical laboratories.

The coagulopathy and thrombocytopenia that can accompany hepatic disease may make lumbar puncture unsafe. If prothrombin time ratios are greater than 1.3 and/or platelet counts are less than 40,000, the physician should be prepared to administer fresh frozen plasma or platelets.

The EEG is abnormal in patients with hepatic encephalopathy, but the abnormalities are nonspecific. Symmetrical frontal slow waves that spread posteriorly are seen. Triphasic slow waves, commonly attributed to hepatic encephalopathy, may occur in patients with head injury, subdural hematomas, uremia, cerebral anoxia, and electrolyte abnormalities. Psychometric testing, although not particularly helpful in diagnosing hepatic encephalopathy, provides a semiquantitative means of following response to therapy. Easy bedside evaluations include trail-making (Reitan number connection) and tests using block designs or star constructions.

Differential Diagnosis

Since the neuropsychiatric manifestations of hepatic encephalopathy are nonspecific, it is important to rule out other causes of encephalopathy in patients with hepatic disease. Toxins, metabolic abnormalities, and structural lesions can cause similar clinical features. In patients with impaired liver function, cerebral depression caused by the use of sedatives, narcotics, or tranquilizers should be considered. The use of benzodiazepines should be avoided in patients with hepatic encephalopathy because of the increased sensitivities to these agents. The delirium of alcohol withdrawal may be confused with an agitated delirium of hepatic encephalopathy, and a recent history of alcohol abuse may help one make the necessary differentiation. Hypokalemia or hyponatremia are commonly seen in patients with cirrhosis and may produce a coma that can be rapidly reversed with electrolyte correction. Encephalopathy secondary to hypoxia, hypoglycemia, and uremia should also be considered.

Focal neurologic signs may occur, but these are unusual in patients with hepatic encephalopathy and should prompt a search for structural abnormalities. An EEG is essential to rule out subclinical status epilepticus. There are no characteristic computed tomographic (CT) changes of the brain. Patients with a subclinical stable lesion (head trauma, chronic subdural hematoma, stroke) may develop focal neurologic signs or symptoms when hepatic encephalopathy develops. Whenever a patient with hepatic encephalopathy develops focal neurologic signs, it is essential that CT scanning of the head be performed to exclude underlying structural disease (e.g., tumor or abscess). Meningitis should also be considered, especially in patients with alcoholic cirrhosis. Subarachnoid and intracerebral hemorrhage are not uncommon in patients with hepatic encephalopathy and are seen in 11 percent of autopsied patients after orthotopic liver transplantation.

PATHOGENESIS

Multiple hypotheses have been proposed to explain the pathogenesis of hepatic encephalopathy, but a specific cause is not known. Over the last several decades, several agents, including ammonia, short-chain fatty acids, mercaptans, phenols, false neurotransmitters (octopamine), and recently gamma-aminobutyric acid (GABA) have been proposed as candidate "toxins." No single agent is likely to be completely responsible for the disease.

Ammonia is the most commonly incriminated toxin. Its role as an important agent of hepatic encephalopathy is supported by the observation that encephalopathy develops in patients who have elevated ammonia concentrations from urea cycle enzyme defects but who have otherwise normal livers. Often patients with hepatic encephalopathy have elevated arterial ammonia levels. However, hepatic encephalopathy can clearly occur in the presence of normal blood and CSF ammonia levels. In addition, therapies that reduce plasma levels of ammonia ameliorate hepatic encephalopathy. Hyperammonemia is associated with seizures and may contribute to the encephalopathy of primary hyperammonemic disorders. The glutamine concentration is markedly increased in the CNS, probably reflecting brain ammonia detoxification. Although glutamine is inactive, it is an important precursor of amino acid neurotransmitters, including glutamate, aspartate, and GABA.

Hepatic encephalopathy can be rapidly reserved in animals and humans by benzodiazepine antagonists. Benzodiazepines produce their effects in the CNS by modulation of the inhibitory neurotransmitter GABA. New theories on the neurochemical etiology of hepatic encephalopathy suggest that increased inhibitory GABA tone, perhaps secondary to the use of endogenous benzodiazepines or benzodiazepine-like material, is responsible for the encephalopathy of hepatic failure.

TREATMENT

Recognition of Precipitating Causes

Treatment requires that the precipitating causes be addressed (Table 2). Agitated patients are often misdiagnosed as having insomnia rather than early encephalopathy and are treated with sedatives. Excessive diuretic therapy may cause a hypokalemic alkalosis. Hypokalemia causes increased renal ammonia production, and alkalosis favors the diffusion of ammonia into the CNS. Intravascular volume depletion from diuretic therapy reduces renal blood flow and increases the blood urea nitrogen concentration. This excess urea diffuses into the gut, leading to increased ammonia production by bacterial ureases. Bacterial infections can precipitate encephalopathy and are often not suspected because patients with chronic liver disease are frequently hypo-

Table 2 Precipitants of Hepatic Encephalopathy

Drugs
Sedatives
Tranquilizers
Narcotics
Diuretics
Electrolyte imbalance
Hyponatremia
Hypokalemic alkalosis
Hypoxia
Hypovolemia
Excessive nitrogen load
Gastrointestinal hemorrhage
Excess dietary protein
Azotemia
Constipation
Infection

thermic. Cultures of blood, urine, CSF, and ascites, if present, should be obtained for all cases of unexplained encephalopathy.

Specific Therapies

The therapy for hepatic encephalopathy is based on the premise that substances in the gastrointestinal tract are acted upon by intestinal bacteria and converted to "toxins" that are absorbed into the blood (Table 3). These toxins bypass the liver via collateral circulation, enter the brain, and presumably induce encephalopathy. Based on these principles, therapy is directed at (1) decreasing the colonic substrate for these putative comagenic toxins, (2) reducing the bacteria capable of producing these toxins, (3) diminishing the influx of these compounds into the CNS, and (4) decreasing the effect these compounds have on neurotransmitter activity and metabolism.

Reduction of Gastrointestinal Protein and Toxins

Reduction of dietary protein is a simple method for reducing gastrointestinal protein and should be the first step in therapy. Protein intake can be withheld for the first 1 to 2 days, and is gradually increased in increments of 10 g per day. Dietary intake should not be less than 40 g per day chronically, as negative nitrogen balance ensues with increased risk of infection and with diminished hepatic regeneration. Patients with hepatic encephalopathy secondary to gastrointestinal hemorrhage, constipation, or large protein loads should be treated with tap water enemas and lactulose to evacuate nitrogenous substrates.

Lactulose is the mainstay of therapy to prevent or diminish hepatic encephalopathy. Its cathartic action increases ammonia elimination. Bacterial metabolism of lactulose acidifies the colonic contents and converts ammonia to its ionized and less absorbable form. Lactulose may be administered orally or as retention enemas in obtunded patients. For patients with recurrent hepatic encephalopathy, lactulose can be used chronically (30 ml taken orally 3 times per day). In patients refractory to dietary protein restriction and lactulose therapy, the oral antibiotics neomycin and metronidazole have been used to promote colonic bacteriostasis.

Reduction of Gastrointestinal Bacteria

In patients who cannot be managed with dietary protein restriction and lactulose therapy, the elimination of gastrointestinal bacteria may prove useful. The premise of this therapy is that diminution of gastrointestinal flora diminishes the production of ammonia and other possible toxins. Neomycin can be taken orally in a dose of 1 to 2 g every 6 hours.

Table 3 Management of Hepatic Encephalopathy

Therapy
1. Eliminate predisposing factors:
   a. Sedatives, tranquilizers, analgesics
   b. Fluid/electrolyte dysfunction. (Correct hypokalemia/alkalosis, hyponatremia.)
   c. Gastrointestinal bleeding, commonly seen secondary to varices. (Determine if bleeding is occurring by nasogastric aspiration of stomach and stool heme monitoring. If there is gastrointestinal bleeding, frequent bowel movements need to be produced to help cleanse gut of proteinaceous blood—e.g., by repeated enemas.)
      Normalize intravascular volume (to prevent prerenal azotemia).
2. Dietary protein restriction
   a. Begin with protein-free diet (must provide enough calories to inhibit proteolysis—e.g., 10% D/W or nasogastric glucose + lipids; one should try to provide 1,500–2,000 cal/day; avoid hyperalimentation, as this will provide excess amino acids).
   b. With improvement, increase diet protein to 20 g/day and increase protein by 10 g/day increments every 2–3 days until maximum protein total is reached; for outpatients, maximum is usually 50 g/day.
   c. Administer cathartics to eliminate gut protein (e.g., oral magnesium citrate [200 ml] or sorbitol [50 g in 200 ml water).
   d. Administer vitamin supplementation: folate (1 mg/day), vitamin K (10 mg/day), thiamine, and multivitamins.
3. Diminish gastrointestinal ammonia absorption by using either:
      Neomycin (1 g p.o. q.i.d.; complicated by candidal gut overgrowth and malabsorption).
                                          or
      Lactulose (synthetic disaccharide that is not digested in the upper gastrointestinal tract) 10–30 ml p.o. or by retention enema t.i.d.
Monitoring
1. Stage patient.
2. Check arterial ammonia.
3. EEG.
4. CSF glutamine.

Chronic management/prevention
1. Prescribe low-protein diet (usually 50 g/day).
2. Administer vitamin supplementation: folate, vitamin K, multivitamins.
3. Administer lactulose (10–30 ml p.o. t.i.d. (at least one soft bowel movement/day).

Only small amounts of this drug can be absorbed, however, and since it is excreted primarily in urine, its use should be avoided in patients with renal insufficiency. Even in patients with normal renal function, prolonged therapy can produce ototoxicity and nephrotoxicity.

Alternatives to neomycin include metronidazole (250 mg taken orally three times per day), which has side effects that include leukopenia, peripheral neuropathy, metallic taste, and disulfiramlike reaction. Other bacteriostatic therapies include those using oral tetracycline or ampicillin.

Other Therapies

Because there have been so many theories concerning hepatic encephalopathy, several unproven therapies have been tried. These include levodopa and the dopamine agonist bromocriptine, both of which have arousal properties. In controlled clinical trials, these agents failed to produce reliable clinical benefits.

Because patients with hepatic encephalopathy have abnormal plasma and CSF amino acid concentrations, it has been suggested that the increased plasma aromatic amino acids producd in these patients may interfere with normal neurotransmitter synthesis. To that end, trials with solutions enriched with branched-chain amino acids, which compete with aromatic amino acids for transport into the CNS, have been tried. The results of these studies are mixed and controversial. For a variety of reasons, including the excessive cost of these solutions, the high osmolarity and fluid load, and the marginal benefit, this therapy is not routinely recommended.

An important, rare subset of patients with hepatic encephalopathy includes those suffering from inherited urea cycle defects (e.g., ornithine transcarbamoylase deficiency). In these patients, primarily children, accumulation of ammonia is believed to be responsible for the encephalopathy, and attempts to lower serum ammonia have proven useful. Infusions of sodium benzoate and sodium phenylacetate (as much as 0.25 g per kilogram per day of each) may be employed to control potentially fatal hyperammonemia successfully. Alternative therapies include the use of arginine or citrulline, depending on the specific enzyme deficiency.

Flumazenil (RO 15-1788) is a benzodiazepine receptor antagonist widely used in Europe. It is reported to reverse hepatic encephalopathy, eliminate relapsing encephalopathy, and allow the resumption of normal protein intake in patients with chronic hepatic failure. This agent is now being further evaluated in the United States, although it is not yet available.

PREVENTION

Preventative measures help minimize recurrent encephalopathy. Stool softeners reduce constipation and the use of outpatient lactulose serves both as a laxative and a means of eliminating gastrointestinal ammonia absorption. To anticipate the possibility for gastrointestinal hemorrhage, frequent stool Hemoccult can be employed, with the patient mailing test cards to their physician. Obviously, the use of sedatives (especially benzodiazepines) and narcotics should be avoided in patients with hepatic disease. The regular use of multivitamins, especially thiamine, should be encouraged.

FULMINANT HEPATIC FAILURE

Unlike chronic hepatic disease, fulminant hepatic failure (FHF) is associated with a high mortality rate (>50 percent). FHF is associated with a variety of hepatic insults including viral hepatitis, poison, chemical or drug exposure (e.g., acetaminophen), and ischemic hepatitis. Hyperammonemia as well as hypoglycemia, hypoxia secondary to cardiac failure, pulmonary infections, and uremia associated with hepatorenal syndrome all contribute to the encephalopathy. Intensive medical and neurologic management has, however, made inroads to decreasing overall mortality. In these patients, particular attention should be paid to electrolytes, acid-base balance, glucose, coagulation defects, and pulmonary, cardiac, and renal status. These patients may also develop coagulopathy, hypotension, hypoxia, pulmonary edema, hypoglycemia, and pancreatitis, and need to be monitored in an intensive care setting with central venous pressure monitoring as well as standard intensive care unit cardiac monitoring. Constant vigilance for infections must be maintained.

Cerebral Edema in Fulminant Hepatic Failure

Although this encephalopathy appears similar to that associated with chronic hepatic disease, the underlying mechanisms and the treatment may be quite different. Most importantly, FHF is associated with lethal cerebral edema, and that is the major extrahepatic lesion found at autopsy. Because papilledema may not be seen, there are no good clinical indices for cerebral edema. Sudden deterioration of consciousness, hyperactive reflexes along with plantar reflexes, and decerebrate/decorticate posturing may suggest increased intracranial pressure (ICP), but these can also be seen in patients with metabolic encephalopathy. Abnormal pupillary light responses and oculocephalic ("doll's eye" maneuver) reflexes may be reversible; however, abnormal oculovestibular reflexes (cold caloric test) carry a poor prognosis. CT may reveal slitlike ventricles or other signs of an increased ICP. ICP transducers have been used by some to help monitor ICP, but their use may cause significant intracranial bleeding. Standard therapies aimed at controlling ICP, such as hyperventilation and furosemide therapy, can be employed. Mannitol has been used to reduce elevated pressure, but in patients with an ICP greater than 60 mm Hg, it may be deleterious. Mannitol should be used only when ICP transducers are in place. There is no proven value for the use of steroids.

Treatment

In addition to controlling ICP, one must still pay attention to the underlying hepatic abnormalities. Given the large number of metabolic problems, the approach to FHF is not as effective as that used for chronic hepatic disease. Most patients are obtunded or comatose, and therefore little dietary protein is ingested. Lactulose can be used to remove nitrogen waste from the gut initially, but can produce complicating electrolyte disturbances secondary to excessive diarrhea. Other therapies such as total body washout, charcoal hemoperfusion, and hemodialysis have not proved reliable. When available, orthotopic liver transplantation may be the most important therapeutic option.

SUGGESTED READING

Jones EA, Gammal SH. Hepatic encephalopathy. In: Arias IM, Jakoby WB, Popper H, et al, eds. The liver: biology and pathobiology. 2nd ed. New York: Raven Press, 1988:985.

Lockwood AH. Hepatic encephalopathy: experimental approaches to human metabolic encephalopathy. CRC Crit Rev Neurobiol 1987; 3:105–133.

Rothstein JD, Herlong FH. Neurological manifestations of hepatic disease. Neurol Clin 1989; 7:563–578.

Zieve L. Hepatic encephalopathy. In: Schiss O, Schiff ER, eds. Diseases of the liver. Philadelphia: JB Lippincott, 1987:925.

MITOCHONDRIAL ENCEPHALOMYOPATHY

OREST HURKO, M.D.
PATTI L. PETERSON, M.D.

The mitochondrial encephalomyopathies are a group of clinically and genetically heterogeneous disorders that result from dysfunction of the electron transport chain. When mitochondrial oxidative phosphorylation is compromised, the production of adenosine triphosphate (ATP) is impaired significantly. Energy-dependent ionic balance fails, leading to an increase in intracellular calcium, with precipitation of degradative lipolytic and proteolytic effects. In addition, toxic-reduced intermediates (e.g., lactate) accumulate, and partial reduction of oxygen produces toxic-free radicals. These consequences can be deadly to cells. Tissues that are ordinarily most dependent on oxidative metabolism are at greatest risk for permanent damage. The treatment of these disorders is based on avoidance of exacerbating factors and provision of drug therapy that allows continued energy production and ameliorates these degradative processes and toxic effects.

In theory, dysfunction of the electron transport chain can result from mutations affecting any of its constituent 70 polypeptides (13 of which are encoded by mitochondrial DNA and the remainder by nuclear genes) or their associated cofactors. Since oxidative metabolism is crucial for most cells, survival of the individual is possible only if there is enough energy to sustain cellular function. A mutation affecting all of an individual's mitochondria, as in Leber's optic atrophy, only partially disrupts oxidative metabolism. For those patients with massive deletions of mitochondrial DNA and complete disruption of the activity of a crucial component of the electron transport chain, survival is possible owing to the existence of some normal mitochondria. In either case, the reserve of oxidative activity is diminished and cellular activity above a critical threshold may result in tissue damage.

There is great potential for clinical variability (Table 1) since some of the nuclear-encoded subunits exist as tissue-specific isozymes, each presumably under the control of a separate, mutable gene. Each cell contains hundreds of copies of a mitochondrial DNA, only some of which may be mutants, and the proportions of mutant and normal mitochondrial DNA can vary widely in different tissues from the same individual. Although attempts have been made to correlate a given clinical phenotype with a dysfunction at a particular site (i.e., the biochemical site of a partial block) along the electron transport chain, it appears to correlate more strongly with the degree of impairment of oxidative metabolism in affected tissues. This view is supported by our observation of similar biochemical dysfunction in disparate phenotypes, the presence of "overlap" syndromes in certain patients, and the occasional presence of several seemingly different clinical phenotypes within a given family. For this reason, our approach to diagnosis and treatment of the various mitochondrial encephalomyopathies is based on an assumption that many of the phenotypic differences between these patients are quantitative rather than qualitative.

DIAGNOSIS

Analysis of Skeletal Muscle

The diagnosis of these disorders is best made by morphologic, biochemical, and molecular analysis of biopsied skeletal muscle. Ideally, a 3- to 4-g muscle specimen is taken from the vastus lateralis and divided for testing and establishment of muscle cultures, (which can be useful for confirmatory studies.) Morphologic studies of frozen sections include the Gomori trichrome stain for "ragged red" fibers and the more sensitive oxidative stains (NADH, succinate dehydrogenase, and cytochrome oxidase). Specimens can be fixed and embedded for electron microscopy to permit detection of subtle mitochondrial abnormalities, as in Leber's optic atrophy.

Biochemical testing is useful for establishing the diagnosis, to aid prognosis (more severe deficiencies have a poorer prognosis), and for localizing the defect to a particular respiratory complex, which can aid formulation of a rational therapy. Ideally, polarographic studies (with an oxygen electrode) of isolated mitochondria should be performed on at least 2 g of fresh muscle tissue (not frozen). If local facilities for such analysis are not accessible, or if the available muscle mass does not permit a biopsy of this size, a 1-g specimen can be frozen for later enzymatic and spectrophotometric analysis. In

Table 1 Phenotypes Associated With Dysfunction of the Electron Transport Chain

Infantile lactic acidosis
Leigh's disease
Chronic progressive external ophthalmoplegia (CPEO), including the Kearns-Sayre Syndrome
Mitochondrial encephalomyopathy, lactic acidosis, and strokelike episodes (MELAS)
Myoclonic epilepsy and ragged-red fibers (MERRF)
"Ragged red" fiber myopathy
Infantile bilateral striatal necrosis (IBSN)
Leber's hereditary optic atrophy (LHOA)
Others

some instances, biochemical diagnosis is possible in cultured fibroblasts or myoblasts; unfortunately, this is frequently not the case. Clinically useful molecular analysis is currently limited to the detection of gross deletions in mitochondrial DNA (an analysis that requires 100 mg of frozen muscle) or of the point mutation responsible for one form of Leber's optic atrophy (a test that can be accomplished using 5 ml of venous blood collected in EDTA or acid-citrate-dextrose [ACD], but not heparin, tubes). Research is underway to allow detection of other types of nuclear and mitochondrial DNA mutations in other types of tissue.

Clinical Testing

Less invasive laboratory testing is useful in the initial assessment of the patient and as a means of following the efficacy of treatment. Venous levels of the closely related metabolites lactate, pyruvate, and alanine are frequently elevated. Care must be taken to avoid spurious elevations by drawing the sample after release of the tourniquet and ensuring prompt delivery of the specimen to the laboratory on ice. Since the normal levels of these metabolites vary with exercise, it is best to use fasting specimens taken in the morning or those drawn after a standardized exercise protocol. Where available, tests of oxygen consumption can be performed during standardized exercise protocols or 31-P nuclear magnetic resonance (NMR) spectroscopy may be used to assess high energy phosphate content of muscle. These tests are particularly useful for monitoring response to therapy.

Since these disorders can affect multiple organ systems, the workup should include the following:

1. Electroencephalography and magnetic resonance imaging (MRI) (to look for unrecognized abnormalities).
2. Audiometry and brain stem auditory–evoked potentials (to search for sensorineural deafness).
3. Ophthalmoscopy, visual-evoked potentials, and electroretinography (to assess retinal and optic nerve function).
4. Nerve conduction tests and electromyography (to evaluate peripheral nerve involvement).
5. Electrocardiography (to detect cardiac conduction defects).
6. Tests of endocrine function (to look for hormonal insufficiency—most commonly, thyroid hormone and parathormone).
7. Measurement of urinary amino acids (to detect De Toni-Fanconi syndrome) and measurement of urinary protein excretion and creatinine clearance (to assess glomerular and renal function).
8. Tests of liver function.

Other clinical testing should be undertaken to consider differential diagnoses appropriate to the given clinical syndrome. In the case of infantile lactic acidosis, one must rule out nongenetic causes such as septic shock and severe heart failure, and genetic disorders such as those involving gluconeogenesis (e.g., deficiencies of glucose-6-phosphate dehydrogenase, fructose-1,6-diphosphatase, phosphoenolpyruvate carboxykinase, pyruvate carboxylase, or multiple biotin-dependent carboxylases), defects of the pyruvate dehydrogenase complex, and organic acidurias, which can be associated with mild elevations of lactic acid. Systemic carnitine deficiency should be considered when appropriate. Proton MRI alterations of basal ganglia should prompt consideration of Wilson's disease (copper being a component of cytochrome oxidase, the rate-limiting enzyme of the electron transport chain), Hallervorden-Spatz syndrome, Huntington's disease, hypoxia, or carbon monoxide intoxication. Chronic progressive external ophthalmoplegia must be distinguished from centronuclear myopathy, thyroid disease, myasthenia gravis, Whipple's disease, olivopontocerebellar atrophy, progressive supranuclear palsy, and Niemann-Pick disease (type D). MELAS (mitochondrial encephalopathy, lactic acidosis, and strokelike episodes) should also be distinguished from embolic, occlusive, or inflammatory disease of cerebral vessels.

TREATMENT

Nonspecific Therapies

As the pathophysiologic mechanisms underlying these disorders are better understood, rational therapies can be formulated. Since it appears that clinically apparent tissue damage in these disorders occurs only when demand for high-energy phosphates exceeds the capacity of oxidative phosphorylation, care is taken to limit metabolic stress. Patients are cautioned not to exercise to the point of excessive fatigue, so that lactic acidosis (and, rarely, myoglobinuria) are avoided. Adequate hydration should be maintained. Similarly, seizures, whether focal or generalized, are treated aggressively since regional cortical hyperactivity during an ictus may lead to a permanent infarction. Carbamazepine (Tegretol) is given for seizures with a focal onset, and valproate (Depakene, Depakote) is given for primary generalized seizures. Clonazepam (Klonopin) is effective in the treatment of patients with disabling myoclonus. Unless parenteral therapy is necessary, phenytoin (Dilantin) and phenobarbital are avoided because of their inhibitory effect on the electron transport chain. Fever is treated aggressively with acetaminophen (not aspirin, owing to its deleterious effects on mitochondrial function), and when indicated, antibiotics are prescribed early (chloramphenicol and tetracycline are avoided, however, as they are inhibitors of mitochondrial protein synthesis). Extremes of environmental temperature should be avoided when possible. Blood sugars should be monitored for evidence of glucose intolerance, and fasting should be avoided.

In most of the syndromes encountered by neurologists, systemic levels of lactic acid are not sufficiently high to warrant treatment with bicarbonate. However, in patients with infantile lactic acidosis, and, occasionally, those presenting with the Leigh's phenotype, sodium bicarbonate treatment may be necessary for the maintenance of acid-base balance. Supplemental oxygen in patients with adequate cardiopulmonary function is usually unnecessary; indeed, such therapy may be harmful, as it may exacerbate the production of toxic-free radicals.

Specific Therapies

Specific treatment for mitochondrial encephalomyopathies involves provision of the following:

1. Electron shuttling agents (i.e., agents that have an affinity for electrons and that can be used to bypass a block in the electron transport chain).
2. Blocking agents and antioxidants (i.e., agents that block degradative lipolytic and proteolytic effects and free radical scavengers).
3. Cofactors for components of the electron transport chain, concentration or affinity of which may require pharmacologic doses of these compounds for maximal activity.

Ideally, the biochemical defect underlying each patient's disorder should be delineated precisely. This information is used to tailor a specific therapy, and the results of treatment are assessed in a controlled trial with appropriate biochemical and physiologic monitoring. However, because many of the agents that have been found to be effective in the treatment of certain patients have a low potential for side effects, we consider their empirical use appropriate in those patients who do not have access to centers conducting controlled clinical trials. Those patients who respond to therapy usually do so fairly rapidly, with most noting improvement within days to weeks. It is often difficult to assess the results of therapy because of the frequent occurrence of spontaneous improvement, particularly in MELAS patients, and long-term follow-up is therefore necessary. Some patients with a significant degree of acidosis may benefit from carnitine replacement therapy if their serum level is low.

Electron Shuttles

Electron shuttles currently in clinical use include paired menadione (vitamin K_3) and ascorbic acid (vitamin C). This combination can be used to bypass a block in electron flow caused by a deficiency of complex III. In the United States, vitamin K_4 (menadiol) is available as a parenteral preparation in dosages of 5, 10, and 37.5 mg, and in 5-mg tablets (menadiol sodium diphosphate [Synkayvite]). For adults we have administered 1 to 2 5-mg tablets twice per day in conjunction with 1 g of ascorbate twice per day, although others have found better responses with larger dosages. Vitamin K_3 can interfere with the action of warfarin and can paradoxically increase prothrombin times in patients with pre-existing liver disease, to whom the medication should not be given.

Blocking Agents

Blocking agents are used to disrupt degradative processes. Currently, only steroids are available to block the phospholipases that are activated by elevation of intracellular calcium content. Steroids induce the formation of an antiphospholipase compound. Unfortunately, steroids have many other effects, some undesirable and some, undoubtedly, not yet recognized. We use methylprednisolone (Medrol) because its antiphospholipase effect appears to be more potent than that of other glucocorticoids. It is reserved for those patients in metabolic crisis, in which case 80 mg administered via intravenous piggyback daily is given, and then is tapered, usually within 1 week, based on clinical improvement and lactic acid levels. Maintenance doses may be necessary and usually range from 2 to 4 mg every other day to 16 mg daily. Only the lowest effective dose should be used. Patients who do not respond to other forms of therapy may also benefit from a trial of glucocorticoids. In our experience, patients with a deficiency of complex I are the most likely to respond to this therapy. If no improvement is seen within 1 to 2 weeks, it is doubtful that the drug will be beneficial. Extreme care must be taken to monitor the blood glucose, as some of these patients develop diabetes mellitus that requires treatment with insulin. Evaluation of a synthetic steroid that lacks the side effects of available glucocorticoids is currently underway.

Free radical scavengers may also be effective in the treatment of patients with mitochondrial encephalomyopathies. Drugs such as ascorbate (vitamin C) at a dosage of 1 mg twice per day, tocopherol (vitamin E) at a dosage of 200 IU twice per day, and coenzyme Q10 (ubiquinone) are useful. Coenzyme Q10 is the natural electron shuttle between respiratory complexes I (NADH-CoQ reductase) and II (succinate dehydrogenase) to complex III (cytochrome c reductase). It is available in capsules or tablet form and can be obtained from most health food stores, with prices varying widely. In adults, we administer 30 to 75 mg per day in two or three divided doses. As this compound does not cross the blood-brain barrier, its chief use is in the amelioration of cardiac and skeletal muscle dysfunction. We are unaware of any untoward side effects from these doses.

Cofactors

Enzyme cofactors have been reported anecdotally to be effective in some patients and are worthy of future trials. Riboflavin, a cofactor for respiratory complex I, is used at a dosage of 100 mg daily. Thiamine (vitamin B_1), a cofactor for several mitochondrial enzymes not in the electron transport chain, including pyruvate dehydrogenase and pyruvate carboxylase, has been found useful in some children presenting with a Leigh's phenotype when given in large doses ranging up to 600 mg three times per day. Niacin (nicotinic acid; vitamin B_2) is a precursor in the synthesis of NAD and NADP, compounds that serve as soluble electron transporters. We have used this at a dosage of 50 mg per day. Biotin, an essential cofactor for several carboxylases, is given at a dosage of 20 mg per day.

Treatment of many of these patients remains empiric and must be individualized for each patient. In patients for whom controlled clinical trials are unavailable, we recommend empirical treatment with a "cocktail" of these vitamins. In those syndromes with a prolonged natural history, efficacy is difficult to assess clinically, and we find it useful to rely on easily quantifiable parameters, such as the generation of venous lactate after exercise or the recovery of high-energy phosphates by 31-P NMR spectroscopy of skeletal muscle during standardized exercise protocols. When such testing is not available, we recommend those empiric treatments that have a low potential for side effects, as described earlier in this chapter.

SUGGESTED READING

Arts W, Scholte H, Bogaard J, et al. NADH-CoQ reductase deficiency: successful treatment with riboflavin. Lancet 1983; 1:581–582.

Eleff S, Kennaway NG, Buist NRM, et al. 31-P NMR study of improvement in oxidative phosphorylation by vitamins K_3 and C in a patient with a defect in electron transport at complex III in skeletal muscle. Proc Natl Acad Sci USA 1984; 81:3529–3533.

Ogasahara S, Yorifuji S, Nishikawa Y, et al. Improvement of abnormal pyruvate metabolism and cardiac conduction defect with coenzyme Q10 in Kearns-Sayre syndrome. Neurology 1985; 35:372–377.

Peterson PL, Martens ME, Lee CP. Mitochondrial encephalomyopathies. Neurol Clin 1988; 6:529–544.

Przyrembel H. Therapy of mitochondrial disorders. J Inherited Metab Dis 1987; 10(suppl 1):129–146.

NUTRITIONAL DISEASE

WERNICKE'S ENCEPHALOPATHY AND ALCOHOL-RELATED NUTRITIONAL DISEASE

PETER L. CARLEN, M.D., FRCPC
JACK NEIMAN, M.D., Ph.D.

Chronic alcoholism predisposes to nutritional deficiencies for several reasons. When alcoholics go on a binge, frequently their only source of caloric intake is alcoholic beverages. The calories of alcoholic beverages are considered "empty" because alcoholics can ingest large quantities of calories in the form of alcohol and usually not show the expected weight gain, and because liquor, wine, and beer contain only insignificant amounts of vitamins and minerals and no other nutrients. Alcoholism per se is often associated with poor economic conditions, which also contributes to inadequate dietary intake. Impaired appetite secondary to alcohol-related gastrointestinal and liver disorders can also be a factor. Alcoholism can cause secondary malnutrition or deficient nutrient utilization through gastrointestinal damage causing maldigestion or malabsorption of nutrients, by energy wastage, and by decreased utilization of nutrients at the cellular level.

There are several diseases found in alcoholics that are attributed to nutritional deficiencies (Table 1). These are classified into probable and possible nutritional diseases. In this chapter, each disease entity is discussed in turn, and then a more general approach to the management of these alcoholic patients is presented. In addition to treating any specific nutritional deficiency, the physician is needed to assist alcoholics in altering their lifestyle and maintaining abstinence. To treat these alcoholism-related diseases, it is important to recognize the syndromes and the underlying alcoholism problem, sometimes difficult to spot in non-skid–row types, who, in fact, comprise the majority of alcohol abusers in the western world.

PROBABLE ALCOHOLISM-RELATED NUTRITIONAL DISEASES

Wernicke's Encephalopathy

Wernicke's encephalopathy (WE) is an underdiagnosed entity occurring mainly in chronic alcoholics, but also in other disease states including renal failure, renal dialysis, chronic bowel disease, persistent vomiting, or with intravenous hyperalimentation. It has a characteristic presentation of ophthalmoplegia, mental disturbance, and ataxia. The only signs that clearly differentiate WE from the acute alcoholic withdrawal state are the ophthalmoplegia found in WE and the tremulous-hyperexcitable state found in acute alcohol withdrawal. These two syndromes can coexist, however, and not all patients with WE have ophthalmoplegia. Nystagmus is common but is also part of alcohol withdrawal, as is ataxia. The ataxia associated with alcohol withdrawal is probably related to vestibular and cerebellar dysfunction. These patients can be hypothermic, presumably from hypothalamic involvement. The mental disturbance is usually a global confusional state with apathy and drowsiness, which can blend into an amnestic state characteristic

Table 1 Alcoholism-Related Nutritional Diseases of the Nervous System

Probable
    Wernicke's encephalopathy
    Korsakoff's syndrome
    Alcoholic cerebellar degeneration
    Alcoholic pellagra encephalopathy
    Vitamin B_6 deficiency
    Tobacco-alcohol amblyopia
    Alcoholic neuropathy

Possible
    Alcoholic cerebral atrophy (dementia)
    Marchiafava-Bignami disease
    Central pontine myelinolysis
    Alcoholic myopathy

of Korsakoff's amnesia. Confabulation is sometimes present. Often there is an associated peripheral neuropathy. It is thought that WE, as it becomes chronic, can persist as a Korsakoff's syndrome (KS). The topography of the pathologic changes are the same. The mammillary bodies are always involved. The other most consistently involved areas are the thalamus (especially the medial dorsal nuclei), hypothalamus, midbrain, pons, medulla, and midline cerebellar vermis. There is a symmetric, paraventricular distribution of lesions ranging from tissue necrosis to moderate neuronal and myelinated fiber loss with gliosis. In acute WE, there may be microhemorrhages.

Some classify WE as a medical emergency, since the danger of not treating this disease as soon as possible is the development of a chronic and possibly nonreversible KS. WE is due to thiamine (vitamin B_1) deficiency. With thiamine administration, there is a gratifyingly quick recovery from ophthalmoplegia within hours, followed by a clearing of the confusional state. Patients are slower to recover from nystagmus and ataxia. Although normally only a few milligrams of thiamine are required per day, much higher doses are used to treat WE, in part because cellular utilization of the vitamin may be impaired. Thiamine hydrochloride is initially given in a dose of 100 mg IV or IM followed by long-term administration of a multivitamin compound that includes all B vitamins and vitamin A, and a balanced diet. One must avoid giving patients susceptible to WE a sugar load before administering thiamine, since the increased glucose metabolism increases the central nervous system requirement for thiamine and can precipitate WE per se.

Korsakoff's Syndrome

KS is characterized by a memory deficit that is out of proportion to other cognitive functions. It can follow WE, but often there is no apparent history of WE. Superficially, these patients sometimes appear to converse and reason normally. However, they have limited insight into their condition and cannot remember events or comments that occurred even seconds or minutes previously. They have marked retrograde and anterograde amnesia. Their spontaneity and initiative are diminished.

Treatment consists of a nutritional diet and placing these patients in a properly supervised living situation. It is most important to follow up KS cases because some patients (10 to 25 percent) recover quite remarkably over several weeks to months and therefore may not require institutionalization.

Alcoholic Cerebellar Degeneration

Some alcoholics present primarily with a syndrome of ataxia of gait. Characteristically there is little impairment of finger-nose testing. Heel-shin testing is sometimes affected.

Alcoholic cerebellar degeneration is clinically considered a nutritionally related problem of chronic alcoholism, and it is frequently associated with a peripheral neuropathy. It can be seen both pathologically and clinically to coexist with WE and usually resolves with thiamine treatment. It can be chronic, however, and may not respond to thiamine administration. We have noted evidence of cerebellar atrophy on computed tomographic (CT) scans of alcoholics with no correlation to the degree of measured ataxia using the Heath Rails Test. In fact, the measured ataxia correlated better with the degree of supratentorial atrophy on CT scanning. Hence there may be more than one site of neuroanatomic damage to account for alcoholism-related ataxia. Finally, in acute alcohol withdrawal, there may be a profound ataxia syndrome that slowly resolves over weeks to months with maintained abstinence and an adequate diet.

Alcoholic Pellagra Encephalopathy

Pellagra is a nutritional disease associated with niacin deficiency. The hallmarks are dermatitis, diarrhea, and dementia. Pellagra can occur with malnutrition or secondarily with gastrointestinal tract disease, malignant carcinoid, isoniazid, G-mercaptopurine, 5-fluorouracil, or puromycin treatment. Pellagra encephalopathy has also been reported in chronic alcoholics, often coexisting with other alcohol-related encephalopathies in the same patient. Pathologically one finds swollen neurons with eccentric nuclei and loss of Nissl particles in the cerebral cortex, reticular formation, pontine nuclei, and dentate nuclei. The major neurologic findings are a fluctuating confusional state that can progress to coma, hypertonus, and startle myoclonus. Severe deterioration and even death can be precipitated by thiamine and pyridoxine administration without niacin. Alcoholics often do not have the associated pellagra dermatitis or diarrhea. However, it is prudent to ensure that all encephalopathic alcoholics receive niacin in addition to other vitamins. The routine multivitamin therapy used in the western world to treat alcoholics is probably the reason that this disease is relatively uncommon today. There is some question as to whether all the symptoms and signs of alcoholic pellagra encephalopathy can be ascribed to niacin deficiency alone. Hence the treatment should be multivitamins that include niacin and an adequate nutritional diet.

Vitamin B_6 Deficiency

Pyridoxine (vitamin B_6) is converted to pyridoxal 5-phosphate (PLP) primarily in the liver. The level of PLP is often low in chronic alcoholics, especially those with liver disease. Its deficiency can be associated with a peripheral neuropathy and neuromuscular irritability, in addition to dermatitis, stomatitis, immune suppression, and a sideroblastic anemia. It is rare to find only pyridoxine deficiency in alcoholics, since this disease is usually associated with other nutritional deficiencies. Its treatment is multiple B vitamins and a nutritious diet.

Tobacco-Alcohol Amblyopia

This syndrome is characterized by bilateral decreased visual acuity, symmetric scotomata, impaired color vision, and usually normal fundi. There is uncertainty in the literature as to whether alcohol or tobacco alone can cause amblyopia. Patients are usually both alcohol abusers and heavy smokers. Concomitant vitamin deficiencies and liver disease are probably the most important causative factors, although the specific pathogenesis has not yet been elucidated. The formerly cyanide-vitamin B_{12} hypothesis has been debunked. Vitamin A deficiency, which is associated with night blindness, is not uncommon in alcoholics, especially in those with liver disease. It could play a role in the tobacco-alcohol amblyopia. The recommended treatment is an adequate diet, multivitamin administration, and most important, maintained abstinence from alcohol.

Alcoholic Neuropathy

Almost all chronic alcoholics have a peripheral neuropathy to some degree, as evidenced by depressed ankle jerks and decreased vibration and cold sensation in the lower limbs. Usually these signs are not associated with sensory complaints. However, some alcoholics, particularly those with apparent dietary deficiency, do complain of weakness, paresthesia, and pain. These symptoms usually present insidiously. The weakness is often associated with distal wasting, which is usually more apparent in the lower limbs. The pain usually consists of a dull constant ache in the feet or legs, but brief lancinating pains can also occur. Patients may also complain of "burning feet" characterized by painful paresthesia, which is worsened by pressure on the soles and thus makes walking difficult. The cranial nerves are almost never involved, but an autonomic neuropathy and orthostatic hypotension can occur. Pathologically one sees a noninflammatory degeneration of the peripheral nerves with destruction of both myelin and axons. The evidence points to nutritional deficiency and alcohol toxicity as the major causative factors. The specific pathogenesis, however, has not yet been pinpointed. Treatment consists of alcohol abstinence, a nutritional diet, and administration of B vitamins. Symptomatic recovery can take several weeks to months because of the prolonged nature of nerve regeneration. As an aside, it should be noted that alcoholics are subject to pressure nerve palsies (ulnar, radial, peroneal) because of a probable subclinical neuropathy and the tendency of the patient to fall asleep in awkward positions when intoxicated, putting undue and prolonged pressure on the peripheral nerve.

POSSIBLE ALCOHOLISM-RELATED NUTRITIONAL DISEASES

Cerebral Atrophy (Dementia)

On CT or magnetic resonance imaging (MRI) scan, diffuse cerebral atrophy with cortical sulcal widening and enlarged ventricles is a common finding in most chronic alcoholics. There is a weak correlation between the degree of cerebral atrophy and cognitive impairment. Chronic alcohol intake in experimental animals is associated with some cerebral degenerative changes and decreased brain protein synthesis. Malnutrition in humans is associated with cerebral atrophy and cognitive changes. The exact relationship of chronic alcohol intake with alcoholism-related nutritional deficiencies, cerebral atrophy, and cognitive deficits is unclear. Alcoholics can develop a severe global dementia which some have distinguished from KS since more than memory is significantly impaired. However, recent pathologic evidence suggests that all autopsied alcoholics with a global dementia in fact have the pathology of KS. These alcoholics do not appear to have more cerebral cortical atrophy than patients with KS.

Practically speaking, it is important to follow these patients for several months after alcohol withdrawal since some show a marked improvement in their dementia syndrome. This can be associated with some reversibility in their cerebral atrophy and a concomitant increase in their mean cerebral tissue density on CT scan. We have seen several patients who were slated for nursing homes because of their dementia and who, over a few weeks, had improved to the point where chronic institutionalization was no longer necessary. It is presumed that a nutritious diet and lack of alcohol intake was helpful in these cases. However, many chronic alcoholics with a global dementia do not improve, and a small percentage continue to decline even with alcohol abstinence. Clearly other causes of encephalopathy and dementia must be considered. In alcoholics, the greatest danger is subdural hematoma, since its incidence among patients who have atrophied brains and a tendency to fall and suffer head injuries is inordinately high.

Marchiafava-Bignami Disease

This is a rare disease characterized by demyelination and destruction of the corpus callosum and is found in severe chronic alcoholics. Clinically, the presentation is quite variable, but often this pathology is associated with a frontal-lobe or dementia syndrome or with seizures, stupor, and coma.

Central Pontine Myelinolysis

This is another relatively rare entity pathologically defined by a noninflammatory demyelination of the basis pontis. Evidence of this disease can be seen on CT or MRI scans without significant accompanying clinical signs. It is often associated with other alcoholism-related encephalopathies such as Wernicke's encephalopathy, pellagra encephalopathy, or withdrawal seizures. When severe, it presents as a flaccid quadriparesis, dysarthia, and dysphagia. Recently, central pontine myelinolysis has been demonstrated to develop in patients with rapid correction of a significant hyponatremia. Hence in alcoholics with a low serum sodium, which can be associated with seizures and encephalopathy, judicious and slow correction of this metabolic defect is required. We would also advise a nutritious diet and multivitamin administration.

Alcoholic Myopathy

Many chronic alcoholics, especially those who appear malnourished or who have liver disease, present with diffuse proximal muscle weakness, wasting, and increased serum muscle enzymes. Both type I and type II muscle fibers are involved in light microscopic examination. Weakness usually resolves with adequate diet and abstinence. However, some patients may have a subacute or chronic, severe proximal myopathy that resolves only slowly. A few alcoholics develop an acute myopathy with rhabdomyolysis and myoglobinuria, sometimes followed by acute renal failure.

TREATMENT OF ALCOHOL ADDICTION

It is all well and good to diagnose and treat the nervous system disease caused by alcohol abuse. However, if the patient recovers, it is essential to address the underlying problem of the disease—namely, alcohol addiction. This is an extremely complex and difficult subject often ignored by the physician. Addiction management is now a legitimate, important, and difficult area of research. There are a wide variety of treatments available to choose from, depending on one's location and the socioeconomic stratum of the patient. With an alcoholic patient, it is first necessary to identify the problem. Today, many patients abuse other psychoactive drugs in addition to alcohol. Once the alcohol (and other drug abuse) problem is identified, it is important to discuss its consequences for the patient, and when relevant, for the patient's family.

The next step is to match available therapeutic options with the patient in an attempt to achieve behavioral modification such that the patient avoids alcohol abuse. This might sound obvious, but it is frequently overlooked. The recidivism rate is high among alcohol and drug abusers. In most North American communities, Alcoholics Anonymous is available. This organization, like many other programs, believes in total abstinence and uses a form of group therapy. There are also many different types of private and public treatment facilities, but detailed descriptions of these are beyond the scope of this chapter.

SUGGESTED READING

Carlen PL, Wilkinson DA. Reversibility of alcohol-related brain damage: clinical and experimental observations. Acta Med Scand 1987; 717 (suppl):19–26.

Krumsiek J, Kruger C, Patzold U. Tobacco-alcohol amblyopia neuro-ophthalmological findings and clinical course. Acta Neurol Scand 1985; 72:180–187.

Serdaru M, Hausser-Hauw C, LaPlante D, et al. The clinical spectrum of alcoholic pellagra encephalopathy. Brain 1988; 111:829–842.

Victor M. Neurologic disorders due to alcoholism and malnutrition. In: Baker AB, Baker LH. Clinical Neurology Vol. 2 (revised edition). Philadelphia: JB Lippincott, 1982:1.

SUBACUTE COMBINED DEGENERATION AND OTHER VITAMIN B$_{12}$ DEFICIENCY–INDUCED DISORDERS

BARBARA J. MARTIN, M.D.
MARK J. BROWN, M.D.

Vitamin B$_{12}$ (cobalamin) deficiency can lead to myelopathy, encephalopathy, and optic and peripheral neuropathy. Therapy should begin only after one of the syndromes known to result from vitamin B$_{12}$ deficiency has been demonstrated and it has been established that the deficit exists. Accurate laboratory diagnosis of viatmin B$_{12}$ deficiency may be confounded by premature treatment. Therapy consists of lifelong parenteral vitamin B$_{12}$ administration and, when possible, treatment of underlying or associated conditions.

SUBACUTE COMBINED DEGENERATION OF THE SPINAL CORD

The manifestations of vitamin B$_{12}$ deficiency–induced subacute combined degeneration reflect the underlying dorsal and lateral spinal cord white matter abnormalities. Symptoms characteristically begin with paresthesia in the feet, with relative sparing of the hands and arms. Disproportionate vibratory and proprioceptive function loss in the legs and trunk is also characteristic, and small fiber modalities may be affected. Rarely, a thoracic sensory level suggests a segmental spinal cord disorder. Sensory symptoms may be followed by leg weakness and an ataxic or spastic gait. The plantar responses are typically extensor, and pathlolgic hyperreflexia may occur; however, when there is an associated neuropathy, ankle jerks and other reflexes may be depressed. Somatosensory-evoked potentials may indicate central nervous system disease, although signs of an associated axonal neuropathy may predominate in this test.

The characteristic early histologic finding in vitamin B$_{12}$ deficiency–induced subacute combined degeneration is intra-myelin edema, followed by myelin sheath vacuolization. At this point, the process is likely to be reversible. Myelin breakdown follows, and lesions enlarge and coalesce to give a patchy spongiform appearance. The dorsal columns of the cervical and upper thoracic cord are most likely to be affected, with less severe involvement of the lateral and ventral white matter. Chronic lesions are characterized by axonal loss and fibrillary gliosis.

The differential diagnosis of subacute or chronic dorsal and lateral spinal cord dysfunction includes multiple sclerosis and tabes dorsalis. Lyme disease and human immunodeficiency virus (HIV) or human T-cell lymphotropic virus (HTLV)-1 may be considerations, especially if the peripheral nervous system is involved. Friedrich's ataxia patients may have hyporeflexia with extensor plantar responses. Prolonged nitrous oxide exposure may produce a clinical syndrome indistinguishable from subacute combined degeneration secondary to vitamin B$_{12}$ deficiency.

SUBACUTE DEGENERATION OF THE BRAIN

Encephalopathy commonly accompanies subacute combined degeneration of the spinal cord, and appears to have the same neuropathologic basis. Brain myelin lesions and axonal loss are similar to those described for the spinal cord.

Neuropsychological manifestations of the encephalopathy range from mild personality and mood changes to severe dementia. Paranoia and hallucinations may occur, but psychosis is very rare. The severity of the encephalopathy and myelopathy may differ from patient to patient. Vitamin B$_{12}$ encephalopathy can occur without other evidence of nervous system disease. However, because mild dementia and psychiatric disorders are common in the general population and vitamin B$_{12}$ tests are requested frequently, the association between dementia and low levels of vitamin B$_{12}$ may sometimes be coincidental.

PERIPHERAL NEUROPATHY

Peripheral neuropathy is frequently associated with subacute combined degeneration, although neuropathy makes a relatively small contribution to the symptomatology. Distal paresthesias, a symmetric stocking-glove sensory deficit, and orthostatic hypotension can be ascribed to either neuropathy or myelopathy; however, when looked for, hyporeflexia and depressed sensory potential amplitudes often confirm peripheral nervous system involvement. Although peripheral nerve demylination has been reported, more recently studies have demonstrated a predominance of axonal degeneration in biopsied sural nerves. This suggests that the mechanism of pathogenesis is different from that of the central nervous system lesions.

OPTIC NEUROPATHY

Ocular signs and symptoms can occur with subacute combined degeneration. The explanation for the reported severe disc edema, optic atrophy, and bilateral centrocecal scotomas is not clear. There are few neuropathologic reports of well-studied clinical cases, and the nature of the optic neuropathy remains uncertain. Nerve fiber layer hemorrhages are presumably related to the hematologic disorder. Ophthalmoplegia has been reported, but the association may be coincidental.

Tobacco-alcohol amblyopia presents with signs and symptoms similar to those of the optic neuropathy associated with subacute combined degeneration. Both are characterized by loss of visual acuity, dyschromatopsia, centrocecal scotomata, and optic disc pallor. Tobacco-alcohol amblyopia is believed to be secondary to vitamin B-complex deficiency, but is more likely linked to a deficiency of vitamin B_1 than a deficiency of viatmin B_{12}.

PATHOPHYSIOLOGY OF VITAMIN B_{12} DEFICIENCY IN THE NERVOUS SYSTEM

Vitamin B_{12} is a necessary coenzyme for the conversion of propionic acid to succinic acid through the intermediate metabolite methylmalonic acid. Vitamin B_{12} deficiency alters methylmalonic acid metabolism, resulting in abnormal fatty acid synthesis, presumably leading to abnormal myelin and other cell membranes. Serum levels and urinary excretion of methylmalonic acid are elevated with vitamin B_{12} deficiency, and this is used as a supportive diagnostic test. Vitamin B_{12} is also a necessary coenzyme for methionine synthetase which converts homocysteine to methionine by methylation. Serum homocysteine levels may be elevated in patients with neurologic manifestations of vitamin B_{12} deficiency. Notably, excess exposure to nitrous oxide, which inhibits methionine synthetase, can lead to a spinal cord syndrome indistinguishable from subacute combined degeneration.

LABORATORY DIAGNOSIS

The coexistence of anemia, macrocytosis, and neutrophil hypersegmentation strongly supports the diagnosis of vitamin B_{12} deficiency, but neurologic and hematologic manifestations may occur independently. The initial diagnostic step is measuring the serum vitamin B_{12} level through the use of a competitive binding radio-assay, which has supplanted the older bioassay. Serum is added to radio-labeled vitamin B_{12} bound to highly purified intrinsic factor; serum vitamin B_{12} displaces the labeled vitamin B_{12} from the intrinsic factor. The serum concentration is inversely proportional to the remaining bound vitamin B_{12} and can be calculated from the residual radioactivity of the complex. The sensitivity of this assay is approximately 98 percent with less than 0.1 percent false-positives.

Normal serum vitamin B_{12} levels are usually greater than 200 ng per liter although this varies among laboratories. Early vitamin B_{12} deficiency is indicated by levels of 160 to 200 ng per liter. Values for the elderly are consistently lower than those of younger patients, but are routinely greater than 150 ng per liter. Both serum methylmalonic acid and homocysteine levels may be elevated in subacute combined degeneration. These tests currently have limited availability, but may be used to confirm the diagnosis of vitamin B_{12} deficiency when results of standard tests are indeterminate. (Serum homocysteine levels may also be elevated with folate deficiency.) The laboratory diagnosis of vitamin B_{12} deficiency may be obscured by the widespread and nonspecific use of supplemental vitamin B_{12} in clinical practice. The administration of vitamin B_{12} within a week of the test may lead to misleading results and may warrant further studies.

CAUSES

Pernicious anemia (intrinsic factor deficiency) is by far the most important cause of vitamin B_{12} deficiency in the United States. The detection of antibodies to intrinsic factor is highly specific, and blocking antibodies are detected in approximately 50 to 60 percent of patients with pernicious anemia, with only rare false-positives. False-positives have resulted when another radioactive tracer, such as technetium, has been administered previously. False-negative results may be seen when supplemental vitamin B_{12} has been given within 1 week of testing. Causes of intrinsic factor deficiency other than pernicious anemia include atrophic gastritis, stomach neoplasia, and gastrectomy.

The Shilling test is the definitive method for diagnosing intrinsic factor deficiency. During the first stage of this test, radio-labeled oral vitamin B_{12} absorption is impaired, resulting in diminished urinary excretion of the isotope. If vitamin B_{12} excretion is demonstrably low, the second stage of the Shilling test should be performed. This consists of giving intrinsic factor orally along with labeled vitamin B_{12}, after which excretion is increased. Impaired urinary vitamin B_{12} excretion during both stages of the test is found in patients with malabsorption states, intrinsic factor–blocking antibody, severe renal insufficiency, and poor specimen collection. Twenty-five percent of patients with untreated true vitamin B_{12} deficiency show a "malabsorption" picture with the two-stage Shilling test. After prolonged vitamin B_{12} replacement therapy, the majority of these patients display improved vitamin B_{12} absorption and demonstrate repeat test results consistent with pernicious anemia. Pernicious anemia may be associated with other autoimmune diseases such as hypothyroidism. Approximately 20 percent of patients of Lambert-Eaton syndrome have intrinsic factor–blocking antibody without pernicious anemia, most likely reflecting altered autoimmunity in the pathogenesis of this illness.

The customary Western diet generally provides adequate amounts of vitamin B$_{12}$ (approximately 2.5 μg per day). Poor diet and extreme vegetarianism, on the other hand, pose a risk for vitamin B$_{12}$ deficiency. Malabsorption of vitamin B$_{12}$ occurs with diseases such as sprue or inflammatory bowel diseases affecting the ileum, as well as with simple ileal resection. The fish tapeworm *Diphyllobothrium latum* creates a vitamin B$_{12}$ deficient state by competing for vitamin B$_{12}$ within the host's intestine. The blind loop syndrome is attributed to significant bacterial colonization in the small intestine with diversion of vitamin B$_{12}$ from host absorption. Pregnancy may predispose toward vitamin B$_{12}$ deficiency if increased vitamin B$_{12}$ demands are not met with adequate intake. Coexisting folate deficiency should be considered in this context. Impaired B$_{12}$ absorption from the gut may occur in conjunction with the usage of aminoglycosides, aspirin, colchicine, and chloramphenicol, as well as with excessive alcohol intake.

TREATMENT

The treatment of vitamin B$_{12}$ deficiency should consist solely of intramuscular or subcutaneous vitamin B$_{12}$ administration. Because of their limited absorption and high cost, oral vitamin B$_{12}$ preparations with or without intrinsic factor are unacceptable alternatives, except for the rare vegetarian with dietary deficiency. Cyanocobalamin is currently the least expensive preparation available.

Initial treatment consists of 1,000 μg parenteral vitamin B$_{12}$ daily or every other day for several weeks followed by weekly injections for 1 to 2 months. Thereafter, the same dose should be given monthly for life. Some have advised that initial dosages of greater than 30 μg daily afford little therapeutic advantage. However, we recommend continuing the higher dose because the extent to which vitamin B$_{12}$ stores are repleted is directly related to the parenteral dose, and a higher dose poses no additional risk for the patient. Adverse effects of replacement are largely limited to the pain of intramuscular injection with allergic reactions reported very rarely. The hematologic response to vitamin B$_{12}$ may be brisk, occurring at a tempo independent from that of the nervous system response.

Treatment with folate without vitamin B$_{12}$ replacement is strictly contraindicated for patients with megaloblastic anemia with or without neurologic symptoms and signs. It is well known that the anemia of vitamin B$_{12}$ deficiency responds to folate therapy, possibly via the mobilization of stores, while the neurologic symptoms of subacute combined degeneration may surface during this time or worsen if already present.

The success of treatment is related to the duration of neurologic dysfunction before therapy. Patients who have had symptoms for less than 3 months show the greatest improvement, and patients treated within weeks of onset may have a full recovery. Those treated after the first 3 to 6 months of symptoms have a less successful outcome. However, recent data indicate that all patients receive some benefit from replacement regardless of the duration of illness.

SUGGESTED READING

Agamanolis DP, Victor M, Harris JW, et al. An ultrastructural study of subacute combined degeneration of the spinal cord in vitamin B$_{12}$-deficient rhesus monkeys. J Neuropathol Exp Neurol 1978; 37:273–299.

Beck WS. Cobalamin and the nervous system, editorial. N Engl J Med 1988; 318; 1752–1754.

Lindenbaum J, Healton EB, Savage DG, et al. Neuropsychiatric disorders caused by cobalamin deficiency in the absence of anemia or macrocytosis. N Engl J Med 1988; 318:1720–1728.

Pant SS, Asbury AK, Richardson EP Jr. The myelopathy of pernicious anemia: a neuropathological reappraisal. Acta Neurol Scand 1968; 44 (suppl 35).

PERIPHERAL NERVE DISEASE

ACUTE INFLAMMATORY POLYNEUROPATHY

DAVID R. CORNBLATH, M.D.
DANIEL F. HANLEY, M.D.

Acute inflammatory polyneuropathy (AIP), commonly known as the Guillain-Barré syndrome, is an acute demyelinating disorder of the peripheral nervous system that affects individuals of all ages. Currently it is the most common acute neurologic disease leading to paralysis or respiratory failure within days. In two-thirds of patients, the disorder follows within 1 to 3 weeks a "viral" infection. AIP is also associated with several systemic disorders, including Hodgkin's disease, lymphoma, lupus erythematosus, and human immunodeficiency virus (HIV) infection. The disease typically begins with paresthesia in the hands or feet, but rapidly evolves to involve the motor system, with weakness usually progressing in an ascending fashion. Hyporeflexia or areflexia is always seen at some point in the course of the disease. Occasional patients have the rare Miller-Fisher variant of the disease (which includes ataxia, areflexia, and ophthalmoplegia), with preserved strength. The Miller-Fisher variant is considered part of the spectrum of AIP, and the treatment is the same as that for AIP.

DIAGNOSIS

Because of the reports of AIP occurring after the swine-influenza vaccine, standardized diagnostic criteria were developed by the National Institute of Neurologic Communication Disorders and Stroke. It is important to note that these criteria were developed primarily for epidemiologic and medicolegal purposes in response to the AIP-like syndrome associated with swine influenza vaccination, and thus may not include all cases that experienced neurologists would accept as AIP. Weakness and areflexia are required for diagnosis. Supportive features include progression after onset, relative symmetry, sensory and cranial nerve involvement, autonomic dysfunction, absence of fever at onset, and improvement after a nadir has been reached. Features that suggest an incorrect diagnosis include marked persistent asymmetry of weakness, persistent bowel or bladder dysfunction, significant bowel or bladder dysfunction at onset, cerebrospinal fluid (CSF) pleocytosis (>50 mononuclear cells per cubic millimeter), CSF polymorphonuclear cells, and a sharp sensory level. Disorders that may mimic AIP include conditions associated with hexacarbon abuse, porphyria, diphtheria, heavy metal intoxication, and botulism.

EVALUATION

In most patients, a relatively confident diagnosis can be made based on clinical criteria alone. Because of the clinical implications, however, diagnosis should be confirmed by a series of laboratory studies that can usually be completed within 1 to 2 days after admission to hospital. Evaluation serves 3 purposes: (1) to confirm the clinical diagnosis, (2) to eliminate other disorders, and (3) to look for associated diseases accompanying AIP. Blood studies should include a screening hematologic and biochemical battery, determinations of antinuclear antibodies (ANA) and antibodies to both hepatitis and HIV, and blood sent to a central laboratory for acute viral titers to be followed by a blood specimen obtained 2 weeks later for convalescent titers. Urine should be collected for evaluation of porphyria and heavy metal intoxication. CSF should be evaluated for glucose, protein, cell count, and VDRL. In classic AIP, there is little if any value in obtaining CSF for evidence of infection or for measuring of oligoclonal bands, myelin basic protein, or immunoglobulin synthesis. Early in the disorder, spinal fluid protein content may be normal, and for diagnostically difficult cases, it may be necessary to repeat the spinal fluid evaluation 7 to 14 days into the illness. Electrophysiologic studies are particularly important because, in addition to their use in diagnosis, they also have prognostic value (detailed later in this chapter). These studies should include sensory conduction studies, motor conduction studies including F-wave latencies, H-reflex latencies, and electromyography. Like the CSF protein level, routine electrophysiologic studies may rarely be normal early in the course of the disease.

THERAPY

All patients with AIP should be hospitalized. The disorder is highly variable, and in a seemingly well individual, the disease may rapidly progress over a period of hours to respiratory failure. Currently we admit most patients to a regular hospital bed near the nursing station. Those patients with respiratory embarrassment, bulbar weakness, or difficulty handling secretions are best managed in an intensive care unit. One cannot be cavalier about predicting the rate of progressive respiratory impairment for an individual patient.

Plasmapheresis

Three controlled studies comprising more than 450 patients now convincingly demonstrate that plasmapheresis is the treatment of choice for AIP. We use the plasmapheresis protocol developed in our initial studies of AIP: a set of 5 exchanges, each approximately 40 to 50 ml per kilogram, over a period of 7 to 14 days for a total volume exchange of 200 to 250 ml per kilogram. Our standard replacement fluid has been "plasma protein fraction." There is no advantage to fresh-frozen plasma. If possible, the use of a continuous-flow plasmapheresis machine is preferred. In approximately one-half of the patients undergoing pheresis, this can be readily accomplished through the use of peripheral venous access. In many patients, however, the large volumes and high flow rates required by continuous-flow plasmapheresis machines necessitate the placement of central venous catheters. These should be placed only by experienced clinicians and must be watched closely for signs of infection or thrombosis. We usually use a Shiley double-lumen catheter via the femoral venous route. One must pay careful attention to antiseptic technique. The catheter is discontinued after 3 days of use. The large lumenal diameter of these catheters has the additional advantage of allowing for the rapid infusion of fluid if hypotension occurs during pheresis.

One of the most frequently asked questions about plasmapheresis is who should undergo this procedure? We pherese those individuals who are unable to walk and who are able to tolerate plasmapheresis. Individuals whose disease appears to be rapidly progressing but who are still able to walk also undergo pheresis. It is unknown whether there is a lower limit to the age at which one should pherese a patient. Pregnancy is not a contraindication to

pheresis if AIP supervenes during the course of the pregnancy. Individuals with antibodies to hepatitis or HIV can be pheresed safely. It is our practice to assume that all patients have antibodies to hepatitis and HIV until proven otherwise, so that appropriate precautions are taken in all patients. For patients with the Miller-Fisher variant, we follow the same guidelines for the use of plasmapheresis as in patients with more typical AIP.

Supportive Care

Prior to the advent of plasmapheresis therapy, the best therapy consisted of best medical and nursing supportive care. This includes attention to impending respiratory distress, frequent vital signs including measurement of respiratory parameters such as vital capacity and negative inspiratory force, maintenance of adequate nutrition, ongoing surveillance for the presence of infection, and particular attention to difficulties that arise in individuals who have had prolonged bedrest, such as orthostatic hypotension, atelectasis, and the development of decubitus ulcers.

Respiratory Therapy/Intubation

The majority of AIP patients do not require mechanical ventilation. However, because the illness is both unpredictable and reversible, mechanical ventilation should be used at the earliest sign of respiratory embarrassment. Both physicians and nurses perform frequent assessments of all aspects of ventilation (airway patency, mechanical effort, and gas exchange). Impairment of any of these 3 vital functions is an indication for artificial ventilation. We consider the inability to swallow secretions the major indicator of pharyngeal muscle dysfunction. Tidal volume and respiratory rate are the best indicators of mechanical effort. A tidal volume of less than 15 ml per kilogram of body weight or a respiratory rate 20 breaths per minute or greater are most often followed by complete respiratory failure. Systemic arterial hemoglobin desaturation ($\leq$90 percent saturation) via pulse oximetry or hypoxia/hypercapnia on arterial blood gas chemistry are equally important indicators of poor gas exchange. We attempt to identify all AIP patients with ventilatory failure before they achieve this degree of physiologic compromise.

Elective endotracheal intubation is best performed in anticipation of further decline rather than during rapidly progressive hypoxia and hypotension. We prefer to use ventilators that have "pressure support" capabilities, as this method of rate-supported and pressure-supported ventilation offers the ideal flexibility of ventilation settings for encouraging early diaphragmatic training and recovery. We extubate patients when their secretions can be well managed by swallowing, when cough and gag reflexes are present, when mechanical ventilatory effort is sustained at low respiratory rates and high tidal volumes, and when there is little or no parenchymal lung disease to impair gas exchange.

Autonomic Instability

Autonomic instability is frequently seen in patients with AIP. This may take the form of cardiac arrhythmias, hypertension or hypotension, pupillary dilatation, and sweat disturbances. The usual tendency is to rush to treat these manifestations of the disorder. Most are transitory, however, and are rarely life-threatening. Over-vigorous treatment of hypertension may be followed by potentially more threatening severe hypotension resulting from either overtreatment or increased sensitivity of blood pressure control mechanisms caused by the disease. Most patients tolerate their autonomic dysfunction.

Occupational and Physical Therapy

Some patients recover quickly from the disorder, requiring little bedrest or having a short recovery phase. However, the majority have a period of bedrest followed by a slower recovery phase. Early consultation with occupational and physical therapists regarding the maintenance of muscle tone and joint mobility is mandatory. The use of splints for both hands and feet may be useful in preventing contractures. Occupational therapists are particularly helpful for patients who have difficulty communicating and swallowing.

Pain

Pain may be particularly problematic at the onset of the disease. In most patients, it is centered in the lower back without radicular radiation. While the use of narcotic analgesics may depress respiration, one should not hesitate to use narcotics for controlling the pain. These patients generally receive narcotics for a short time and do not become addicted. During the recovery phase, occasional patients develop "neuritic pain," which responds best to tricyclic antidepressants or anticonvulsants. Tricyclic antidepressants have the added benefit of promoting sleep when nocturnal pain is prominent.

Psychological Support

Because the majority of individuals who develop AIP were previously healthy, they experience a great deal of psychic trauma in dealing with the fact that they have an acute devastating illness. Reassuring the patient that the disease is self-limited and that recovery usually occurs is helpful, but many patients are not convinced by this. It is more useful to have patients who have recovered visit currently ill patients in the hospital. Maintaining open lines of communication through the use of communication boards is extremely helpful and reasurring to the patient, who is frequently fearful of abandonment (by physicians and nurses). Rarely do patients need active psychiatric intervention or require major psychotropic drugs.

PROGNOSIS

Our prospective studies have elucidated important factors regarding the long-term prognosis (e.g., the ability to walk independently 6 months after the onset of the disease). Four of these are factors over which the physician has no control. These are the patient's age, the duration of the illness before treatment ($\leq$7 days versus >7 days), respirator status (i.e., whether the patient is supported by a respirator), and mean distal motor amplitude ($\leq$20 versus >20 percent of the lower limit of normal). A sample calculation of mean distal motor amplitude is shown in Table 1.

The only variable effecting prognosis over which the physician has influence is treatment. Our studies demonstrated that the prognosis was statistically improved by the use of plasmapheresis, even in the face of poor prognostic variables for the patient's age, the duration of the illness before treatment, respirator status, and mean distal motor amplitude.

In general, the prognosis for this illness is good. Most individuals make a complete or near-complete recovery. Residual signs and symptoms are frequent but rarely interefere with functional activities. In a subgroup, the disorder is more devastating and results in severe and permanent disability.

Table 1 Sample Calculations of Mean CMAP Amplitude From Distal Stimulation (Distal CMAP Amplitude)

Nerve	Values	Laboratory Normal	Percentage of the Lower Limit of Normal
Peroneal	500	2,000	25
Tibial	200	2,000	10
Median	5,000	4,000	125
Ulnar	4,000	4,000	100
Total			260
Mean distal CMAP amplitude			65

CMAP=compound muscle action potential.
Republished with permission from Cornblath, DR, Mellits ED, Griffin JW, et al (The GBS Study Group). Motor conduction studies in Guillan-Barré syndrome: description and prognostic value. Ann Neurol 1988; 23:354–359.

After the acute hospitalization, many patients are transferred to specialized rehabilitation centers for more intensive occupational and physical therapy than can be given in acute-care hospitals.

SUGGESTED READING

Ad Hoc NINCDS Committee. Criteria for the diagnosis of Guillain-Barré syndrome. Ann Neurol 1978; 3:565–566.

Cornblath DR, Mellits ED, Griffin JW, et al (The GBS Study Group). Motor conduction studies in Guillain-Barré syndrome: description and prognostic value. Ann Neurol 1988; 23:354–359.

French Cooperative Group on Plasma Exchange and Guillain-Barré Syndrome. efficiency of plasma exchange in Guillain-Barré syndrome: role of replacement fluids. Ann Neurol 1987; 22:753–761.

The Guillain-Barré Syndrome Study Group. Plasmapheresis and the acute Guillain-Barré syndrome. Neurology 1985; 35:1096–1104.

McKhann GM, Griffin JW, Cornblath DR, et al (GBS Study Group). Plasmapheresis and Guillain-Barré syndrome: prognostic factors and the effect of plasmapheresis. Ann Neurol 1988; 23:347–353.

Osterman PG, Ludemo G, Pirskanem R, et al. Beneficial effects of plasma exchange in acute inflammatory polyradiculoneuropathy. Lancet 1984; 2:1296–1299.

PATIENT RESOURCE

The Guillain-Barré Syndrome Support Group International is a patient-based organization providing information to individuals with AIP. The organization has chapters in the United States, Australia, Canada, Great Britain, and West Germany.

GBS Syndrome Support Group
P.O. Box 262
Wynnewood, PA 19096
Telephone: (215) 642–6855.

CHRONIC NEUROPATHY

DANNY F. WATSON M.D., Ph.D.

DIAGNOSIS

Accurate etiologic diagnosis is vitally important for the primary treatment of a neuropathy; furthermore, many neuropathies are manifestations of systemic diseases that require treatment in their own right. Diagnostic efforts are appropriately directed to the identification of treatable disorders, despite the relatively frequent occurrence of neuropathies for which no specific treatment is available. Although a comprehensive review of the diagnosis of neuropathies is beyond the scope of this chapter, some principles that guide the diagnostic approach should be discussed.

The least specific pattern of neuropathy is distal degeneration of the longest axons of all fiber types (myelinated and unmyelinated, sensory, motor and autonomic) with subsequent dying-back to more proximal levels as the disease progresses. This pattern can be produced by a wide range of disorders, since any derangement in the complex processes of synthesis and transport of macromolecules from nerve cell bodies to their terminals produce distal axonal degeneration. By contrast, if a neuropathy differs from this common pattern (e.g., a primarily demyelinating neuropathy, a neuropathy with disproportionate involvement of the upper extremities, or a neuropathy with a single functional modality involved), there are fewer possible diagnoses and the chance of identifying a specific treatment is greatly enhanced. Recognition of special patterns of neuropathy requires that one obtain a careful history of the tempo and spatial distribution and perform a thorough examination of the function of different fiber classes: motor, large fiber sensory (vibration and joint position sense), small fiber sensory (pin and temperature), and autonomic (sympathetic and parasympathetic). Further characterization by nerve conduction testing and electromyography can be helpful in making these distinctions and may also prove valuable in identifying patients with discrete focal lesions of multiple nerves (a pattern with relatively few causes) as opposed to true polyneuropathy.

Systematic consideration of broad categories of etiologies helps the clinician avoid the pitfall of focusing on esoteric possibilities while forgetting more common ones. A list of common etiologies of neuropathy for which there exists some specific therapeutic intervention is shown in Table 1.

PRIMARY TREATMENT

The treatment of immune-mediated neuropathies is considered elsewhere in this text. The treatment of toxic and metabolic neuropathies is conceptually straightforward; the offending toxin is removed or the metabolic disorder is controlled. A few specific management problems are common enough to warrant comment.

Diabetes

In a patient with diabetes, identification of new onset neuropathy calls for careful re-evaluation of diabetic control. Mild reversible changes in nerve

Table 1 Major Treatable Causes of Polyneuropathy

Toxic
  Medications
    Amiodarone
    Cisplatin
    Colchicine
    Dapsone
    Gold salts
    Hydralazine
    Isoniazid
    Metronidazole
    Misonidazole
    Nitrofurantoin
    Pyridoxine
    Vincristine
  Environmental exposure
    Lead
    Mercury
    Thallium
    Acrylamide
    Hexacarbons
    Kepone
  Intentional exposure
    Alcohol
    Nitrous oxide
    Arsenic

Metabolic
  Diabetes
  Nutritional deficiency
    Thiamine
    Pyridoxine
    Niacin
    Cobalamin (vitamin B_{12})
    α-tocopherol (vitamin E)
  Uremia
  Porphyria
  Endocrine
    Hypothyroidism
    Acromegaly
    Hyperparathyroidism
  Refsum's disease

Paraneoplastic

Immune-mediated

conduction velocities and slight associated paresthesias may resolve with adequate diabetic control. Diabetic lumbosacral plexopathy often undergoes significant improvement over some months, aided by good control of diabetes. More frequently, adequate diabetic control is useful for slowing the rate of progression of the weakness and numbness, but little improvement occurs. Very tight control, such as that which may be achieved with subcutaneous "insulin pump" therapy, has been disappointing with regard to neuropathy; good control by conventional means should be pursued. Pancreatic transplantation may offer some advantages over insulin therapy, but there are still too few patients with adequate long-term follow-up. There are reports of modest improvement occurring in patients with diabetic neuropathy who have received aldose reduc-

tase inhibitors; however, the overall ratio of risk to benefit is not clearly favorable on the basis of studies to date.

Alcohol

Abstention from alcohol or even moderation of alcohol intake can produce considerable long-term improvement in patients with distal pain and weakness; however, this may take many months to several years. When obvious malnutrition is a conjoined cause, the response to vitamin repletion may occur more quickly, with improvement beginning within a few weeks. Because of the associated distal axonal degeneration, some residual weakness and sensory disturbance usually remain in alcohol-related neuropathies.

Paraproteinemia

Among patients with paraproteinemia leading to chronic axonal polyneuropathy, only a small proportion undergo a significant clinical improvement of their neuropathy with the use of plasma exchange and/or oral cytotoxic agents; however, it remains impossible to predict in advance which patients will improve. Usually the therapy must be intensive and achieve sustained reduction of circulating paraprotein levels. Decisions to initiate such treatment must be highly individualized with regard to the degree of potential benefit as compared with the potential risks of cytotoxic agents.

Paraneoplastic Syndromes

Stabilization of or improvement in paraneoplastic neuropathies may occur after effective surgical or chemotherapeutic treatment of the malignancy. Because of the demonstrated immunologic basis for certain other paraneoplastic neurologic syndromes, there is interest in treatment with corticosteroids or other immunosuppressive regimens. These treatments are experimental, however, and must not be viewed as established therapies.

SECONDARY COMPLICATIONS

Loss of Protective Sensation

Patients with altered sensation in the hands and especially in the feet should take precautions to avoid the trauma and sustained mechanical pressure that underlie "trophic" ulcers. If sensation is significantly impaired, the patient should change shoes (to redistribute pressure points) and inspect the feet several times per day. Persistent redness or breaks in the skin should be viewed with alarm and should lead to prompt measures to avoid all pressure until there is improvement. Procedures that break the skin should be avoided; well-intentioned orthopedic and podiatric procedures often lead to a wound that does not heal in the severly denervated foot. In order to avoid serious burns, the feet should not be immersed in bath water until the temperature is felt with a more normally innervated part of the body.

Altered Gait

Severe loss of proprioception is nearly as disabling as loss of motor power, and at its worst forces a patient to rely on a wheelchair. For lesser degrees of sensory difficulty, attempts at improving sensory feedback, such as use of a light cane and judicious placement of night-lights between the bed and bathroom, may be helpful. Foot drop may lead to an exaggerated steppage gait that predisposes to falls and degenerative joint disease of the hips and lower back. Appropriate ankle-foot orthoses may prove very helpful for foot drop, although they interfere with the patient's ability to point the foot downward and thereby may cause difficulty in walking down stairs and stepping down from curbs. Mechanical stabilization of weakened ankles, which is usually obtained with high-topped shoes, may improve steadiness of gait and may help prevent recurrent ankle sprains.

Pain

Unpleasant paresthesias are a common experience during the early stages of sensory neuropathy; fortunately, only a minority of patients experience significant chronic pain. In a few instances, a specific treatable cause of the pain can be remedied—for example, focal compression of the tibial nerve at the ankle. More frequently, chronic medical treatment for pain is required.

Narcotic analgesics are of limited usefulness, in part because neuropathic pains seem especially resistant to ordinary doses of narcotics, and in part because tolerance soon reduces the modest degree of relief obtained acutely. Anticonvulsants and tricyclic antidepressants are the mainstays of treatment. Carbamazepine may be helpful for a variety of neuropathic pain syndromes. Side effects of acute atoxia, drowsiness, and nausea are reduced when the dose is gradually increased from 100 mg twice daily to 200 mg three times daily over 10 days, thereby improving patient acceptance. Further adjustments can be made to achieve the same range of serum concentrations as those used in the treatment of epilepsy (8 to 12 mg per liter for most laboratories). Monitoring for hepatocellular injury or bone marrow dysfunction should be instituted early in the course of treatment. Maximum benefit at a single dose level is generally achieved in a few days. Phenytoin is a good second choice if carbamazepine is effective but is poorly tolerated.

If carbamazepine is not effective, or for selected patients who experience pain that is predominantly superficial and burning in quality or those patients with depression complicating the pain syndrome, desipramine hydrochloride administered at a dosage increased from 25 mg daily to 100 mg daily may prove helpful; usually 25 mg is added to the daily dose each week during initiation. Amitriptyline causes significant side effects in a greater proportion of patients than desipramine hydrochloride, but its sedative properties can prove useful for the not-unusual patient whose painful feet cause misery chiefly on retiring for the night. The effects of antidepressants tend to accrue gradually over several weeks and also wear off slowly, so that some patients appreciate the benefit only when neuropathic pains recur in full force a few weeks after the medication has been discontinued. In addition to the usual precautions and contraindications for tricyclic antidepressant use, the presence of a significant autonomic component to the neuropathy should be viewed as a relative contraindication. Constipation, urinary retention, and orthostatic hypotension are likely to become intolerable, and if the QT interval is already prolonged because of the autonomic neuropathy, tricyclic antidepressants might in principle predispose to serious cardiac arrhythmias.

Cardiac anti-arrhythmic drugs, especially mexiletine, have some ability to reduce neuropathic pains. Typical dosages are 150 to 200 mg three times daily.

Autonomic Dysfunction

Constipation, urinary retention, dry mouth, and other manifestations of cholinergic deficit seldom have a satisfactory long-range response to oral bethanecol or cholinomimetic drugs, although such drugs may prove helpful acutely. Diarrhea caused by abnormal gastrointestinal motility may be helped by metoclopramide; in addition, diarrhea sometimes results from bacterial overgrowth (initially because of stasis of enteric contents) and may be improved by occasional courses of antibiotics such as tetracycline. Erectile dysfunction can be managed by penile implants or, in selected cases, by injection of papaverine hydrochloride into the corpora cavernosa to produce erection.

Generally orthostatic hypotension is first managed by modest volume expansion through generous salt intake and mineralocorticoids such as fludocortisone. Tight elastic stockings must usually be extended to the proximal thighs or (ideally) to the abdomen to be effective. These are difficult for many patients to use, especially if the patient has weakness and hand incoordination. In young patients without significant coronary or peripheral vascular disease, ergotamines such as dihydroergotamine mesylate at a dosage of 0.5 to 1.0 mg intramuscularly daily or ergotamine tartrate at a dosage of approximately 1 mg taken orally twice daily may be helpful.

In the treatment of autonomic dysfunction, one must also avoid the therapeutic misadventures that ensue when slight supine hypertension is mistakenly treated in a patient with marked postural drop, or when sympathomimetic or anticholinergic medications act on partially denervated end-organs without effective reflex control of blood pressure and heart rate.

SUGGESTED READING

Bannister R, ed. Autonomic failure: a textbook of clinical disorders of the autonomic nervous system. New York: Oxford University, 1988.
Dyck PJ, Thomas PK, Lambert EH, Bunge RP, eds. Peripheral neuropathy. Philadelphia: WB Saunders, 1984.
Schaumburg HH, Spencer PS, Thomas PK, eds. Disorders of peripheral nerves. Philadelphia: FA Davis Company, 1983.

BRACHIAL NEURITIS

AUSTIN J. SUMNER, M.D.

Effective treatment of brachial neuritis, usually a painful and frequently disabling disorder, depends to a large extent on early diagnosis, which can be difficult for even an experienced neurologist to make. It is a diagnosis of elimination of conditions that can produce acute pain, weakness, wasting, and sensory disturbance around the shoulder girdle. Brachial neuritis is also called neuralgic amyotrophy, Parsonage-Turner syndrome, brachial plexus neuritis, and multiple neuritis of the shoulder girdle.

The disorder has a peak incidence in middle life between the ages of 20 and 40 years, but children with the disorder and elderly patients are commonly encountered. The clinical picture is characteristic. There is usually a sudden onset of pain that is localized to the shoulder and upper arm and has a deep-aching quality. There may also be pain around the elbow when the anterior interosseus nerve or other forearm nerves are involved. Muscles around the shoulder may be tender to palpation and because movement is painful, the arm is often held splinted against the side in a position of shoulder adduction, internal rotation, and elbow flexion. The severe pain usually lasts less than 2 weeks. although in 20 percent of patients it may last longer. The cessation or amelioration of pain is associated with the onset of paralysis of one or more of the shoulder girdle muscles.

PAIN MANAGEMENT

Pain management often requires the use of narcotic analgesics. For most patients, middle-level narcotics such as oxycodone hydrochloride (Percodan, Percocet, Tylox) or acetaminophen (Tylenol #4) in a dose of one or two tablets taken regularly at 4- to 6-hour intervals is effective. Those with more severe pain may require strong narcotics such as hydromorphone (Dilaudid hydrochloride), 2 to 4 mg taken orally every 4 to 6 hours, or morphine, 10 mg taken orally every 4 hours. The key to effective pain management is regular dosage to maintain adequate blood levels. I have seldom found intramuscular administration to be necessary in these cases. One should bear in mind that oral dosage must be somewhat higher than that used for parenteral administration because of the more limited gastrointestinal absorption. The likelihood of addiction to these narcotics is minimized because analgesic medication is clearly required and is given regularly for relatively short periods. The initial drowsiness lasts for no more than 48 hours. Some patients also respond to treatment with corticosteroids. I use oral prednisone, beginning with a daily dose of 80 mg which is tapered at 3-day intervals to 60 mg, 40 mg, and 20 mg, and is then discontinued on Day 12. There is no good evidence that corticosteroid use influences the prognosis, but it does seem to produce more rapid resolution of the painful phase of the illness. It is of course important to have eliminated subdiaphragmatic inflammatory conditions, infiltrative lesions of the brachial plexus, and cervical intraspinal lesions before embarking on this course of symptomatic treatment. Early pain relief should be combined with physical therapy to maintain a good range of passive movement at the shoulder, thus reducing the incidence and severity of adhesive capsulitis or "frozen shoulder," which is a frequent complication when deltoid, supraspinatus, and infraspinatus muscles are paralysed.

PATHOGENESIS

Muscle paralysis usually develops fairly suddenly. Currently it is believed that the deep aching pain can be attributed to nerve trunk pain caused by lesions within the major nerve branches arising from the brachial plexus. These lesions are believed to be inflammatory or vascular in nature, causing acute axonal degeneration within the involved nerve. Lesions are patchy. However, it is important to appreciate that the precise pathology and pathogenesis of this condition are still unknown. The nerves that show a particularly high susceptibility to involvement are (1) the long thoracic nerve to serratus anterior, (2) the suprascapular nerve supplying the supraspinatus and infraspinatus muscles, (3) the axillary nerve to the teres minor and deltoid muscles, (4) the radial nerve, and (5) the musculocutaneous nerve to biceps. However, there are many additional nerves that are occasionally involved, such as the branches to the trapezius, pectoralis major, and teres major muscles, or the dorsal scapular nerve to the rhomboid muscle. The anterior interosseus branch of the median nerve is frequently affected, while median, posterior interosseus, lateral antebrachial cutaneous, ulnar, accessory, phrenic, and recurrent laryngeal nerve involvement have all been encountered. Brachial neuritis is truly an idiopathic mononeuritis multiplex of the upper extremities. Disturbance of sensation is not a prominent feature of brachial neuritis. When present, it most commonly involves the axillary cutaneous distribution. The outer aspect of the forearm in the distribution of the lateral antebrachial cutaneous nerve is also often affected. Partial loss within the median cutaneous innervation of the digits is less commonly encountered, and occasionally, lesions within such small cutaneous branches as the palmar cutaneous branch of the median can be demonstrated. These cutaneous lesions were formerly interpreted as indicating radicular lesions, but the sharply demarcated margins and the electrodiagnostic studies are most consistent with peripheral nerve lesions rather than root lesions. Bilateral involvement is rarely simultaneous, but sequential involvement of the contralateral extremity, almost always producing an asymmetric pattern of lesions is not uncommon. It is usually a monophasic illness, although recurrent attacks do occur in some patients. A recurrent familial form of the disorder is rarely encountered. Clearly the detailed assessment of the complex combinations of neurogenic lesions that can be encountered frequently calls for neurologic and especially electrodiagnostic evaluation.

Brachial neuritis usually affects otherwise healthy adults without any recognizable predisposing cause. Sometimes, however, it occurs in circumstances that may lead to confusion regarding the diagnosis. For instance, it is encountered after surgical operations, after childbirth, and after recovery from serious multiple trauma. It has been associated historically with vaccination, but this has been a rare occurrence in recent epidemiologic studies. An association with mycoplasma pneumoniae, Epstein-Barr virus, brucellosis, versiniosis, human immunodeficiency virus (HIV) infection, and the use of intravenous heroin has been described. Brachial neuritis has been seen in association with systemic Sjögren's syndrome and as a side effect of interferon treatment.

PROGNOSIS

The prognosis is generally good. Two processes contribute to the recovery of strength in paralysed muscles. The first is collateral reinnervation from surviving intact axons supplying the involved muscle. This is a remarkably efficient process, with some motor units increasing their tension outputs as much as twentyfold. Thus if electromyographic examination demonstrates the presence of some surviving motor units within muscles at the height of the deficit, the prognosis for early improvement in strength is good. Through collateral reinnervation, as few as 10 percent of the motor unit population produce near-normal strength over a period of 3 to 6 months. Completely denervated muscles, on the other hand, have a more guarded prognosis. Recovery in this case is dependent on axon regrowth to the muscle, a process not always effective in restoring good function. The rate of reinnervation in these circumstances is similar to that associated with regrowth after nerve crush or transsection. Electrical stimulation has no useful role in the treatment of paralyzed muscles during this period before reinnervation. However, there is a useful role for physical therapy in the maintenance of joint mobility and the prevention of contractures. Passive exercises should be emphasized during the period before reinnervation, but as movement is restored, graduated active exercises hasten the recovery. Improvement in function may continue for as long as 2 to 3 years after a severe attack. A word of caution, however: patients who have made good functional recovery from brachial neuritis may decompensate later in life by a process similar to the postpolio syndrome.

SUGGESTED READING

Dillin L, Hoagland FT, Scheck M. Brachial neuritis. J Bone Joint Surg 1985; 67:878–883.

England JD, Sumner AJ Neuralgic amyotrophy: an increasingly diverse entity. Muscle-Nerve 1987; 10:60–68.

Favero KJ, Hawkins RH, Jones MW Neuralgic amyotrophy J Bone Joint Surg 1987; 69:195–198.

BELL'S PALSY

JAMES W. ALBERS, M.D., Ph.D.
MARK B. BROMBERG, M.D., Ph.D.

The name of Sir Charles Bell is associated with idiopathic acquired facial mononeuritis, although he was not the first to describe the clinical syndrome and his initial description in 1821 included facial nerve mononeuropathies of any cause, including trauma. Because a variety of disorders are associated with facial mononeuropathy, the initial step in management is exclusion of the 20 to 25 percent of patients with facial palsy who have an identifiable etiology. Included are patients with known trauma (skull fracture, surgical), infection (acute and chronic otitis media, herpes zoster or Ramsay Hunt syndrome, granulomatous disease), or neoplasm (meningeal infiltration, meningioma, parotid gland tumor, neurolemmoma).

ANATOMIC FEATURES

The facial nerve is predominately a motor nerve that innervates all muscles of facial expression, as well as the stapedius, the posterior belly of the digastricus, and the styloid muscles. Sensory components of the facial nerve include taste sensation from the anterior two-thirds of the tongue, proprioceptive information from muscles innervated by the facial nerve, and exteroceptive sensation from a portion of the external auditory canal. The facial nerve also carries parasympathetic fibers to the salivary and lacrimal glands, as well as to mucous membranes of the oral and nasal cavities. The motor division of the facial nerve is separate from the sensory and parasympathetic fibers (nervus intermedius), although the two join together within the facial canal.

ETIOLOGY

The etiology of idiopathic Bell's palsy is, by defintion, unknown. There are several proposed pathophysiologic explanations that may have relevance to therapy. One relates to local compression of the nerve within the confines of the facial canal. It has been proposed that a similar mechanism is involved in carpal tunnel syndrome, and many although not all of the same predisposing factors are common to both (pregnancy, advancing age, hypothyroidism, diabetes mellitus). The ''compression'' in Bell's palsy is believed to be related to localized epineural edema, resulting from some initial lesion that progresses in a self-perpetuating fashion. It has

been proposed that mast cell degranulation in the epineural tissue results in additional edema, increased pressure, and focal nerve damage. The initial lesion may have multiple etiologies, including ischemia (e.g., vasoconstriction induced by exposure to cold), a localized immune-mediated response that becomes self-perpetuating because of the confines of the facial canal, or direct viral involvement of the facial nerve (e.g., reactivation of herpes simplex virus). All proposed explanations are speculative.

CLINICAL EVALUATION

Motor functions of the facial nerve are easily examined. The face is inspected while the patient is at rest and during activation for asymmetry. This may consist of unequal palpebral fissures, loss of the nasal labial fold, incomplete blinking, or absence of normal wrinkling. Individual facial muscles can be activated by asking the patient to smile, grimace, forcefully close the eyes, wrinkle the forehead, expose the teeth, purse the lips, or puff out the cheeks with the lips closed. Muscles such as the orbicularis oculi, orbicularis oris, and frontalis can be tested against manual resistance to reveal mild weakness. It is usually not difficult to differentiate between central and peripheral facial weakness. Neurons innervating the frontalis muscle receive bilateral upper motor neuron input. Therefore unilateral supranuclear lesions can be easily differentiated from facial nerve lesions by demonstrating sparing of the frontalis muscle. Combined motor and visceral involvement also establishes facial paralysis as having peripheral origin. Taste sensation can be examined on the anterior portion of each half of the tongue, although localizing the site of damage along the nerve by determining which sensory or parasympathetic function is spared has limited clinical application in the evaluation of idiopathic Bell's palsy. Establishing a diagnosis of Bell's palsy depends on the exclusion of identifiable underlying abnormalities. A thorough neurologic examination occasionally demonstrates equivocal or minimal findings implicating involvement of other cranial nerves. While evidence of a generalized cranial polyneuritis does not necessarily exclude the diagnosis of Bell's palsy, such findings should certainly intensify the search for an underlying disorder. Inspection of the tympanic membrane to search for the characteristic vesicular lesions associated with herpes viruses should also be performed.

LABORATORY STUDIES

Laboratory studies are of limited value in establishing a diagnosis of Bell's palsy, but they can demonstrate some underlying disorder that may be associated with facial mononeuropathy. Cranial computed tomography or magnetic resonance imaging is obtained only when there is suspicion of a posterior fossa mass.Evaluation of cerebrospinal fluid (CSF) is not usually performed in the routine evaluation of Bell's palsy, but it is useful in the evaluation of suspected inflammatory disorders, granulomatous disease, or meningeal carcinomatosis. The presence of elevated protein, leukocytosis, and hypoglycorrachia should prompt appropriate cultures and evaluation of cytology. A mild lymphocytosis, with or without elevated protein, is a nonspecific finding and has been reported in typical Bell's palsy. Specific tests are available to quantify abnormalities not easily tested during the clinical examination. Some are of purported use in identifying the site of the facial nerve lesion. Included are tests for lacrimation (Schirmer test), stapedial reflex, electrogustometry, and submaxillary salivary secretion. Overall, such studies are not highly reliable and add little to the clinical evaluation in most situations. In patients with suspected corneal abrasion, slit-lamp examination with fluorescein confirms lesions.

ELECTRODIAGNOSIS

Several types of peripheral dysfunction can be identified in Bell's palsy, including slowed or blocked conduction and partial or complete axonal degeneration. In Bell's palsy, unlike most other clinical "entrapment" mononeuropathies, the facial nerve cannot be directly stimulated proximal to the presumed lesion. It is possible, however, to study the distal segment of the nerve, stimulating the facial nerve near the styloid foramen and recording from any muscle of facial nerve innervation (e.g. the orbicularis oculi, orbicularis oris, nasalis, frontalis muscles). Proximal conduction also can be evaluated via blink reflex studies, whereby a trigeminal sensory nerve is percutaneously stimulated, resulting in reflex activation of the facial nerves. Needle electromyography (EMG) of facial muscles has a more limited role in Bell's palsy. EMG may demonstrate the presence of motor unit action potentials under volitional control in patients without any clinical evidence of facial nerve function. This may have limited prognostic implications (discussed below), and such a finding does demonstrate the anatomic continuity of the facial nerve.

In order to evaluate the use and utility of electrodiagnostic studies in the treatment of Bell's palsy, it is useful to consider the temporal changes that occur with sudden focal nerve injury. After nerve transection, stimulation distal to the lesion results in a normal compound muscle action potential (CMAP) for several days, with eventual disappearance of the response in 5 to 7 days (Fig. 1). It is

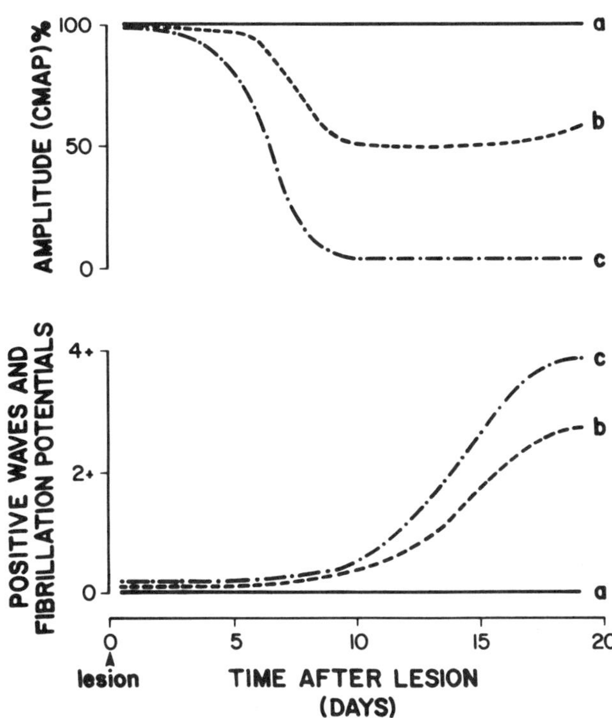

Figure 1 Representation of electrodiagnostic findings after facial nerve lesions of varying severity, plotted against time. A=conduction block only; B=conduction block and partial axonal degeneration; C=complete axonal degeneration. *Top,* Compound muscle action potential (CMAP) amplitude as percentage of contralateral, unaffected side. *Bottom,* Presence and degree of abnormal spontaneous activity (fibrillation potentials and positive waves) recorded during needle EMG.

only after this that evidence of axonal damage can first be detected in the form of positive waves and fibrillation potentials recorded by needle EMG. It can be argued that the precise time course of axonal degeneration in Bell's palsy is unknown, and it is possible that degeneration of all fibers progresses over a substantial time period, thereby permitting the clinician performing the EMG evaluation to recognize the first signs of denervation. However, in most patients with evidence of extensive axonal degeneration, the CMAP disappears within 1 week of onset, and patients with a more protracted course with evidence of cumulative axonal degeneration over a longer period of time are uncommon. Although needle EMG is a highly sensitive indicator of axonal degeneration, it is of limited use in estimating the magnitude of denervation because injury of only a few axons results in positive waves and fibrillation potentials (see Fig. 1). Since localized conduction block does not interfere with the evoked response after stimulation distal to the lesion, the CMAP amplitude can be used to estimate the extent of axonal degeneration only after the initial 7-day period. In a partially or completely paralyzed muscle, a preserved evoked response after 7 days reflects intact but blocked fibers. CMAP amplitude therefore provides a much more accurate estimate of the magnitude of axonal degeneration than can be obtained by needle EMG. Some recommend that evoked response studies be performed daily and that therapeutic decisions such as those regarding the need for surgical decompression be based on the results. As described above, electrodiagnostic findings of axonal degeneration reflect irreversible denervation that occurred days before the disappearance of the evoked response. We perform electrodiagnostic studies only in patients with a suspected pre-existing lesion or severe clinical involvement that has not demonstrated any evidence of improvement 7 to 10 days after onset. The reason for performing studies in the latter situation is to predict prognosis, not to modify treatment. Once the CMAP is substantially reduced (less than 10 percent of the contralateral side), intervention of any type is not likely to be helpful. Studies performed within 72 hours of onset cannot be used to establish prognosis, although, in certain situations they may have value in identifying an underlying abnormality that may have been present before the clinical onset of paralysis.

CLINICAL FEATURES

The incidence of Bell's palsy is approximately 20 to 25 per 100,000 individuals; the incidence is lower for young adults but increases with age. For those over 60 years of age, the incidence is approximately 30 to 35 per 100,000 individuals. Bell's palsy is slightly more common in females younger than 50 years of age; among individuals older than 50 years of age, it is more common in males. There is no racial predilection. Bell's palsy is almost always unilateral, and involvement of the right or left sides is equal. In the rare patient with bilateral facial involvement (reported to occur in as many as 0.5 percent of patients with Bell's palsy), it is our experience that there is commonly an identifiable underlying illness, such as Guillain-Barré syndrome, myasthenia gravis, sarcoidosis, carcinomatous meningitis, or Lyme disease. There may be seasonal variation, with a slighlty higher incidence during the winter, and localized clustering of patients has been reported, suggesting a possible associated infectious etiology. An antecedent respiratory tract infection is frequently reported. A history of an immediately preceding exposure to cold or drafts is common, and textbook descriptions of Bell's palsy over the past 100 years almost always list exposure to cold as a frequent antecedent event. Pregnancy (third trimester), diabetes mellitus, and hypothyroidism are also believed to be associated with a higher incidence of Bell's palsy than expected

in the general population. Recurrent Bell's palsy has been reported in as many as 10 percent of patients. A positive family history in approximately 8 percent of patients with Bell's palsy seems higher than what the overall incidence would predict, and several families have been described to have recurrent Bell's palsy in association with isolated oculomotor nerve palsies.

The onset of Bell's palsy is subacute, developing rapidly over hours to days. Occasionally it develops overnight. Mild pain in or behind the ear is common at onset, as is a subjective sensation of "numbness" of the involved side of the face. This may relate to the loss of facial tone, although some believe that Bell's palsy consists of predominant facial nerve involvement in association with a cranial polyneuritis, including involvement of the trigeminal nerve. In our experience, overt clinical involvement of other cranial nerves is uncommon. Usually facial weakness is first apparent when the patient directly observes it in a mirror or notes that he is having difficulty drinking or holding liquids in the mouth or in eating, because food tends to collect between the cheek and gums. Occasionally someone else first notices the facial asymmetry. Because of decreased blinking, tearing on the involved side is common, although lacrimation may become defective. Rarely, other symptoms such as diminished taste, low-tone hyperacusis (from stapedius weakness), or xerostomia are initial or accompanying symptoms. Progression is rapid, and most patients reach the nadir of clinical involvement within several days, although there are reports of progression over 1 to 2 weeks.

PROGNOSIS

Approximately 75 percent of patients with Bell's palsy experience complete recovery, most within 2 to 3 weeks. An additional 15 percent experience satisfactory recovery but may have mild facial asymmetry, a residual impairment demonstrable on clinical testing, or abnormal reinnervation. Five to ten percent of patients have poor recovery at 4 months, with persistent neurologic impairment and cosmetic disfigurement. In time, some of these patients experience slowly progressive improvement. In addition to residual weakness, another form of poor recovery relates to aberrant facial nerve reinnervation, resulting in facial synkinesis, characterized by involuntary activation of one set of facial muscles during activation of other facial muscles. Examples include contraction of all or multiple ipsilateral facial muscles when the patient attempts to purse his lips, or involuntary lower facial movements during eye blinking. Another type of aberrant reinnervation results in lacrimation while eating (crocodile tears), presumably caused by regenerating fibers intended for the salivary glands inadvertently reinnervating the lacrimal glands.

Although none is absolute, multiple factors have been associated with poor prognosis, including severity at onset, prolonged interval to initial improvement, advanced age, hyperacusis, any underlying illness associated with neuropathy, hypertension, and the presence of severe pain. Although treatment remains controversial, there is agreement that clinical findings alone give limited prognostic information, and electrodiagnostic evidence of complete axonal degeneration is associated with poor prognosis. Unfortunately, none of the clinical signs or laboratory tests predict in which patients the disorder will progress to complete denervation, the information we would like to know at onset. In our experience, the results of electrodiagnostic testing at the nadir of involvement are the most reliable indicators of poor prognosis. Patients who develop evidence of extensive axonal degeneration (discussed below) have a poorer prognosis than patients who do not. Partial or complete preservation of the CMAP amplitude, as well as the presence of any voluntary motor unit action potentials on needle EMG indicate anatomic continuity of the facial nerve and partial axonal preservation. When present at least 72 hours after clinical nadir, these findings suggest a better prognosis than when axonal degeneration is complete. If CMAP amplitude remains greater than 10 percent of the contralateral response at that time, recovery is likely to occur and sequelae are inversely proportional to the amplitude; the greater the amplitude, the more rapid the recovery and the less the sequelae. Distal latency measurements appear to be of limited prognostic value, and prolonged latency early in the course of Bell's palsy is usually associated with reduced CMAP amplitude. Blink reflex studies can be used to demonstrate proximal facial conduction slowing. Return of an initially absent response indicates survival of some axons, suggesting a good prognosis. Partial denervation is extremely common in Bell's palsy, and its presence on needle EMG does not necessarily affect prognosis adversely.

TREATMENT

Patients should be reassured that, although the symptoms associated with Bell's palsy are frightening, the outcome is usually favorable. They should also be told that the problem is not related to a stroke, a common interpretation. They should be told that the facial weakness is the most apparent difficulty, although other symptoms may be observed, including decreased tearing, decreased salivation, altered taste, and sensitivity to or alteration of loud sounds in the ear on the affected side. A simple aid reported to reduce dysarthria consists of instructing the patient to elevate the corner of the upper lip with the index finger while talking. This simple maneuver may make speech intelligible in patients with severe dysarthria from facial weakness.

The combination of poor eye closure and decreased tearing may allow the cornea to become excessively dry and potentially results in corneal ulceration and decreased vision. Fortunately, this is a rare complication because of preserved Bell's phenomenon (upward deflection of the ocular globe with attempted eye closure). Nevertheless, whenever the cornea is without protection, or whenever excessive corneal dryness or ocular irritation exists, the use of artifical tears as needed while awake and of an eye ointment at bedtime reduces the likelihood of corneal damage. The eye can also be kept moist by manually closing the eye periodically. It may be helpful to use eyeglasses during the day or to protect the involved eye with an eye shield. Simply taping a gauze over the involved eye may be counterproductive because poor eye closure can result in direct corneal abrasion from the protective pad.

Corticosteroids are commonly prescribed for the treatment of Bell's palsy in patients in whom the medication is not contraindicated. The basis for their use is related to reduced nerve edema or perhaps to decreased inflammation. Nevertheless, the use of corticosteroids remains controversial and there are studies both promoting and refuting the purported beneficial response. In a disorder with a 90 percent recovery rate, anecdotal experience cannot be used to prove efficacy of treatment. In addition, the incidence of adverse effects must be very low. In controlled evaluations, prednisone has been associated with early reduction of postauricular pain, more full recovery, and less severe complications of aberrant reinnervation. Because of the short duration of treatment, complications associated with prednisone use are rare. The most common complications are transient and include indigestion, loss of control of diabetes or onset of hyperglycemia, insomnia, activation of duodenal ulcer, and behavioral changes. Pregnancy is not an absolute contraindication to the use of prednisone.

Most would agree that if prednisone is to be effective it must be administered within the 1st week after onset of neurologic symptoms. A variety of protocols exist. Commonly, prednisone is initiated at 60 mg (or 1 mg per kilogram) per day in a single morning dose. If improvement is observed or if mild weakness does not progress over 4 or 5 days, the medication is tapered over the next 7 to 10 days. If improvement is not observed and involvement is severe, prednisone is continued for approximately 10 days and then tapered as described above. In patients at risk, blood pressure, blood glucose, and electrolytes should be monitored at the time of reevaluation.

Surgical decompression of Bell's palsy was first proposed 50 years ago, but it is rarely recommended today. Nevertheless, the surgical literature contains recommendations for immediate surgical decompression when the CMAP on the involved side reaches 5 to 10 percent of the contralateral response. It is argued that decompression prevents further degeneration by releasing the compression of the swollen facial nerve within the facial canal. There is controversial evidence suggesting satisfactory return of facial movements in patients so treated. When the CMAP decreases to less than 5 percent of the contralateral side, proponents note that surgical decompression has no adverse effect on subsequent regeneration. Our main concern with such a recommendation is that the measure on which the surgical decision is based provides information on the status of the facial nerve several days before the testing, and not at the actual time of testing. It is our experience that there is no indication for acute surgical decompression in patients with uncomplicated Bell's palsy.

For patients with severe residual impairments at least 1 year after onset, several surgical procedures exist including hypoglossal-to-facial anastomosis and cross-face nerve and muscle grafts to improve eye closure, provide lower facial expression (leva-tor), and orbicularis oris function. Our experience with the latter procedure has been limited, but results have not been dramatic and only limited function has been demonstrated in most patients. There also are corrective surgery procedures for protection of the cornea and cosmetic purposes.

In our experience, the role of physical therapy and electrical stimulation of facial muscles is limited. Experimental studies have demonstrated that intermittent percutaneous electrical stimulation of denervated muscle does reduce residual impairment, but the small initial difference between treated and untreated groups rapidly disappears after reinnervation begins.

SUGGESTED READING

Adour KK, Wingerd MA, Bell Dn, et al. Prednisone treatment for idiopathic facial paralysis (Bell's palsy). N Engl J Med 1972; 287:1268–1272.

Esslen E. The acute facial palsies: investigations on the localization and pathogenesis of meatolabyrinthine facial palsies. New York: Springer-Verlag, 1977.

Katusic SK, Beard M, Wiederholt WC, et al. Incidence, clinical features, and prognosis in Bell's palsy: Rochester, Minnestoa, 1968–1982. Ann Neurol 1986; 20:622–627.

Wolf SM, Wagner JH, Davidson S, Forsythe A. Treatment of Bell palsy with prednisone: a prospective, randomized study. Neurology 1978; 28:158–161.

ENTRAPMENT NEUROPATHY

ASA J. WILBOURN, M.D.
PATRICK J. SWEENEY, M.D., FACP

Although the terms "entrapment neuropathy" and "compressive neuropathy" are often used interchangeably, they are not synonymous. A compressive neuropathy results when sustained pressure is applied to a localized region of the nerve. Most often this pressure derives from an external source and is transmitted through the tissues (including skin) overlying the nerve. However, occasionally pressure arises internally, such as from an expanding hematoma or neoplasm. An entrapment neuropathy, on the other hand, is one caused by constriction or mechanical distortion of the nerve within a fibrous or fibro-osseous tunnel, or by a fibrous band. In these situations, the source of injury is internal, and focal nerve compression may be less important in symptom production than nerve angulation and stretching.

MEDIAN NEUROPATHY AT OR DISTAL TO THE WRIST (CARPAL TUNNEL SYNDROME)

Although the characteristic clinical presentation of chronic entrapment of the median nerve beneath the transverse carpal ligament was first recognized only about 40 years ago, carpal tunnel syndrome (CTS) is the most common entrapment neuropathy by far and the most frequently encountered nontraumatic focal peripheral nerve lesion.

The initial step in the treatment of CTS is to confirm, by electrodiagnostic studies, that it is actually present. While its symptoms are often described as "characteristic" and frequently seem so, we have seen experienced clinicians confuse CTS with other entities (particularly C-6 or C-7 radiculopathies) often enough that such confirmation is warranted. When electrodiagnostic evaluation consists not only of the routine median motor and sensory nerve conduction studies (NCS), but also of median and ulnar (for comparison) palmar NCS, the procedure is highly sensitive for CTS. Electromyographic (EMG) studies are particularly important in patients with "atypical" CTS presentations. Frequently in these patients, either another focal neurogenic lesion is detected (e.g., a radiculopathy or a more proximal median nerve lesion) or, much more often, the studies are normal. Since CTS operations performed in patients of the latter group are likely to be failures, in our experience, the electrical data are helpful in management. Another useful benefit of electrodiagnostic studies in suspected CTS is that they identify those patients in whom CTS, while present, is not occurring in isolation but instead is superimposed on a generalized peripheral polyneuropathy, which can result in a very different diagnostic and therapeutic approach.

A variety of treatments are available for CTS. Wrist immobilization in the neutral position by an Ace bandage or a volar splint may offer considerable relief, by limiting flexion and extention movements at the wrist. Unfortunately, this compromises the functional use of the hand (which is often the dominant hand), thus limiting its use to periods of sleep. Also, symptom relief may be incomplete, symptoms often recur when splinting is discontinued, and few patients follow this regimen indefinitely. A short course of either nonsteroidal anti-inflammatory agents or diuretics helps some patients, but the symptoms frequently reappear after variable periods of time, and these medications cannot be given to some patients with CTS (e.g., pregnant women). A cortisone injection into the carpal tunnel is often beneficial, presumably because it decreases inflammation in the tendon sheaths. This treatment usually proves to be temporary, however, with relapses occurring after 2 to 3 months, and it is not without some risk. No attempt should be made to perform this procedure without first doing so under the direct supervision of an experienced clinician. We have seen patients whose median nerves were destroyed by the injudicious use of cortisone injections by clinicians unfamiliar with the technique. Also, only a limited number of injections (probably 3 or less) should be attempted, and the patient should be reassessed at intervals. If the condition is worsening, clinically or electrically, this therapeutic approach should be abandoned. The most consistently helpful treatment by far (and the only one that usually provides permanent symptom relief) is sectioning of the transverse carpal ligament. This alleviates symptoms in more than 90 percent of patients, and most of the surgical failures are associated with inappropriate patient selection or improper surgical techniques. Patients in the former group are commonly those with atypical clinical findings and/or normal electrodiagnostic studies. Unsatisfactory surgical techniques generally result in incomplete sectioning of the ligament, and are usually associated with transverse or ''micro'' surgical wrist scars. A repeat operation by another surgeon is usually successful.

The clinical findings in these patients are generally more helpful in selecting surgical candidates than are the electrical findings. The symptoms, at least during the initial stages of the disorder, are caused primarily by small fiber involvement, while the electrical changes reflect only large myelinated nerve fiber compromise. Clinical signs of progression include pain increasing in frequency and occupying greater portions of the 24-hour day, (e.g., occurring more and more often during the wake cycle as well as during the sleep cycle), persistent sensory loss in a median nerve distribution (with subsequent finger clumsiness), and lateral thenar wasting. Lateral thenar wasting should be taken as an indication for prompt surgical intervention because it is a sign of a far-advanced problem. Many physicians consider certain electrical abnormalities to be indications for surgical treatment, since they, too, generally reflect advanced disease. These include (1) unelicitable median sensory nerve action potentials, (2) markedly prolonged median motor distal latency, (3) low-amplitude or unelicitable median motor compound muscle action potential, and (4) fibrillation potentials in the median-innervated thenar muscles.

Although CTS is sometimes self-limited (particularly in pregnant women and patients who have used their hands excessively for a restricted period of time), more often it is static or progressive. Hence if CTS does not appear serious enough to mandate therapy when it is first recognized, provision should be made for periodic reassessment. We have seen several patients over the years whose initially mild CTS ultimately culminated in total axon loss lesions, with permanent residuals, because they were not re-evaluated appropriately.

ULNAR NEUROPATHY AT THE ELBOW

Although these lesions have been recognized for much longer than CTS, in the majority of patients, their exact location along the ulnar nerve is unclear. For years, ulnar neuropathies at the elbow were attributed to nerve compromise at the ulnar groove. More recently, however, the cubital tunnel area, which lies immediately distal to the ulnar groove, has been implicated. To add to the confusion, some physicians are now referring to all ulnar neuropathies that occur at the elbow as ''cubital tunnel syndrome,'' although there is no proof that even the majority of lesions actually occur at this site. Those within the groove are typically compressive or stretch lesions. By contrast, lesions within the cubital tunnel may be caused by either entrapment or external compression; both mechanisms may even be operative in the same patient. Electrodiagnostic studies are less sensitive for ulnar neuropathy at the elbow than for CTS. Although they are usually abnormal (a major exception being chronic lesions manifested solely as intermittent paresthesias), a focal demyelinating component (e.g., focal slowing, differential slowing, conduction block), detectable along the ulnar nerve and allowing localization to the elbow segment, is found in only about half of the patients. In the remaining patients, the lesions are "pure" axon loss in character and the EMG localization becomes much less precise. Hence the more severe ulnar neuropathies are more likely to be poorly localized by EMG examination.

With many ulnar neuropathies, the source of symptom production is as unclear as the lesion site. Some physicians attribute the symptoms to excessive elbow flexion/extension alone (somewhat comparable to carpal tunnel syndrome). Splinting the elbow region, particularly while the patient is asleep, with a removable rigid cast has been tried but is ineffective in many patients. In some patients a definite history of excessive elbow leaning can be elicited; they should be encouraged to cease this practice and be given elbow protection (elbow protectors worn by hockey or football players can be very helpful and can be obtained at any sporting goods store). A brief trial of a nonsteroidal anti-inflammatory drug occasionally relieves symptoms. If the symptoms are progressive, and particularly if a bony deformity is present at the elbow, surgical intervention should be considered. However, several aspects of the treatment of ulnar neuropathies stand in contrast to that of CTS: (1) several different surgical procedures are used to treat ulnar neuropathy at the elbow (depending largely on exactly where the particular surgeon believes the lesion is located), including medial epicondylectomy, cubital tunnel decompression, and nerve transposition; (2) the surgical success rate for ulnar neuropathies is much less predictable than that for CTS, although usually the milder the lesion, the better the result; and (3) the operations for ulnar neuropathies are not without risk. We have seen a few patients who had only sensory symptoms preoperatively, with little to no evidence of axon loss. However, after undergoing the operation, they had very severe axon loss ulnar neuropathies, presumably reflecting nerve infarction caused by stripping of nutrient arteries from the nerve while it was being prepared for transposition.

RADIAL NEUROPATHY AT THE SPIRAL GROOVE

These upper extremity nerve lesions are not commonly encountered. Those lesions not caused by obvious trauma rarely are due to nerve entrapment. Instead, they are usually caused by external compression. Because the type of pathophysiology at the lesion site is a major consideration in therapy, the electrodiagnostic evaluation is an important component of the initial assessment of these lesions. Since almost all patients present with extensor forearm muscle weakness (i.e., wrist and finger drop),

the responsible process must be axon loss or demyelinating conduction block or a combination of both (demyelinating focal slowing and differential slowing are not associated with clinical weakness). These can be readily differentiated from one another if the appropriate studies are performed, thereby permitting early accurate prognostication and appropriate therapy. The most informative study is the radial motor NCS, with nerve stimulation at the elbow area and immediately distal and proximal to the spiral groove, while one records with a surface electrode over the proximal extensor forearm muscles. Radial neuropathies caused by external pressure (the so-called "Saturday night palsies") are usually demyelinating conduction block lesions and tend to resolve completely within approximately 6 to 8 weeks. Occasionally, however, they are axon loss in type, similar to those seen with midshaft humeral fractures and radial nerve injection injuries. Nonetheless, even these usually recover satisfactorily, although they are much slower in tempo because the nerve fibers must regenerate distally from the lesion site. Regeneration can be ascertained by electrodiagnostic studies several weeks before it is clinically evident, through needle electrode examination of the closest "target" muscle(s) distal to the injury site (i.e., the brachioradialis and extensor carpi radialis). A few motor unit potentials (MUPs) of low amplitude, with markedly increased duration and highly polyphasic in configuration ("reinnervation" MUPs) are seen in those muscles on attempted voluntary activation several weeks before enough reinnervation has occurred to produce a visible muscle twitch. If reinnervation is not progressing, (i.e., if "reinnervation" MUPs are not seen in the target muscles during 2 or 3 examinations, performed at 4-week intervals, with the first being performed at the time reinnervation was expected), surgical exploration is mandatory.

With all types of radial neuropathy at the spiral groove, sensory symptoms tend to be minimal and are overshadowed by the motor deficit, which results in wrist and finger drop. The latter should be treated with splinting, although the functional use of the hand is significantly impaired. For those relatively few patients with permanent axon loss radial neuropathies (i.e., those in whom no clinical or EMG evidence of reinnervation is present after approximately 1 year), reconstructive tendon transfers should be considered.

THORACIC OUTLET SYNDROME

At least 2 types of "neurogenic" thoracic outlet syndromes (TOS) have been described, but only one is noncontroversial. It is a rare entrapment lesion, limited to young and middle-aged females. It presents with weakness and wasting of the hand (particularly the lateral thenar eminence) and sometimes of the medial forearm, along with long standing aching pain along the medial forearm. Neck radiographs show a rudimentary cervical rib or at least an elongated C-7 transverse process (the lower trunk of the brachial plexus is stretched and angulated over a translucent band extending from the tip of this anomaly to the first rib). EMG examination is almost pathognomonic, showing a highly chronic, axon loss, lower-trunk brachial plexopathy. Appropriate treatment is sectioning of the band via a supraclavicular surigcal approach.

''Neurogenic'' TOS is also diagnosed in a great number of patients (particularly women) who do not have the characteristic radiographic or EMG features described above. Frequently workman's compensation claims or personal injury lawsuits for minor automobile accidents are pending. For these patients, conservative therapy is indicated. Unfortunately, many of them undergo first rib removal or some other type of TOS surgery. This not only produces fleeting symptom relief in many (probably the majority), but also causes severe axon loss, lower-trunk brachial plexopathies in some.

PERONEAL NEUROPATHY AT THE FIBULAR HEAD

This is the most common mononeuropathy of the lower extremity. Most of these lesions are caused by compression or stretching of the common peroneal nerve fibers at the fibular head; entrapment is rarely the cause. Because these neuropathies characteristically present with foot drop (i.e., weakness of the tibialis anterior muscle), the pathophysiological process is either axon loss, demyelinating conduction block, or a combination of both. Clinically, it is difficult to distinguish between them, since each can produce any gradation of weakness, from mild to complete. Yet their prognosis with regard to time and degree of recovery is quite different. Hence, just as with radial neuropathies, electrodiagnostic studies (particularly peroneal motor NCS while recording from tibialis anterior) are of major importance in assessing these lesions. They not only reveal the pathophysiology at the lesion site, but also document that the cause of the patient's foot drop is a peroneal mononeuropathy, rather than a more proximal lesion, such as a sciatic neuropathy, sacral plexopathy, or particularly an L-5 radiculopathy. Any one of these would result in a different diagnostic and therapeutic regimen. Compressive peroneal neuropathies tend to be associated with recent, significant weight loss (>10 kg), chronic leg crossing, and/or major illness that causes prolonged hospitalization.

The most appropriate therapy is preventing additional nerve compression. In the hospital setting, this requires that adequate protection for the nerve at the fibular head be assured by proper padding and positioning. If the patient is a chronic leg-crosser, this habit must be discouraged. Because it is typically an unconscious act, merely advising the patient to stop crossing his legs is not sufficient. Instead, he should be instructed to tell his friends and close acquaintances to inform him each time they observe him doing this. Avoiding leg crossing can result in rapid resolution of symptoms in those patients with demyelinating conduction block. Hence during a subsequent visit, the patient often reports that his foot drop is improving while he simultaneously expresses displeasure concerning the number of times he has been told to uncross his legs by his associates and family members. Even when the nerve lesion is caused by traction, surgical nerve repair is rarely indicated. If the traction is mild and produces primarily demyelinating conduction block, recovery is relatively rapid and complete. Conversely, if the traction is severe enough to produce axon degeneration, the nerve segment affected is often so extensive as to preclude successful surgical repair. Nonetheless, if only for medicolegal reasons, a neurosurgical opinion should be obtained for any patient with an axon loss lesion that is not showing clinical or EMG improvement after 6 months.

Because most of these lesions are painless and produce few sensory complaints, the major disability is foot drop. This is corrected relatively easily by means of a dorsiflexor foot splint; of particular value are the light-weight, plastic foot splints that fit in the shoe. (However, these cannot be used with high-heeled shoes.) Orthopedic tendon transfers should be offered to those patients with permanent lesions, although many patients consider such surgery unnecessary.

MEDIAL/LATERAL PLANTAR ENTRAPMENT NEUROPATHY (TARSAL TUNNEL SYNDROME)

Although chronic entrapment of the terminal portions of the posterior tibial nerve—tarsal tunnel syndrome (TTS)—is well described in the literature, its incidence is uncertain. This entity is not the ''CTS of the foot''; its electrical characteristics and response to surgical treatment are markedly different from those seen with CTS. As with all other compressive/entrapment neuropathies, other causes for the patient's symptoms (which in this case is predominantly or solely foot pain and paresthesia) must be excluded. Unilateral TTS can be confused with primary arthritic bone spurs in the foot, ischemic monomelic neuropathy, tibial neuropathies, sciatic neuropathies primarily affecting the tibial fibers, and sacral plexopathies affecting primarily the S-1, S-2 tibial fibers and, most often, S-1,

S-2 radiculopathies. Bilateral TTS is most often confused with peripheral polyneuropathies and bilateral S-1, S-2 radiculopathies (cauda equina lesions).

Electrodiagnostic studies can be of help in the differential diagnosis. Although this syndrome has been reported to produce a characteristic electrodiagnostic pattern (slowing along the medial and/or lateral plantar nerves in a manner analogous to that of CTS), these findings can be demonstrated only rarely in patients referred to the EMG laboratory with a diagnosis of TTS. Much more often, when the lesion cannot be localized to a more proximal location, the EMG examination either is normal or demonstrates only axon loss in the distribution of one or both of these nerves. Because often the studies are performed in patients who have already undergone multiple unsuccessful TTS surgical procedures, there is no way to determine whether these electrical abnormalities antedated the operations or were caused by one or more of them. Since, in our experience, TTS surgery so often proves to be unsuccessful (i.e., the patient reports not only that the symptoms were unrelieved, but actually increased with each operation) possibly the best therapy a neurologist can provide for suspected TTS, once other diagnostic possibilities have been excluded, is avoidance of surgery. Those patients who have undergone multiple unsuccessful operations can present difficult management problems. Analgesics usually provide only temporary (if any) benefit, and carbamazepine (Tegretol), while helpful, seldom produces complete relief.

SUGGESTED READING

Dawson DM, Hallett M, Millender LH. Entrapment neuropathies. Boston: Little, Brown, and Co., 1983.

Gilliatt RW, Harrison MJG. Nerve compression and entrapment. In: Absury AK, Gilliatt RW, eds. Peripheral nerve disorders: a practical approach. Stoneham MA: Butterworths, 1984: 243.

Katirji MB, Wilbourn AJ. Common peroneal mononeuropathy: a clinical and electrophysiological study of 116 lesions. Neurology 1988; 38:1723–1728.

Stewart JD. Focal peripheral neuropathies. New York: Elsevier, 1987.

NEUROMUSCULAR JUNCTION AND MUSCLE DISEASE

MYASTHENIA GRAVIS

KLAUS V. TOYKA, M.D.

Myasthenia gravis (MG) is an autoimmune disease of the neuromuscular junction that is caused by an antibody-mediated immune attack against nicotinic acetylcholine receptors (AChR). The formation of autoantibodies may be caused indirectly by hyperactive T-helper lymphocytes or by reduced activity of suppressor cells. The exact mechanism of the disordered immunoregulation is incompletely understood. It has been speculated that the thymus may be a site at which the pivotal break in self-tolerance occurs.

The immunologic diagnostic tests and immunosuppressive treatment of MG are based on these immunopathologic concepts.

EVALUATION OF PATIENTS WITH MG

The diagnosis of MG is based on the typical clinical presentation, which includes muscle weakness of ocular, bulbar, truncal, and limb muscles. Muscle fatigue on exertion is usually present. If MG is suspected, pharmacologic testing with a cholinesterase (ChE) inhibitor such as edrophonium chloride (Tensilon) will show marked improvement of muscle strength in a typical patient. Equivocal test results may be seen in some patients with otherwise typical MG. In these patients, the diagnosis must be supported by antibody measurements.

The most sensitive and specific test for MG is the demonstration of circulating autoantibodies to AChR in the serum. Elevated titers can now be shown in several laboratories in more than 95 percent of patients with generalized MG. This applies to the modified double immunoprecipitation assay originally described by Lindstrom, which uses crude human muscle AChR. Other tests using nonhuman AChR or enzyme-linked immunosorbent assay (ELISA) methods are less sensitive, and the titers may differ substantially. The test should be ordered in every patient with unexplained weakness or fatigue. A minority of patients with otherwise typical myasthenia may have titers in the normal range. In some laboratories, additional test methods are available for these patients. Absolute antibody titers do not correlate with severity of MG. In most patients, serial titers correlate with weakness in the individual.

Traditionally neurologists confirm the diagnosis by electrophysiologic testing. On repetitive stimulation of motor nerves, a typical fatigue reaction (decrement) can be recorded from proximal muscles in 70 percent of patients with generalized weakness. Single-fiber electromyography is more sensitive but is not specific for MG; it can be performed only by experienced examiners. In my opinion, it should be reserved for the "difficult patient," such as those with ocular myasthenia and antibody-negative cases.

Every patient is checked for thymic abnormalities by chest computed tomography (CT) or magnetic resonance imaging (MRI). In my patients with thymic hyperplasia, I have seen the enlargement on either scan in roughly 50 percent of patients preoperatively. With thymomas, the rate of discovery is usually higher but depends on the tumor size and type of malignancy.

MG may be associated with other autoimmune disorders that may have passed undiagnosed. A laboratory screen for other circulating autoantibodies, thyroid hormones, and diabetes mellitus should be done. Tuberculosis should be formally excluded if immunosuppressive treatment is planned.

MONITORING DISEASE ACTIVITY

Patients with MG should be seen at regular intervals, ranging from every 2 weeks in the more severely affected patient after the initiation of immunosuppressive treatment to every year in stable patients. I follow Drachman's suggestion of asking the patient to keep a diary in which one or two prominent clinical symptoms are recorded. Whenever possible, this self-testing should include a quantitative measurement such as a record of the length of time that the head can be lifted in the supine position and the length of time that the arms can be outstretched while standing.

Repeated tests for autoantibodies to AChR are needed only in patients with unexplained deterioration—in particular, when immunosuppressive drugs have been discontinued or the dose has been reduced. In my experience, rising antibody titers in immunosuppressed patients mean that the patient's condition may deteriorate after a lag phase of as long as 3 months.

TREATMENT MODALITIES

Most experts agree that patients with severe generalized myasthenia gravis should be treated vigorously with immunosuppressive drugs in combination with ChE inhibitors, and with plasmapheresis during critical deteriorations. Neither of these treatments has been studied by a prospective, double-blind, placebo-controlled trial, with the exception of cyclosporin A. The treatment of ocular MG and of the mildly or moderately affected patient is controversial. An important consideration is how much the physician and the patient expect from the treatment. In my experience, it has been possible in virtually every newly diagnosed patient to induce remission or near-remission. The only common exception is the elderly myasthenic patient with other severe disorders such as coronary artery disease, kidney failure, obstructive lung disease, strokes, and other life-threatening conditions; in these patients, treatment may improve myasthenic signs but may not result in general improvement.

I always discuss the possible outcome and the risks of treatment in great detail with the patient. Some patients prefer to have mild residual symptoms rather than to risk developing adverse reactions from immunosuppressive drugs. Most patients wish to be free of disease and to live a normal life, even if this requires having to take drugs for long periods.

Cholinesterase Inhibitors

Pharmacologic ChE inhibitors are the first-line treatment for almost all patients with symptomatic MG (Fig. 1). They enhance neuromuscular transmission by increasing effective transmitter concentrations and thus prolong the ligand (ACh)-receptor interaction. The compound most often used is pyridostigmine bromide (Mestinon), which is taken orally in 60-mg tablets. The average dose is 60 mg every 4 hours during the daytime. Action starts approximately 30 minutes after ingestion and lasts for about 4 to 6 hours, although the half-life is much longer. This regimen can be adjusted to the patient's needs. The intervals at which the drug is taken can be

shortened to every 3 hours. Timing can be adjusted such that one single dose of 60 mg is given 30 to 60 minutes before major meals. A sustained-release tablet containing 180 mg of the drug is available (Mestinon Timespan). One such tablet taken at bedtime may be given to patients with marked weakness in the early morning. The maximum dosage of ChE inhibitors usually should not exceed 90 mg every 3 hours except over the short-term. The need for a steady increase of the dose of ChE inhibitors should alert the physician to the possibility of progressive deterioration.

ChE inhibitors can precipitate asthma. Other side effects are usually limited and reversible. I have rarely seen persistent diarrhea, but when I do, I treat it with atropine (0.2 to 0.5 mg) or by diphenoxylate hydrochloride with atropine (Lomotil) once or twice daily.

When stable remission has been achieved, I recommend that ChE inhibitors be withheld for a day or two. If no symptoms of MG recur, the patient may not need the drug anymore. Patients with double vision or severe ptosis may not respond satisfactorily to any dose of ChE inhibitors.

Thymectomy

Thymectomy is always indicated in patients with thymoma and is sometimes followed by x-irradiation, depending on the tumor type.

Performing thymectomy in patients with thymic hyperplasia without thymoma is still controversial. In some centers, every patient is treated with thymectomy, and in others, only those with more severe disease who are also treated with immunosuppressive medication undergo this procedure. Even patients with pure ocular myasthenia are treated in this way at one institution. In a large clinical series, thymectomy has been shown to lead to marked improvement in roughly one-third of patients and to moderate improvement in another one-third. There is no controlled trial comparing thymectomy with immunosuppressive medication in terms of efficacy and adverse reactions.

I recommend thymectomy in conjunction with ChE inhibitors for all patients with mild MG who are between the ages of 6 and 60 years. If symptoms of MG persist for more than 3 months after thymectomy or if the patient's condition deteriorates, I discuss the possibility of immunosuppressive medication with the patient. For patients with moderate or marked MG, I recommend thymectomy only after pretreatment. For those younger than 15 years of age, this may be a short series of plasmapheresis. In older patients, I try to induce remission by immunosuppressive drugs first and have them thymectomized after reducing or stopping immunosuppression within the following 6 to 9 months. Plasmapheresis has also been used in older patients.

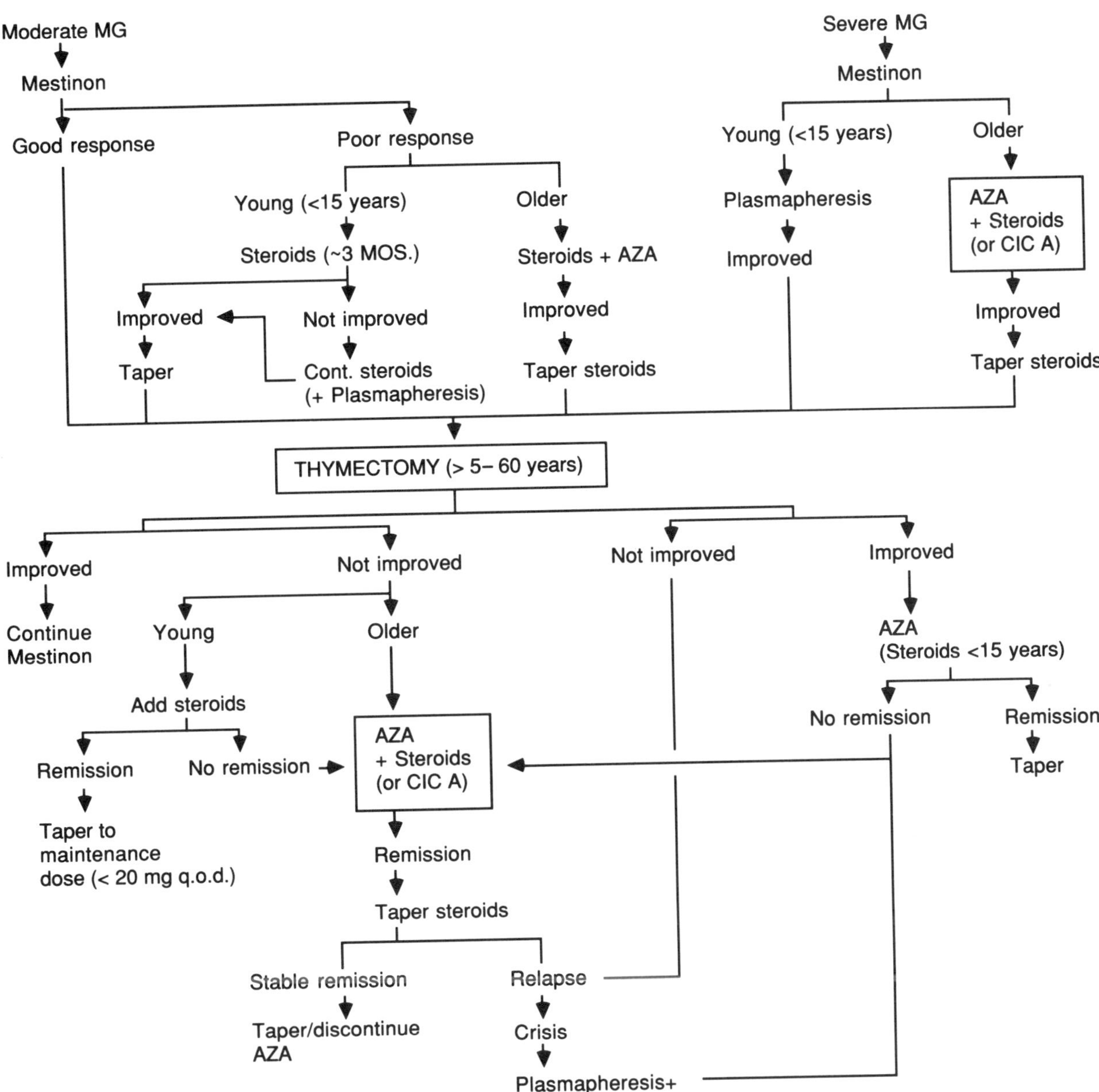

Figure 1 Steps in management of moderate and severe generalized MG. "Remission" includes near-remission; "moderate" includes at least two test items of the clinical MG score grade 2; "severe" incldues at least two test items or one vital sign (e.g., vital capacity) grade 3.

AZA=azathioprine; steroids=glucocorticosteroids; CIC A=cyclosporine.

Most experts recommend that thymectomy be performed early in the course of the disease.

The operation should be performed in a center that has experienced thoracic surgeons and a consulting neuromuscular physician available. If patients have been pretreated successfully, postoperative complications are virtually zero, as is mortality. Our patients are observed in an intensive care unit for 24 to 48 hours even though they all breathe spontaneously. Before the operation, patients are switched from oral pyridostigmine to intravenous neostigmine (Prostigmin) given via an infusion pump at 0.15 to 0.3 mg per hour. Sixty mg of pyridostigmine is roughly equivalent to 0.5 to 0.75 mg Prostigmin IV. Oral treatment can be given as soon as the patient is allowed to drink.

Immunosuppression

Before or after thymectomy, immunosuppressive drugs are now generally administered to patients not satisfactorily controlled by ChE inhibitors. In my opinion, the antimetabolite cytotoxic drug azathioprine is the first choice long-term drug for proper control of moderate, marked, and severe MG. To speed up recovery I generally give it in conjunction with corticosteroids for a few months until near-remission is achieved. Steroids are then gradually reduced and administered on alternate-day schedules until a dose of 20 mg or less every other day has been reached. In patients with stable remission or near-remission for more than 6 months, discontinuing the drug or decreasing the dose can be tried (see below). Long-term treatment with immunosuppressive drugs requires continual medical attention by physicians with experience in such treatment. Patients not followed in this way are at risk for developing potentially dangerous adverse reactions unnoted.

Corticosteroids

In patients with generalized moderate to marked MG, corticosteroids are used in conjunction with azathioprine, 60 to 100 mg per day, in a single morning dose. In young patients with mild generalized myasthenia, I occasionally use a short course of steroids alone if thymectomy has not improved myasthenic weakness satisfactorily within 3 months. Corticosteroids in high doses may transiently exacerbate myasthenic signs. Therefore Drachman has suggested slowly increasing doses of prednisone. In my experience, this is now rarely needed in the modern setting of available treatment modalities.

Steroids produce many unpleasant and serious side effects. It has been my experience that patients are reluctant to accept steroids if they know of another treatment. The most important side effects are cataracts, gastrointestinal ulcers, severe hypertension, and unusual bacterial or parasitic infections. Osteoporosis may be a problem in elderly patients even if the duration of high-dose treatment is restricted to a few months. Gastrointestinal discomfort is best dealt with by drinking skim milk during the day. I do not recommend antacids such as Maalox because they may interfere with intestinal absorption of drugs and mineral salts. A prescription of calcium gluconate, vitamin D supplements, and sodium fluoride may help prevent osteoporosis. If a patient has a history of recurrent ulcers or develops an ulcer during this treatment I now use ranitidine (Zantac). In patients with diabetes mellitus, I try to avoid administering corticosteroids and tend to administer cyclosporin A on a short-term basis instead.

Azathioprine

Azathioprine (Imuran, Imurek) is now the drug of first choice for patients with moderate and severe MG, and is used in conjunction with steroids and plasmapheresis for those in myasthenic crisis. In patients with moderate MG, I start with 3 mg per kilogram of body weight per day for several weeks and reduce this to 2.5 mg per kilogram thereafter. In patients with severe MG, one can start with 3.5 to 4 mg per kilogram and taper the dose gradually. A simple way of monitoring is to check total white blood cell (WBC) count, which should decrease to 3,500 to 4,000 per microliter. The lymphocyte count should be between 900 and 1,200 per microliter. If the WBC count is reduced to less than 3,200, the medication should be discontinued for a few days and treatment continued after it returns to more than 3,500. The long-term dose can be adjusted by checking these numbers. In patients receiving azathioprine plus steroids, the WBC count is two to three times as high and the above-mentioned counts can be used only after steroids have been discontinued. Another measure of drug effects is mean corpuscular volume of red cells (MCV), which is usually mildly elevated during long term treatment.

Adverse Reactions

In rare patients (less than 1 percent of my series), an acute idiosyncratic reaction including vomiting, fever, skin reactions, and general malaise has occurred. In this situation, the drug should be discontinued immediately. More commonly, milder gastrointestinal discomfort is reported. Splitting the dose into three divided doses, taking the drug after meals, and reducing the dose temporarily usually resolves these problems. Elevation of liver enzymes up to three times the baseline is also common and is reversible after the dose has been reduced. There is some evidence that long-term medication carries an increased risk of developing malignancies. In contrast to that of organ transplant patients, the risk seems to be very low in patients with MG. One estimated risk figure is four times the incidence compared with that of the general population. Theoretically, patients receiving azathioprine should be prone to serious infection. In my experience, however, this has rarely been a problem. Azathioprine is potentially teratogenic and mutagenic. I advise patients to use contraceptive measures during treatment and at least 6 months after its completion.

Cyclosporin A (Cyclosporine)

Cyclosporin A is the only immunosuppressive drug that has proved useful in a prospective, double-blind, placebo-controlled trial. This compound is more selective than azathioprine. It suppresses the activation and proliferation of T-helper lymphocytes. Cyclosporin A requires less time to act than azathioprine. This compound resembles corticosteroids in this regard. Because of its multiple and in part serious adverse reactions it is a third-choice drug. I use it in patients with marked or severe MG in conjunction with azathioprine when patients cannot take steroids (e.g., those with diabetes mellitus) or if azathioprine has induced idiosyncratic reactions. Whenever possible, cyclosporin A should be discontinued within the first 6 months of treatment. I do not use it in patients with a creatinine level of more than 1.5 mg per 100 ml. The starting dose is 5 mg per kilogram of bodyweight per day. This dose is corrected by measuring the trough level in whole blood or in plasma. Pharmacologic levels depend on the assay used (presently 40 to 60 ng per milliliter in plasma using a monoclonal antibody radioimmunoassay kit; one should check with a local laboratory.).

The major side effect of this drug is nephrotoxicity. This correlates with duration of treatment and with dose. If the creatinine level increases by 50 percent over baseline values or to more than 1.5 mg per 100 ml during treatment, the dose should be reduced or the drug discontinued. A more sensitive indicator is the measurement of creatinine clearance. There are many other adverse reactions, including arterial hypertension, tremor, hirsutism, and hepatic function abnormalities, which are usually reversible after cessation of treatment. The drug must be discontinued when idiosyncratic or allergic reactions develop. The risk of late malignancies is not firmly established. In patients with autoimmune disease, the risk may be similar to that carried by azathioprine.

Plasmapheresis

In therapeutic plasmapheresis, the plasma is separated from blood cells by centrifugation or, more commonly, by plasma filtration. All antibodies and other soluble factors are removed. Plasma is replaced by albumin-electrolyte solutions. Sometimes high-dose immunoglobulin G is added. Its main indication is myasthenic crisis. Less commonly it has been used for severe refractory MG and before an elective operation such as thymectomy is performed. Plasmapheresis should be carried out only in specialized centers because the number of serious adverse reactions is inversely correlated with experience. Most commonly one plasma volume is exchanged four to five times over a period of 6 to 8 days. Alternatively, one and a half plasma volumes can be exchanged three times every other day. There is practically no age limit for this treatment if the patient is in good general health. In my experience, it is only the elderly patient with multiple organ disease who carries a high risk for developing severe complications. Virtually all patients also receive combined immunosuppression with azathioprine and corticosteroids (or cyclosporin A) beginning at the time of plasma exchange. This is

done to reduce antibody rebound and to prevent relapses.

A new alternative to plasmapheresis is selective immunoadsorption by tryptophan-linked polyvinylalcohol gels. This procedure is now licensed in Europe. We have treated 15 patients with this new procedure and found its efficacy virtually identical to that of plasmapheresis. No substitution with heterologous protein solutions is required.

Myasthenic Crisis

Myasthenic crisis is a neurologic emergency, with the patient unable to swallow and breathe. Progressive deterioration of muscle strength that cannot be improved with ChE inhibitors can result in rather sudden decompensation. Therefore any patient who is having difficulty breathing or swallowing should be tested for vital capacity and swallowing immediately. If the previous dosage of medication with ChE inhibitors has not exceeded 120 mg every 3 hours, the patient may receive 0.5 mg Prostigmin IV as a bolus injection and be admitted to the hospital immediately. Ventilatory support should be available during transfer. If the vital capacity drops to less than 1.5 L in males and 1.2 L in females, intubation and assisted ventilation should be provided. If the vital capacity cannot be measured accurately, artificial respiration is needed when arterial oxygen decreases to less than 85 mm Hg and arterial carbon dioxide increases to more than 45 mm Hg. In my experience, it is now rare that patients have been treated with excessive overdoses of ChE inhibitors, which is done to cope with myasthenic weakness but which instead accelerates the critical deterioration (this was formerly called cholinergic crisis).

Often viral infections are precipitating factors of rapid deterioration. Secondary bacterial infection is common if swallowing problems lead to aspiration. Early treatment with appropriate broad-spectrum antibiotics is indicated. After the infectious organism has been identified, the antibiotic regimen can be tailored more specifically. I see no restriction for aminoglycoside antibiotics under these circumstances.

Patients with myasthenic crisis receive the same respiratory support as patients with other breathing disorders. At my institution, patients with atelectases are treated invasively by bronchoscopy. Once patients are no longer receiving ventilation, they should not be treated with breathing devices that force them to breathe against a pressure gradient, as this will lead to early fatigue of respiratory muscles.

Specific Treatment of MG

I continue to administer ChE inhibitors (Prostigmin) to patients at pharmacologic doses of 0.2 to 0.4 mg per hour because some muscle groups may still respond satisfactorily. Others have recommended a "drug holiday" during artificial respiration.

Virtually every patient in myasthenic crisis is now treated with plasmapheresis and high-dose corticosteroids (150 to 1,000 mg prednisone or methylprednisolone) for the 1st week. The use of corticosteroids is controversial in patients with bacterial infection or septicemia. I add high-dose immunoglobulin G preparations (7 S globulin, 10 to 15 g per day) and immunoglobulin M (19 S globulin, 5 to 10 g per day) to substitute for losses during plasmapheresis. Immunoglobulin G has been shown to unspecifically downregulate formation of AChR antibodies, presumably by a Fc-mediated negative feedback mechanism. With immunoadsorption, this may not be necessary. A few days later, azathioprine is added to the regimen.

CHILDHOOD MYASTHENIA

Neonatal transitory myasthenia develops in 15 percent of newborns within a few days after birth. All newborn babies have circulating AChR antibodies if the mother has them. They may develop signs of MG regardless of whether the mother is symptomatic. I advise patients to schedule delivery in a specialized center where pediatricians and neurologists have experience with this condition. When a neonate develops sucking difficulties and muscle hypotonicity, Prostigmin is given intravenously (0.02 to 0.06 mg or more). The pharmacologic response supports the diagnosis. Later, oral pyridostigmine (Mestinon) can be given at a dosage of 2 to 10 mg every 4 hours. Weakness gradually wears off over the next weeks.

Childhood Autoimmune MG

In prepubescent patients, ChE inhibitors are the first-line drug and immunosuppressive agents are given with great care. Most physicians recommend thymectomy after the patient is 5 years of age. In myasthenic crisis, plasmapheresis may be performed with preloading albumin and immunoglobulin solutions. After puberty, treatment is essentially that given to adult patients. I recommend azathioprine for older children only in exceptional cases of severe and otherwise refractory MG.

OCULAR MG

This is often a difficult diagnosis to make. Only 50 to 60 percent of patients with clinically definite ocular MG have AChR antibodies. Several clinical signs need to be present to support the diagnosis, including lid twitch, ocular quiver movements, fatigue on sustained tonic deviation, pseudointernuclear ophthalmoplegia, and unequivocal response to ChE inhibitors. In the antibody-negative patients, other orbital or retro-orbital disorders that can masquerade as myasthenia need to be ruled out. In some centers, a low-dose curare test is performed. Single-fiber electromyography may detect subclinical disease in limb muscles. The majority of patients do not respond satisfactorily to treatment with ChE inhibitors. I recommend a short course of corticosteroids, starting with 30 to 50 mg per day until remission has been achieved, and then taper this to the lowest possible maintenance dose. The indication for azathioprine and thymectomy is still controversial.

ADDITIONAL REMARKS

If elective surgery is required, the patient is treated as before thymectomy. In view of the effective treatments now available, myasthenia rarely poses a problem for the anesthesiologist and surgeon. If an emergency operation has to be performed in a patient with still marked or severe signs of MG, succinylcholine or very low doses of curare—like muscle relaxants (less than 10 percent of the regular dose)—can be used if any relaxation is required at all.

I recommend that my patients become members of the National Muscular Dystrophy Association and obtain a medical ID indicating their diagnosis and medication. Several therapeutic agents have a potential for depressing neuromuscular transmission including beta-blockers, aminoglycoside antibiotics, chinidine, procainamide, and other antiarrhythmic compounds, as well as tranquilizers. In properly treated patients with at most mild signs of MG, I have not seen any problems with these drugs. Myasthenic patients are advised to contact our institution or any other specialized center immediately if uncommon problems arise. I do not recommend that patients receiving immunosuppressive drugs take trips to Third World countries because precautions such as live vaccines are contraindicated and a neuromuscular specialist may not be available. For other trips abroad, the patient is provided with name and address of the closest specialized center.

A small subgroup of patients remains that can be called "difficult" for various medical and psychological reasons. These patients often seek advice at many specialized centers. I strongly advise these patients to authorize the physicians to exchange their medical documents and opinions before profound changes in treatment are made, particularly if signs of MG are mild or absent. A similar recommendation applies to patients who have been misdiagnosed as having MG and are receiving treatment for MG.

SUGGESTED READING

Drachman DB, ed. Myasthenia gravis: biology and treatment. Ann NY Acad Sci 1987; 505:1–909.

Heininger K. Toyka KV, Gaczkowski A, et al. Selective removal of pathogenic factors in neurologic disease. Plasma Ther Transfus Technol 1986; 7: 351–357.

Hohlfeld R, Michels M, Heininger K, et al. Azathioprine toxicity during long-term immunosuppression of generalized myasthenia gravis. Neurology 1988; 38:258–261.

Hohlfeld R, Toyka KV, Besinger U, et al. Myasthenia gravis: reactivation of clinical disease and of autoimmune factors after discontinuation of long-term azathioprine. Ann Neurol 1987; 17:238–242.

Kissel JT, Levy RJ, Mendell JR, Griggs RC. Azathioprine toxicity in neuromuscular disease. Neurology 1986; 36:35–39.

Mertens HG, Hertel C, Reuther P, Ricker K. Effect of immunosuppressive drugs (azathioprine). Ann NY Acad Sci 1981; 377:691–699.

Michels M, Hohlfeld R, Hartung H-P, et al. Myasthenia gravis: discontinuation of long-term azathioprine. Ann Neurol 1988; 24:798.

National Institute of Health. The utility of therapeutic plasmapheresis for neurologic disorders. JAMA 1986; 256: 1333–1337.

Tindall RSA Rollins JA, Phillips JT, et al. Preliminary results of a double-blind, randomized, placebo-controlled trial of cyclosporine in myasthenia gravis. N Engl J Med 1987; 316:719–724.

PATIENT RESOURCES

Myasthenia Gravis Foundation
Suite 909
53 W. Jackson Blvd.
Chicago, Illinois 60604
(Provides information.)

Muscular Dystrophy Association
710 Seventh Avenue
New York, New York 10019
Telephone: (212) 586-0808
(Provides patient services).

European Alliance of Muscular Dystrophy Associations
Association de Myopathes de France (AMS)
13, Place Rungis
F-75650 Paris Cedex 13
Telephone: (33) 145651300
(Provides names and addresses of national European associations.

ACUTE VENTILATORY FAILURE IN NEUROMUSCULAR DISEASE

CECIL O. BOREL, M.D.
MARC MALKOFF, M.D.
DANIEL F. HANLEY, M.D.

Ventilatory performance depends on effective skeletal muscle activity. Ventilatory failure is the major cause of death in patients with neuromuscular disorders. Although the extent of respiratory involvement depends on the type, distribution, and duration of neuromuscular disease, respiratory function does not directly parallel the extent of general muscle weakness. Thus, essential respiratory functions such as inspiration, cough, and airway patency must be assessed and managed specifically.

PATHOPHYSIOLOGY

Ventilation requires muscle activity for inspiration. Expiration is independent of muscle contraction because expiratory forces are generated from the recoil of the chest wall. Negative intrathoracic pressure (relative to atmospheric pressure) is generated mainly by the contraction of the intercostal muscles and the diaphragm. Gas exchange, particularly excretion of carbon dioxide, is dependent on alveolar air flow, which is a function of both minute ventilation and the ratio of dead space to tidal volume. Dead space is the portion of tidal volume necessary to fill the parts of the respiratory system not participating in gas exchange and is a fixed volume. As tidal volume decreases, the relative proportion of dead space increases relative to the decreasing alveolar ventilation, limiting the ability of the lungs to excrete carbon dioxide.

When inspiratory effort is compromised by neuromuscular disease, the initial result is an insidious loss of ability to increase minute ventilation at times of increased demand. Sepsis, fever, starvation-refeeding, and increased alveolar dead space all demand an increase in minute ventilation. As demands are increased, normal or partially impaired inspiratory musculature begins to tire as a consequence of overuse, leading to further exacerbation of ventilatory insufficiency. Tachypnea is the usual response to unfulfilled ventilatory demand. Unfortunately, tachypnea increases the proportion of dead space ventilation to tidal volume and the relative amount of time spent in inspiration. Since diaphragmatic nutrient blood flow occurs in expiration, increasing the time spent in inspiration may exacerbate the fatigue of compromised inspiratory musculature. Patients sometimes rest fatiguing inspiratory musculature by alternating patterns of breathing between weakened and accessory groups, even at the expense of decreased tidal volume and carbon dioxide excretion. In chronic neuromuscular diseases associated with hypoventilation, the normal response to hypercarbia may become blunted, allowing carbon dioxide retention. These patients may have altered ventilatory drive. Finally, the patient's ability to excrete carbon dioxide is lost, and frank ventilatory insufficiency leads to respiratory acidosis and death.

Although expiration is a passive process, resulting from the elastic recoil of the stretched chest wall and diaphragm to expel air, active forced exhalation is crucial to clear secretions and foreign objects from the respiratory tract. Weakening the muscles of forced exhalation results in an impaired ability to cough as well as some loss of diaphragmatic efficiency, with bulging of the abdomen during diaphragmatic contraction on inspiration. When cough is impaired, secretions accumulate in the most dependent portion of the lung, leading to collapse of alveoli, subsegments, and even entire lobes. Collapsed segments are not ventilated. Pulmonary vasoactive responses may decrease perfusion to the unventilated segments, but this compensation is incomplete. Oxygen in unventilated alveoli is absorbed quickly, so that further perfusion of blood through these regions cannot load oxygen. The result is dilution of oxygenated blood from ventilated alveoli with blood low in oxygen from the collapsed alveoli. This dilution process lowers the total oxygen content of arterial blood and is described as the process of intrapulmonary shunt. Retained airway secretions are fertile media for bacterial colonization and pneumonia. Infection leads to further alveolar congestion, shunting, and hypoxemia. The patient's decreased ability to cough from any form of neuromuscular disease can have profound implications for recovery from ventilatory failure. Alveolar collapse may progress to hypoxemia, tissue hypoxia, and death.

Patients with neuromuscular illness frequently complain of difficulty swallowing, chewing, or speaking. The degree of upper airway dysfunction is difficult to evaluate in the neuromuscular patient. The risks of aspiration of gastric contents and position-dependent airway obstruction are well known in neuromuscular disease patients whose laryngeal and glottic muscles have been weakened.

When these muscles are weakened, recurrent aspiration and airway obstruction to air flow become major forms of morbidity.

PATIENT ASSESSMENT AND ACUTE INTERVENTION

Ventilatory failure is the inability to maintain minute ventilation, oxygenation, or airway integrity (Table 1). Patients who meet criteria for ventilatory failure should be transferred to a critical care unit, undergo endotracheal intubation, and begin mechanical ventilation.

The inability to oxygenate is an early manifestation of ventilatory failure. Arterial blood gas determinations and pulse oximetry offer a means of monitoring oxygenation and are important assessment tools when ventilatory function is compromised. Chest x-ray studies reveal the presence of atelectasis or infiltrate, which may worsen hypoxemia. Clinical signs of hypoxemia are late indicators of ventilatory insufficiency.

Paradoxical movement of the abdomen and rib cage, use of the accessory muscles of ventilation, and an increase in the respiratory rate portend ventilatory failure due to respiratory muscle weakness. Bedside spirometry measures respiratory volumes and pressures and provides indirect measurements of respiratory muscle strength. Tidal volume, functional vital capacity, inspiratory force, and expiratory force are among the values obtained. A functional vital capacity of 10 to 15 ml per kilogram and both inspiratory force and expiratory force greater than 25 mm Hg generally correlate with adequate ventilatory strength. Daily measurements are used to track changes in respiratory muscle function.

Transdiaphragmatic pressure is a direct measure of diaphragmatic strength. A specially designed nasogastric tube with balloons in the gastric fundus and esophagus is used for the measurements and feeding. Since the diaphragm is the major inspiratory muscle, changes in transdiaphragmatic pressure correlate with changes in respiratory muscle

---

Table 1 Assessment of Ventilatory Performance in Patients with Neuromuscular Disease

Oxygenation Status
No Failure:	oxygen saturation >97% on room air, Po_2 >75, absence of atelectasis on chest x-ray film
Borderline:	oxygen saturation <98% on any supplemental O_2, Pco_2/FiO_2 <100, presence of subsegmental atelectasis
Failure:	oxygen saturation <95% on any supplemental O_2, Po_2 < 55 torr on any FiO_2, major atelectasis, or infiltrate

Ventilation: Forced Vital Capacity
No Failure:	> 15 ml/kg
Borderline:	10 ml/kg to 15 ml/kg
Failure:	<10 ml/kg—ventilatory muscle

Airway Integrity
No Failure:	Eats and drinks normally, no difficulty articulating
Borderline:	Cannot handle fluids well but can manage with oral suction; noticeable speech impairment
Failure:	Obstruction of airway in certain positions, intermittent aspiration of secretions

performance. During weaning, the critical diaphragmatic strength, defined as the ratio of transdiaphragmatic pressure of an average breath to the maximal transdiaphragmatic pressure, declines. Fatigue is likely to occur when the value of this ratio approaches 0.40.

Ventilatory drive must be assessed in all patients. Some patients with neuromuscular disease have been shown to have altered responses to hypercapnia. The altered responses do not corrlecate closely with static pressures and other indirect measures of respiratory strength. Hypercapnia is worse at night but can be corrected with voluntary hyperventilation. Although some patients have complaints of daytime somnolence and early morning headaches, many are asymptomatic. Pressure generated by airway occlusion for 100 msec (P100) has been suggested to reflect central ventilatory output. This measurement, however, is dependent upon respiratory muscle (especially diaphragmatic) strength. The fraction of time in inspiration to the total time of breathing is less dependent upon strength and also reflects ventilatory drive.

Airway integrity depends on the adequacy of the gag and cough reflexes. A small sip of water may be used as a bedside assessment of swallowing capability. The inability to maintain airway integrity leads to airway obstruction and aspiration from pooled secretions.

MEDICAL MANAGEMENT

Medical management involves treatment of underlying lung pathology, infection, malnutrition, and correction of electrolyte abnormalities.

Reducing the work of ventilation assists the weaning process. Since increased work of breathing is a major factor in ventilatory failure when parenchymal lung disease is present, decreasing airway resistance and minimizing the extraneous work of breathing improve ventilartory ability. Pneumonia increases respiratory work by reducing lung compliance (forcing the inspiratory muscles to develop more force to generate the same tidal volume).

The treatment of any infection assists the weanning process in several ways. Infection induces a catabolic state. Nitrogen wasting occurs from all skeletal muscles, including the diaphragm. Muscles compensate by reducing the number of sarcomeres, leading to loss of strength and increased fatigability. The catabolic state produces a rise in carbon dioxide production, which also requires an increase in minute ventilation. Finally, the catabolism of infection limits the efficient use of nutrients.

Nutritional support is important in maintaining muscle strength and structure. The changes described in muscle during infection also occur during starvation. Autopsy studies show a reduction in diaphragmatic mass that correlates with body weight. Maintaining adequate nitrogen intake corrects and reverses this process. Routine measurements of 24-hour urinary nitrogen excretion are useful in adjusting protein intake to account for nitrogen utilization. Both commercial and modular enteral feeding preparations will achieve a positive nitrogen balance. If enteral delivery of protein is not tolerated or is insufficient, we use parenteral nturition to satisfy nutrient requirements.

Electrolyte imbalance and deficiency states can also contribute to muscle weakness and weaning difficulties. Hypophosphatemia is a common problem in nutritionally depleted patients and a well-documented cause of reversible muscle weakness. Hypomagnesemia has also been reported to cause mild respiratory weakness. Although iron and potassium depletion have not been reported to cause diaphragmatic weakness, they have been reported to cause limb muscle weakness. Routine monitoring and supplementation avoid these problems.

We attempt to augment normal respiratory drive. Sedatives and narcotics are decreased as much as possible. Abnormalities of blood pH are corrected, especially metabolic alkalosis, because the compensatory respiratory acidosis is achieved by hypoventilation. We correct metabolic alkalosis by replacing chloride and removing bicarbonate and acetate from intravenous and nutritional fluids. If this is unsuccessful, volume expansion with chloride and diuresis with acetazolamide are used to induce mild metabolic acidosis. In order to avoid compensation for either hyper- or hypocarbia, normocapnia is maintained by appropriate minute ventilation.

THERAPY OF NEUROMUSCULAR DISEASE

Plasma Exchange

Patients with myasthenia gravis who are difficult to wean from mechanical ventilation benefit from plasma exchange. Preoperative plasma exchange in patients with severe myasthenia gravis undergoing thymectomy reduces the need for postoperative mechanical ventilation, decreases time to extubation, and decreases the length of stay in intensive care. Plasma exchange decreases the time of mechanical ventilation when used early in the course of patients with Guillain-Barré syndrome. Plasma exchange therapy is now routinely used to treat patients with these neuromuscular diseases who require ventilatory support.

Myasthenic Crisis

Rapid deterioration of neuromuscular and respiratory functions may occur as a result of infection, stress, or overdose with anticholinesterase drugs. Endotracheal intubation and mechanical ventilatory support are often required before the cause of myasthenic crisis can be determined and treated. Although crisis may be the result of inadequate anticholinesterase therapy, satisfactory recovery is not often acheived by increasing the dose of these drugs. Instead, anticholinesterase drugs should be decreased after ventilatory support is initiated to avoid contributing to cholinergic side effects. These side effects are also characterized by respiratory and bulbar muscle weakness, excessive salivation, and abdominal cramps. Atropine or glycopyrrolate ameliorates the vagal symptoms rapidly, but muscular strength returns slowly as the anticholinesterase drug is metabolized. Plasma exchange effectively increases muscle strength, facilitates weaning from mechanical ventilation, and allows reintroduction of anticholinesterases at lower dosages after cholinergic crisis.

MANAGING MECHANICAL VENTILATION

Weaning involves strategies designed to decrease and discontinue ventilatory support. The decision to begin the weaning process depends on assessments of respiratory drive and muscle strength.

Respiratory muscle fatigue is often a problem during this period. Nocturnal rest, allowing sleep and recovery, may be used throughout weaning. Diaphragmatic and accessory muscle training with appropriate rest periods is also helpful in increasing respiratory muscle strength. Aminophylline has been reported to increase diaphragmatic strength and endurance, but at present we reserve this drug for patients with concurrent reactive airway problems.

We use both pressure support ventilation (PSV) and intermittent mandatory ventilation (IMV) modes of respiratory support. Weaning failures are usually related to fatigue and not to method of support. Consequently, we withdraw ventilatory support from either mode in proportion to the return of ventilatory performance. The patient is rested if clinical signs of fatigue or carbon dioxide retention are encountered.

In patients with an intact respiratory drive, we prefer the pressure support mode of ventilatory assistance. The ventilatory assistance is adjusted to an inspiratory pressure that supports a respiratory rate of less than 25 breaths per minute and a tidal volume of greater than 5 ml per kilogram. The "triggering" pressure for assisted breaths should be easily attained, ranging between 2 and 6 cm H_2O. Increasing pressure support can be used to ease tachypnea, increase tidal volume, and reduce the resistance of the airway circuit to the patient. We usually add 5 cm H_2O or more of positive end-expiratory pressure (PEEP) and sighs to prevent atelectasis. Arterial blood gases are monitored as needed. If arterial access is limited, pulse oximetry and end-tidal carbon dioxide monitors may suffice.

Once the patient becomes stable on the above regimen, we wean by reducing the pressure support 2 to 5 mm Hg and observing respiratory rate and tidal volume. We follow similar parameters to assess the need for rest periods. Pressure support is raised 2 to 10 mm Hg to allow rest and encourage sleep. Atelectasis is treated by a combination of chest physical therapy, increased PEEP, and increased pressure support. When a pressure support of 5 cm H_2O is tolerated well, the patient no longer needs ventilartory assistance. We have found that this method is well tolerated by patients. It allows for inspiratory muscle training continuously by encouraging inspiratory muscle effort. The major problems with this method are inability to trigger breaths due to weakness, changes in lung compliance, and ventilatory drive dysfunction.

IMV is an important mode of ventilatory support and may be used in conjunction with PSV. Patients who lack sufficient ventilatory drive need this mode of mechanical ventilatory support. We wean IMV support by gradually decreasing the daytime rate and allowing nocturnal rest. Normocarbia is maintained. End-expiratory pressure is generally set at 5 cm H_2O and adjusted as clinically indicated by degree of atelectasis, shunting, or arterial hypoxemia. Pressure support may be added to overcome the resistance of the airway circuit during spontaneous breathing. We generally wean the IMV rate to less than 4 breaths per minute before weaning pressure support. Strict IMV weaning suffers from two disadvantages. First, patients may "buck" the volume-cycled breaths, raising peak airway pressures and risking barotrauma and patient discomfort, or the unassisted breaths may be inefficient and rapidly lead to ventilatory muscle fatigue. Second, unassisted breaths require a high inspiratory force to overcome airway resistance and trigger the ventilator's demand valve.

When the patient is breathing easily on a pressure support of 5 mm Hg or an IMV rate of 2 breaths per minute or less, we attempt a trial of T-piece ventilation. A continuous positive airway pressure valve of 2.5 to 7.5 cm may be added to maintain expiratory lung volumes and prevent atelectasis. Repsiratory rate and clinical signs of respiratory distress are used as indicators of success or failure. Arterial blood gas measurements or pulse oximetry and end-tidal carbon dioxide are monitored. We generally monitor patients for signs of respiratory distress for at least 24 hours after the discontinuation of mechanical ventilation.

LONG-TERM AIRWAY MANAGEMENT

We prefer to proceed to tracheostomy when we believe the patient will need ventilation or airway protection for longer than 30 days. Tracheostomy offers advantages in allowing easier pulmonary toilet, negative pressure ventilation, and avoidance of risk of long-term endotracheal intubation. Pitt (TM Mallincrodt Co) speaking tracheostomy tubes facilitate speech without increasing the risk of aspiration. Cuffed tracheostomy tubes are used to prevent aspiration. We reserve uncuffed tubes for those patients who require long-term tracheostomy, such as patients requiring negative pressure ventilation or long-term pulmonary toilet who have little risk of aspiration.

Secretion management requires airway suctioning, coughing, and deep breathing. We add bronchial lavage with either saline or bicarbonate if secretions are tenacious. We reserve postural chest percussion and drainage for patients with infiltrates or atelectasis and who appear to clear more secretions after treatment. We have also used "prophylactic" percussion and intermittent positive-pressure breathing in selected patients who appear to need prolonged pulmonary toilet. We believe that two or three sessions of percussion daily may be effective in clearing secretions from infiltrates.

The ability to manage secretions is required before the artificial airway can be removed. Artificial airway devices should be removed in a controlled environment. Endotracheal tubes are removed by personnel experienced in intubation techniques. The trachea and pharynx are suctioned. Then the cuff is deflated. The tube is quickly removed, and the patient is encouraged to cough. We use a similar process to remove cuffed tracheostomy tubes. The risks of removal of these devices include aspiration, laryngospasm, and tracheal collapse from secondary tracheomalacia.

SUGGESTED READING

MacIntyre N. Respiratory function during pressure support ventilation. Chest 1986; 89:667–683.
Newsome Davis J, Loh L. Alveolar hypoventilation and respiratory muscle weakness. Bull Eur Physiopathol Respir 1979; 15:45–51.
Rochester DF. Malnutrition and the respiratory muscles. Clin Chest Med 1986; 7:91–99.
Sporn PHS, Morganroth ML. Discontinuation of mechanical ventilation. Clin Chest Med 1988; 9:113–126.
Tobin MJ. Respiratory muscles in disease. Clin Chest Med 1988; 9:263–286.

LAMBERT-EATON MYASTHENIC SYNDROME

DONALD B. SANDERS, M.D.

The Lambert-Eaton myasthenic syndrome (LEMS) is a rare condition, frequently associated with cancer of the lung. It probably occurs more frequently than is recognized, since the diagnosis may not be made unless the appropriate electrodiagnostic tests are performed on the population at risk.

In 1953, Anderson and colleagues reported abnormal neuromuscular transmission in a 47-year-old man with oat cell carcinoma of the lung. The patient had primarily proximal muscle weakness with reduced tendon stretch reflexes. He had prolonged apnea following surgery during which succinylcholine was given, and he was later shown to be abnormally sensitive to the effects of curare and decamethonium. There was some improvement in strength after the administration of edrophonium and oral neostigmine. This patient demonstrates many of the features now known to be characteristic of LEMS.

In 1957, Eaton and Lambert described the clinical and electrodiagnostic features of the syndrome that now bears their names. In 1968, Elmqvist and Lambert reported that the microphysiology of LEMS studied in intercostal muscle biopsy differed from that of myasthenia gravis (MG).

CLINICAL FEATURES

LEMS usually begins in later life, although it has been reported in children. Males and females are equally affected, and about half the patients have a malignancy when the disease begins or develop cancer later. Weakness is the major symptom and the proximal muscles are predominantly affected, especially in the legs. Oropharyngeal and ocular muscles may be mildly affected but not to the degree seen in MG. On examination, the weakness is usually relatively mild, and in some patients strength may improve initially after exercise and then weaken with sustained activity. Edrophonium (Tensilon) or neostigmine (Prostigmin) may produce improvement in strength, but this is rarely as dramatic as in MG. Tendon reflexes are reduced or absent but can frequently be brought out or increased by activity of the appropriate muscles or by tapping the tendon repeatedly. Dry mouth is a frequent symptom, resulting from autonomic dysfunction. Other manifestations of autonomic dysfunction include impotence in males and hypotension in occasional patients.

In many patients, LEMS is discovered when prolonged paralysis follows the use of neuromuscular blocking agents during surgery. Clinical worsening has been described following administration of aminoglycoside antibiotics, magnesium, calcium channel blockers, and iodinated intravenous contrast agents.

Although LEMS is similar to MG in many ways, the clinical presentations of the two conditions are usually quite distinct. The weakness in LEMS is rarely life-threatening, and in most cases the differential diagnosis would include cachexia, polymyositis, or other paraneoplastic neuromuscular disease. In some patients, clinical and electrodiagnostic features overlap with those of MG. When acetylcholine-receptor antibodies are elevated or lung cancer is present, the distinction between these two diseases is clear, but in other patients the response to treatment and the ultimate course of the disease may determine the diagnosis. Since both diseases respond to many of the same treatments, the ultimate diagnosis may be moot in patients with mixed features.

About half the patients with LEMS have an underlying malignancy, and in 80 percent of cases this is a small cell carcinoma of the lung. The cancer may be discovered years before or after the symptoms of LEMS begin.

ELECTRODIAGNOSIS

The diagnosis of LEMS may be confirmed by demonstrating characteristic findings on electromyographic studies: the size of the compound muscle action potential recorded with surface electrodes is low and falls further with repetitive stimulation of the nerve at frequencies between 1 and 5 Hz. During stimulation at frequencies from 20 to 50 Hz, the compound muscle action potential increases in size and becomes at least twice the size of the initial response. Brief maximal voluntary contraction of the muscle also is followed by a transient increase in the compound muscle action potential size. These findings are not present in all muscles in all patients with LEMS and may occasionally be seen in patients with MG; thus the electromyogram does not distinguish between these two conditions in all patients.

PATHOPHYSIOLOGY

Intracellular recordings demonstrate that there is a presynaptic abnormality of acetylcholine release at the neuromuscular junction in LEMS. In most if not all patients, LEMS probably results from an autoimmune process directed against calcium channels on the nerve terminal.

TREATMENT

Before treatment is begun, MG must be excluded. If acetylcholine receptor antibodies are present in the serum, the patient should be treated as having MG no matter what the clinical or electromyographic findings. When the diagnosis of LEMS has been confirmed, an extensive search for underlying malignancy should be carried out, including especially x-ray studies and computed tomographic scan of the chest. If any findings are suspicious, bronchoscopy should be performed. Initial treatment should be directed toward any tumor present, since the weakness may improve with effective cancer therapy and, in some patients, no further treatment may be necessary for the LEMS. If no tumor is found, the search for an occult malignancy should be repeated periodically, the frequency of these evaluations being determined by the patient's cancer risk factors.

In most patients with LEMS, the weakness is relatively mild and does not affect vital muscles to the degree that MG does. In patients with cancer, LEMS is usually not the major therapeutic concern, nor does it represent the major threat to life. In patients with LEMS who do not have cancer, aggressive treatment of LEMS is more readily justified.

No one treatment approach is suitable for all patients with LEMS. Therapy must be tailored to the individual, based on the severity of weakness, underlying disease(s), life expectancy, and response to previous treatment. The treatment plan that follows may serve as a general guide but should be modified as indicated by the specific situation (Fig. 1).

Cholinesterase inhibitors do not usually produce significant improvement in LEMS, although they may provide dramatic relief from weakness and autonomic symptoms in occasional patients. Pyridostigmine (Mestinon) (30 or 60 mg every 6 hours) is the preferred drug and should be given to all patients with LEMS for several days to determine how much benefit, if any, it produces.

The *aminopyridines* improve neuromuscular transmission by facilitating the release of acetylcholine from the motor nerve terminal. 4-Aminopyridine produces marked improvement in strength in LEMS, but therapeutic doses produce seizures and central nervous system hyperactivity. 3,4-Diaminopyridine has even greater effects on the neuromuscular junction and also reverses the autonomic dysfunction in LEMS. This drug does not enter the central nervous system as readily as 4-aminopyridine, and side effects are minimal at therapeutic levels. 3,4-diaminopyridine is given orally in doses of 5 to 15 mg, three to four times daily. The effects are markedly augmented by the concurrent administration of pyridostigmine. Some patients find that the best response occurs when 30 to 60 mg of pyridostigmine are taken 30 minutes after each dose of 3,4-diaminopyridine. Side effects are usually negligible, consisting of transient perioral and digital paresthesias after doses higher than 10 to 15 mg. Seizures have been produced by doses of 100 mg per

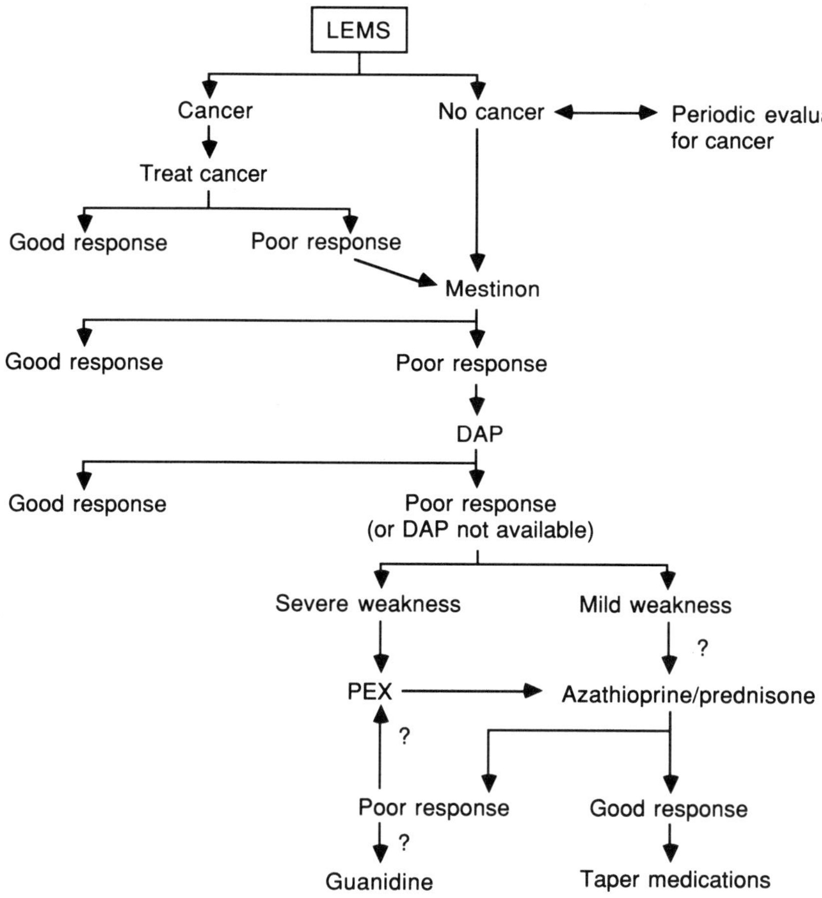

Figure 1 An approach to the treatment of LEMS. DAP = 3,4-diaminopyridine; PEX = plasma exchange.

day, and asthma attacks may be induced in patients with asthma. Gastrointestinal hyperactivity, with cramps and diarrhea, may occur when 3,4-diaminopyridine is taken with pyridostigmine and can be minimized by reducing the dose of the latter. 3,4-Diaminopyridine promises to be a safe and effective treatment for LEMS but is not yet available for general clinical use in the United States. Clinical trials of this drug are currently being carried out at several institutions in this country.

If pyridostigmine is not effective and the patient has relatively mild weakness, it must be determined whether aggressive immunotherapy is justified. If so, azathioprine or prednisone (or prednisolone) may be given, alone or in combination. I begin azathioprine at 50 mg per day and increase the dose 50 mg per day every 3 days to a total dose of 150 to 200 mg per day. A complete blood count and a liver function test should be performed once a week for the first month, then once a month for 6 months after beginning azathioprine and every 3 months thereafter as long as the patient takes this medication. About 25 percent of patients have some sort of untoward reaction to azathioprine, but in most this can

be managed without discontinuing the drug altogether. If hepatic dysfunction occurs, the dose should be reduced by 50 or 100 mg per day and liver function monitored weekly until normal. If liver dysfunction persists, the dose should be reduced further or the drug discontinued. After several weeks, the dose may be increased again by 25 or 50 mg per day, without recurrence of liver dysfunction in most patients. If the white blood cell count falls below 4,000 per mm^3 and demonstrates a trend to continue falling, the dose should be reduced by 50 mg per day, every week until this count if stable. If the white blood cell count falls below 3,000 per mm^3, azathioprine should be withheld until the count rises above 4000 per mm^3; it then should be recommenced at a dose lower than that given before the count fell and thereafter slowly increased. Most patients develop a mild macrocytic anemia when azathioprine is given at effective therapeutic doses, but this alone does not require treatment or adjustment of the dose. If a dose of 150 mg per day cannot be tolerated despite these maneuvers, azathioprine is not likely to be of benefit, and alternative therapy should be considered. About 10 percent of patients develop a skin eruption or serum-sickness syndrome (fever, prostration) after beginning azathioprine, in which case the drug must be discontinued.

Prednisone (or prednisolone) should be given in high daily doses initially (60 to 80 mg per day) until improvement is seen; then the dose should be changed to 100 to 120 mg every other day to minimize side effects. The dose should then be tapered over many weeks or months to the lowest level that maintains the improvement. The rate at which the dose is tapered is determined by the risk of side effects. All patients develop some side effects if a high dose of prednisone is given long enough. Weight gain, a cushingoid appearance, hypertension, diabetes, cataracts, and osteoporosis are the major complications seen with this treatment. These effects are reversible as the dose is reduced and become minimal at doses less than 20 mg of prednisone every other day. However, if the dose is reduced rapidly, weakness recurs. Prednisone may be given with azathioprine if either is not effective alone. It may take several weeks for benefit to become apparent and months to achieve maximal benefit. If azathioprine and prednisone are given together, it may be possible to reduce and ultimately discontinue prednisone after maximal improvement has occurred.

Plasma exchange may also produce striking improvement in some patients with LEMS, although the results are usually not as marked as in MG. Unless the patient is also receiving immunosuppressive agents, the improvement induced by plasma exchange is temporary. When weakness is severe, plasma exchange may be used initially and prednisone and/or azathioprine added after improvement begins. As in MG, intermittent courses of plasma exchange may be necessary to maintain improvement in some patients. One course of plasma exchange consists of 6 to 9 exchanges, depending on the patient's response. At each exchange, we remove one plasma volume (55 m per kilogram body weight), up to a maximum of 3 L. The plasma volume removed is replaced with lactated Ringer's solution containing approximately 200 ml of 25 percent albumin solution per 1,000 ml, and exchanges are performed three times a week.

Guanidine has a mechanism of action similar to that of 3,4-diaminopyridine, increasing the release of acetylcholine and producing temporary improvement in strength. Unfortunately, this drug frequently produces severe side effects, and I consider using it only as a last resort in patients with severe weakness who have failed to respond satisfactorily to all the above approaches. Guanidine is given orally, beginning at a dose of 5 to 10 mg per kilogram per day, divided throughout the waking hours. The dose may be increased to a maximum of 50 mg per kilogram per day, depending on the clinical response. Dose increases should be made no more frequently than every 3 days, since the maximal response to a given dose may not be seen for 2 to 3 days. Side effects are frequent and include bone marrow depression, renal tubular acidosis, chronic interstitial nephritis, cardiac arrhythmia, hepatic toxicity, pancreatic dysfunction, peripheral paresthesias, ataxia, confusion, and alterations of mood. Deaths attributable to the drug have been reported. Frequent blood tests of hematologic, hepatic, and renal functions must be performed as long as patients are taking guanidine. In all patients, the demonstrated beneficial response to treatment with this drug must constantly be balanced against the risk of the treatment.

MEDICATIONS/SITUATIONS TO AVOID

Any drug that impairs neuromuscular transmission may exacerbate the weakness in LEMS (Table 1). It is not uncommon for patients with the disease to come to clinical attention when prolonged weakness or apnea follows administration of neuromuscular blocking agents during anesthesia. Aminoglycoside antibiotics and antiarrhythmics are also common offenders. These medications should be given with caution, and only if there is no suitable alternative. There are isolated reports of LEMS becoming worse after administration of a number of drugs, including magnesium and intravenous iodinated radiographic contrast agents. In general, any new medication should be given to patients with LEMS with caution. Whenever there is a deterioration in clinical status in such a patient, you should determine if a new medication was recently begun. To assure that medical personnel are aware of these possible effects, I affix a drug alert card to the front of the medical record of my patients with MG and LEMS (Table 1).

Table 1 Drug Alert Notice to Be Affixed to the Medical Record

The following drugs produce worsening of weakness in most patients with abnormal neuromuscular transmission. They should be used only if absolutely necessary, and such patients should be monitored closely for any exacerbation of symptoms:

Succinylcholine or D-tubocurarine (or equivalent)
Quinine, quinidine, or procainamide (Pronestyl, Procan)
Aminoglycoside antibiotics, especially gentamicin, kanamycin, neomycin, or streptomycin
Propanolol (Inderal)
Timolol eyedrops (Timoptic)

Many other drugs have been reported to exacerbate the weakness in some patients. Therefore, whenever any new medication is begun, the patient should be observed closely for worsening of symptoms.

The weakness of LEMS may be worse when the ambient temperature is elevated or when the patient is febrile. Patients should avoid hot showers or baths. Systemic illness of any sort may cause transient worsening of weakness in patients with LEMS.

SUGGESTED READING

Henriksson KG, Nilsson O, Rosen I, Schiller HH. Clinical, neurophysiological and morphological findings in Eaton Lambert syndrome. Acta Neurol Scand 1977; 56:117–140.

Ingram DA, Schwartz MS, Traub M, et al. Cancer-associated myasthenic (Eaton-Lambert) syndrome: Distribution of abnormality and effect of treatment. J Neurol Neurosurg Psychiatry 1984; 47:806–812.

Jenkyn LR, Brooks PL, Forcier RJ, et al. Remission of the Lambert-Eaton syndrome and small cell anaplastic carcinoma of the lung induced by chemotherapy and radiotherapy. 1980; Cancer 46:1123–1127.

Lundh H, Nilsson O, Rosen I. Novel drug of choice in Eaton-Lambert syndrome. J Neurol Neurosurg Psychiatry 1983; 46:684–687.

Newsom-Davis J, Murray NMF. Plasma exchange and immunosuppressive drug treatment in the Lambert-Eaton myasthenic syndrome. Neurology 1984; 34:480–485.

O'Neill JH, Murray NM, Newsom-Davis J. The Lambert-Eaton myasthenic syndrome. A review of 50 cases. Brain 1988; 111:577–596.

PATIENT RESOURCES

Research, patient care clinics, and information about nerve and muscle diseases, inluding LEMS.

The Muscular Dystrophy Association of America
810 Seventh Avenue
New York, NY 10019

Information about local chapters and neuromuscular transmission disorders, including LEMS.

The Myasthenia Gravis Foundation
Suite 909 53 W. Jackson Boulevard
Chicago, IL 60604

MUSCULAR DYSTROPHY

ALLEN D. ROSES, M.D.

DUCHENNE'S MUSCULAR DYSTROPHY

Duchenne's muscular dystrophy (DMD) offers one of the major clinical treatment problems to clinicians seeing patients with neuromuscular diseases. Because it affects approximately 1 in 3,000 live male births, it is a relatively common genetic disease. Together with the childhood spinal muscular atrophies, DMD represents the most severe and relentlessly progressive of the crippling neuromuscular diseases. There is no cure and no treatment currently available to stop the progression of the disease. There are, however, palliative measures that can significantly alter the comfort and functional abilities of the patients. The major advances to date are in the areas of disease prevention through accurate carrier detection, genetic counseling, and programs of prenatal diagnosis.

Symptomatic Treatment

During the initial years after a patient is diagnosed, there is little intervention that can or should be done other than a program of passive exercises, including stretching of the Achilles tendon and extension of the ileotibial band. Once the patient is recognized as having DMD, provisions should be made at home and at school for his integration into normal patterns of activity for as long as possible. The family should be counseled concerning the need to treat their son as much like any other child as they can, since these are the most normal years that he will experience.

A popular misconception is that there is no treatment at all for DMD. As in so many other diseases that are terminal and relentless, there is much that can be done for the patient to prolong useful function. As the patient is periodically followed, a stage is reached when walking becomes more difficult, and this sometimes appears as a balance problem associated with a shift of the center of gravity. It is at this time that clinicians should be aware of the effect on gait that hip, knee, and/or ankle contractures may be having. As long as useful muscle strength is still present at the joints, consultation with an experienced orthopedic surgeon can be most useful. Frequently contracture release procedures that do not put the patient to bed for days can be performed at this time. The result is often months and up to several years of useful ambulation. Eventually ambulation is limited by muscle strength rather than awkwardly enforced postures due to contractures. Tendon releases can be performed a second or third time when contractures limit ambulation or interfere with the use of lightweight braces in order to prolong the time the patient may remain in the upright position.

Later, when the patient relies on a wheelchair, other therapeutic concerns become quite important.

Two objectives during this period are proper wheelchair fitting and posture alignment to try to avoid the development of scoliosis. Surgical treatment of scoliosis should be considered at this time if it has begun to develop. The posture of DMD patients in wheelchairs is relatively easy to assess but can be difficult to manage. Some simple manipulations can be most helpful. Fitting the chair with a table top so that the patient can perform certain functions in front of him and lean forward symmetrically may help to produce an antero-posterior kyphosis. Kyphosis is a preferred posture, since scoliosis inevitably inhibits breathing and may compromise cardiovascular functioning. Later in the course of the disease scoliosis can have serious deleterious effects on the positioning of bedridden patients. Care in the wheelchair fit and attention to the posture of the patients when they first need the chair and thereafter can avoid later severe difficulties that can significantly affect pulmonary function.

Scoliosis can make the patient's life miserable, complicating his ability to function in the wheelchair. Orthopedic surgical procedures have been developed in recent years that are associated with shorter postoperative hospitalizations. In the hands of surgeons experienced in scoliosis surgery of patients with DMD, significant functional, respiratory, and cardiovascular benefits can be achieved.

Genetic Counseling

The range of diagnoses associated with problems with dystrophin, the molecule at the site of the genetic defect in DMD, is expanding to include less severe diseases. New treatment protocols involving myoblast transplantation are being piloted in order to determine whether function can be maintained or restored by adding cells able to make dystrophin the affected tissue. These and other attempts to normalize the expression of muscle in DMD may change therapy options dramatically.

Fewer than 5 percent of DMD carriers have significant weakness and a late occurring myopathy. The significant burden on possible carriers is the uncertainty of their genetic status and the decision not to have children afflicted with DMD. With the discovery of the gene for DMD, it is now possible to diagnose many DMD carriers with 100 percent accuracy (deletion analysis) and many others with 98 to 99 percent accuracy (linkage analysis). Although the social and economic machinery has yet to catch up to the scientific capabilities, prevention of DMD in families known to be at risk is possible. In our clinic, which is associated with a molecular genetic research laboratory, we make every effort to ascertain and offer testing to all at-risk females. The therapeutic benefit of a woman's knowing her genetic status and being able to plan her reproductive choices is a major triumph for clinical medicine,

resulting in the birth of many normal males who would have previously been aborted.

In the simplest case, the affected male is tested with specific fragments of the dystrophin cDNA in order to document a deletion of part of the gene. With careful testing, more than 50 percent (approximately 68 percent in our clinic) of affected males show a deletion. Using this information, the family of the affected male can be tested to determine whether at-risk females carry the deletion on one of their X chromosomes. When a woman carrying a deletion becomes pregnant, determination of a male fetus at the time of chorionic villus biopsy (8 to 9 weeks) no longer automatically leads to the decision of abortion. If the male fetus carries the deletion, he is affected; if the cDNA probe detects no deletion; a normal male is diagnosed. Thus, many more male babies have populated family trees of DMD patients than had been the case during the previous 20 years. It is not yet well documented, but clinics involved in these determinations seem to be seeing a greater proportion of normal as opposed to affected male fetuses, possibly because of very early fetal wastage.

Third-party insurance carriers and disease-oriented service agencies have not yet come to terms with the support of genetic testing that can prevent the disease. Many families pay for these tests themselves. In our clinic, local families who cannot afford testing are supported by assistance from the Duke Hospital Women's Auxiliary.

In more complicated cases when a deletion of the affected male cannot be documented, a series of polymorphic DNA markers can be used to determine grandmaternal or grandpaternal chromosomes. Tracking of the chromosome type that went to the affected male allows accurate approximations to be made concerning carrier and fetal status. Thus, in DMD families accurate carrier diagnosis is frequently possible, altering the perception and acceptance of the carrier state dramatically.

MYOTONIC MUSCULAR DYSTROPHY (DM)

DM is the most common inherited neuromuscular disease affecting both adults and children. Of all the diseases affecting humans, DM exhibits the most variable expressivity and age of onset. It is apparent in large pedigrees that elderly individuals can carry the gene and transmit it to their progeny without having any diagnostic phenotypic expression, yet in the same family there can be instances of congenital DM. The basis for this variability is still unknown, but heterozygotes can therefore be affected in any of the organ systems at any age. Other than myotonia and weakness of skeletal muscle, the most significant clinical problems are those associated with cardiac dysfunction, personality problems, sleep disorders, and cataracts.

Symptomatic Treatment

Myotonia of DM is seldom severe and usually requires no treatment. At some point in their disease, some patients may have symptomatic myotonia of their hands or jaw muscles, but unlike in congenital myotonia, treatment with phenytoin, procainamide, or quinidine is rarely necessary. As the disease progresses, myotonia is less symptomatic. There is no treatment for the slow, progressive dystrophy of skeletal muscle, but it should be recognized that crippling dystrophy affects only a minority of gene carriers. As a rule, the younger the age of onset of myotonia and dystrophy, the more likely that symptomatic weakness will develop. The time frame of progressive weakness is 2 to 4 decades. A patient presenting with teenage myotonia and weakness may be expected to remain ambulatory into middle age; a patient with presentation of symptoms in the thirties can be expected to remain ambulatory into the fifties or beyond.

The initial pattern of weakness that requires treatment usually involves extension of the foot. Use of lightweight orthotics can significantly improve ambulation for many years. A small minority of the total gene carriers mapped in large pedigrees (probably less than 10 percent) eventually exhibit muscular weakness severe enough to require a wheelchair.

By far the most common problem associated with DM is the personality characteristics. Heterozygotes are often indifferent but can be hostile, reticent, suspicious, mildly retarded, and/or exhibit a remarkable stubbornness. Frequently the socioeconomic status of heterozygotes within a sibship is significantly lower than nonaffected siblings as a result of their difficult personalities. Recent psychological studies have suggested that DM may be a genetic model for sociopathic personality disorder. Frequently heterozygotes exhibit hypersomnolence and may sleep up to 20 hours per day; patients with these symptoms may rarely leave their homes. If such patients are not employed, their withdrawal from society may not be diagnosed or understood. From a medical point of view, my appreciation of the extent of this problem has resulted from home visits for genetic studies, since these patients rarely make or keep clinic appointments. When hypersomnolence becomes a problem for an affected individual who is employed, treatment with melthylphenidate (Ritalin) or dextroamphetamine (Dexedrine) may be helpful. In some cases, imipramine or amitryptyline has provided some effective relief, although there is no rationale for the use of either drug in this situation.

The most serious manifestations of the disease are the cardiac complications. During genetic studies of large family trees, it becomes obvious that sudden death at any age in patients without previous heart disease is a real phenomenon. I have become aware of numerous cases of sudden death of high school athletes in members of DM pedigrees who were undiagnosed at the time of death. The cause of death often is undocumented, but cardiac conduction abnormalities have been demonstrated to be progressive once they are found. I have followed patients over 2 decades and documented electrocardiographic progression from first-degree heart block to complete heart block. Since bradycardia is often present, complete heart block in DM often results in a rate less than 30 beats per minute with syncope. This may well be a mechanism of sudden death in some patients.

As a rule electrocardiograms (ECGs) are obtained in all heterozygotes in a family, whether or not symptoms are present. Individuals with first-degree heart block are followed at 6-month intervals and later at 1-year intervals if they are stable for several years. If the block becomes more prolonged at follow-up or a more severe rhythm disturbance develops, additional studies are warranted. We have performed serial His–ventricular conduction studies in such patients and documented the prolongation of conduction to a delay time requiring cardiac pacemaker implantation. Over the years, there have been several patients whose demand pacemakers have become activated and, when they were evaluated under cardiology laboratory conductions, they were found to have idioventricular rates that were not compatible with maintaining consciousness. Periodic ECGs should therefore be performed on cooperative gene carriers whether or not any symptoms of DM are present. I have seen complete heart block start with prolonged conduction time at age 8 and at age 57 progressing to death at 15 and to pacemaker implantation at age 62, respectively. I have no doubt that cardiac conduction problems expressed at any age and can be recognized by follow-up studies. However, the first symptom may be sudden death.

Genetic Counseling

Genetic testing by linkage techniques is available for DM families. It is interesting that the most frequent use of linkage markers for diagnostic purposes is by siblings of affected individuals for their own diagnosis, usually when they are interested in starting families. Some of these individuals are pre-symptomatic heterozygotes with no phenotypic expression; others are normal. Both benefit from genetic testing. Heterozygotes can elect prenatal diagnostic testing, whereas the normal individuals can go on to have families without risk of DM. Multiple tightly linked probes are available and, with the cooperation of other family members, particularly those known to be affected with DM, 99 percent accurate diagnosis is often possible. The use of these tests by known affected individuals is far less than that of patients known to have other genetic family traits, such as Huntington's disease, DMD, or cystic fibrosis. The lack of interest in or concern for transmission of the disease probably reflects the peculiar personality disorder associated with DM.

OTHER MUSCULAR DYSTROPHIES

Treatment of other muscular dystrophies, such as the autosomal dominant or autosomal recessive limb-girdle dystrophies, the facioscapulohumeral dystrophies, scapuloperoneal dystrophy, and other rare forms of disease is symptomatic. These diseases rarely progress at a rate as rapid as DMD, and most of the treatment principles are developed from those used to treat DMD.

Two rare forms of muscular dystrophy deserve separate mention—oculopharyngeal muscular dystrophy and humeroperoneal muscular dystrophy (Emery-Dreifuss disease). The dangers associated with each can be serious and are frequently a result of lack of recognition of the disease. Oculopharyngeal muscular dystrophy is a rare progressive disease that is inherited as an autosomal dominant trait and is frequently confused with myasthenia gravis. It begins with ptosis and eye movement signs and involves the swallowing function. Aspiration leading to choking and/or pulmonary complications is common in this rare disease. The use of feeding tubes or a feeding gastrostomy may become necessary in severe cases. I have followed one patient for many years who functions well by using a feeding tube several times a day for nourishment; he still enjoys chewing and tasting "real food," although it is necessary for him to spit it out because he cannot safely swallow it.

Recognition of the problem is important. One of my patients was thought to have myasthenia gravis and had been treated with acetylcholinesterase inhibitors. She developed increased secretions because of the side effects of high doses of ineffective drugs, which led to severe aspiration pneumonitis. Conversely, I have seen several patients with myasthenia gravis with early ocular and dysphagic symptoms who developed a disfiguring lower facial "dystrophy" associated with a fixed snarl as well as speech and swallowing problems. Without a positive family history for the disorder, the diagnosis of oculopharyngeal dystrophy may lead to delay of proper and effective treatment of myasthenia gravis. One patient who was believed to have oculopharyngeal dystrophy had progression of her speech and swallowing difficulties over several years. In 1978, when antiacetylcholine receptor tests became available, we entertained the diagnosis of myasthenia gravis for this patient despite lack of electromyographic support (single-fiber electromyography was not yet available). The patient underwent a thymectomy and was found to have a hyperplastic thymus. Progression of her disease stopped, and marked improvement of her ocular and swallowing functions occurred over time. There was some improvement in her facial movement. Plastic surgery was later performed to correct the fixed snarl. She has done well for a decade without other medications.

Emery-Dreifuss disease is an X-linked recessive muscular dystrophy that manifests with weakness and wasting involving the scapulohumeroperoneal distribution. Contractures at the elbow, the back of the neck, and the Achilles tendon are common. Patients may develop a life-threatening cardiac arrhthymia, particularly atrioventricular block. Complete heart block can develop, and fatal "heart attacks" at a relatively young age are common in family histories. The cardiac conduction abnormalities can develop before muscular signs and symptoms become obvious and at any time thereafter. It is therefore important to periodically screen the ECGs of individuals at risk. Pacemaker implantation is effective and should be performed early, since the conduction abnormalities are progressive. Demand cardiac pacemakers prevent sudden cardiac death and allow many years of functional activity to patients whose muscular symptoms may be obvious but not crippling. Recognition of the diagnosis provides the rationale for lifetime cardiac monitoring for a treatable arrhthymia.

SUGGESTED READING

Bregman AM. Living with progressive childhood illness: Parental management of neuromuscular disease.Soc Work Health Care 1980; 5:387.

Brooke MH. A clinician's view of neuromuscular diseases. 2nd ed., Baltimore: Williams & Wilkins, 1986.

Emery AEH. Duchenne muscular dystrophy. Oxford: Oxford University Press, 1987: 156–163.

Moorman JR, Coleman RE, Packer DL, et al. Cardiac involvement in myotonic muscular dystrophy. Medicine 1985; 64: 371–387.

Siegel IM, Plastic molded knee-ankle-foot orthosis in the management of Duchenne muscular dystrophy. Arch Phys Med Rehabil 1975; 56:322.

PATIENT RESOURCE

The Muscular Dystrophy Association maintains an outpatient clinic network spread throughout the United States. There are clinics in large medical centers with extensive resources as well as smaller clinics staffed by knowledgable physicians. The Muscular Dystrophy Association periodically rewrites information pamplets for patients and families concerning a wide range of neuromuscular diseases.

Muscular Dystrophy Association
810 Seventh Avenue,
New York, New York 10019
Telephone: (212) 586-0808.

POLYMYOSITIS

RUP TANDAN, M.D., M.R.C.P.

Polymyositis (PM) and dermatomyositis (DM) are nonsuppurative inflammatory myopathies in which the muscle damage is immune-mediated. In DM, there is an associated skin rash over the face, hands, and sometimes elsewhere. About one-third of all cases of inflammatory myopathy constitute pure PM, another third are pure DM, one-fifth of patients have PM or DM with associated connective tissue disease (such as scleroderma or rheumatoid arthritis), 10 percent of patients have childhood DM with vasculitis, and about 10 percent have DM or PM in association with a neoplasm.

CLINICAL FEATURES

In adult patients, evaluation usually reveals weakness and tenderness of limb-girdle muscles, weakness of neck flexor and trunk muscles, typical skin rash (in DM cases only), and features of associated collagen vascular disease where this is the case. Reflexes are usually well preserved and often brisk. Extraocular muscles are unaffected. In childhood DM cases, there is often associated vasculitis. DM in patients over the age of 60 has a high association with underlying neoplasm, usually of the lung, breast, ovary, intestinal tract, or hemopoietic tissue.

Although the diagnosis of DM is not difficult because of the characteristic skin rash, clinically PM has to be distinguished from other causes of the limb-girdle syndrome, such as the muscular dystrophies (myotonic, facioscapulo-humeral, and Becker's muscular dystrophy), spinal muscular atrophies, metabolic myopathies, and endocrine myopathies.

LABORATORY EVALUATION

Hematologic, biochemical, electrophysiologic, and histologic studies confirm the clinical suspicion of an inflammatory myopathy. The erythrocyte sedimentation rate is moderately elevated in about two-thirds of patients, but other hematologic indices are normal. Serum levels of muscle enzymes are usually elevated, with a decreasing sensitivity of creatine kinase, aldolase, glutamic oxaloacetic transaminase, lactic acid dehydrogenase, and glutamic pyruvate transaminase. Rheumatoid factor and antinuclear antibodies in high titer are seen in about one-third of cases, particularly in patients with PM or DM with associated connective tissue disease.

There is some indication to suggest that serum myoglobin estimation more closely parallels the extent of muscle damage and recovery than do muscle enzyme levels.

Electromyography should be performed, as results are abnormal in almost half the patients with inflammatory muscle disease. It reveals increased insertional activity (irritability), fibrillations, and positive sharp waves in addition to myopathic motor unit potentials of low amplitude and increased polyphasia that recruits easily. These changes are usually more pronounced in the proximal limb muscles, but in some patients electromyographic abnormalities are more revealing or only present in the paraspinal muscles.

Muscle biopsies in inflammatory myopathy show the typical pathologic features in about two-thirds of patients. It is important not to perform biopsy on muscles that have recently been subjected to electromyography or used for intramuscular injections, because inflammatory changes and muscle fiber damage can be produced by needle insertion. It is also important to select muscles for biopsy that are clinically moderately weak, as the histology of profoundly weak muscles may only reveal end stage nondiagnostic changes, whereas the histologic appearance of muscles with near-normal strength may be normal. Moreover, since the pathologic process in inflammatory muscle disease is patchy not only between muscles but also within a single muscle, it is advisable to biopsy two clinically affected muscles (deltoid or biceps *and* one of the vastus muscles). The diagnostic yield is also improved by serially sectioning the biopsy specimen and by taking a sufficiently large piece of muscle for adequate study. Some investigators have used computer-assisted tomographic scanning, magnetic resonance imaging, isotope scintigraphy, or ultrasonography of muscle in the hope of identifying lesions prior to biopsy so as to improve the diagnostic yield. However, experience with these procedures is limited. In my opinion, careful selection of clinically affected muscles, a biopsy from two sites, and serial sectioning of muscle usually suffice for documenting the features of inflammatory myopathy.

The histology of PM/DM is characterized by inflammatory cell infiltration in the endomysium and perimysium, consisting of lymphocytes, plasma cells, and macrophages. The infiltrating cells are activated T lymphocytes, both of the helper-inducer and cytotoxic-suppressor types, which are accompanied by macrophages in PM and B cells in DM. Muscle fiber necrosis, phagocytosis, and regeneration are frequently seen. Prominent perifascicular atrophy, vasculitis, endothelial cell necrosis, and capillary loss are characteristic of childhood DM but may be seen in adult DM and PM. Although muscle fiber atrophy is frequent, especially of type 2 fibers, hypertrophy rarely occurs. Patients who have limitation of movement because of muscle pain and particularly those on steroid therapy show prominent type 2 fiber atrophy. The muscle biopsy also helps to diagnose inclusion body myositis and eosinophilic myositis, conditions that are often difficult to differentiate from PM clinically. In inclusion body myositis, characterisitc rimmed vacuoles with basophilic granules are seen in hematoxylin and eosin-stained cryostat sections in fibers of both types, and these contain typical membranous osmiophilic whorls. Intramuscular or intracytoplasmic tubulofilamentous inclusions in some instances resembling the nucleocapsids of paramyxoviruses confirm the diagnosis. Eosinophilic myositis shows the appearances of a myositis but with an inflammatory infiltrate consisting predominantly of eosinophils.

SEARCH FOR UNDERLYING MALIGNANCY IN ADULT DERMATOMYOSITIS PATIENTS

Adult patients with DM have a higher probability of harboring an underlying neoplasm, and thus physicians should be alert for this association. A thorough clinical examination (including rectal and breast examination), chest x-ray film, sputum analysis for cytologic study urinalysis, stool guaiac testing for occult blood, and a hemogram are usually sufficient to diagnose most neoplasms. Further directed radiologic investigation is only indicated in the presence of specific symptoms and signs. An undirected investigative approach, with costly radiologic procedures, is usually unrewarding and is unwarranted.

TREATMENT OF INFLAMMATORY MYOPATHIES

Several studies in the last two decades have shown that treatment of moderately severe or severe PM or DM initially with daily glucocorticoid therapy is beneficial in the majority of cases. After appropriate investigations and confirmation of the diagnosis, treatment with 60 to 100 mg per day of oral prednisone, which can be given in divided doses, should be initiated. Improvement in strength usually begins within 2 to 4 weeks, although this may be delayed for up to 3 months in some patients and is accompanied by a decrease in creative kinase and erythrocyle sedimentation rate. Patients with childhood DM and acute or subacute adult PM/DM improve more rapidly than those with chronic PM. With improvement in the clinical condition, the daily dose of prednisone is reduced by 5 mg every 2 to 4 weeks until it comes down to 40 mg daily. The patient's progress is best monitored by clinical muscle strength grading or by following muscle torque with a dynamometer and by serial sedimentation rate and serum creative kinase estimations. Patients who show no improvement in strength before 3 to 6 months of high-dose, daily prednisone therapy need constant and regular follow-up and encouragement. With continued improvement, further reduction in the dose of prednisone can be made either by changing to 80 mg on alternative days and tapering by 5 mg every 2 weeks, or by reducing the alternate-day dose of prednisone (ie, 40 mg one day and 35 mg the next day for 2 weeks, then 40 mg one day and 30 mg the other day for 2 weeks, and so on. Patients who are mildly affected may benefit from the use of alternate-day prednisone from the very outset, with an effect almost as good as with daily dosing but with the advantage of a decreased incidence of side effects. The dose of prednisone should be reduced until either it is discontinued or clinical or biochemical signs of a relapse appear. If a relapse occurs, the dose of prednisone should be increased until the disease activity is again controlled.

The use of daily high-dose prednisone carries the risk of side effects for which patients need to be closely monitored. Some of these include weight gain, cushingoid appearance, exacerbation or precipitation of a diabetic state or hypertension, upper gastrointestinal distress or bleeding from a peptic ulcer, hypokalemia, aseptic necrosis of the femoral head, atrophy of the skin, and increased susceptibility to infections. Therefore the patient's blood pressure, weight, serum electrolytes, and glucose level should be closely followed during treatment with high-dose prednisone. Use of regular antacids with meals or histadine receptor antagonists (cimetidine or ranitidine) protect the upper gastrointestinal mucosa from ulceration and bleeding. Supplementation with calcium, 0.5 g per day, and vitamin D, 50,000 U weekly, minimizes osteopenia. Potassium replacement is necessary in patients receiving high-dose corticosteriods, especially because hypokalemia can itself produce weakness and thus delay recovery. The use of antihypertensive therapy is required in some patients.

In patients whose disease does not respond to treatment with high-dose prednisone for 3 to 6 months, the risks of continued high-dose therapy with corticosteroids almost always outweigh the benefits. In this instance and in those patients in whom the response to corticosteroids is inadequate, the addition of an immunosuppressive agent is usually beneficial. Personal experience suggests that patients with severe or long-standing disease benefit more if therapy with prednisone and immunosuppressive agents is initially instituted simultaneously. We have found azathioprine, 2.5 to 3.5 mgs per kilogram body weight daily in divided doses, to be helpful as additional therapy in such patients. Cyclophosphamide, cyclosporin A, and other alternative immunosuppressive agents can be used. We reserve the use of methotrexate (5 to 40 mg weekly) for young patients, particularly females, because of its relative safety from gonadal suppression and genotoxic effects, which are produced by azathioprine and cyclophosphamide. The aim of immunosuppressive therapy with azathioprine or cyclophosphamide is to decrease the absolute lymphocyte count to between 700 and 800 cells per mm^3 while maintaining the hemoglobin above 12 g per deciliter, the total white blood cell count above 3,000 cells per mm^3, and the platelet count above 125,000 per cubic millimeter. Methotrexate is effective at doses that do not produce lymphopenia.

Weekly complete blood counts initially are necessary to monitor cytotoxic therapy in patients in order to establish a safe and effective dose, but later counts can be done at intervals of 2 to 4 weeks. Apart from bone marrow suppression, alopecia, gastrointestinal dysfunction, and damage to the testes and ovaries produced by immunosuppressive agents, azathioprine is also hepatotoxic, cyclophosphamide may produce hematuria as a result of hemorrhagic cystitis, and methotrexate may produce liver fibrosis. Thus, liver function tests and urine analysis are necessary, where appropriate, in order to recognize toxicity early. The occurrence of liver fibrosis in patients taking methotrexate can be minimized by weekly single-dose intravenous therapy or intermittent oral therapy. An increased incidence of internal malignancy, most commonly of the lymphopoietic system, is a rare hazard of immunosuppressive therapy.

Treatment with prednisone alone or in combination with immunosuppressive agents may have to be continued for several years in some patients, but a yearly attempt to withdraw therapy must be made, particularly in patients who are stable, in order to see if the disease is still active. Eventually about 75 percent of patients can discontinue therapy, although active disease continues in the remainder for more than 5 years.

Steroid-induced myopathy can occur in patients on high-dose prednisone therapy, making it difficult to differentiate from ongoing active disease. Clinical deterioration in a patient on high-dose long-term prednisone, without an increase in the serum creative kinase level, should raise suspicion of steroid-induced myopathy. Often the diagnosis can be confirmed clinically by reducing the dose of prednisone; if the muscle weakness and serum creative kinase level increase, this suggests continuing or active inflammatory muscle disease, but if the muscle weakness decreases, this suggests a steroid-induced myopathy. The diagnosis of steroid-induced myopathy is further supported by a normal creative kinase level, absence of features of muscle membrane irritability on electromyogram and lack of inflammatory infiltration but considerable type 2 fiber atrophy in a muscle biopsy specimen. Thus, some patients who pose this diagnostic problem may require an additional muscle biopsy to help resolve the issue. Nevertheless, steroid myopathy and active PM/DM may coexist, but this therapeutic dilemma can be best resolved by decreasing the dose of prednisone and adding or increasing the dose of immunosuppressive agent.

Lack of or diminished effect of therapy in inflammatory muscle disease is most commonly due to an inadequate dose of corticosteroids or to rapid dose reduction to a low level. Inclusion body myositis and eosinophilic myositis usually show a less favorable response to corticosteroids than do PM and DM. Relapse of the weakness can also occur with a rapid taper of the drug, requiring return to the next higher level dose. Serum creative kinase levels are useful in following patients on treatment during reduction of the dose of prednisone, since a rise in level usually suggests an incipient relapse. These relapses are often more difficult to treat than the original disease presentation. Patients with PM/DM associated with collagen vascular diseases are usually more disabled at diagnosis and consequently show a less favorable outcome. Paraneoplastic DM usually responds to corticosteriods and may be "cured" if the tumor is removed.

The role of physical therapy in the management of patients with inflammatory muscle disease is vital in preserving range of movement, maintaining muscle strength, and preventing the development of contractures without jeopardizing muscle fiber regeneration. During the acute phase with severe inflammatory disease, passive range of motion should be carried out two or three times daily to prevent soft tissue contractures. During recovery, when the inflammation is less severe, slow-paced activity should be encouraged and occupational therapy should be initiated to help patients in the activities of daily living.

PROGNOSIS IN THE INFLAMMATORY MYOPATHIES

Most patients with inflammatory myopathy improve on prednisone alone or in combination with immunosuppressive agents. Many patients recover full function, although mild, nondisabling weakness of the limb-girdle muscles may remain. About 50 percent of patients recover within 5 years and can discontinue therapy; about 30 percent have inactive disease but with residual muscle weakness; and about 20 percent require continued treatment with persistence of the disease. The prognosis, in general, is worse in adults, blacks, patients severely affected at initial presentation, patients with PM/DM and associated malignancy, and patients with significant dysphagia that predisposes to aspiration pneumonia.

The overall 5-year survival rate is about 75 percent and even higher in childhood cases. Even though recent therapeutic approaches have undoubtedly improved the outcome, the mortality in PM/DM is still about four times that in the general population. Death is usually from pulmonary, renal, or cardiac complications. Although the morbidity and mortality from PM/DM and the therapy employed to treat these diseases are significant, it is generally believed that these diseases are treatable and in many cases can be cured. It is thus imperative to diagnose and treat them early and vigorously.

SUGGESTED READING

Bradley WG, Tandan R. Inflammatory diseases of muscle. In: Kelley WN, Harris ED, Ruddy S, Sledge CB, eds. Textbook of rheumatology 3rd ed. Philadelphia: WB Saunders, 1989: pp 1263–1287.
Bunch TW. Prednisone and azathioprine for polymyositis: Long-term follow-up. Arthritis Rheum 1981; 24:45–48.
Herrikson KG, Sandstedt P. Polymyositis—treatment and prognosis. A study of 107 patients. Acta Neurol Scand 1982; 65: 280–300.
Hochberg MC, Feldman D, Stevens MB. Adult onset polymyositis/dermatomyositis—an analysis of clinical and laboratory features and survival in 76 patients with a review of the literature. Semin Arthritis Rheum 1986; 15:168–178.
Uchino, M, Araki S, Yoshida O, et al. High single-dose alternate day corticosteroid regimen in treatment of polymyositis. J Neurol 1985; 232:175–178.

PATIENT RESOURCES

Muscular Dystrophy Association
810 Seventh Avenue
New York, New York 10019

Patient services offered include the following:
Orthopedic aids (braces, crutches, splints, walkers, wheelchairs)
Aids for daily living (grab bars, shower and bathtub seats, raised toilet seats)
Influenza inoculations
Transportation
Education and accessibility
Community resources

PERIODIC PARALYSIS

THERA P. LINKS, M.D.
HANS J.G.H. OOSTERHUIS, M.D., Ph.D.

Patients suffering from periodic paralysis have attacks of transient flaccid weakness of the extremities and trunk muscles. These attacks vary in intensity and duration. In severe attacks, the tongue and throat muscles may be involved and rarely the respiratory muscles; the eye muscles are never affected. During the attacks, muscle fibers become inexcitable to either direct or indirect stimulation. Serum potassium levels usually change in relation to the attacks; the classification in Table 1 is based on this phenomenon.

The molecular base of the membrane inexcitability in the different types of periodic paralysis is unknown, as is the exact mechanism of any of the treatment modalities used (except for the correction of serum potassium levels).

If a positive family history is known to the patient or to the physician, the diagnosis of a familial hypokalemic (less frequently hyperkalemic) periodic paralysis is easily confirmed by measuring serum potassium levels. In the absence of a family history, other diagnoses may be considered if a first episode of flaccid limb muscle weakness has occurred (Table 2). In general, these conditions have a more insidious onset than the periodic paralysis and they are accompanied by other signs and symptoms. The secondary forms of hypokalemic paralysis can be surmised if the patient's history reveals the use of laxatives or diuretics or gastrointestinal disturbances.

HYPOKALEMIC PERIODIC PARALYSIS

In this disorder, paralytic attacks begin in the first or second decade of life, increase in frequency during early adult life, and become less frequent or

Table 1 Classification of the Periodic Paralyses*

Hypokalemic Periodic Paralysis
Primary:
familial
sporadic
Secondary:
to urinary and/or gastrointestinal potassium loss (laxatives, diuretics)
to intoxication by barium salts
Hyperkalemic Periodic Paralysis
Primary:
familial
sporadic
Secondary:
to renal or adrenal insufficiency to diuretics
Paramyotonia Congenita
Serum potassium level during attacks is variable
Thyrotoxic Periodic Paralysis
Serum potassium level during attacks is normal or low

*In normokalemic periodic paralysis, the appearance is based on description of some kinships. The clinical value of this entity is not yet clear.

Table 2 Differential Diagnosis of Acute Limb Muscle Weakness (Without Sensory Signs) Not Including the Periodic Paralyses.

	History	*Clinical Picture*
Paralysis from tick bite	Tick bite	First weakness of the legs, later of the arms and the bulbar (respiratory) muscles
Paralysis from snake bite	Snake bite	First weakness of the ocular and bulbar muscles and weakness in the region of the bite, later of respiratory muscles
Paroxysmal myoglobinuria (Meyer-Betz)	Occasionally familial	Malaise, fever, vomiting, muscle pain, limb paralysis, elevated creatine kinase level, myoglobinuria
Rhabdomyolysis	Various conditions, e.g., trauma, drug abuse, excessive exertion	Dependent on various conditions; myoglobinuria, creatine kinase level elevated
Myasthenia gravis	Fever, provocation by medication, e.g., intravenous benzodiazepines	Limb muscles, eye muscles, and bulbar muscles are affected
Poliomyelitis (seldom coxsackie or echoviruses)	Fever, meningeal irritation	Weakness usually asymmetric
Botulism	Consumption of suspicious food	Ocular, bulbar weakness, autonomous signs
Conversion	History of acute emotion?	Reflexes preserved

cease after the fifth decade. Men are affected more seriously and more frequently than women. If untreated, these attacks may last from half a day to 7 days; very rarely, respiratory paralysis or cardiac arrhythmias lead to death. Hypokalemic periodic paralysis typically occurs as a dominant autosomal disease, although sporadic cases may occur. A permanent myopathy is not unusual in older patients, even in those who do not experience attacks. In an affected family, the present and *future* patients can be identified by a reduced muscle fiber conduction velocity.

Preventive Therapy

In patients with hypokalemic periodic paralysis, some changes in lifestyle can prevent paralytic attacks. These individuals have to restrict their daily carbohydrate and sugar intake and avoid heavy carbohydrate meals, especially in the evening. They also have to avoid exposure to cold and over-exertion. Some patients can prevent an attack that would be precipitated by excercise or a heavy carbohydrate meal by taking a late evening dose of 20 to 40 mEq potassium chloride. Sometimes an incipient attack can be prevented by mild exercise; the patient can "walk off" the attack. In our personal experience, some patients can diminish their problem by eating fruit (an orange contains about 4 mEq potassium per 100 g). Theraputic agents and/or medications include (1) *carbonic anhydrase inhibitors,* (2) *potassium-sparing diuretics,* (3) *beta blockers,* and (4) *potassium salts* (Table 3).

Carbonic Anhydrase Inhibitors

Acetazolamide. Acetazolamide, a carbonic anhydrase inhibitor, is the most useful and common drug in preventing attacks of hypolcalemic periodic paralysis. It may also increase the muscle strength and decrease the muscle stiffness in patients with weakness unrelated to attacks and not caused by permanent myopathy. Whether long-term treatment with acetazolamide reduces or prevents permanent late-onset myopathy is unknown. The way in which this agent is effective is still unclear. Acetazolamide inhibits the reabsorption of sodium, potassium, and

Table 3 Preventive Treatment in the Periodic Paralyses

Hypokalemic periodic paralysis
Acetazolamide 3 × 125 mg (max 1,200 mg)
Dichlorophenamide 2 × 50 mg (max 150 mg)
Potassium salts 15–50 mEq
Amiloride 2 × 5 mg (max 20 mg)
Triamterene 3 × 50 mg (max 200 mg)
Spironolactone 2 × 25 mg (max 100 mg)
Propranolol 2 × 40 mg (max 240 mg)
Hyperkalemic periodic paralysis
Acetazolamide 3 × 125 mg (max 1,200 mg)
Chlorothiazide 250 mg (max 500 mg)
Hydrochlorothiazide 25 mg (max 100 mg)
Hyperkalemic periodic paralysis with Myotonia
Tocainide 3 × 400 mg
Paramyotonia congenita
Tocainide 3 × 400 mg
Thyrotoxic periodic paralysis
Propranolol 3 × 20–40 mg

bicarbonate ions in the renal tubules, which results in a significant potassium loss in the urine. A mild metabolic acidosis occurs in most patients, which may be the mechanism of action. Its possible influence on the glucose-insulin metabolism and consequently on stabilizing the muscle membrane is another unclarified hypothesis.

A starting dose of 125 mg acetazolamide two to three times a day is preferred (in children half this dose is needed). The first effects on the frequency of attacks can be shown after 1 or 2 days, but an increase in the interictal strength takes place over a longer period (7 to 14 days). If the expected beneficial effect does not appear, the dosage can be increased 125 mg per dose up to a maximal daily dose of 1,000 to 1,200 mg. If a single dose is increased, the late evening dose is preferred, followed by the morning dose.

The most common side effects are paresthesias, dysgeusia, fatigue, and the formation of renal calculi. The paresthesias appear in the fingers, toes, and around the mouth, especially during transition from cold to warm temperatures, with a duration of some minutes. Most of the side effects decrease in severity after weeks of use. The risk of formation of renal calculi (family history of stones) makes it necessary to advise an adequate daily fluid intake.

Dichlorophenamide. This agent is another carbonic anhydrase inhibitor, with an inhibitory action of the enzyme 30 times greater than that of acetazolamide. Because of the induction of chloride excretion in the urine, this agent does not change the plasma pH; therefore the mechanism of action is even more puzzling.

The starting dose is 50 mg twice a day, with an increase to 50 mg 3 times a day if there is only a partial effect. If there is no response at this dosage, the medication should be discontinued. Side effects are the same as those for acetazolamide. Although the carbonic anhydrase inhibitors are the drugs of choice, in some cases it can be useful to have some alternatives, although in the treatment of hypokalemic periodic paralysis efficacy varies from patient to patient.

Potassium-Sparing Diuretics

The effect of potassium-sparing diuretics is possibly caused by a contribution to a permanent rise in plasma potassium level, which may be protective against a paralytic attack. Hyperkalemia can occur with or without using potassium salts, especially in older patients with impaired renal function; therefore regular control of electrolytes, blood urea nitrogen, and serum creatinine concentrations is necessary.

Amiloride. Amiloride directly interferes with tubular electrolyte transport, especially in the distal tubules. It should be given twice daily, 5 mg, increasing until a maximal daily dose of 20 mg is reached. Side effects include gastrointestinal disturbances, rashes, and disturbances of renal function (the last especially when it is administered in combination with nonsteroid, anti-inflammatory drugs).

Triamterene. Triamterene directly interferes with tubular electrolyte transport, especially in the distal renal tubules. The dosage is 50 mg, three times daily. If necessary, it is possible to increase to a maximal dose of 200 mg daily. Side effects are the same as those for amiloride.

Spironolactone. Spironolactone, an antagonist of aldosterone, acts in the distal renal tubules, decreasing the sodium reabsorption and sparing potassium. The specific drug regimen is 25 mg twice a day; if necessary it can be increased to 25 mg three times daily. The total dose should not exceed 100 mg. Side effects are gynecomastia, impotence, menstrual irregularities, gastrointestinal symptoms, and rashes.

Beta Blockers

Some case reports show a beneficial effect of beta blockers in reducing paralytic attacks. This effect could be ascribed to the inhibition of the activation of the sodium-potassium pump by catecholamines, which prevent a net shift of potassium to the intracellular space.

With propranolol, a nonselective beta blocker, 40 mg is given two or three times a day. If necessary, the dose can be doubled. Side effects include bronchospasm, bradycardia, hypotension, and cold and cyanotic extremities.

Potassium Salts

Potassium salts are widely used by patients with paralytic attacks. Although the intracellular shift of the potassium ions during an attack is not prevented, most likely the supply of extra potassium keeps the muscle membrane excitable. Based on our personal experience, potassium salts are only a supplemental therapy. Acetazolamide is still the drug of choice. However, some patients practically stay free of attacks while taking only potassium salts, in doses varying from 40 to 50 mEq divided over one day or only 15 mEq when symptoms are present.

Therapy of Acute Attacks

If total paralysis of the extremities is present without difficulties in deglutition or respiration, oral sips of potassium chloride solution can be given, 15 to 30 mEq (in children 10 to 14 mEq) over 30- to 60-minute intervals (the release from potassium chloride tablets is too slow). Often a patient will have taken several of these doses at home. (In patients using potassium-sparing diuretics or with renal function disturbances, serum potassium levels may rise rapidly after oral administration of potassium chloride.) If no improvement appears after four or five oral doses or if nausea or diarrhea accompanies the oral potassium chloride intake, intravenous administration is necessary. This also is preferable in patients with acute attacks of paralysis, difficulties in swallowing, and impaired respiration. In this situation, serial measurement of potassium and continued electrocardiographic monitoring are necessary. When using a peripheral vein, the concentration of the potassium chloride should not exceed 40 mEq per liter. Five percent mannitol is the preferred diluent; saline (0.9 percent) may be used, but not glucose. Infusion must be continued until the serum potassium level is normal and the patient's strength returns. Several hours of observation are necessary, during which potassium and muscle strength should be measured because sometimes the paralysis will return.

Patients with periodic paralysis who undergo surgery in which general anesthesia is required can develop paralytic attacks after the operation. Perioperative complications have not been reported. The anesthesiologist should use saline instead of 5 percent glucose, should prevent a decrease in the patient's temperature, and should monitor the patient for a longer period than usual.

HYPERKALEMIC PERIODIC PARALYSIS

This disease is transmitted as an autosomal dominant agent with high penetrance in both sexes. Attacks begin in the first or second decade and are often brief (10 to 20 minutes) but sometimes can last up to several days. Myotonic and nonmyotonic forms of hyperkalemic periodic paralysis can be distinguished. Myotonia can occur in the face, tongue and finger extensor and thenar muscles between attacks.

Preventive Therapy

The frequency of paralytic attacks can be lowered by many small meals of high carbohydrate content and avoidance of fasting. Exposure to cold and overexertion should also be avoided.

Drug treatment includes (1) acetazolamide, (2) thiazide diuretics, and (3) tocainide (see Table 3).

Acetazolamide. As in the hypokalemic form, of periodic paralysis, this drug has been found to be the most effective treatment. Its mechanism of action in hyperkalemic periodic paralysis can possibly be ascribed to the kaliuresis. However, because it is not the most effective kaliuretic diuretic, some other mechanism may play a role. Often patients with hyperkalemic periodic paralysis require a lower dose than those with hypokalemic periodic paralysis, but

paresthesias occur more frequently in the former group.

Thiazide Diuretics. These drugs are also effective in hyperkalemic periodic paralysis probably because of the effect of kaliuresis. Specific drug regimens include chlorothiazide, 250 mg daily, or hydrochlorothiazide, 25 mg daily (children 6 months and older should receive chlorothiazide 20 mg per kilogram and hydrochlorothiazide 2 mg per kilogram daily, in two equal doses, but should not exceed the adult dosage). The lowest dose of diuretic required should be used. The serum potassium concentration should not fall below 3.7 mEq per liter.

Side effects include increased fasting blood glucose and uric acid levels, hypokalemia, hyponatremia, hypercalcemia, and occasionally blood dyscrasias.

Tocainide. Tocainide is an antiarrhythmic drug that blocks sodium channels and is useful in treating myotonic hyperkalemic periodic paralysis and in preventing the weakness and myotonia in paramyotonia congenita. It does not prevent hyperkalemic weakness. A dose of 400 mg 3 times daily is used. Side effects include gastrointestinal effects, blood dyscrasias, rash, and fever.

Acute Attacks

Acute attacks of weakness are often so brief that no treatment is necessary. Prompt ingestion of carbohydrates containing beverages at the first onset of weakness usually aborts the attack. Intravenous glucose is necessary only for prolonged and serious weakness. Sometimes a combination of oral glucose 1 to 2 g per kilogram with 10 to 20 U insulin subcutaneously is helpful. Paralytic attacks also respond favorably to beta-adrenergic agents. The mechanism of action may involve a beta-adrenergic–mediated increase of potassium transport via the sodium potassium pump. Case reports have appeared about the effective use of salbutamol (inhalation of 200 to 400 μg every 15 minutes) and metaproterenol (inhalations of 1.3 mg every 15 minutes for three doses. Calcium gluconate 0.5 to 2.0 g given intravenously has terminated attacks in some cases but has not been effective in others.

PARAMYOTONIA CONGENITA

This rare condition has an autosomal dominant inheritance and is characterized by myotonia and periods of weakness, both of which are provoked by exposure to cold and to a lesser degree by prior exercise. The onset is in childhood. Serum potassium levels may be elevated but also may be normal or even decreased.

Tocainide may reduce the myotonia and weakness (see Hyperkalemic Periodic Paralysis). Potassium-sparing diuretics can be useful in preventing paralytic attacks (see Hypokalemic Periodic Paralysis and Table 3).

THYROTOXIC PERIODIC PARALYSIS

This disease resembles hypokalemic periodic paralysis in clinical appearance and often in changes in serum potassium concentration. However, 95 percent of the cases are sporadic and occur among Orientals. The male:female ratio is 6:1, and the onset is usually in adult life. The most important part of therapy is the treatment of the hyperthyroidism and maintenance of the euthyroid state.

Preventive Treatment

Patients should avoid high carbohydrate intake, muscle cooling, or extreme exercise. Effective medications include (1) propranolol, at a dosage of 20 to 40 mg three times daily, which probably inhibits beta receptor–mediated actions of the thyroid hormones, (side effects are listed under Hypokalemic Periodic Paralysis), and (2) spironolactone (for details see Hypokalemic Periodic Paralysis and Table 3). In most of the reported cases, acetazolamide had a negative effect, and oral use of potassium does not prevent attacks of weakness.

Acute Attacks

The treatment of an acute attack of thyrotoxic periodic paralysis is the same for the hypokalemic form.

PERIODIC PARALYSIS WITH CARDIAC ARRHYTHMIA

In this disorder, treatment of the potentially fatal arrhythmia is of more importance than treatment of the paralytic attack. In these cases, tests to provoke the weakness (e.g., intravenous glucose and insulin) should not be used. Imipramine is the drug of choice in controlling cardiac arrhythmia, and low doses of acetazolamide are sometimes useful.

NORMOKALEMIC PERIODIC PARALYSIS

Although this is considered a distinct nosologic entity, no convincing therapeutic approach has been described. It is currently held that the therapy of choice is the same as for hyperkalemic periodic paralysis, but sometimes treatment with acetazolamide is not successful.

SUGGESTED READING

Gould RJ, Steeg CN, Eastwood AB, et al. Potentially fatal cardiac dysrhythmia and hyperkalemic periodic paralysis. Neurology 1985; 35:1208–1212.

Links TP, Zwarts MJ, Oosterhuis HJGH. Improvement of muscle strength in familial hypokalemic periodic paralysis with acetazolamide. Neurol Neurosurg Psychiatry 1988; 51:1142–1145.

Meyer-Lehnert H, Kramer HJ, Heck I, et al. Schwere periodische hypokaliämische Lähmung. Dtsch Med Wochenschr 1987; 112:1173–1177.

Streib EW. Paramyotonia congenita: Successful treatment with tocainide. Clinical and electrophysiologic findings in seven patients. Muscle Nerve 1987; 10:155–162.

Zwarts MJ, Van Weerden TW, Links TP, et al. The muscle fiber conduction velocity and power spectra in familial hypokalemic periodic paralysis. Muscle Nerve 1988; 11:166–173.

CRAMPS

RICHARD T. MOXLEY III, M.D.

Skeletal muscle cramps may be generalized or occur in a limited region of the body. Patients with common causes of cramps, such as peripheral vascular disease, benign postexercise cramps, or idiopathic cramps in the elderly, are frequently not seen by neurologists. More typically, the neurologist sees patients with denervating conditions or myopathic disorders that have produced either cramps or myalgia or a combination of these two problems. A muscle cramp develops suddenly, is painful, appears more often in a portion of a muscle than the entire muscle group, causes visible and palpable contraction, begins and ends with intermittent twitching movements in the muscle, and often is provoked by only a slight movement involving the muscle with the cramp. Cramps can almost always be terminated immediately with passive stretching of the muscle. Subsequently that area of the muscle may remain sore, and there may be an associated rise in serum creatine kinase level. The precise pathogenic mechanism responsible for a muscle cramp is unknown. It is postulated that distal portions of the neuron are triggered in some fashion to produce spontaneous firing, and the electrical activity spreads to adjacent neurons by ephaptic transmission. During the cramp, electromyographic recordings show irregular, high frequency bursts of motor unit potentials. This electrical appearance contrasts with a muscle contracture that is electrically silent. Muscle contractures are clinically similar to cramps and occur in conditions such as hypothyroidism and rare metabolic disorders such as McArdle's disease.

Muscle pain, myalgia, may coexist in patients with muscle cramps but is a separate complaint. Myalgia is a sensation of pain and is thought to be mediated by group III (small myelinated) and group IV (unmyelinated) afferent fibers. These pain fibers are felt to be activated by mechanical factors (trauma, increased myofascial tension, increased tenseness of muscles, Parkinson's disease) or by other conditions that promote the release of chemicals such as bradykinin, serotonin, and histamine, which are known to activate nocireceptors. Inflammatory disorders, vascular-ischemic conditions, and neuropathic disorders may lead to the release of these chemicals, causing muscle pain.

DIAGNOSIS

The diagnosis-treatment outline shown in Table 1 provides a listing of the different problems that might cause muscle cramps in a restricted region or generalized cramps. It should be emphasized that most individuals with frequent muscle cramps are medically normal. Neurologists typically see patients with neuropathic disorders and occasionally patients with rare metabolic diseases who manifest muscle cramps. In the patients suspected of having a

Table 1 Diagnosis of Muscle Cramps (Potential Causes)

Frequently Occurring in Legs and/or Arms	*Restricted to One Region*

Vascular disease
(as indicated under causes restricted to one region
	Vascular disease
	  Small vessel—medical treatment of cause
	  Large vessel—surgical evaluation

Radiculopathy, peripheral neuropathy
(as indicated under causes restricted to one region)
	Local compression neuropathy (for example)
	  Carpal tunnel syndrome:
	    Splint + rest, if ineffective—surgical evaluation

Amyotrophic lateral sclerosis, Postpolio syndrome
(as indicated under causes restricted to one region)
	Compartment syndrome (for example)
	  Anterior compartment of leg:
	    Rest; evaluate compartment pressure before and after
	      exercise; surgical evaluation

Electrolyte disturbances
(hypoadrenalism, dehydration, diuretic therapy, chronic
  diarrhea/vomiting, hemodialysis):
  Evaluate serum electrolytes
  Institute corrective treatment
	Radiculopathy, mononeuropathy:
	  Establish cause
	    Initial therapy: rest, analgesia
	    Chronic therapy: individualized physiotherapy and
	      exercise; consider anticramp drug treatment

Uremia:
  Obtain renal function tests
  Dialysis often effective therapy
  Restless legs?:
    Drug therapy
	Amyotrophic lateral sclerosis, postpolio syndrome:
	  Initial therapy
	    Rest and patient assessment
	    Anticramp drug medication
	  Chronic therapy
	    Individualized exercise program
	    Patient supervision
	    As necessary, anticramp drug therapy

Hypothyroidism:
  Thyroid function tests
  Replacement therapy
	Overuse syndromes (for example)
	  Cubital tunnel (violinists, pianists):
	    Rest; patient evaluation;
	    Surgical evaluation

Drug-induced (lithium, cimetidine, salbutamol, clofibrate, danazol): Remove offending drug or reduce dosage	

Nocturnal (benign) cramps:
  Exercise and stretching
  Drug therapy	

Rare metabolic diseases
(usually provoked by exercise)
  Creative kinase level (often elevated)
  Muscle biopsy
  Muscle function tests
    (Lactate release—McArdle's disease)
    NH_3 release—myoadenylate deaminase deficiency):
  Institute dietary therapy and individualized exercise
    program	

metabolic disease of muscles, it is necessary to perform muscle biopsy, electrodiagnostic studies, and functional tests of muscle metabolism (exercise with measurements of lactate and ammonia production). These tests help to identify certain rare myopathic disorders that cause muscle cramps (myophosphorylase deficiency, myoadenylate deaminase deficiency, and mitochondrial disorders).

TREATMENT

Successful treatment of muscle cramps requires distinguishing a cramp from other problems, such as muscle pain and muscle spasm. Muscle pain and muscle spasm often are alleviated only by treatment of the specific disorder responsible for these symptoms. The following section contains an outline of a general approach to the treatment of muscle cramps. This is followed by recommendations for treatment of specific conditions associated with muscle cramps.

General Treatment of Muscle Cramps

The mainstays of treatment for cramps are muscle stretching, rest, and physical therapy tailored to the specific cause of the muscle cramping. Often a patient receives a warning that a cramp is imminent. Fasciculations may appear intermittently throughout the day in a portion of the muscle susceptible to a cramp. Preventive therapy should involve stretching of this muscle as well as rest. In the case of the calf musculature, it is helpful to perform stretching exercises for at least 10 to 15 minutes prior to bedtime and to place a pillow, a rolled blanket, or even a footboard under the feet so that they may be partially dorsiflexed during sleep. Specific instructions for the technique of stretching muscles involved should be provided by the physician, along with the consultation of a physical therapist. It is helpful to have a physical therapist develop an individualized program of muscle stretching, range of motion exercise, and a graduated exercise program for patients with focal or generalized neuropathies that are disabled by cramping. Usually this requires a minimum of three or four sessions with the therapist. During these sessions, the patient and the spouse can be instructed in the stretching techniques and muscle massage. An effective regimen for stretching the gastrocnemius and soleus muscle groups, which are frequently the target of idiopathic and neurogenic muscle cramps, is to stand facing a wall, approximately 3 to 4 feet away, and to lean against the wall with outstretched arms. During this movement the heels should be kept on the floor, the knees locked, and the back straight. This can be performed for 2 to 3 minutes at a time and provide a sustained stretch of the calf muscles. Several repetitions may be performed with 1-minute periods of rest in-between. These stretching exercises should be performed immediately prior to bedtime or before a long period of inactivity if the patient tends to develop cramps under these circumstances during the day. For individuals who are too weak to stand or are otherwise handicapped, a variety of techniques can be developed with the help of a physical therapist. For example, a towel or lightweight dishcloth can be used to loop over the foot so as to maintain it in a dorsiflexed position with a pull of the patient's arms.

Decreased use of certain stimulant medications is often helpful in controlling muscle cramps. Elimination of coffee intake and decreased use of antiasthmatic therapy (theophylline, beta-adrenergic agents) may be helpful. Cigarette smoking or chewing tobacco may predispose to muscle cramps. Neostigmine treatment in patients with amyotrophic lateral sclerosis or other chronic neurogenic disorders often worsens muscle cramps. Some of the medications known to provoke muscle cramps are shown in Table 1. To the degree possible, these should be eliminated or the dosage reduced.

TREATMENT OF CRAMPS CAUSED BY SPECIFIC CONDITIONS

Denervating Disorders (Radiculopathy, Mononeuropathy, Amyotrophic Lateral Sclerosis, Peripheral Neuropathy, and Postpolio Syndrome)

Successful treatment of muscle cramping associated with the conditions listed above requires the general treatment program described in the previous section. Patients with amyotrophic lateral sclerosis and postpolio syndrome particularly benefit from individualized, physical therapy programs. These programs often include mat exercises to stretch and strengthen muscles. This mat work usually is needed two or three times a week. It is helpful to intersperse 2 or 3 days of swimming or pool exercises with the mat program. This type of individualized exercise program allows anticramp medications to be reduced in dosage or completely discontinued. The other neuropathic disorders listed above often do not require drug therapy to control cramps.

Muscle cramping attributable to neurogenic disorders frequently responds to carbamazepine. The patient is started on 200 mg as a morning and evening dose, and the dose is gradually increased by initially increasing the evening and then the morning dose by 200-mg steps. A midafternoon dose is added after the patient has been able to tolerate doses of 400 mg in the morning and 400 mg in the evening. The usual effective dose of carbamazepine is one that produces anticonvulsant levels of drug in the plasma. Low therapeutic anticonvulsant levels are often sufficient to prevent muscle cramps in patients who are responsive to drug treatment. After achieving effective control of the cramps for a period of 2 to 3 months it is often helpful to determine if continued treatment is needed. The midday dose is discontinued first, and gradually the morning and finally the evening dose is decreased. Treatment with carbamazepine is preventive and requires regular doses. The same is true for phenytoin, which in my experience is not as effective as carbamazepine. The general guidelines for phenytoin are similar to those for carbamazepine. One would give a total daily dose that is sufficient to maintain drug levels in the low therapeutic range for anticonvulsant efficacy.

Control of muscle cramps in conditions such as amyotrophic lateral sclerosis and postpolio syndrome may be achieved with very low doses of diazepam. Despite the lethargy and habituation that are significant side effects of this medication, it is often possible to avoid these with the intermittent use of 5 mg to 2.5 mg of diazepam once or twice daily. Often the judicious use of low doses of diazepam with an individualized exercise program permits the patient to take the drug only a few times a week. In patients with amyotrophic lateral sclerosis, their associated upper motor neuron signs may predispose them to cramps in association with a muscle spasm. In these patients, it may be helpful to consider concomitant use of baclofen. Treatment should be started at low doses, using half of a 10-mg tablet three times daily. The dosage should be increased by one-half of a tablet every 2 weeks. The evening dose would be increased first, then the morning, and then the midday dose. This pattern usually prevents the development of significant drowsiness and allows the early identification of any weakness produced by the loss of spasticity. Baclofen therapy should be discontinued slowly over a few weeks in order to avoid abrupt withdrawal symptoms, such as hallucinations and seizures.

Hypothyroidism

Replacement therapy is almost uniformly successful in controlling muscle cramps and other muscle pain in hypothyroid individuals. However, it is necessary to monitor closely the thyroid-stimulating hormone and creatine kinase plasma concentrations when determining the appropriate dosage of thyroid replacement. Occasionally end-organ resistance to the hormone develops and there is relative intracellular hypothyroidism despite normal circulating levels of total and free thyroxine. Muscle cramps disappear once the correct replacement dosage has been achieved. This dosage will lower thyroid-stimulating hormone concentration to the low or immeasurable range. To achieve this may require giving doses of thyroid hormone that elevate thyroxine levels to the upper limit of normal. Increases in the dose of thy-

roid hormone in hypothyroid patients should be made very cautiously in 25- to 12.5-μg steps. The doses can usually be advanced at 2-to 3-week intervals without difficulty. Careful monitoring of anginal symptoms is important in older patients with longstanding hypothyroidism.

Uremia and Restless Legs Syndrome

Muscle cramps are common in a variety of electrolyte disturbances and in patients with both acute and chronic uremia The muscle spasms that occur in acute uremia are felt to be caused by toxins related to the renal failure and not by advanced damage to peripheral nerves. These cramps usually respond to dialysis and other measures to reverse renal failure. However, a subset of patients with uremia develop restless legs syndrome, as do certain individuals with no known associated medical conditions. As a part of the restless legs syndrome, patients have muscle cramps that often respond dramatically to treatment with clonazepam, 0.5 mg taken at bedtime. Carbamazepine given in the fashion described above is also effective but would be a second choice. It is helpful to be certain that no anemia exists in the uremic patient. Correction of the associated anemia often is helpful in relieving the muscle cramps.

Benign, Nocturnal Cramps and Familial Cramps

Autosomal dominant familial cramps as well as benign nocturnal cramps are difficult to treat with drugs and are most effectively controlled by physical therapy and stretching exercises. Patients suffering from autosomal dominant hereditary muscle cramps usually must avoid prolonged sitting in one position and sudden movements. These patients frequently develop severe cramps during yawning or stretching. These cramps can be alleviated by avoiding long periods of inactivity and rest. In patients with hereditary muscle cramps, the specific drugs mentioned above for neurogenic cramps can be tried, but they are almost uniformly unsuccessful.

Patients with benign, nocturnal muscle cramps are often older, and these cramps are responsive to single doses of quinine sulfate, usually 300 mg at bedtime. Despite the concern that quinine may be acting primarily as a placebo, I would recommend it as the first choice for benign cramps in the elderly. Clonazepam in a dose of 0.25 mg or 0.5 mg is a second choice.

Overuse and Compartment Syndromes

Overuse syndromes usually involve the upper extremities, especially the forearm musculature, and are almost always relieved by placing the limb at rest for a sufficient period of time. This is often difficult to do, however, because the symptoms are related to the patient's occupation or sports interests.

In individuals suffering from compartment syndromes, primarily the anterior compartment of the lower limb, the cramps typically develop during or immediately after prolonged exercise. The affected patients are weekend athletes or recent inductees into aerobics or jogging or individuals with covert hypothyroidism who are at special risk. In patients with anterior leg cramps caused by exercise, it is necessary to measure pressures in the anterior compartment both at rest and after exercise to search for signs of abnormal increase in compartment pressure. Treatment often requires surgical intervention (fasciotomy) to prevent excessive pressure that might lead to necrosis and permanent damage to nerve and muscle tissues. Conservative treatment includes the avoidance of exercise and is often sufficient to eliminate the muscle cramps. However, it is important for long-term management to determine the pressure in the anterior compartment before and after exercise.

Chronic Myalgia with Muscle Spasms

Many of the conditions listed in Table 1 have associated muscle pain with the cramps. In those disorders in which there is no specific treatment, it is also helpful to include analgesic therapy. Often a combination of nonsteroidal anti-inflammatory drug and amitriptyline is effective in ameliorating the pain. Acetaminophen or aspirin, 650 mg every 4 to 6 hours, is useful in controlling the severe muscle pain that may develop shortly after a sustained muscle cramp or following exercise. The use of aspirin should be continued for several days, with the interval between doses gradually increasing to approximately every 8 hours. In individuals with long-standing peripheral nerve damage, such as long thoracic nerve palsy, which often produces chronic muscle spasm in the upper fibers of the trapezius, the long-term use of analgesics in combination with amitriptyline taken at bedtime, 30 to 80 mg, is effective. Amitriptyline is given initially as a single 30-mg nighttime dose. The dose is increased in 10-mg increments every 2 to 3 weeks until a beneficial analgesic effect develops. In some patients it has been helpful to add a calcium channel blocker, which may act to improve circulation to the muscle that has been in prolonged spasm. Nifedipine, 10 mg every 8 to 12 hours, is often effective. In patients with conditions predisposing them to prolonged periods (weeks) of muscle spasm, it is preferable to use a slow release form of verapamil, 240 to 120 mg, as a single daily dose taken with the evening meal. Calcium channel blocker treatment usually is discontinued after the severe muscle spasm disappears. This drug treatment can be reinstituted if severe chronic muscle spasm recurs.

SUGGESTED READINGS

Layzer RB. Muscle pain, cramps and fatigue. In: Engel AG, Banker BQ, eds. Myology. New York: McGraw-Hill, 1986: pp 1907–1924.

Moxley RT. Muscle and "muscle-like" complaints associated with sports. Semin Neurol 1981; 1:323–333.

Rowland LP. Cramps, spasms, and muscle stiffness. Rev Neurol 1985; 141:261–273.

Roy EP, Gutmann L. Myalgia. Neurol Clin 1986; 6:621–636

PSYCHIATRIC CONDITIONS PRESENTING AS NEUROLOGIC DISEASE

HYSTERICAL BEHAVIOR

MARK L. TEITELBAUM, M.D.
PAUL R. McHUGH, M.D.

DEFINITION

Hysteria is the imitation of the behavior of a physically ill person. It appears in two forms.

Acute Hysteria. Acute hysteria is also referred to as conversion disorder. It generally involves the sudden onset of a single neurologic symptom such as sensory loss, a paralyzed limb, or an abnormal gait, for which there is no physical explanation.

Chronic Hysteria. Chronic hysteria is also referred to as somatization disorder or Briquet's syndrome. This condition is characterized by the lifelong complaining to medical personnel about a variety of symptoms involving multiple organ systems for which there is no adequate explanation based on physical disease. Patients with chronic hysteria may intermittently display the typical pseudoneurologic symptoms seen in acute hysteria as well.

PREDISPOSING FACTORS

Genetic Factors. Chronic hysteria tends to run in families. There is an increased prevalence of chronic hysteria in the first-degree female relatives of patients suffering from this disorder. There is also an increased prevalence of antisocial personality disorder among first-degree male relatives of patients suffering from this condition.

Personality Traits. Histrionic personality traits such as self-dramatization, mood lability, and egocentricity may predispose to the development of hysteria. Patients with chronic hysteria, however, seem to have a mixture of both histrionic and obsessional traits of character.

Sociologic Factors Social and cultural factors may also predispose to the development of hysteria. Cultures and social groups that encourage emotional display as opposed to verbal expression of emotion may be predisposing factors.

PRECIPITATING FACTORS

Acute hysteria and exacerbations of chronic hysteria are often precipitated by stressful life events such as bereavement, other losses, separations, physical trauma, or combat. Difficulties in interpersonal relationships is a common precipitating factor in hysteria.

DIFFERENTIAL DIAGNOSIS

Unrecognized Physical Disorder. Physical disorders that have polysymptomatic presentations and a vague and variable course, such as multiple sclerosis, myasthenia gravis, and systemic lupus erythematosus, may readily be confused with hysteria. Ultimately the recognition of characteristic signs on physical examination and confirmatory laboratory tests will distinguish such conditions from hysteria. Hysterical behavior is sometimes associated with physical disorder. Hysterical seizures coexisting with bona fide epilepsy are not uncommon and can produce a confusing picture for the clinician.

Affective Disorder. Depressed patients often present to their primary care physician with a variety of physical complaints for which no adequate physical explanation can be found. Symptoms such as loss of energy, poor appetite, sleep disturbance, headache, indigestion, and constipation may be the initial complaints of a depressed patient. The diagnosis of depression ultimately rests on examination of the patient's mental state and the recognition of the characteristic features of mood disturbance, self-attitude disturbance, and disturbance in the patient's vital sense. A past and/or family history of depression all help to support the diagnosis.

Anxiety Disorder. Patients with anxiety also typically present to their primary care physician with physical complaints for which there is no adequate physical explanation. Symptoms such as fatigue, poor concentration, palpitations, shortness of breath, and sweating can all be seen as caused by anxiety. Here also the diagnosis ultimately rests on both the history and an examination of the patient's mental state. Characteristic symptoms of tension, apprehension, worry, and poor concentration or frank episodes of panic with feelings of impending death or thoughts that one is losing one's mind establish the diagnosis of an anxiety disorder.

EPIDEMIOLOGY

General Population. In the Baltimore epidemiologic catchment area study, the prevalence of chronic hysteria was found to be 0.6 percent.

Medical Population. At The Johns Hopkins University Hospital, the prevalence of acute hysteria among patients seen in consultation by the Psychiatric Consultation–Liaison Service is about 2.5 percent. Among inpatients hospitalized on the Psychiatric Service of The Johns Hopkins University Hospital, the prevalence of acute hysteria is about 0.5 percent.

RECOGNITION AND DIAGNOSIS

Acute Hysteria. The diagnosis of acute hysteria rests upon the recognition of a sign or symptom for which there is no physical explanation that appears in a predisposed individual in the midst of a stressful life situation. The diagnosis ultimately rests on the clinician's being able to make a meaningful connection between the symptom, the particular person, and the provoking life circumstance (Table 1). For example, a young woman arriving at a hospital emergency room with the acute onset of blindness for which no physical explanation can be found might be discovered to be a timid person of histrionic temperament who several hours previously had witnessed a murder and had been re-

quested by the police to testify. In such an instance the patient's blindness can be meaningfully understood as the reaction of this particular person to a particular situation. As in most cases of acute hysteria, the motivation for the behavior is outside the awareness of the patient but often is readily discernible by the physician. The fact that the motivation for the behavior is unconscious distinguishes hysteria from malingering.

Chronic Hysteria. The diagnosis of chronic hysteria rests on the presence of a history of multiple medically unexplained physical complaints beginning before the age of 30 and persisting for several years. To confirm the diagnosis, at the time of examination by the physician, at least 13 symptoms must be included by the patient from a symptom list covering various gastrointestinal, pain, cardiopulmonary, pseudoneurologic, and sexual symptoms (Table 2).

Chronic hysteria may also be screened for in a patient with a history of unexplained physical complaints starting before the age of 30 by establishing the presence of any two of the following symptoms: vomiting other than during pregnancy, pain in the extremities, shortness of breath with physical exertion, amnesia, difficulty in swallowing, a burning sensation in the sexual organs or rectum other than during intercourse, or painful menstruation.

For a symptom to be actually counted as positive, in addition to there being no organic pathology found to explain it, it must have caused the patient to see a physician or take some medication other than an over-the-counter pain drug or have produced some alteration in the patient's life-style. As in acute hysteria, the motivation driving the behavior in chronic hysteria is usually outside the patient's conscious awareness. Issues involving desires for nurturance, love, and attention are frequently involved. In other words, part of the reason why hysteria exists is that there are physician and hospital system in our culture that provide certain privileges to individuals who are sick, including support, attention, and concern.

Table 1 Conversion Disorder (DSM III R Criteria)

1. A loss of or alteration in physical functioning, suggesting a physical disorder.
2. Psychological factors are judged to be etiologically related to the symptom because of a temporal relationship between a psychosocial stressor that is apparently related to a psychological conflict or need and initiation or exacerbation of the symptom.
3. The person is not conscious of intentionally producing the symptom.
4. The symptom is not a culturally sanctioned response pattern and cannot, after appropriate investigation, be explained by a known physical disorder.
5. The symptom is not limited to pain or to a disturbance in sexual functioning.

COMPLICATIONS

Hysteria, especially chronic hysteria, may be complicated by drug dependence or addiction as well as by iatrogenic injury from unnecessary medications, invasive diagnostic tests, or surgical procedures. It has been well documented, in fact, that the prevalence of surgery among patients with chronic hysteria is significantly increased when compared with both healthy and physically ill controls. Chronic hysteria may also be complicated by occupational, social, and marital disruption and by secondary depressive or anxiety symptoms.

Table 2 Somatization Disorder (DSM III R Criteria)

A history of many physical complaints or a belief that one is sickly, beginning before the age of 30 and persisting for several years.

Patient's physical complaints include, at least 13 symptoms from the list below. To count a symptom as significant, the following criteria must be met:

1. No organic pathology or pathophysiologic mechanism (e.g., a physical disorder or the effects of injury, medication, drugs, or alcohol) to account for the symptom or, when there is related organic pathology, the complaint or resulting social or occupational impairment is grossly in excess of what would be expected from the physical findings
2. Symptom has not occurred only during a panic attack
3. Symptom has caused the person to take medicine (other than over-the-counter pain medication), see a physician, or alter lifestyle

Gastrointestinal Symptoms
    Vomiting (other than during pregnancy)
    Abdominal pain (other than when menstruating)
    Nausea (other than motion sickness)
    Bloating (gassy)
    Diarrhea
    Intolerance of (gets sick from) several different foods

Pain Symptoms
    Pain in extremities
    Back pain
    Joint pain
    Pain during urination
    Other pain (excluding headaches)

Cardiopulmonary Symptoms
    Shortness of breath when not exerting oneself
    Palpitations
    Chest pain
    Dizziness

Conversion or Pseudoneurologic Symptoms
    Amnesia
    Difficulty swallowing
    Loss of voice
    Deafness
    Double vision
    Blurred vision
    Blindness
    Fainting or loss of consciousness
    Seizure or convulsion
    Trouble walking
    Paralysis or muscle weakness
    Urinary retention or difficulty urinating

Sexual Symptoms for the Major Part of the Person's Life:
    Burning sensation in sexual organs or rectum (other than during intercourse)
    Sexual indifference
    Pain during intercourse
    Impotence

Female Reproductive Symptoms Judged by the Person to Occur More Frequently or Severely Than in Most Women
    Painful menstruation
    Irregular menstrual periods
    Excessive menstrual bleeding
    Vomiting throughout pregnancy

THE ROLE OF PSYCHIATRIC CONSULTATION

Patients with unexplained physical complaints for whom a diagnosis of hysteria is being entertained should have the benefit of psychiatric consultation. The function of consultation is to aid in the diagnostic process as well as to help in treatment planning. Preparing the patient for psychiatric consultation is an important part of the procress. Patients may be anxious about psychiatric consultation, feel insulted by the physician's suggestion, or experience their physician's suggestion as threatened abandonment of them. Adequate preparation should involve a careful explanation to the patient about the reasons for seeking consultation and sufficient time to discuss the patient's reaction to this suggestion. At this time, appropriate support, further explanation, and reassurance can be given by the physician in order to facilitate the consultation.

TREATMENT OF HYSTERIA

Acute Hysteria. The treatment of acute hysteria is based primarily on (1) persuading patients that their symptoms can be meaningful understood as the outcome of an interaction between their personality and the stressful circumstances they are under, and that although these circumstances have produced sufficient stress or shock to make them ill, they are now at the point where recovery can begin; and (2) suggesting to patients, with or without the use of an injection of amobarbital Amytal Sodium, that some signs of recovery or regaining of function can already be demonstrated and will continue to become evident. Patients with acute hysteria are commonly treated in an inpatient setting, where a series of interviews with a physician with or without the use of amobarbital can be undertaken with the end of persuading the patient that although he or she was made ill by certain circumstances, he or she is now healing and gradually can be encouraged to give up the symptom. It is crucial that the patient be allowed to "save face." In no way should it be communicated to the patient that it is thought his or her suffering is imaginary, "all in the head," or in any way fake. The suffering of the patient with acute hysteria is indeed real and no less genuine an illness than any other, despite the absence of organic pathology. Patients with acute hysteria who fail to respond to such simple measures over a short hospital stay may require transfer to an inpatient psychiatric unit for further treatment over a more extended period of time.

Treatment of Chronic Hysteria. As with acute hysteria, the goal of treatment of chronic hysteria is ultimately to reinterpret patients' illnesses to them in terms of the interaction between their personal vulnerabilities, their life circumstances, and the meaning of their symptom complaints to the physician. This is done with the hope that eventually a dimuntion in symptom complaints may occur, and more direct and satisfying solutions to life problems may be sought with the help of the physician. With chronic hysteria, such a goal may never be attained completely, and more modest goals of simply protecting the patient from unnecessary diagnostic tests, surgical interventions, drug addiction, and unnecessary treatments may be more realistic. Treatment should be built around regularly scheduled appointments. Seeing a patient with chronic hysteria on an as needed basis generally is not helpful and often leads to an increase in symptom complaints. The frequency of appointments varies with the patient's needs and the physician's available time. Through trial and error, the optimal frequency of visits can generally be ascertained. Initially, the focus of each visit generally involves an exploration of symptom complaints, and when new symptoms have appeared, a brief physical examination is performed. The setting of limits on unneeded tests and treatments generally is part of the interaction between physician and patient. When a good relationship between physician and patient exists and trust has developed, such limit-setting can generally be accomplished in a kindly but firm manner that is acceptable to the patient and does not lead to a rupture of the relationship. Over time, the physician can begin to explore more of the patient's personal history, aspects of his or her temperament, and his or her current life circumstances and difficulties in coping that may help enlighten both physician and patient about the meanings of the patient's symptomatic complaints. When such an approach is successful over an extended period of time, symptomatic complaints gradually diminish, only to reappear at times of personal stress, and more and more time at each appointment will be spent by the patient in discussing personal matters relating to his or her life circumstances. Although the majority of patients with chronic hysteria can be effectively managed by their primary physician, those patients with chronic hysteria who develop associated depressive symptoms, particularly if these symptoms are associated with suicidal ideation, severe symptoms of anxiety, or substance dependence or abuse, are best referred to a psychiatrist for treatment.

PROGNOSIS

The prognosis for recovery from an episode of acute hysteria is quite good. The majority of patients recover with appropriate treatment. The prognosis for recovery in chronic hysteria is much more guarded. However, a significant number of these patients can be helped to decrease their utilization of medical resources and thereby to reduce their exposure to unneeded interventions and the attendant risks of complications.

SUGGESTED READING

Lazare A. Conversion symptoms. N Engl J Med 1981; 305:745–748.

Monson RA, Smith CR. Somatization disorder in primary care. N Engl J Med 1983; 308:1464–1465.

Murphy GE. The clinical management of hysteria. JAMA 1982; 247:2559–2564.

Perley MJ, Guze SB. Hysteria—the stability and usefulness of clinical criteria: a quantitative study based on a follow-up period of six to eight years in 39 patients. N Engl J Med 1962; 266:421–426.

Perry JC, Jacobs DJ. Overview: clinical applications of the Amytal interview in psychiatric emergency settings. Am J Psychiatry 1982;139:552–559.

DEPRESSION

J. RAYMOND DePAULO, Jr., M.D.

Depression is a nonspecific term whose meaning varies from a temporary sense of discouragement to a disabling disease state, which until 50 years ago had a high mortality rate in hospitalized patients (from suicide, inanition, and infection). My approach to the diagnosis and management of the clinical syndrome of major depression is discussed.

Despite the general availability of many effective treatments, over 70 percent of people with depression never receive any treatment. Fifty percent fail to seek help, and only half of those who do seek it are diagnosed and adequately treated. Besides the usual clinical reasons for misdiagnosis of any disorder, the diagnosis of clinical depression often is not seriously considered even when its manifestations abound because the physician (and the patient) consider these manifestations to be rational, if painful, responses to life circumstances. In fact, 80 percent of the episodes of severe major depression are associated with patient-reported stressful life events near the onset date. The presence of these life events neither dictates the clinical diagnosis nor predicts drug treatment response. On the other hand, the type and severity of the depressive symptoms do both with great efficiency.

Although no pathology of the brain has been established for most cases of major depression (or manic-depressive illness), a variety of neuropathologies (e.g., stroke, Parkinson's disease, multiple sclerosis have been associated with the syndrome. The majority of affective syndromes *not* associated with clear neuropathologies are probably genetic in origin. The remaining small fraction of cases, which are neither genetic nor neuropathologically based, are caused by endocrine disorders, drugs, or other conditions (Table 1).

Diagnosis is based on the patient history and a mental status examination. The characteristic cross-sectional clinical features of a depressive syndrome are changes in mood, self-attitude, and vital sense. Mood is usually low but is not always experienced as sad. Self-esteem and self-confidence are regularly, often dramatically, diminished, so that a depressed person may feel worthless or useless and often feels hopeless about the future. Suicidal ideas frequently are derived from this cluster of feelings. In addition, a depressed "vital sense" includes feelings of decreased mental and physical capacity. Feelings of lethargy and fatigue are usually matched by a sense of muddled, confused, or slowed thinking. In addition, hallucinations (perceptions without stimuli) and delusions (fixed, false, idiosyncratic ideas) often

are based on the changes in self-attitude and vital sense. Finally, "vegetative" changes in sleeping, eating, and sexual drive are very common (see Table 2).

A longitudinal view of the "typical" depressive syndrome reveals *episodes* of illness interspersed with symptom-free periods. Depression may alternate with manic periods (the bipolar form of affective illness). Although it is episodic, the condition varies enormously from person to person in severity, duration, and frequency of relapses. The mild or "atypical" forms of depression merge imperceptibly with normal moods and can be chronic rather than episodic. They are also usually associated with a tendency to overeat and oversleep and with a high frequency of anxiety disorders, and they often wax and wane with the seasons or endogenous hormonal rhythms.

Manic-depressive illness, i.e., bipolar affective disorder, is an important subtype of affective illness. Perhaps one-third of all patients with major depression have had or will have a severe manic attack at some time. A larger fraction have either a severe mania or a less severe condition (called hypomania) at some time in their lives. The bipolar patients are distinguished from unipolar patients by their responses to antidepressants as well as by symptomatic and potential etiologic differences. An important issue in the treatment of any depression with antidepressive agents is whether a severe manic state might be precipitated. Clearly, the patients at highest risk are those who have had prior manic attacks (Table 3).

Table 1 Common Nongenetic Causes of Major Depressive Syndromes

Neural	*Endocrine*	*Pharmacologic*
Cushing's disease	Cushing's disease	Steroids
Parkinson's disease	Hypothyroidism	Reserpine
Stroke		Propranolol
Multiple Sclerosis		

Table 2 DSM III Revised Criteria for Major Depressive Episode

A. At least five of the following symptoms have been present during the same 2-week period and represent a change from previous functioning:
1. Depressed mood
2. Markedly diminished interest in almost all activities
3. Significant appetite/weight loss or gain
4. Insomnia or hypersomnia
5. Psychomotor agitation or retardation
6. Fatigue or loss of energy
7. Feelings of worthlessness or excessive guilt
8. Diminished ability to think or concentrate
9. Recurrent thoughts of death or suicide

B. Not due to diagnosable brain injury, bereavement, or schizophrenia;

Table 3 DSM III Revised Criteria for Manic Episode

A. A distinct period of abnormally and persistently elevated, expansive, or irritable mood.
B. At least three of the following symptoms are present:
1. Inflated self-esteem or grandiosity
2. Decreased need for sleep
3. More talkative than usual
4. Flight of ideas or subjective experience that thoughts are racing
5. Distractibility
6. Increased activity
7. Excessive involvement in activities that have a high potential for painful consequences
C. Symptoms sufficiently severe to cause marked impairment in occupational functioning, social activites, or relationships
D. Not due to diagnosable brain injury or schizophrenia

The clinical laboratory offers little diagnostic help currently. The dexamethasone suppression test could add diagnostic information in inpatients without evidence of systemic or neurologic medical conditions if the local cortisol assay were standardized for use in diagnosing major depression. Sleep electroencephalography could also be of help, although it is time-consuming, expensive, and requires special facilities for overnight recordings.

Even when major depression is diagnosed and an effective antidepressant medication is given, the dosage prescribed is often inadequate. Finally, the medication is often stopped by the patient before the beneficial effects can occur. Thus, successful management of depressed patients requires that physicians actively seek out the syndrome and initiate well-directed and persistent treatment efforts.

TREATMENT

Because of our ignorance of the pathophysiology of the affective syndromes, rational treatments are not generally available. Therefore, empirical and empathic treatments are the mainstays of clinical management.

Among empirically validated treatments, the tricyclic antidepressants are the best studied and most widely used. I usually start a depressed patient on the tricyclic antidepressant, nortriptyline. Nortriptyline is the demethylated metabolite of amitriptyline. Like desipramine (the metabolite of imipramine), it is less sedating and less anticholinergic than its parent compound. Nortriptyline also causes less orthostatic hypotension than the other tricyclics.

Finally, a wealth of data have demonstrated that maintaining a steady-state blood level of nortriptyline between 50 and 140 ng per milliliter is the optimal way to achieve the antidepressant response. Somewhere between 65 and 80 percent of depressed patients become symptom-free on this regimen over a 2-month period.

In beginning treatment, I usually instruct the patient to take 25 mg of nortriptyline on the first evening and, if he or she has no adverse effects, to take 50 mg on the second evening. I instruct outpatients to stay on the 50-mg dosage for 2 weeks, at which time clinical reappraisal and a blood test for nortriptyline level is taken. If the patient is noticing brisk improvement, I leave the nortriptyline dose unchanged by note the blood level. If improvement is minimal or less, I adjust the dose, depending on the blood level. As long as the patient is still not feeling improvement, I pursue a level of not less than 90 ng per millileter and not more than 140 ng per milliliter. I keep in mind the ± 20 ng per milliliter day-to-day variation in the tricyclic assay, so that a level of 160 ng/ml does not necessarily mandate a retreat, and a level of 80 ng/ml does not require an increase in dosage. Also recall that a steady-state level is not achieved until 10 to 14 days after the patient has been on the same dose of a tricyclic.

Prior to commencing treatment, I review the American Medical Association's "patient medication instruction sheet" for tricyclics with patients and give it to them for later reference. At each visit thereafter, I review the list of side effects to see which, if any, have been experienced by the patient. The main contraindications for tricyclics are hypotension (orthostatic or otherwise), central nervous system depression (sedation), bladder obstruction, and cardiac conduction defects. The most frequent serious complications are falls in elderly neurologically impaired patients caused by orthostatic hypotension and delirium (especially in depressed stroke and parkinsonian patients) resulting from the central anticholinergic effects of the tricyclics.

After 6 to 8 weeks of therapy with the nortriptyline maintained at a blood level of between 90 and 140 mg per milliliter, I expect substantial improvement. If this has not occurred, generally, I add lithium carbonate (seeking a serum level of 0.6 to 0.9 mEg per liter) to augment the failed tricyclic regimen. Before adding lithium, I check creatinine level and thyroid function and make sure the patient is not on a salt-restricted diet. As before, the American Medical Association's "patient medication instruction sheet" for lithium is a useful focal point for patient education about the medication. After 2 weeks on a lithium regimen of 600 to 1,800 mg per day, the therapeutic enhancement, if any, will be apparent.

An easy to use alternate, antidepressant drug, fluoxetine, can be recommended if nortriptyline is contraindicated or if it has been adequately tried with an unsuccessful outcome. Fluoxetine is a noncyclic compound that is a relatively pure serotonin reuptake inhibitor with quite a long half-life. I usually prescribe it as one 20-mg capsule each morning and do not change the dosage (except if a toxic reaction occurs) until 6 to 8 weeks have elapsed. Probably because of its very long half-life (fluoxetine's half-life is 2 to 3 days and the half-life of non-fluoxetine its metabolite, is 7 to 9 days), it takes longer to start working when given at the usual maintenance dose (20 mg) from the start of therapy. On the positive side, it is usually even better tolerated than the tricyclics. In particular, it has no anticholinergic effects and does not cause orthostatic hypotension or tachycardia.

The only contraindication to fluoxetine is recent use of monoamine oxidase inhibitors. Common side effects are transient insomnia, increased anxiety, and transient mild nausea. There are two significant drug interactions: (1) the excretion of the tricyclics, the benzodiazepines, and related drugs is blocked by fluoxetine; therefore, their serum levels can double or triple when they are coadministered; and (2) monoamine oxidase inhibitors cannot be safely given until 5 weeks after fluoxetine is stopped. In the reverse sequence, avoid starting fluoxetine until 2 weeks after a monoamine oxidan inhibitor is stopped. Never coadminister these drugs.

I recommend that depressed patients who have failed two adequate trials of treatment be referred for specialist psychiatric consultation. Such patients often require hospitalization and electroconvulsive therapy to alleviate the depression.

Special problems posed by depressive syndromes also may arise from primary neurologic disorders (e.g., stroke, Parkinson's disease). These depressive syndromes may be relatively refractory to the usual antidepressants and may require electroconvulsive therapy more frequently than would be otherwise expected.

In addition, these patients may become delirious and suffer other drug toxicities more frequently than non-neurologically impaired depressed cases. Therefore, drug management must be carried out more cautiously in these patients. An excellent discussion of poststroke depression can be found in the 2nd edition of this series.

Duration of Medical Treatment

For patients with serious or subacute neurologic conditions (recent stroke patients), there is a general tendency to keep antidepressant therapy brief. We tend to keep antidepressants at maximal therapeutic levels for only about 6 weeks after the symptoms remit. Similarly, for patients with manic-depressive illness (bipolar affective disorder) who are maintained on lithium therapy, intercurrent antidepressant therapy is continued for about 4 to 6 weeks beyond symptomatic improvement. This is because, in bipolar (even lithium-treated) patients, most antidepressants increase the frequency of manic relapses.

For most patients therapy for even a single depressive episode should continue for 6 to 12 months. For patients with frequently recurrent severe depressions, a well-tolerated effective antidepressant should be continued for at least 2 years and often much longer. In the 30 years of tricyclic use, no long-term adverse consequences have been reported.

When stopping antidepressants in a recovered patient, the dosage should be tapered slowly. My practice is to decrease the dosage by 25 percent per week.

If the drug is being stopped because of toxicity or in order to switch to another antidepressant, the switch can occur much more quickly, except that a monoamine oxidase inhibitor must be stopped for 2 weeks before starting a cyclic antidepressant or fluoxetine, and fluoxetine must be stopped for 5 weeks before starting monoamine oxidase inhibitor.

The reasons for tapering the dosage are two: First and foremost, a significant fraction of patients have transient or sustained relapses of depression during the tapering period. These are milder and more easily controlled with a tapering schedule than with an abrupt halt. Also paradoxical hypomanic responses sometimes occur with abrupt cessation of antidepressants. Second, a few patients experience a distressing somatic "cholinergic" rebound with abrupt cessation of tricyclics. The symptoms are usually acute gastrointestinal distress with periodic nausea and vomiting, especially at mealtimes. If left untreated, this condition can last for several weeks. It can be relieved by temporarily reinstituting a small dose of the tricyclic.

Psychological Management

Empathic treatments are those directed to the suffering of the ill person (rather than to the disease). Most forms of psychotherapy are derived from the empathic traditions, but even the most routine "doctoring" procedures (taking a complete history, doing a thorough examination, and providing, in a reassuring manner, the diagnosis, prognosis, and treatment plan) can provide enormous relief and hope to a depressed patient.

These patients regularly believe they cannot be diagnosed or treated, and they are often convinced that their prognosis is hopeless. I tell all depressed patients what my diagnosis is, how confident I am of it, and why (or why not). I tell them that the diagnosis means that their suffering is caused by an as yet undefined bodily (i.e., brain) disorder. I discuss etiologic issues briefly (e.g., genetic, neural injury, endocrinopathy) and then describe the prognosis for recovery, which is already excellent in most cases and how this may be improved dramatically with early antidepressant treatment.

We discuss what patients should expect from

treatment: for the first 2 weeks, this is mostly side effects. After that, they should notice improved energy and concentration (as well as normalization of sleep and appetite patterns). Last, they will notice gradually improving feelings of self-confidence and self-esteem.

I discourage patients from making any major life decisions during this 2-month period except for the decision to seek and accept treatment. I have seen many depressed patients change spouses, jobs, and locations in an attempt to "fix" their problem under the assumption that it must be environmental in origin.

Management of Suicide Issue

Major depression is the most powerful predictor of suicide. Fifteen percent of patients hospitalized for major depression or manic-depressive illness eventually end their lives by suicide; many more think about it, make plans to do it, and attempt suicide. Patients who have depressive delusions (especially males) are at the highest risk and should be hospitalized. All depressed patients should be asked if they have thoughts of, plans of, or any prior attempts at suicide, and if so, this makes them more or less likely to attempt it in the immediate to short-term future. These same questions should be asked at follow-up visits so that the patient routinely reports on them positively or negatively.

When patients are not delusional and are having persisting suicidal thoughts that they cannot dismiss, some management plan must be made with them (and their families) to minimize the risk and to alert the physician promptly to the need for hospitalization should it arise. These plans are always individual and usually hinge on either a very dutiful and dependable patient or the active participation of the family. Most patients who have suicidal thoughts do not want to act on them and either will manage these unwanted thoughts themselves or will be grateful to you for helping them to work out a simple plan for reporting increasing suicidal thoughts and seeking short-term protection with family, friends, or if necessary in the hospital.

SUGGESTED READING

Crowe RR. Electroconvulsive therapy: a current perspective. N Engl J Med 1984; 311:163–167.
Folstein MF, Robinson R, Folstein S, McHugh PR. Depression and neurological disorders: new treatment opportunities for elderly depressed patients. J Affective Disord 1985; 9:S11–14.
Gold P, Goodwin F, Chrousos G. Medical progress: clinical and biochemical manifestations of depression. N Engl J Med 1988; 319:348–353, 413–420.
Lipsey JR, Robinson RG, Pearlson GD, et al. Nortriptyline treatment of post-stroke depression: a double-blind study. Lancet 1984; 1:297–300.

PATIENT RESOURCES

There are a number of organizations an publications that may be helpful for your patients.

Associations

Voluntary organizations that offer support groups, publications, and newsletters are as follows:

Depression and Related Affective Disorders Association
Meyer 4-181
The Johns Hopkins University Hospital
Baltimore, Maryland 21205

National Depression and Manic Depressive Illness Association
Merchandise Mart
Box 3395
Chicago, Illinois 60654

National Foundation for Depressive Illness
P.O. Box 2257
New York, New York 10016
Telephone 1-800-248-4344

Literature

Books

DePaulo JR, Ablow K. How to cope with depression. New York: McGraw-Hill, 1989.
Papolos D, Papolos J. Overcoming depression. New York: Harper & Row, 1987.

Pamphlets

Single copies of all pamphlets listed below are available at no cost from the source listed.

Facts about: depression
Facts about: manic-depressive disorders
Facts about: teen suicide
Facts about: Mental health of the elderly

Published by the American Psychiatric Association. Write to American Psychiatric Association 1400 K Street, N.W., Washington, DC 20005.

Depression: What you need to know
Helpful facts about depressive disorders
National education program on depressive disorders

Published by the National Institutes of Mental Health, U.S. Department of Health and Human Services. Write D/ART, National Institutes of Mental Health Room 15-C-05, 5600 Fisher Lane, Rockville, Maryland 20857.